Second Edition

Appleton & Lange's Review for the
PHYSICIAN ASSISTANT

Second Edition

Appleton & Lange's Review for the
PHYSICIAN ASSISTANT

Editor

Patrick J. Cafferty, PA-C
Neurosurgical Associates of Western Kentucky
Paducah, Kentucky

APPLETON & LANGE
Norwalk, Connecticut

Copyright © 1994 by Appleton & Lange
A Simon & Schuster Company
Copyright © 1991 by Appleton & Lange
A Publishing Division of Prentice Hall

96 97 98 / 10 9 8 7 6 5 4 3

Prentice Hall International (UK) Limited, *London*
Prentice Hall of Australia Pty. Limited, *Sydney*
Prentice Hall Canada, Inc., *Toronto*
Prentice Hall Hispanoamericana, S.A., *Mexico*
Prentice Hall of India Private Limited, *New Delhi*
Prentice Hall of Japan, Inc., *Tokyo*
Simon & Schuster Asia Pte. Ltd., *Singapore*
Editora Prentice Hall do Brasil Ltda., *Rio de Janeiro*
Prentice Hall, *Englewood Cliffs, New Jersey*

Acquisitions Editor: Jamie Mount
Production Service: Rainbow Graphics, Inc.

Library of Congress Catalog Card Number: 94-071833

ISBN 0-8385-0065-X

9 780838 500651

90000

PRINTED IN THE UNITED STATES OF AMERICA

Contributors

Joan Alfiero, PA-C
Clinical Coordinator, AIDS Program
Yale New Haven Hospital
New Haven, Connecticut

Mary S. Andresen, MS, PA
Assistant Professor in Pediatrics
Child Health Associate Program
University of Colorado
Denver, Colorado

James T. Barker, PA-C
Private Practice, Psychiatry
Lexington, Kentucky

Patrick J. Cafferty, PA-C
Neurosurgical Associates of Western Kentucky
Paducah, Kentucky

William K. Chapman, Jr., PA-C
Private Practice, Internal Medicine
Stockton, California

Charles J. Currey, MHA, PA-C
Assistant Professor
College of Health Related Professions
Physician Assistant Program
University of Florida
Gainesville, Florida

Kathleen L. Dolce, MS, CHA, PA-C
Instructor in Pediatrics
Child Health Associate Program
University of Colorado
Denver, Colorado

Mariann Doyle, PA-C
Private Practice, Occupational Medicine
Bardstown, Kentucky

Kevin T. Fitzpatrick, PA-C
Trauma and Surgical Intensive Care Research
Duke University Medical Center
Durham, North Carolina

Robert W. Jarski, PhD, PA-C
Associate Professor
Director of Clinical Research Program
School of Health Sciences
Oakland University
Rochester, Michigan

Peter Juergenson, PA-C
Lecturer in Internal Medicine
Yale University School of Medicine
New Haven, Connecticut

Janet Stayer Kozel, PA-C
Lecturer in Psychiatry
University of Kentucky Physician Assistant Program
Lexington, Kentucky

James B. Labus, PA-C
Peachtree Neurosurgery
Atlanta, Georgia

Janet Ann Leone, PA-C
Private Practice, Gastroenterology
Greensboro, North Carolina

Janet Rigberg Mayes, PA-C
Department of Surgery
University Hospitals of Cleveland
Cleveland, Ohio

Denyse Mahoney, PA-C
Department of Obstetrics and Gynecology
Booth Memorial Medical Center
Flushing, New York

Judy Mochizuki, MA, PA-C
Instructor in Pediatrics
Child Health Associate Program
University of Colorado
Denver, Colorado

Ricky D. Miller, PA-C
Emergency Department
Sand Lake Hospital
Orlando Regional Medical Center
Orlando, Florida

Judy Mochizuki, PA-C
Instructor in Pediatrics
Child Health Associate Program
University of Colorado Health Sciences Center
Physician Assistant
Mercy Family Practice Residency Program
Family Medicine Center
Denver, Colorado

Diane R. Nielsen, PA-C
Instructor in Pediatrics
School of Medicine
University of Colorado Health Sciences Center
Physician Assistant
Department of Pediatrics
University Hospital
Denver, Colorado

Doris Rapp, PharmD, PA-C
Associate Professor
University of Kentucky Physician Assistant Program
and College of Pharmacology
Lexington, Kentucky

H. Tim Reynolds, PA-C
Division of Dermatology
Department of Medicine
University of Kentucky Medical Center
Lexington, Kentucky

William D. Reynolds, PA-C
Emergency Department
Sand Lake Hospital
Orlando Regional Medical Center
Orlando, Florida

Linford J. Stillson, D.O.
Resident
Maine Medical Center
Portland, Maine

Amy Susan Winicov, PA-C
Gastroenterology
LeBauer, Weintraub, Brodie, Patterson and Associates
Greensboro, North Carolina

Kelly Werkmeister, PA-C
Department of Physician Assistant Studies
College of Allied Health Professions
University of Kentucky
Lexington, Kentucky

Contents

Preface

The Physician Assistant profession continues to grow at a rapid pace and recently passed the 25-year milestone. With the present desire for health care reform it is imperative that PAs maintain the high ground in ethics, particularly in ensuring continued competency amongst the members of the profession. With this in mind, we have revised this text to include updates in the various specialties. The original format has been maintained and each topic has been reviewed to include updated reference material. In response to suggestions from students, educators, and colleagues, we have expanded the cardiology section with better ECGs and have also increased the number of questions on antibiotics in the pharmacology section. The section on infectious disease was supplemented with questions and answers on drug-resistant TB and male sexually transmitted disease. In addition, a new section for gastroenterology is included in Chapter 4.

We have tried to make this review book a useful tool for exam preparedness and have appreciated the comments and constructive criticism brought to our attention. The future of this book depends on you, and we hope to incorporate your concerns in future revisions.

I would like to thank my wife, Karen, as well as our children, Patrick and Brigid, for their patience and understanding during the long and late hours spent working on this project. In addition, I would like to thank all of you for your support and confidence and wish you much success on the examination.

Patrick J. Cafferty, PA-C

Introduction

This book has been designed as a study aid to review for the Physician Assistant National Certification and Recertification Examination. Here, in one package, is a comprehensive review resource with more than 1000 questions presented in the same format as those seen in the national examinations. Each of these questions is answered with referenced, paragraph-length answers. In addition, the final section of the book is a 200-question Practice Test for self-assessment purposes. The entire book has been organized by specialty area to help evaluate your areas of relative strength and weakness and further direct your study effort with the available references.

ORGANIZATION

This book is divided into 8 chapters. Chapters 1 through 7 review the major areas of medicine using the question-and-answer format. Chapter 4, Internal Medicine, is subdivided into 8 sections covering its subspecialties. The final chapter is a 200-question Practice Test.

This introduction provides information on question types, methods for using this book, and specific information on the National Certifying and Recertifying Examinations.

QUESTIONS

The National Certifying Examinations contain four different types of questions. In the past, about 40% of these have been "one best answer–single item" questions; 45% were "multiple true–false or K type"; 10% were "one best answer–matching set"; and 5% were "comparison-matching set" questions. In some cases, a group of two or three questions may be related to a situational theme. In addition, some questions have illustrative material (graphs, x-rays, tables) that require understanding and interpretation on your part. Finally, some of the items are stated in the negative. In such instances, we have

printed the negative word in capital letters (eg, "All of the following are correct EXCEPT"; "Which of the following choices is NOT correct"; and "Which of the following is LEAST correct").

One Best Answer–Single Item Question

This type of question presents a problem or asks a question and is followed by five choices, only **one** of which is entirely correct. The directions preceding this type of question will generally appear as below:

DIRECTIONS (Questions 1 through 7): Each of the numbered items or incomplete statements in this section is followed by answers or by completions of the statement. Select the ONE lettered answer or completion that is BEST in each case.

An example for this item type follows:

1. An obese 21-year-old woman complains of increased growth of coarse hair on her lip, chin, chest, and abdomen. She also notes menstrual irregularity with periods of amenorrhea. The most likely cause is

    (A) polycystic ovary disease
    (B) an ovarian tumor
    (C) an adrenal tumor
    (D) Cushing's disease
    (E) familial hirsutism

In this type of question, choices other than the correct answer may be partially correct, but there can only be one *best* answer. In the question above, the key word is "most." Although ovarian tumors, adrenal tumors, and Cushing's disease are causes of hirsutism (described in the stem of the question), polycystic ovary disease is a much more common cause. Familial hirsutism is not associated with the menstrual irregularities mentioned. Thus, the *most* likely cause of the manifestations described can only be "(A) polycystic ovary disease."

One Best Answer–Matching Sets

These questions are essentially matching questions that are usually accompanied by the following general directions:

DIRECTIONS (Questions 2 through 6): Each group of items in this section consists of lettered headings followed by a set of numbered words or phrases. For each numbered word or phrase, select the ONE lettered heading that is most closely associated with it. Each lettered heading may be selected once, more than once, or not at all.

Any number of questions (usually two to six) may follow the five headings.

Questions 2 through 4

For each adverse drug reaction listed below, select the antibiotic with which it is most closely associated.

    (A) tetracycline
    (B) chloramphenicol
    (C) Clindamycin
    (D) cefotaxime
    (E) gentamicin

2. Bone marrow suppression

3. Pseudomembranous enterocolitis

4. Acute fatty necrosis of liver

Note that, unlike the single-item questions, the choices in the matching sets questions *precede* the actual questions. As with the single-item questions, however, only **one** choice can be correct for a given question.

Any number of questions (usually two to six) may follow the four headings.

Questions 5 and 6

    (A) polymyositis
    (B) polymyalgia rheumatica
    (C) both
    (D) neither

5. Pain is a prominent syndrome

6. Associated with internal malignancy in adults

Note that, as with the other matching-set questions, the choices precede the actual questions. Once again, only **one** choice can be correct for a given question.

Multiple True–False or K-Type Questions

These questions are considered the most difficult (or tricky), and you should be certain that you understand and follow the directions that always accompany these questions:

DIRECTIONS: For each of the items in this section, ONE or MORE of the numbered options is correct. Choose answer

    (A) if only (1), (2), and (3) are correct.
    (B) if only (1) and (3) are correct.
    (C) if only (2) and (4) are correct.
    (D) if only (4) is correct.
    (E) if all are correct.

This code is always the same (ie, (D) would never say "if (3) is correct"), and it is repeated throughout this book in a summary box (see below) at the top of any page on which multiple true–false item questions appear.
    A sample question follows:

7. The superficial perineal space contains which of the following?

    (1) crura of the clitoris
    (2) the deep transverse perineal muscle
    (3) the ischiocavernosus muscle
    (4) the anal sphincter

You first need to determine which choices are right and wrong, and then which code corresponds to the correct numbers. In the example above, (1) and (3) are both structures contained in this space, and therefore (B) is the correct answer to this question.

Answers, Explanations, and References

In each of the sections of this book, the question sections are followed by a section containing the answers, explanations, and references for the questions. This section (1) tells you the answer to each question; (2) gives you an explanation and reviews the reason the answer is correct, background information on the subject matter, and the reason the other answers are incorrect; and (3) tells you where you can find more in-depth information on the subject matter in other books and journals. We encourage you to use this section as a basis for further study and understanding.

    If you choose the correct answer to a question, you can then read the explanation (1) for reinforcement and (2) to add to your knowledge of the subject matter (remember that the explanations usually tell not only why the answer is correct, but often also why the other choices are incorrect). **If you choose the wrong answer** to a question, you can read the explanation for an instructional review of the material in the question. Furthermore, you can note the reference cited (eg, Pritchard, p. 250), look up the complete source in the references at the end of the chapter (eg, Cunningham FG: *Williams Obstetrics,* 19th ed. Norwalk, CT., Appleton & Lange, 1993), and refer to the pages cited for a more in-depth discussion.

Practice Test

The 200-question Practice Test at the end of the book covers and reviews all the topics covered in Chapters 1 through 7. The questions are grouped according to question type (one best answer–single item, one best answer–matching sets, comparison–matching sets, then multiple true–false items or type K questions), with the subject areas integrated. Specific instructions for how to take the Practice Test are given later.

The Practice Test is followed by a subspecialty list that will enable you to analyze your areas of strength and weakness and thereby focus your review. For example, by checking off your incorrect answers, you may find that a pattern develops in that you are incorrect on most or all of the pediatric questions. In this case, you could note the references (in the Answers and Explanations section) for your incorrect answers and read those sources. You might also want to purchase a pediatric text or review book to do a much more thorough review. We think you will find this subspecialty list very helpful and we urge you to use it.

HOW TO USE THIS BOOK

There are two logical ways to get the most value from this book. We will call them Plan A and Plan B.

In **Plan A,** you go straight to the Practice Test and complete it according to the instructions given. Using the subspecialty list, analyze your areas of strength and weakness. This will be a good indicator of your initial knowledge of the subject and will help to identify specific areas for preparation and review. You can now use the first seven chapters of the book to help you improve your relative weak points.

In **Plan B,** you go through Chapters 1 through 7 checking off your answers, and then comparing your choices with the answers and discussions in the book. Once you have completed this process, you can take the Practice Test and see how well prepared you are. If you still have a major weakness, it should be apparent in time for you to take remedial action.

In Plan A, by taking the Practice Test first, you get quick feedback regarding your initial areas of strength and weakness. You may find that you have a good command of the material, indicating that perhaps only a cursory review of the first nine chapters is necessary. This, of course, would be good to know early in your exam preparation. On the other hand, you may find that you have many areas of weakness. In this case, you could then focus on these areas in your review—not just with this book, but also with appropriate textbooks. It is, however, unlikely that you will not study prior to taking the National Boards (especially since you have this book). Therefore, it may be more realistic to take the Practice Test after you have reviewed the first seven chapters (as in Plan B). This will probably give you a more realistic type of testing situation, as very few of us merely sit down to a test without studying. In this case, you will

have done some reviewing (from superficial to in-depth), and your Practice Test will reflect this study time. If, after reviewing the first seven chapters and taking the Practice Test, you still have some weaknesses, you can then go back to the first of these chapters and supplement your review with the reference texts.

SPECIFIC INFORMATION ON THE EXAMINATIONS

The official source for all information on the Certification or Recertification process is the National Commission on Certification of Physician Assistants, Inc. (NCCPA), 2845 Henderson Mill Road, N.E., Atlanta, Georgia 30341. This organization is comprised of representatives from the major organizations of medicine, including the American Academy of Physician Assistants and the Association of Physician Assistant Programs. Their function is to formulate and administer the annual certification examination and to provide the means for recertification.

Eligibility requires completion or near completion of a Physician Assistant or Surgeon's Assistant program that is accredited by the American Medical Association's Committee on Allied Health and Accreditation. Details regarding registration are available from the NCCPA.

The examination consists of several portions; the first is the general examination. This is a 200-question examination addressing all aspects of Physician Assistant education, including anatomy, physiology, history taking, physical examination, laboratory and radiographic interpretation, as well as treatment modalities. The extended-core written examinations include surgery and primary care. Each of these are 150 questions in length and focus on that specialty. The examinee must choose one of these extended-core exams; however, for an additional fee you may take both extended-core exams. The score of the examination is a composite of your performance on the general and clinical skills portions. Tips for improving your score on the written exam are provided in the following section. The future of the recertification examination is not clear as of this revision. Plans for an alternative pathway for recertification are in the trial phase and may provide practicing PAs with a choice for recertification.

CLINICAL SKILLS PROBLEMS

The final component of the National Board Examination is a series of clinical scenarios in which the physician assistant examinee is asked to demonstrate his or her ability to correctly perform a problem-oriented physical examination. There has been discussion over the usefulness of this portion of the examination and the need for standardization. No specific changes in format have been announced, although we believe this will continue to be an important component of the future NCCPA exam.

In the present format, the examinee will be provided with three problems. Two of these will be examinations limited to 10 minutes, whereas one will be a 20-minute exam that frequently will involve a neurologic assessment. The examinee is expected to interpret the organ system or systems involved in the scenario and correctly perform a series of physical examination maneuvers related to the potential problems presented in this scenario. There is no requirement of obtaining historical information and there is limited communication between the examinee and the simulated patient. The patient can respond to simple commands, for example, "Does this hurt?" and directions to perform various physical examination maneuvers. The method used for scoring the clinical skills problems is a simple check sheet for the completion both accurately and in appropriate sequence of physical examination maneuvers related to the presenting problem. There are no penalties or point deductions for performing excessive or unwarranted physical examination maneuvers during the allotted time. Hence, the examinee would be best advised to perform all appropriate maneuvers within their allotted time. It is the responsibility of the examinee to provide all equipment appropriate to the examination, and this should be assembled far in advance of the examination date. Please see Table 1–1 for a checklist of suggested equipment. A sample clinical scenario would be the following: *A 47-year-old white female with a history of hypertension complains of lightheadedness and it is noted that she fell to the ground, striking her head with a resultant brief loss of consciousness.*

It is clear that this is a complicated presentation involving syncope as well as a closed head injury. The patient would need to be evaluated for her level of consciousness and associated neurologic deficits. In addition, one would need to evaluate the underlying cause of her syncopal episode. This would include evaluation of the carotid vessels for bruits, careful auscultation of the

TABLE 1–1. RECOMMENDED EQUIPMENT

1. Otoscope and ophthalmoscope
2. Flashlight or penlight
3. Tongue depressors
4. Ruler and flexible tape
5. Thermometer
6. Watch with a second hand
7. Sphygmomanometer
8. Stethoscope
9. Reflex hammer
10. Tuning fork
11. Safety pins
12. Test tubes containing scents for the neurologic exam
13. Cotton
14. Paper and pen or pencil
15. Latex or vinyl gloves

heart for evidence of murmurs or clicks as well as other evidence of cardiac pathology. Care must be taken to also include in your assessment the acquisition of vital signs, a frequently overlooked portion of the physical examination. In this particular patient scenario, one would wish to include checking the orthostatic blood pressure and/or blood pressure in both arms. While conducting the examination, there are occasionally points when you will be observing certain findings, and it would be prudent to talk through the examination, both as a reminder to yourself and to help point out to the examiner exactly what you are looking or listening for. This will avoid any misconceptions as to what you might have been observing.

We hope that through careful use of this book, whether through Plan A or Plan B, you find this text a useful and beneficial study guide.

Test-Taking Skills— Tips and Techniques

Machine-scorable written exams measure not only medical knowledge but also test-taking skills. Through examples, practice, and explanations, this section is designed to help the physician assistant student or graduate use appropriate methods for answering the types of written questions found on standardized Board exams. Information on preparing for Board exams will also be included.

To pass written Board exams, three conditions are generally necessary: (1) knowing about or recognizing the medical information contained in the questions; (2) using appropriate test-taking skills; and (3) avoiding situations that are likely to cause mistakes or impede performance. Test anxiety is an example.

Standardized exams can be intimidating and result in test anxiety. However, remembering that most test questions were created by well-intentioned clinicians can help keep the exam's purpose in perspective. In addition, multiple-choice questions are limited in what they can evaluate; they generally assess only fundamental cognitive knowledge. Test-wise individuals use strategies that enable them to perform their best in responding to questions on fundamental knowledge.

The fact is, written tests—even at their "state-of-the art" best—are crude evaluation devices (Snelbecker, 1985; Maatsch, 1983). Multiple-choice questions cannot reflect a clinician's total fund of medical skills. For example, patient rapport and the mechanics of examining patients are not accurately measured through multiple-choice questions. Multiple-choice questions can, however, successfully measure certain cognitive or knowledge skills. Machine-scored exams have limited assessment capabilities. Test taking is a discrete skill that is different from clinical skills, and expert clinicians are not necessarily expert test takers.

Test takers should master the skill of test taking the same way he or she has mastered the skill of physical examination. This may be accomplished by practicing the methods suggested in this section while answering the questions that follow in the text.

This section primarily presents information based on objective studies and sound psychological theories of test taking, perception, and recall (Snelbecker, 1985; U.S. Department of Education, 1986; DeCecuo and Crawford, 1974; Carman, 1984; Phipps, 1983). The section is organized in four sections: (1) what to do when preparing for the exam; (2) what to do during the exam; (3) illustrative questions; and (4) do's and don'ts that bring together the strategies explained in the previous three sections.

Objectives

In this section the student or graduate physician assistant will

1. identify proven techniques from the psychology of learning and educational measurement that will enhance test performance;
2. identify information from testing theory that will help avoid "careless" errors; and
3. practice using clues to help identify correct and incorrect responses to exam questions.

WHAT TO DO WHEN PREPARING FOR THE EXAM

Getting into Practice

To develop test-taking skills, you must actively practice what you will be doing on the test, that is, answering multiple-choice questions. Reading and reviewing texts is rarely enough. To become proficient in suturing wounds, you not only read about suturing, but you practice suturing. Some physician assistants have not taken a written exam in weeks, months, or years. Do not attempt to sit for Board exams without practicing answering multiple-choice questions any sooner than you would suture a facial laceration without having sutured skin in weeks, months, or years. Responding to questions similar to those encountered on the Boards is invaluable for exam preparation. The present text is designed for this purpose.

Areas to Emphasize

Direct your studying to the primary care areas with which you are least familiar. Although you may enjoy studying the areas relating directly to your practice, the task at hand is to pass the Boards. This is best accomplished by achieving a fundamental knowledge of each medical discipline appearing on the exam.

Write several of your own test questions. Those who do so frequently comment that their questions were surprisingly similar to those on the boards. This is probably so because only a limited amount of knowledge is amenable to the written exam format. In addition to identifying clinical information that is likely to be tested, you will gain valuable insight into the logic of test item construction that in turn helps in selecting correct answers.

Scheduling Preparation Time

Using a calendar, schedule specific periods for test preparation, setting aside specific times for reviewing and answering multiple-choice questions. Regular preparation over several months is preferred to cramming; studying just before the exam is usually nonproductive.

For the recertification exam, the amount of preparation needed depends largely upon your practice setting. If your knowledge in primary care family medicine is current, you probably need less preparation than a physician assistant in a subspecialty practice. Although an attempt is made to compare a physician assistant's practice profile to board scores by discipline, primary care knowledge will enhance test performance. A certain knowledge level in primary care is assumed. In addition, preparation in specialty disciplines is encouraged for graduates sitting for specialty Board exams.

The usual learning aids, such as the use of mnemonics, are highly recommended. The reader is referred to appropriate references (Carman, 1984; Phipps, 1983) for general information about study skills. The remainder of this section will address specific information about the Board exams.

WHAT TO DO DURING THE EXAM

Physical Needs

Find a seat with few or no distractions, avoiding places near doorways and thoroughfares. Repeated interference can hinder your test performance. Take your watch in case a clock is not easily visible. Nonsmokers should ascertain through the proctor that they will have a smoke-free environment.

Speak with the proctor about any reasonable and specific needs you may have. Consider the proctor your advocate. He or she is there (usually voluntarily and with pay) to provide a favorable testing environment. It is the proctor's responsibility to provide it.

Consider nutritional and other personal needs. It is recommended that a heavy meal not be eaten within 2 hours prior to the exam. You may wish to bring with you a complex carbohydrate snack, packaged drinks, and other supplies, such as tissues and cough drops. Keep food and drinks handy for breaks if consuming them during the exam is restricted. Get adequate sleep and rest before the exam.

Time Allowance

Before beginning each section of the exam, calculate the amount of time you can spend on each question. Never go over the calculated time limit on your first attempt at each question. If you do not know an answer, come back to it at the end. When calculating your time allotment, allow for a few extra minutes at the end so you can return to skipped items. Your subconscious will process those items while you work on the other questions. Also, hints often appear in other test items.

Time is usually not an obstacle in the Board exam; you probably will have more time than needed.

Attitude

During the test, maintain a positive, confident attitude. Remind yourself that you prepared as best you could, and use some other effective techniques such as those described below.

Do not become discouraged by questions you cannot answer. Many test items are, by design, those having been answered incorrectly by a large number of test takers. Test questions having a predetermined discrimination level are retained for use in future exams. If too many test takers answer a particular test item correctly, it is not used again. Therefore, most of the items you will be answering are those that many test takers have failed. So keep in mind that there will be a number of questions you are not expected to answer correctly.

Also be aware that numerous experimental questions are found on most standardized exams. Experimental questions are those being field tested, and they are not counted in your score. Because you do not know which items these are, assume that any absurd question is experimental. Try not to become irate or unnecessarily concerned about any question.

Self-coaching and imaging techniques (Greenberg, 1987; Pelletier, 1977; Hiebert et al, 1983) may be helpful for all test takers. Stress management methods (Greenberg; Benson, 1975; Hiebert et al, 1983) may be especially useful for anxious test takers. Most professional athletes and stage performers master and routinely use these techniques to avoid situations likely to interfere with optimal performance.

These techniques will not bring to mind medical knowledge never encountered, but they may help in retrieving learned information and in avoiding exam errors due to extreme stress. Managing stress generally results in improved concentration and the ability to reason logically. The suggested techniques may be learned through special courses and by consulting appropriate references (Greenberg, 1987; Pelletier, 1977; Benson, 1975; Hiebert et al, 1985). Techniques should be learned and practiced several weeks before the exam and used the day of the exam; certain brief imaging procedures may be used for relaxing and improving concentration during the exam.

Concentration

During the exam, think of nothing except the questions in front of you. When working in the operating room, you concentrate on the operative field. Similarly, give the exam your full, serious, and undivided attention. Problems at work or home should be left at the exam room doorstep; your one and only task during the exam period is to answer questions to the best of your ability.

Test Mechanics

Before beginning each section of the exam, read the directions. Formats could change. Never find yourself having answered an entire section incorrectly because you failed to read the instructions.

You are allowed to mark on the test booklet unless instructed otherwise. It has been found that errors can be minimized by marking your answers in the test booklet, and then marking the machine scorable answer sheet after every 20 to 30 questions. This process varies the task, allows some psychological rest and forces you to periodically check for accuracy in marking the correct item number on the answer sheet.

If you do not know the answer to a question, skip it and continue answering the questions you know. Frequently, you will find clues in other questions that will help you answer those you left blank. In addition, your subconscious will have processed the questions you skipped. It has been found that a great deal of information is stored in memory, but information retrieval is often faulty. Methods such as rest and varying mental tasks enhance retrieval. Come back later to the questions you left blank.

Changing Your Answer

Contrary to some popular misconceptions, if you doubt an answer selection and want to change it, it is suggested that you do so. In numerous studies across disciplines examining thousands of changed responses, answers were changed approximately twice as often from incorrect responses to correct ones (Welch and Leichner, 1988; Fabrey and Case, 1985; Shababudin, 1983). If you really have no idea which response is correct and you find yourself purely guessing, perhaps your first instinct is accurate. However, if you have a reason to change your answer, you will probably change from an incorrect to a correct response.

Answering by Elimination

Selecting your answer by the process of elimination increases the probability of choosing the correct response. Using the stem of the question, form a sentence with each choice provided. Be cautioned against selecting the first answer you think is correct; consider all possibilities before making a final selection.

Most test questions have in common the following anatomic features: (1) one choice is easily recognized as an outlyer and incorrect; (2) two choices appear plausible as either slightly off the topic or the opposite of the correct answer (eg, artery versus arteriole, left versus right hemithorax); (3) two choices are correct, but one is better than the other.

The test taker's job is to (1) eliminate the outlyer; (2) identify the two plausible choices and reject them after weighing them against the two that are more likely to be correct; and then (3) select the better answer of the remaining two. Similar to a differential diagnosis, this job is accomplished effectively through the process of elimination.

By using the process of elimination, almost anyone can eliminate the outlyer. In doing so, the probability of selecting the wrong answer by guessing alone is decreased by 20%. If the two plausible but incorrect choices are identified, the test taker then has two remaining items and a 50-50 chance of guessing the correct answer.

Always Triage First

On some exams, points for selecting unnecessarily dangerous, invasive, expensive, or potentially harmful choices are tallied separately. On the exam, as in real life, you are allowed very few such errors. Screen each and every question for potentially harmful or invasive choices. Just as patients are triaged, you should similarly triage each test item encountered. There are three question categories that should be identified.

The first is the "friendly" question—the one that assesses your medical knowledge simply by asking for information. The second category includes those questions designed to trap. Unlike the "friendly" question, the item designed to trap has a preconceived attractor or distractor that may catch the test taker off guard. The third type of question is the one containing a potentially harmful choice. It may refer to a treatment, procedure, finding, or diagnosis.

The third category might not be necessarily tricky, but the test item writer had in mind a possible pitfall that must not be selected. This pitfall should be identified in your triaging. As you read each test item, place it into one of the three categories before selecting your answer.

Detailed examples of each question type are presented under the section, "Illustrative Questions."

About Type K Questions

Type K questions are multiple combination, multiple-choice questions. Memorize the following combination schemes before the exam:

Mark (A) if only (1), (2), and (3) are correct.
Mark (B) if only (1) and (3) are correct.
Mark (C) if only (2) and (4) are correct.
Mark (D) if only (4) is correct.
Mark (E) if all are correct.

This will avoid confusion and loss of time you could put to better use.

When answering questions, form a sentence using the stem with each foil, as you would with single-answer multiple-choice questions. Mark only those you are *sure* are true or false. Then rule out among answers (A) through (E) those that are not possibilities. For example, if you are sure that foil 3 is false, eliminate (A), (B), and (E). By guessing alone, you now have a 50-50 chance of selecting (C) or (D) as the correct answer.

It is especially important to practice using the Type K scheme before the actual exam. In addition, writing several of your own test questions is highly recommended. Valuable insights will be gained by doing so.

Type Ks require that you consider more chance probabilities and answer combinations than single-answer multiple-choice questions. Test takers who learn to play and enjoy the game of answering Type Ks tend to report success. The opposite appears true of those who are hostile toward the format.

Some General Hints
Certain "hints" of test taking apply to most multiple-choice tests. These hints are not, however, as likely to work on standardized exams as on other tests, but they may be useful as a last resort for answering some test items.

The choices "all of the above" or "none of the above" have an increased probability of being correct. If in a single-answer multiple-choice question two alternatives mean exactly the same thing, they probably are both incorrect.

Finally, if you must make a pure guess, (C) is most likely the correct choice. The next most likely choice is (B). Board exam test writers try to guard against these probabilities, but the odds might prove useful to you if all else fails.

ILLUSTRATIVE QUESTIONS

You will encounter the following types of questions on Board exams. Each example presented illustrates a strategy to help identify correct choices. As always, first triage each question and identify its category.

The Oversimplification
Some questions appear tricky because you think "no question could be this simple!" If you really know the answer to a question, answer it without belaboring or looking for booby traps that are not there. The following is an example.

A 22-year-old woman presents with abdominal pain and fever of 2 days' duration. During the digital pelvic exam, she experiences exquisite pain when the cervix is moved. This suggests a diagnosis of

    (A) uterine fibroids

    (B) vaginitis

    (C) peritonitis

    (D) cystitis

    (E) cervical carcinoma

The foil least likely to cause pain, (E), is eliminated. Any of the remaining four are possibilities, but peritonitis of some etiology is usually a safe diagnostic consideration. Do not get bogged down considering the unlikely diagnostic possibilities when an obvious choice is present. The oversimplification in this case was the correct answer, (C).

The Oversimplification That Is Dangerous by Omission
As always, triage questions for traps. In the following question, the correct choice is an oversimplification that is dangerous by omission.

A painless testicular mass is found in an otherwise normal 38-year-old. Which of the following diagnoses should be pursued?

    (A) varicocele

    (B) carcinoma

    (C) furuncle

    (D) torsion

    (E) strangulation

Choices (C), (D), and (E) are ruled out because they usually are painful. (A) and (B), however, usually are painless. Because of its prognosis if left untreated, a testicular mass should be considered cancer until proven otherwise. Not to do so would be considered a life-threatening omission. Although a simple and obvious component of the self-exam and the primary care exam, the correct choice was (B).

Always screen questions for dangerous or critical choices whether harmful by omission or commission. A potentially harmful choice may present as an oversimplification.

Clues from Logic
Sometimes a logical (and correct) answer is contained in the stem, as shown in the following example.

The diagnosis of congenital hip dislocation is made

    (A) in utero

    (B) at birth

    (C) at 6 weeks of age

    (D) at 6 months of age

    (E) fluoroscopically

The term "congenital" means "present at birth." This is when the diagnosis of congenital hip dislocation is made. The correct choice was (B).

Clues from Related Areas
Similar to "Clues from Logic," knowledge about related disciplines can provide additional hints.

An obese 45-year-old woman presents with acute genital pain. Upon examination you find a 2- to 3-cm soft mass in the right labia majora. This is most likely

(A) an inguinal hernia
(B) a femoral hernia
(C) a femoral aneurysm
(D) marked lymphadenopathy
(E) neurofibroma

If the mass were located in the scrotum of an obese man, you would probably not miss the common diagnosis of inguinal hernia. Remembering from developmental anatomy that the labia majora and scrotum are corresponding tissues, (A) would be selected as the correct response, even if the test taker had minimal knowledge about surgical emergencies.

The "Odd" Choice

This test-taking clue is demonstrated by way of two examples. The first example comes from psychiatry.

Which of the following is not a sign of transsexualism?

(A) rejecting one's anatomic sex
(B) sex identity problems during childhood
(C) dressing in clothing of the opposite sex
(D) aversion toward one's own genitalia
(E) sex identity problems during adolescence

Transsexualism is considered pathological because the patient considers a mutilating procedure preferable to living as his/her designated sex. Each choice except (C) implies pathology—rejecting one's own anatomy, sex identity problems, and aversion. The odd choice, (C), has, however, no associated pathology and was the correct response.

The second example follows.

A 65-year-old man complains of burning pain of the distal extremities especially upon exposure to heat. Upon examination, the hands and feet are warm and erythematous. The findings are most consistent with

(A) diabetes mellitus
(B) arteriosclerosis
(C) Raynaud's phenomenon
(D) thromboembolism
(E) erythromelalgia

With the limited amount of information provided in the stem, it is unlikely that you can differentiate precisely among the choices provided. Your only clue is the odd choice. Even if you are unfamiliar with the infrequently seen problem of erythromelalgia, notice that choices A through D are associated with problems causing impaired circulation and cold extremities. "Erythro" or "red" implies increased circulation and warmth. (E), the

odd choice among the options provided, was the correct answer.

Qualifying Words

Test-item stems containing qualifying words such as most, more, usually, often, less seldom, few, etc., will sometimes lead you to the correct answer.

You see in the outpatient clinic a 32-year-old man whom you suspect is suffering from alcohol withdrawal. The most likely finding would be

(A) visual hallucinations
(B) auditory hallucinations
(C) fine motor tremors
(D) major motor seizures
(E) autonomic hyperactivity

Any of the above may be seen with alcohol withdrawal. However, fine motor tremors are the most common by far. The stem contains a qualifying word suggesting (C) as the correct choice.

If a qualifying word appears among the choices presented, it deserves special attention. Words such as *best, entirely, completely, always,* and *all* imply that something is always true; words such as *worst, never, no,* and *none* imply that something is never true. In clinical practice, *always* and *never* are rarely correct.

The Overqualified Choice

To make an answer acceptable, test-item writers sometimes must qualify a choice to the point at which the test taker recognizes the ploy. The following example illustrates the overqualified choice.

In a 66-year-old emphysematous man with a 100-pack-per-year smoking history, clubbing is most appropriately described as

(A) discoloration
(B) a flattened angle between the dorsal surface of the distal phalanx and the proximal nail
(C) an abnormal inwardly curved nail
(D) a pack/year history
(E) a measurably increased eponychium

The overqualified (lengthy) choice, (B), is likely to be correct, as in this example.

However, remember the "Odd Choice" described above! Sometimes the very short "Odd Choice" is correct. You will recognize this variation because it will be attractively precise and succinct. Having at least some knowledge of the item, you will identify it as accurate.

Strange Terms

Choices containing completely unfamiliar words are likely to be distractors. Do not assume that you somehow missed an important chapter of Harrison's or that there was a gap in your education. If the choice appears completely bizarre, the test-item writer was probably scraping the barrel for a distractor.

On a routine peripheral blood smear from a 13-year-old boy, you see a nucleated cell that is filled with bright red granules and is approximately three times the diameter of a typical red blood cell. This should be recognized as a (an)

(A) Franz-Kulig cell

(B) myelocyte

(C) eosinophil

(D) Olson cell

(E) Kuppler cell

Choices A, D, and E are completely fictitious. The test-item writer obviously did not lack imagination. B is familiar—remember basic anatomy or hematology? However, identifying a myelocyte on the peripherial smear is not basic primary care, which the Board exam covers. Hence, physician assistants should recognize the morphology and significance of an eosinophil. The correct response was (C).

"Apple Pie" Choices

There are some responses to which no one would object. Consider the following test question.

When evaluating a 23-year-old woman with vaginal bleeding, the most important clinical information is gained from the

(A) prothrombin time

(B) partial thromboplastin time

(C) CBC and iron studies

(D) physical exam

(E) detailed history

A patient's history provides a clinician's best information and is almost never incorrect. (E) is an "apple pie" choice.

The "apple pie" choice, however, can also be used by test-item writers to set traps.

The most important physical exam component(s) in the emergency evaluation of an unconscious patient is (are)

(A) body symmetry

(B) a carefully performed and prompt neurological exam

(C) the cardiopulmonary exam

(D) vital signs

(E) blood gases

The initial triage of this question would identify it as a "trap" question because of the critical nature of the scenario combined with an incorrect "apple pie" choice. Blood gases are promptly dismissed because they are not physical exam components, for which the stem asks.

(B) appears attractive because of its "apple pie" component. Nevertheless, remember your ABCs of emergency care! The correct response was (D).

Hints from Inconsistencies in Terminology

Grammar inconsistencies between the stem and a choice (e.g., tense, number, gender) are usually recognized by expert educational evaluators who screen Board exam test questions. You will, therefore, seldom encounter this type of "hint" on Board exams, although it will be found more frequently in classroom situations. Hints due to inconsistencies in terminology are more frequent than other types of hints because expert test-item reviewers frequently lack a medical background. Therefore, you may benefit from recognizing inconsistencies in terminology.

A 19-year-old unconscious motorcycle accident victim with suspected multiple trauma is brought to the emergency room. The most significant physical findings usually will result from

(A) undressing the patient

(B) a prompt neurological exam

(C) interviewing the family

(D) interviewing a witness to the accident

(E) all the above

Choices (C) and (D) can be excluded because they refer to historical, not physical findings. This also excludes foil (E). Because critical, life-saving information across organ systems may be gained from observing the patient, choice (A) was correct. Similarly, choice (E), blood gases, in the previous example was eliminated because it was inconsistent with the information asked for in the stem.

Rank Orders

When given a list of numbers or other rank orders, the correct response most often occurs somewhere between the extremes, as shown in these examples.

A 17-year-old woman presents with a history of pelvic discomfort during menses. Through questioning, you determine that the amount of blood lost during each cycle is normal. The amount of her blood loss would be approximately

(A) 25 mL

(B) 35 mL

(C) 70 mL

(D) 100 mL

(E) 125 mL

Here is the second example.

In reviewing the chart of a 45-year-old man, you notice a past diagnosis of chronic schizophrenia. To be termed *chronic,* this disorder was present for at least

(A) 3 months

(B) 1 year

(C) 2 years

(D) 3 years

(E) 4 years

Most test-item writers try to bury the correct answer somewhere in the middle. (C) was the correct answer in each example.

As with "Hints from Inconsistencies in Terminology," this clue does not work as often on board exams as it does on classroom tests. Educational evaluators try to randomize the position of correct responses as much as possible. However, when in doubt, it is better to avoid the extremes when presented with rank-ordered options.

DO'S AND DON'TS

The following "do's and don'ts" summarize some of the important points made earlier in this section.

DO practice what you will be doing during the exam, that is, answering multiple-choice questions. Answering these questions is a skill different from knowing clinical information. Get into practice for answering multiple-choice questions by actually answering them. This is imperative for the clinician who has not taken a multiple-choice exam recently.

DO direct your studying to the primary care areas with which you are least familiar. Passing the boards is best accomplished by achieving a fundamental knowledge level in each medical discipline assessed on the exam.

DO write your own multiple-choice questions (including Type K). Not only will you gain insights into the mechanics of test-item writing and correctly answering questions, but it is likely that the content of many of your items will resemble those of actual Board exam questions.

DO get adequate sleep and rest before the exam.

DO relate test questions to your own practice and experience. Test-item writers are people who have derived many test questions from their own clinical experience. What would *you* expect a primary care physician assistant to know? Use this mindset to understand the goal of a question and to keep a positive attitude throughout the exam.

DO change your answer if you have a good reason to do so. You are twice as likely to change from an incorrect response to a correct one. However, if you are only playing a hunch with no information about the topic at all, your first "gut" reaction might be correct.

DO triage each and every question before selecting your answer. Evaluate it as a question designed to (1) test knowledge in a "friendly" way; (2) trap by including common pitfalls; or (3) trap by including potentially dangerous choices. In the first case, the apparent oversimplification is probably the correct choice. In questions designed to trap, beware of the "apple pie" choice—ommission or commission. On the test, as in real clinical life, you cannot afford to make many dangerous errors.

DO use the process of elimination. Your job is to find the single best answer. As with a patient's differential diagnosis, this usually is done by *elimination*. Avoid choosing an answer until after you have considered each choice.

DO read the question stem and combine it with each foil to form a sentence. After doing this, use the process of elimination to arrive at the final answer.

DO mark your answers in the test booklet and transfer them to the machine scorable answer sheet after every 20 to 30 questions. This procedure tends to minimize errors and provide psychological rest.

DO consider the proctor your colleague. He or she is there to support you and to facilitate your best performance on the exam. Expect and demand this kind of treatment.

DO leave items blank if you are not sure of the answer. Return to these items when you finish the rest of the exam or at a time when you gain information from other questions.

DO pace yourself, allowing a calculated amount of time per question. In your time allocation, allow for some extra minutes at the end for returning to items left blank.

DO make educated guesses, if you must guess. Use the information provided in this section to help in your decision. By also using your medical knowledge and judgment, your chances will be much improved.

DO be alert for qualifying words such as most, more, usually, often, less seldom, few, etc., which will sometimes lead you to the correct answer.

DO consider choices containing completely unfamiliar words distractors. If the choice appears completely unfamiliar, the answer is probably incorrect.

DO consider "apple pie" choices as probably correct. However, beware that they may also be used to trap.

DO consider choices that are different from the others—the "odd choice." This may involve the choice having the "odd" meaning or the "odd" length—long or short. The overqualified choice is often correct.

DO select item (C) when purely guessing. It is most frequently the correct response on many one-choice-only multiple-choice questions. If you can somehow eliminate (C) as a possibility, (B) is the next most likely choice. This is a "last-ditch" strategy that works more often on classroom tests than on Board exams.

DO select "all the above" or "none of the above" as a last-ditch strategy. When appearing as choices, they are likely to be correct.

DO read all instructions for each section of the exam. Be aware of any change in format.

DO use the hints in this chapter pertaining to single-answer multiple-choice questions for answering Type K questions. As with other formats on the Board exam, triage each item and beware of dangerous or potentially harmful responses—choosing even a few incorrectly may result in failing the exam.

DO avoid situations that might put you in an unfavorable mindset before the exam. For example, if you anticipate heavy highway traffic, arrive at the exam site a day early. If disturbances bother you during an exam, come early and select a seat in a far corner of the testing room. Let nothing interfere with your best possible performance on the day of the exam.

DO consider taking the exam a positive experience. Keep your motivation high through self-coaching and imaging techniques. Use recommended stress management techniques, especially if you are anxious when taking tests.

DO plan to reward yourself for a good performance after the exam. This facilitates a positive attitude.

DON'T cram at the last minute. This kind of preparation will not be adequate for an exam that covers mostly primary care breadth rather than depth.

DON'T eat a large meal within 2 hours of the beginning of the exam. Be well nourished, but not full.

DON'T think of anything except the exam in front of you. Think of it as your "operative field." Concentrate on giving your best possible performance.

DON'T become irate over seemingly absurd questions. Answer them to the best of your ability, realizing that they probably are experimental questions that will not affect your score. Other test takers probably will also consider them absurd.

DON'T guess randomly. Even if you are completely unsure of the answer to a question, use the hints suggested in this section to increase the probability of "guessing" the correct response. Make educated, not random guesses.

DON'T leave any item blank at the end of the exam. Unanswered items generally will be counted wrong. However, it is better to leave an item blank than to choose an incorrect response involving a dangerous, invasive, or otherwise potentially harmful item.

REFERENCES

Benson H. *The Relaxation Response.* New York: Avon Books; 1975.

Carman RA. *Study Skills: A Student's Guide for Survival,* 2nd ed. John Wiley: New York; 1984.

DeCecco JP, Crawford WR. *The Psychology of Learning and Instruction,* 2nd ed. Englewood Cliffs, NJ: Prentice Hall; 1974.

Fabrey L, Case SM. Further support for changing multiple-choice answers. *J Med Educ.* June 1985: 488–490.

Greenberg JS. *Comprehensive Stress Management,* 2nd ed. Dubuque, IA: Wm. C. Brown; 1987.

Hiebert B, Cardinal J, Dumka L, Marx RW. Self-instructed relaxation: A therapeutic alternative. *Biofeedback Self-Regul.* December 1983: 601–617.

Maatsch, JL. *The Predictive Value of Medical Specialty Examinations: Final Report.* Washington, D.C.: National Center for Health Services Research, Contract No. HS-02-038-04; 1983.

Pelletier KR. *Mind as Healer, Mind as Slayer.* New York: Dell; 1977.

Phipps R. *The Successful Student's Handbook: A Step-by-Step Guide to Study, Reading and Thinking Skills.* Seattle, WA: University of Washington Press; 1983.

Shababudin SH. Pattern of answer changes to multiple-choice questions in physiology. *Med Educ.* March 1983: 316–318.

Snelbecker GE. *Learning Theory, Instructional Theory and Psychoeducational Design.* Lanham, MD: University Printers of America; 1985.

U.S. Department of Education. *What Works: Research About Teaching and Learning.* Washington, D.C.: U.S. Department of Education; 1986.

Welch J, Leichner P. Analysis of changing answers on multiple-choice examination for nationwide sample of Canadian psychiatry residents. *J Med Educ.* February 1988: 133–135.

Robert W. Jarski, PhD, PA-C

CHAPTER 1

Surgery
Questions

DIRECTIONS (Question 1): Each of the numbered items or incomplete statements in this section is followed by answers or by completions of the statement. Select the ONE lettered answer or completion that is BEST in each case.

Question 1

1. Which of the following disorders of hemostasis is most commonly seen in the bleeding surgical patient?

    (A) thrombocytopenia
    (B) disseminated intravascular coagulopathy (DIC)
    (C) Von Willebrand's disease (Factor VIII)
    (D) Christmas disease (Factor IX)
    (E) classical hemophilia (Factor VIII)

DIRECTIONS (Questions 2 through 5): Each set of items in this section consists of a list of lettered options followed by several numbered words or phrases. For each numbered word or phrase, select the ONE lettered option that is most closely associated with it. Each lettered option may be selected once, more than once, or not at all.

Questions 2 through 5

Match the following symptoms or signs with the most likely diagnosis.

    (A) neurogenic shock
    (B) septic shock
    (C) insulin shock
    (D) hypovolemic shock
    (E) cardiogenic shock

2. Lower extremity paresthesias

3. Muffled heart sounds

4. Fracture of the femur

5. Tachycardia and warm skin

DIRECTIONS (Questions 6 and 7): Each of the numbered items or incomplete statements in this section is followed by answers or by completions of the statement. Select the ONE lettered answer or completion that is BEST in each case.

Questions 6 and 7

6. Which of the following symptoms are LEAST likely to be associated with carcinoma of the breast?

    (A) nipple retraction
    (B) erythema or skin discoloration
    (C) skin dimpling
    (D) breast pain
    (E) axillary lymphadenopathy

7. Mammography is indicated

    (A) annually in all women of child-bearing age
    (B) annually in women more than 35 years of age
    (C) at 40 years of age and then annually after the age of 50
    (D) to evaluate a palpable breast mass
    (E) none of the above

vascular etiology (handwritten)

DIRECTIONS (Question 8): For each of the items in this section, ONE or MORE of the numbered options is correct. Choose answer

    (A) if only (1), (2), and (3) are correct,
    (B) if only (1) and (3) are correct,
    (C) if only (2) and (4) are correct,
    (D) if only (4) is correct,
    (E) if all are correct.

Question 8

8. Which of the following is/are of historical importance in evaluating the patient with a breast mass?

    (1) use of oral contraceptives
    (2) age of the first childbirth
    (3) family history of breast cancer
    (4) history of benign breast mass

DIRECTIONS (Questions 9 through 15): Each of the numbered items or incomplete statements in this section is followed by answers or by completions of the statement. Select the ONE lettered answer or completion that is BEST in each case.

Questions 9 through 15

9. Diffuse abdominal pain that is "wave-like" and associated with vomiting is most likely

    (A) pancreatitis
    (B) peptic ulcer disease
    (C) appendicitis
    (D) bowel obstruction
    (E) cholelithiasis

10. Abdominal pain that is sudden in onset and severe is NOT associated with

    (A) perforated peptic ulcer
    (B) ureteral colic
    (C) biliary colic *insidious, p prandial* (handwritten)
    (D) ruptured abdominal aneurysm
    (E) pancreatitis

11. If intestinal obstruction is suspected, which radiologic procedure is indicated initially?

    (A) barium enema
    (B) abdominal ultrasound
    (C) abdominal CAT scan
    (D) flat and upright abdomen
    (E) upper GI series with small bowel follow through

12. "Pain out of proportion" with physical findings is associated with which diagnosis?

    (A) perforated peptic ulcer
    (B) peritonitis
    (C) mesenteric occlusion
    (D) Crohn's disease
    (E) cecal volvulus

13. Which nervous structure is at greater risk during thyroidectomy?

    (A) cervical sympathetic chain
    (B) recurrent laryngeal nerve *- tracheoesophageal groove bilaterally* (handwritten)
    (C) vagus nerve
    (D) superior laryngeal nerve
    (E) inferior laryngeal nerve

14. The most useful diagnostic test in the preoperative evaluation of a solid thyroid mass is

    (A) ultrasound *- cystic* (handwritten)
    (B) thyroid function test *most ca. still euthyroid* (handwritten)
    (C) needle aspiration
    (D) radioactive scan *- shows "cold" nodules, but benign nodules also cold.* (handwritten)
    (E) needle biopsy

15. Which thyroid malignancy has the best prognosis following surgical excision?

    (A) follicular carcinoma *44-86%* (handwritten)
    (B) papillary carcinoma *99% · 10 yr.* (handwritten)
    (C) medullary carcinoma
    (D) anaplastic carcinoma
    (E) lymphoma

DIRECTIONS (Questions 16 through 21): For each of the items in this section, ONE or MORE of the numbered options is correct. Choose answer

    (A) if only (1), (2), and (3) are correct,
    (B) if only (1) and (3) are correct,
    (C) if only (2) and (4) are correct,
    (D) if only (4) is correct,
    (E) if all are correct.

Questions 16 through 21

16. Which of the following might be associated with thyroid carcinoma?

    (1) hoarseness
    (2) dysphagia
    (3) palpable mass
    (4) Delphian node

17. Which factor is most significant as a precursor to thyroid carcinoma?

—(1) family history of medullary thyroid cancer
(2) history of hyperthyroidism
—(3) irradiation of the neck
(4) history of goiter

18. Primary hyperparathyroidism is NOT caused by

(1) parathyroid adenoma
(2) hyperplasia of the parathyroid
(3) carcinoma of the parathyroid
»(4) vitamin D deficiency

19. The most common cause(s) of hypoparathyroidism is/are

(1) idiopathic – V. rare, would occur before 14 yrs.
(2) metastatic carcinoma ↑ serum ca⁺
(3) renal failure ↑ serum ca⁺⁺
→ (4) surgery

20. Which of the following is/are branches of the superior mesenteric artery?

(1) right colic artery
(2) left colic artery
(3) middle colic artery
(4) sigmoid artery

21. Characteristic features of the colon include

(1) taenia coli
(2) valvulae conniventes
(3) haustra
(4) ligament of Treitz

DIRECTIONS (Questions 22 through 26): Each set of matching questions in this section consists of a list of lettered options followed by a set of numbered words or phrases. For each numbered word or phrase, select the ONE lettered option that is most closely associated with it. Each lettered option may be selected once, more than once, or not at all.

Questions 22 through 26

Match the following sign/symptom with the most commonly associated form of colitis:

(A) Crohn's colitis
(B) ulcerative colitis

22. Discontinuous involvement

23. Transmural involvement

24. Bleeding

25. Anal fissures

26. Abdominal mass

DIRECTIONS (Questions 27 and 28): Each of the numbered items or incomplete statements in this section is followed by answers or by completions of the statement. Select the ONE lettered answer or completion that is BEST in each case.

Questions 27 and 28

27. Antibiotic-induced colitis results from overgrowth of

(A) *Bacteroides fragilis*
(B) *Escherichia coli*
(C) *Clostridium tetani*
(D) *Clostridium difficile*
(E) *Bacteroides vulgatus*

28. Treatment of pseudomembranous colitis consists of

(A) steroids
(B) sulfasalizine
(C) ampicillin 500 mg PO qid
(D) vancomycin 500 mg PO qid
(E) colectomy

DIRECTIONS (Questions 29 through 32): For each of the items in this section, ONE or MORE of the numbered options is correct. Choose answer

(A) **if only (1), (2), and (3) are correct,**
(B) **if only (1) and (3) are correct,**
(C) **if only (2) and (4) are correct,**
(D) **if only (4) is correct,**
(E) **if all are correct.**

Questions 29 through 32

29. Radiographic finding(s) in Crohn's colitis include

(1) cobblestoning
(2) fistulization
(3) stenosis
(4) calcium deposits

30. Complications of ulcerative colitis include

(1) toxic megacolon
(2) hemorrhage
(3) perforation
(4) carcinoma

31. Initial treatment of colitis includes

    (1) azulfidine
    (2) ACTH
    (3) prednisone
    (4) surgical resection

32. Surgical management of ulcerative colitis includes

    (1) ileostomy
    (2) abdominoperineal resection
    (3) total colectomy
    (4) regional resection

DIRECTIONS (Questions 33 through 37): Each of the numbered items or incomplete statements in this section is followed by answers or by completions of the statement. Select the ONE lettered answer or completion that is BEST in each case.

Questions 33 through 37

33. Bleeding from diverticulosis is

    (A) rare
    (B) indolent
    (C) often the only symptom
    (D) associated with abdominal pain
    (E) never life-threatening

34. The diagnostic procedure of choice for massive lower GI bleeding is

    (A) CT scan
    (B) colonoscopy
    (C) barium enema
    (D) arteriography
    (E) radionucleotide imaging

35. Which is NOT a complication of diverticulitis?

    (A) obstruction
    (B) perforation
    (C) fistula
    (D) carcinoma
    (E) bleeding

36. Which of the following have NO malignant potential?

    (A) polyposes coli
    (B) tubular adenoma
    (C) villous adenoma
    (D) familial polyposis
    (E) juvenile polyposis

37. Anal fissure is NOT associated with

    (A) Crohn's disease
    (B) tuberculosis
    (C) trauma
    (D) diabetes
    (E) syphilis

DIRECTIONS (Questions 38 through 46): For each of the items in this section, ONE or MORE of the numbered options is correct. Choose answer

    (A) if only (1), (2), and (3) are correct,
    (B) if only (1) and (3) are correct,
    (C) if only (2) and (4) are correct,
    (D) if only (4) is correct,
    (E) if all are correct.

Questions 38 through 46

38. Indications for hemorrhoidectomy include

    (1) pain
    (2) bleeding
    (3) prolapse
    (4) thrombosis

39. Diverticulitis frequently presents as

    (1) pain
    (2) fever
    (3) anorexia
    (4) vomiting

40. Screening for carcinoma of the colon should include

    (1) hemoccult
    (2) barium enema
    (3) colonoscopy
    (4) carcinoembryonic antigen (CEA) titers

41. Esophageal achalasia consists of

    (1) relaxation of lower esophageal sphincter
    (2) absence of esophageal peristalsis
    (3) gastroesophageal reflux
    (4) contraction of lower esophageal sphincter

42. Therapy for esophageal achalasia consists of

    (1) esophagomyotomy
    (2) vagal denervation
    (3) esophageal dilation
    (4) Nissan fundoplication (antireflux procedure)

43. Which of the following are important in the diagnosis of esophageal motility disorders?

    (1) manometry
    (2) endoscopy
    (3) contrast radiography
    (4) CT scanning

44. Complications associated with diaphragmatic hernias include

    (1) volvulus
    (2) obstruction
    (3) ischemia
    (4) carcinoma

45. The diagnosis of acute pancreatitis is based on

    (1) elevated amylase
    (2) elevated calcium
    (3) history and physical
    (4) abdominal radiographs

46. Treatment of pancreatitis consists of

    (1) IV fluids
    (2) nasogastric suction
    (3) analgesics
    (4) exploratory laparotomy

DIRECTIONS (Questions 47 through 52): Each of the numbered items or incomplete statements in this section is followed by answers or by completions of the statement. Select the ONE lettered answer or completion that is BEST in each case.

Questions 47 through 52

47. The complications of gastroesophageal reflux include all the following EXCEPT

    (A) bleeding
    (B) Barrett's esophagus
    (C) esophageal contractures
    (D) esophageal ulceration
    (E) Mallory–Weiss syndrome

48. The earliest feature of esophageal carcinoma is

    (A) dyspnea
    (B) hematemesis
    (C) pain
    (D) dysphagia
    (E) weight loss

49. The main duct emptying the pancreas is

    (A) ampulla of Vater
    (B) duct of Sylvius
    (C) duct of Wirsung
    (D) duct of Santorini
    (E) ampulla of Laffaye

50. The most common complication of acute pancreatitis is

    (A) pseudocyst
    (B) abscess
    (C) diabetes
    (D) steatorrhea
    (E) chronic pancreatitis

51. Diagnosis of chronic pancreatitis has been easier with the advent of

    (A) CT scan
    (B) ultrasound
    (C) MRI (magnetic resonance imaging)
    (D) ERCP (endoscopic retrograde cholecystopancreatography)
    (E) radionucleotide imaging

52. Treatment of a pancreatic pseudocyst consists of

    (A) observation
    (B) total pancreatectomy
    (C) endoscopic cannulation and drainage
    (D) internal drainage
    (E) percutaneous drainage under CT scan

DIRECTIONS (Questions 53 through 56): For each of the items in this section, ONE or MORE of the numbered options is correct. Choose answer

    (A) if only (1), (2), and (3) are correct,
    (B) if only (1) and (3) are correct,
    (C) if only (2) and (4) are correct,
    (D) if only (4) is correct,
    (E) if all are correct.

Questions 53 through 56

53. Classic findings in a patient with chronic pancreatitis might include

    (1) diabetes
    (2) steatorrhea
    (3) weight loss
    (4) fever

54. Symptoms of carcinoma of the pancreas may include

    (1) pruritis
    (2) epigastric pain
    (3) weight loss
    (4) jaundice

55. In the Whipple procedure (pancreaticoduodenectomy), which of the following is/are removed?

    (1) head of the pancreas
    (2) gallbladder
    (3) duodenum
    (4) spleen

56. Normal splenic function consists of

    (1) hematopoiesis
    (2) production of tissue thromboplastin
    (3) vitamin K synthesis
    (4) erythrocyte sequestration

DIRECTIONS (Questions 57 through 61): Each set of matching questions in this section consists of a list of lettered options followed by a set of numbered words or phrases. For each numbered word or phrase, select the ONE lettered option that is most closely associated with it. Each lettered option may be selected once, more than once, or not at all.

Questions 57 through 61

Match the following hernias to their definitions.

    (A) an organ is involved in the hernia
    (B) unreducible
    (C) ischemia
    (D) patent tunica vaginalis
    (E) Hesselbach's triangle

57. Strangulated hernia

58. Incarcerated hernia

59. Direct hernia

60. Indirect hernia

61. Sliding hernia

DIRECTIONS (Questions 62 through 64): Each of the numbered items or incomplete statements in this section is followed by answers or by completions of the statement. Select the ONE lettered answer or completion that is BEST in each case.

Questions 62 through 64

62. The most common type of hernia in females is

    (A) indirect hernia
    (B) direct hernia
    (C) femoral hernia
    (D) ventral hernia
    (E) spigelian hernia

63. Which of the following is the most common tumor of the brain?

    (A) glioblastoma
    (B) meningioma
    (C) astrocytoma
    (D) metastases
    (E) acoustic neuroma

64. A 29-year-old male presents with complaints of severe low back and leg pain following a sneeze. His pain extends from the buttocks posteriorly to the sole of the foot. On examination you note an absent ankle jerk and weakness of plantar flexion. The most likely diagnosis is

    (A) spinal cord tumor
    (B) S1 radiculopathy
    (C) L5 radiculopathy
    (D) pulled hamstring
    (E) spondylolysis

DIRECTIONS (Questions 65 through 69): For each of the items in this section, ONE or MORE of the numbered options is correct. Choose answer

    (A) if only (1), (2), and (3) are correct,
    (B) if only (1) and (3) are correct,
    (C) if only (2) and (4) are correct,
    (D) if only (4) is correct,
    (E) if all are correct.

Questions 65 through 69

65. Complications of hernia repair include

    (1) testicular edema
    (2) recurrence
    (3) bleeding
    (4) ilioinguinal nerve damage

66. Which is/are symptom(s) of a brain tumor?

    (1) headache
    (2) loss of vision
    (3) seizure
    (4) hemiparesis

67. Which of the following statements about melena are true?

    (1) Melena usually indicates upper gastrointestinal tract bleeding.
    (2) The tarry color is a result of the production of the acid hematin by the action of gastric acid on hemoglobin.
    (3) As little as 50 mL of blood may produce melena.

(4) Only blood is capable of producing black stools.

68. Which of the following are true regarding proximal gastric ulceration?

   (1) Stress is often a precipitating factor.
   (2) Incidence increases with age.
   (3) Acid hypersecretion is an associated factor.
   (4) In the United States gastric ulcers are much less common than duodenal ulcers.

69. Which of the following would be most likely to decrease gastric acid production?

   (1) parietal cell vagotomy
   (2) antrectomy
   (3) proximal gastrectomy
   (4) pyloroplasty

DIRECTIONS (Questions 70 through 73): Each of the numbered items or incomplete statements in this section is followed by answers or by completions of the statement. Select the ONE lettered answer or completion that is BEST in each case.

Questions 70 through 73

70. The most common abnormal physiologic mechanism of duodenal ulcer formation is

   (A) increased secretion of gastric acid
   (B) rapid gastric emptying
   (C) fasting hypergastrinemia
   (D) hyperpepsinogenemia
   (E) deficient duodenal buffers

71. A 70-year-old female presents with massive melena and associated hypotension which is corrected with IV fluid and blood. Which of the following should be done first to determine the source of gastrointestinal bleeding?

   (A) a lower gastrointestinal barium enema
   (B) sigmoidoscopy
   (C) colonoscopy
   (D) radionucleotide imaging
   (E) selective arteriography

72. A 60-year-old diabetic male presents with a bleeding duodenal ulcer. He is treated with nasogastric suctioning, saline lavage, and blood transfusions as needed. However, he continues to bleed actively and requires more than 12 U of blood in the first 24 hours. Prior to this he was otherwise healthy. The treatment of choice is

   (A) systemic infusion of vasopressin (pitressin)
   (B) angiographic catheterization of the gastroduodenal artery and gelfoam embolization
   (C) proximal gastric vagotomy
   (D) oversewing the ulcer, bilateral truncal vagotomy and pyloroplasty
   (E) bilateral truncal vagotomy, antrectomy and Billroth II gastrojejunostomy

73. The treatment of choice for a 50-year-old male with biopsy-documented gastric lymphoma would be

   (A) wide local excision
   (B) chemotherapy
   (C) subtotal gastrectomy and radiotherapy
   (D) subtotal gastrectomy
   (E) radiotherapy

DIRECTIONS (Questions 74 through 77): For each of the items in this section, ONE or MORE of the numbered options is correct. Choose answer

   (A) if only (1), (2), and (3) are correct,
   (B) if only (1) and (3) are correct,
   (C) if only (2) and (4) are correct,
   (D) if only (4) is correct,
   (E) if all are correct.

Questions 74 through 77

74. Most gallstones contain

   (1) cholesterol
   (2) calcium
   (3) bile pigments
   (4) oxalates

75. Gallstone formation has been associated with

   (1) hemolytic disease
   (2) aortic valve replacement
   (3) use of birth control pills
   (4) ileal resection

76. Which of the following statement(s) regarding the use of HIDA isotope scans to define gallbladder functions is/are correct?

   (1) They can be used to define obstruction of the extrahepatic ducts.
   (2) They are seldom effective when the patient's serum bilirubin level is higher than 3.5 mg per 100 mL.
   (3) They are the diagnostic tools of choice for defining acute cholecystitis secondary to cystic duct obstruction.
   (4) Their toxicity is approximately the same as that of IV cholangiography.

77. Which of the following statement(s) regarding sclerosing cholangitis is/are true?

    (1) It produces a clinical and laboratory picture of extrahepatic jaundice.

    (2) It occurs more frequently in males than females.

    (3) It has been seen in association with ulcerative colitis.

    (4) It is thought to result from trauma during the passage of gallstones.

DIRECTIONS (Questions 78 through 83): Each of the numbered items or incomplete statements in this section is followed by answers or by completions of the statement. Select the ONE lettered answer or completion that is BEST in each case.

Questions 78 through 83

78. Lithogenic bile is characterized by a low ratio of concentration of

    (A) cholesterol to bile salts

    (B) cholesterol to lecithin and bile salts

    (C) cholesterol to lecithin

    (D) bilirubinate to cholesterol

    (E) lecithin and bile salts to cholesterol

79. The major stimulus for gallbladder emptying is mediated by

    (A) stimulation of the sympathetic system

    (B) release of cholecystokinin

    (C) stimulation of the parasympathetic (vagal) system

    (D) release of secretin

    (E) secretion of hydrochloric acid

80. The treatment of radiolucent gallstones with chenodeoxycholic acid for 2 years results in a complete dissolution in what percentage of patients?

    (A) less than 5%

    (B) 15%

    (C) 25%

    (D) 35%

    (E) greater than 40%

81. In patients with asymptomatic gallstones who were treated without surgery, symptoms developed in

    (A) less than 10%

    (B) 20%

    (C) 30%

    (D) 40%

    (E) 50%

82. A 40-year-old female complains of recurrent postprandial attacks of colicky right upper quadrant pain. Ultrasonography does not demonstrate gallstones. She presently is pain free. The next diagnostic test should be

    (A) flat plate of the abdomen

    (B) oral cholecystography

    (C) HIDA scan

    (D) CT scan of the gallbladder

    (E) percutaneous transhepatic cholangiography (PCT)

83. A 65-year-old male who has previously undergone cholecystectomy presents in the Emergency Room with jaundice, fever, and right upper quadrant abdominal pain. Initial treatment should be

    (A) antibiotics

    (B) endoscopic sphincterotomy

    (C) percutaneous transhepatic drainage

    (D) T-tube decompression of the common bile duct

    (E) emergency exploratory laparotomy

DIRECTIONS (Questions 84 through 87): Each set of items in this section consists of a list of lettered options followed by several numbered words or phrases. For each numbered word or phrase, select the ONE lettered option that is most closely associated with it. Each lettered option may be selected once, more than once, or not at all.

Questions 84 through 87

    (A) acute cholecystitis

    (B) chronic cholecystitis

    (C) both

    (D) neither

84. Cystic duct obstruction

85. Empyema

86. Requires immediate operation

87. HIDA scan is the specific diagnostic test

DIRECTIONS (Questions 88 through 90): For each of the items in this section, ONE or MORE of the numbered options is correct. Choose answer

    (A) **if only (1), (2), and (3) are correct,**
    (B) **if only (1) and (3) are correct,**
    (C) **if only (2) and (4) are correct,**
    (D) **if only (4) is correct,**
    (E) **if all are correct.**

Questions 88 through 90

88. Which of the following statement(s) about liver anatomy is/are true?

    (1) The caudate lobe involves both the anatomic right and anatomic left lobes.
    (2) The quadrate lobe is within the medial segment of the left lobe.
    (3) The left lobe extends to the right of the falciform ligament.
    (4) The right lobe is divided into the inferior and superior segments.

89. Physiologic functions of the liver include which of the following?

    (1) It is the only site of albumen synthesis.
    (2) During fasting it supplies glucose by glycogenolysis and glyconeogenesis.
    (3) It is the primary site of cholesterol synthesis.
    (4) It actively secretes secondary bile acids.

90. Which of the following statement(s) is/are true about the hepatic arterial supply?

    (1) Normal arterial anatomy is present in only 50% of persons.
    (2) It provides 75% of blood flow to the liver.
    (3) It parallels the portal venous system within the liver.
    (4) The most common variant is right hepatic artery arising from the gastroduodenal artery.

DIRECTIONS (Questions 91 through 96): Each of the numbered items or incomplete statements in this section is followed by answers or by completions of the statement. Select the ONE lettered answer or completion that is BEST in each case.

Questions 91 through 96

91. The most common primary tumor site associated with hepatic metastases is

    (A) pancreas
    (B) stomach
    (C) colon
    (D) breast
    (E) lung

92. Which of the following is/are true regarding the treatment of primary hepatocellular carcinoma?

    (A) Most lesions are amenable to resection with a resulting 5-year survival rate of approximately 30%.
    (B) Most lesions are NOT amenable to partial resection and are best treated with radiation.
    (C) Orthotopic liver transplanation has become the treatment of choice.
    (D) Mean survival of untreated patients is 3 to 4 months from the time of onset of the symptoms.
    (E) Both systemic chemotherapy and hepatic arterial chemotherapy produce a response rate of approximately 60%.

93. The demonstration of an elevated level of alpha-fetoprotein in the serum of an adult suggests the diagnosis of

    (A) metastatic cancer of the liver
    (B) primary cancer of the liver
    (C) focal nodular hyperplasia of the liver
    (D) pyogenic liver abscess
    (E) biliary cirrhosis

94. The most common cause of portal hypertension is related to

    (A) extrahepatic venous outflow obstruction
    (B) intrahepatic portal venous obstruction (presinusoidal)
    (C) increased hepatopedal blood flow
    (D) extrahepatic portal venous obstruction
    (E) intrahepatic-hepatic venous obstruction (postsinusoidal)

95. Which of the following best determines long-term survival following a shunting procedure of an alcoholic patient with cirrhosis of the liver?

    (A) control of ascites
    (B) a low-protein diet
    (C) a low-salt intake
    (D) use of lactulose
    (E) abstinence from alcohol

96. Which of the following criteria in a patient with alcoholic cirrhosis provides the most acceptable indication for portal systemic shunting with the best chance of survival?

    (A) documented varices that have never bled but are large
    (B) documented varices that have bled several times in the recent past and have not responded to endoscopic variceal sclerosis
    (C) documented acutely bleeding varices that have not stopped after 10 U of transfused blood
    (D) large esophageal varices and mild encephalopathy
    (E) very high portal pressure discovered during abdominal surgery

DIRECTIONS (Questions 97 through 101): Each set of items in this section consists of a list of lettered options followed by several numbered words or phrases. For each numbered word or phrase, select the ONE lettered option that is most closely associated with it. Each lettered option may be selected once, more than once, or not at all.

Questions 97 through 101

Select the type of hepatic abscess described best by the following statements.

    (A) amebic liver abscess
    (B) pyogenic liver abscess
    (C) both
    (D) neither

97. Usually single

98. Predominantly involves the right lobe of the liver

99. The cultures are usually sterile

100. Treatment is primarily medical

101. Treatment is primarily surgical

DIRECTIONS (Questions 102 through 109): For each of the items in this section, ONE or MORE of the numbered options is correct. Choose answer

    (A) **if only (1), (2), and (3) are correct,**
    (B) **if only (1) and (3) are correct,**
    (C) **if only (2) and (4) are correct,**
    (D) **if only (4) is correct,**
    (E) **if all are correct.**

Questions 102 through 109

102. True statements regarding benign tumors of the small bowel include:

    (1) They are most often found in the ileum.
    (2) They often produce no symptoms and are difficult to diagnose by either clinical or radiological examination.
    (3) They most commonly present with bleeding and obstruction.
    (4) They obstruct the bowel either by encroachment on the lumen or by causing intussusception.

103. True statements regarding malignant small bowel tumors include:

    (1) Carcinoid is the most common malignancy of the small intestine.
    (2) They account for 2% of all gastrointestinal malignancies.
    (3) Five-year survival is highest with adenocarcinoma followed by lymphoma, and still lower with leiomyosarcoma.
    (4) Wide resection with regional lymphadenectomy is the preferred operation.

104. True statements regarding carcinoid tumors include:

    (1) There is a tendency toward multicentricity.
    (2) The cell of origin is the Kupffer cell.
    (3) Prognosis is related to tumor size, location, and histologic pattern.
    (4) The rectum is the most common site of origin.

105. True statements regarding Meckel's diverticulum include:

    (1) They occur in 50% of the population in one form or another.
    (2) They are true diverticula.
    (3) Diverticulitis is the most common complication.
    (4) Some can be visualized with technetium pertechnetate scans.

106. Which of the following is/are true in acute appendicitis?

    (1) Anorexia is usually present.

    (2) Pain often begins in the periumbilical area.

    (3) Obstipation or diarrhea often occur.

    (4) Vomiting usually precedes pain.

107. Which of the following is/are true regarding acute appendicitis in the elderly?

    (1) Symptoms and physical findings may be minimal.

    (2) It is associated with a high rate of perforation.

    (3) Perforation often results in diffuse peritonitis.

    (4) Perforation is associated with a 50% mortality rate.

108. Which of the following is/are true regarding the pathogenesis of acute appendicitis?

    (1) Fecaliths are identified in most patients with uncomplicated appendicitis.

    (2) Fecaliths are more often found with gangrenous appendicitis than with simple appendicitis.

    (3) When examined carefully, a congenital narrowing of the appendiceal-cecal junction can frequently be identified.

    (4) Luminal obstruction is the most important factor in the development of appendicitis.

109. Which of the following regarding the anatomy of the appendix is/are true?

    (1) In the adult the base of the appendix is located in the posteromedial aspect of the cecum below the ileal cecal valve.

    (2) The position of the tip in acute appendicitis is a function of the source of infection.

    (3) The tenia coli form the outer longitudinal muscle layer.

    (4) The position of the tip is relatively constant and is approximately under McBurney's point.

DIRECTIONS (Questions 110 through 112): Each of the numbered items or incomplete statements in this section is followed by answers or by completions of the statement. Select the ONE lettered answer or completion that is BEST in each case.

Questions 110 through 112

110. In the evaluation of a female patient with right lower quadrant pain, which of the following should be included in the differential diagnosis?

    (A) twisted ovarian cyst or tumor

    (B) diverticulitis of the sigmoid colon

    (C) ruptured ectopic pregnancy

    (D) epiploic appendicitis

    (E) all of the above

111. Which of the following radiological findings are associated with acute appendicitis?

    (A) distended loop of small bowel in the right lower quadrant

    (B) partial filling of the appendix on barium enema

    (C) a gas-filled appendix

    (D) a mass effect in the cecum on barium enema

    (E) all of the above

112. For which of the following patients would nonoperative treatment of appendicitis be appropriate?

    (A) a pregnant woman during her first trimester

    (B) a 35-year-old patient with subsiding symptoms and a right lower quadrant mass

    (C) an elderly patient with coexisting cardiac disease

    (D) a 20-year-old woman with Crohn's disease

    (E) none of the above

DIRECTIONS (Questions 113 through 116): For each of the items in this section, ONE or MORE of the numbered options is correct. Choose answer

(A) if only (1), (2), and (3) are correct,
(B) if only (1) and (3) are correct,
(C) if only (2) and (4) are correct,
(D) if only (4) is correct,
(E) if all are correct.

Questions 113 through 116

113. Which of the following statements are true regarding serum acid phosphatase in prostatic disease?

(1) Acid phosphatase has been useful as a tumor marker in assessing treatment results for prostatic cancer.
(2) Acid phosphatase may be elevated after rectal examination of a normal prostate.
(3) Acid phosphatase that is elevated in a patient with prostatic cancer usually precludes a surgical cure.
(4) Acid phosphatase elevations are specific to prostatic cancer.

114. A male patient in good health presents with an asymptomatic prostate nodule. Biopsy reveals adenocarcinoma. The metastatic work-up is negative. Which one or more of the following therapies may be appropriate?

(1) transurethral prostate resection (TURP)
(2) radical prostatectomy
(3) orchiectomy
(4) local radiotherapy alone

115. A 30-year-old male presents with a nontender hard testicular lump. Appropriate treatment includes which one or more of the following?

(1) determination of serum alpha-fetoprotein and human chorionic gonadotropin levels
(2) incisional biopsy via a scrotal incision
(3) orchiectomy via an inguinal incision
(4) incisional biopsy via an inguinal incision

116. An adolescent male presents with a 3-hour history of severe scrotal pain. The examination reveals scrotal swelling and tenderness that does not permit discrete palpation of the epididymis. The best treatment at this point is

(1) heat, scrotal elevation, and antibiotics
(2) manual attempt at detorsion
(3) analgesics and reexamination
(4) surgical exploration

DIRECTIONS (Questions 117 and 118): Each of the numbered items or incomplete statements in this section is followed by answers or by completions of the statement. Select the ONE lettered answer or completion that is BEST in each case.

Questions 117 and 118

117. A testicular mass in a 25-year-old would most likely be which of the following?

(A) benign tumor
(B) seminoma
(C) teratocarcinoma
(D) choriocarcinoma
(E) embryonal cell carcinoma

118. Urinary tract calculi are most commonly composed of

(A) uric acid
(B) cystine
(C) calcium oxalate
(D) ammonium magnesium phosphate
(E) pure calcium phosphate

DIRECTIONS (Questions 119 through 125): Each set of items in this section consists of a list of lettered options followed by several numbered words or phrases. For each numbered word or phrase, select the ONE lettered option that is most closely associated with it. Each lettered option may be selected once, more than once, or not at all.

Questions 119 through 121

Match the type of joint with its appropriate example.

(A) elbow
(B) skull sutures
(C) pubic symphysis

119. Fibrous joint

120. Fibrocartilaginous joint

121. Diarthrodial joint

Questions 122 through 125

Match the following primary shoulder disorders with their appropriate clinical characteristic.

(A) pain extending along the proximal humeral groove
(B) unrelenting pain not relieved by change in position

(C) limitation of internal rotation and full abduction

(D) surgical repair may be required

122. Subacrominal bursitis

123. Bicipital tendonitis

124. Supraspinatus tendonitis

125. Rotator cuff tear

DIRECTIONS (Questions 126 through 129): Each of the numbered items or incomplete statements in this section is followed by answers or by completions of the statement. Select the ONE lettered answer or completion that is BEST in each case.

Questions 126 through 129

126. Physiologic interruption of nerve conduction caused by a transient incomplete or complete paralysis of a peripheral nerve is

    (A) axonopraxia
    (B) neuropraxia
    (C) axonotmesis
    (D) Wallerian degeneration
    (E) neurotmesis

127. A tear of the lateral meniscus is best diagnosed by a means of

    (A) an accurate history
    (B) physical examination
    (C) arthroscopy
    (D) arthrotomy
    (E) arthrography

128. Regarding chondromalacia of the patella, which of the following statements is true?

    (A) Radiographs show characteristic changes early in the course of the disease.
    (B) The pain is aggravated by knee flexion, kneeling, and descending stairs.
    (C) The progressive nature of the disease warrants early surgical intervention.
    (D) The initial changes usually occur on the lateral aspect of the patella.
    (E) Patellectomy is the only proven form of successful surgical therapy.

129. Which of the following is most sensitive to anoxia?

    (A) peripheral nerves
    (B) striated muscle
    (C) skin

(D) tendon

(E) bone

DIRECTIONS (Questions 130 through 133): Each set of items in this section consists of a list of lettered options followed by several numbered words or phrases. For each numbered word or phrase, select the ONE lettered option that is most closely associated with it. Each lettered option may be selected once, more than once, or not at all.

Questions 130 and 131

    (A) pain in the calf
    (B) pain in the buttock
    (C) both
    (D) neither

130. Aortic occlusion

131. Superficial femoral artery occlusion

Questions 132 and 133

    (A) gangrenous digits
    (B) trophic ulcers
    (C) both
    (D) neither

132. Diabetes mellitus

133. Buerger's disease

DIRECTIONS (Questions 134 through 137): For each of the items in this section, ONE or MORE of the numbered options is correct. Choose answer

    (A) if only (1), (2), and (3) are correct,
    (B) if only (1) and (3) are correct,
    (C) if only (2) and (4) are correct,
    (D) if only (4) is correct,
    (E) if all are correct.

Questions 134 through 137

134. Patients complaining of leg pain and cold feet may show signs of chronic tissue ischemia including

    (1) loss of hair from digits
    (2) atrophy of skin
    (3) brittle nails
    (4) rubor on dependency

135. Which of the following abnormal finding(s) produced by an arterial injury is/are most important?

    (1) paralysis
    (2) pain
    (3) paresthesia
    (4) pallor

136. Congenital arteriovenous fistula

    (1) port wine stain
    (2) massively hypertrophied extremity
    (3) may produce a thrill or bruit
    (4) should be treated aggressively

137. Following arterial repair for trauma of the femoral artery, postoperative pulses are now absent. What is the recommended course of action?

    (1) conservative therapy—wait and see if pulses return
    (2) arteriogram
    (3) anticoagulant therapy
    (4) reexploration and thrombectomy

DIRECTIONS (Questions 138 through 141): Each of the numbered items or incomplete statements in this section is followed by answers or by completions of the statement. Select the ONE lettered answer or completion that is BEST in each case.

Questions 138 through 141

138. Which of the following is/are the best method(s) for the control of bleeding?

    (A) tourniquet
    (B) tourniquet and direct digital pressure
    (C) direct digital pressure
    (D) tourniquet and packing the wound with gauze and applying a pressure dressing
    (E) direct digital pressure and packing the wound with gauze and applying a pressure dressing

139. The following statements about anterior compartment syndrome are true EXCEPT

    (A) it results from the compromise of the outflow of fluid from a closed space
    (B) the elevated intracompartmental pressure affects the tibial artery, the anterior tibial nerve, and the anterior tibial, extensor digitorium longus, peroneus tertius, and extensor hallucis longus muscles
    (C) is best treated by decompression fasciotomy following disappearance of pedal pulses
    (D) must be differentiated from shin splits

    (E) early treatment may result in complete return of function

140. Which of the following ankle brachial indices reflects that of a diabetic with complaints of stocking neuropathy?

    (A) 0.25
    (B) 0.50
    (C) 0.75
    (D) 1.00
    (E) 1.25

141. The most important laboratory examination in arterial occlusive disease is

    (A) arteriography
    (B) B-mode ultrasonography
    (C) Doppler ultrasound
    (D) plethysmography
    (E) magnetic resonance imaging

DIRECTIONS (Questions 142 and 143): Each set of matching questions in this section consists of a list of lettered options followed by a set of numbered words or phrases. For each numbered word or phrase, select the ONE lettered option that is most closely associated with it. Each lettered option may be selected once, more than once, or not at all.

Questions 142 and 143

    (A) the first sign of unrecognized heart disease
    (B) cardioarterial embolization
    (C) both
    (D) neither

142. Thrombi

143. Emboli

DIRECTIONS (Questions 144 and 145): Each of the numbered items or incomplete statements in this section is followed by answers or by completions of the statement. Select the ONE lettered answer or completion that is BEST in each case.

Questions 144 and 145

144. A patient presents with complaints of swollen legs that have become increasingly brown in color. The patient is likely to have

    (A) chronic venous insufficiency
    (B) venous thrombosis
    (C) varicose veins
    (D) lymphedema
    (E) atherosclerotic occlusive disease

145. Which arteriosclerotic aneurysm is most common?

(A) abdominal aortic aneurysm

(B) carotid artery aneurysm

(C) popliteal aneurysm

(D) femoral aneurysm

(E) subclavian artery aneurysm

DIRECTIONS (Question 146): For each of the items in this section, ONE or MORE of the numbered options is correct. Choose answer

(A) **if only (1), (2), and (3) are correct,**

(B) **if only (1) and (3) are correct,**

(C) **if only (2) and (4) are correct,**

(D) **if only (4) is correct,**

(E) **if all are correct.**

Question 146

146. What treatment course should be taken for patients with an embolic event to their lower extremity?

(1) prompt administration of IV heparin

(2) under local anesthesia, removal of emboli with Fogarty balloon catheter through short incisions

(3) fasciotomy

(4) operative angiography

DIRECTIONS (Questions 147 through 158): Each set of matching questions in this section consists of a list of lettered options followed by a set of numbered words or phrases. For each numbered word or phrase, select the ONE lettered option that is most closely associated with it. Each lettered option may be selected once, more than once, or not at all.

Questions 147 and 148

(A) proliferative reaction in the media causing narrowing of the arterial lumen

(B) degenerative changes in the media

(C) both

(D) neither

147. Abdominal aortic aneurysm

148. Atherosclerotic occlusive disease

Questions 149 and 150

(A) impotence

(B) claudication

(C) both

(D) neither

149. Abdominal aortic aneurysm

150. Aortoiliac occlusive disease

Questions 151 through 153

For each set of symptoms, select the associated disorder.

(A) painless, cold cyanosis of the hands and feet

(B) red, warm, painful extremities

(C) persistent mottled reddish-blue discoloration of the skin of the extremities

151. Livedo reticularis

152. Erythromelalgia

153. Acrocyanosis

Questions 154 through 156

(A) recurrent episodes of vasoconstriction in the upper extremities initiated by exposure to cold or emotional stress

(B) secondary manifestation of a more serious disorder of the vascular system

(C) both

(D) neither

154. Raynaud's phenomenon

155. Raynaud's disease

156. Buerger's disease

Questions 157 and 158

(A) edema and redness of the affected part without necrosis of the skin

(B) formation of blisters

(C) both

(D) neither

157. First-degree frostbite injury

158. Second-degree frostbite injury

DIRECTIONS (Questions 159 and 160): Each of the numbered items or incomplete statements in this section is followed by answers or by completions of the statement. Select the ONE lettered answer or completion that is BEST in each case.

Questions 159 and 160

159. The best temperature range for rewarming cold exposed tissue should be

    (A) 25°–30°C
    (B) 32°–36°C
    (C) 40°–44°C
    (D) 48°–52°C
    (E) 55°–60°C

160. The following statements about Buerger's disease are correct EXCEPT:

    (A) The distribution of arterial involvement is the same as that of atherosclerosis.
    (B) The distribution of disease in the lower extremity is similar to the typical arterial involvement in the diabetic.
    (C) Early in the course of the disease, the superficial veins undergo recurrent superficial thrombophlebitis.
    (D) It is most often seen in men who are between the ages of 20 and 40.
    (E) A history of at least a 20-cigarette-per-day habit is present.

DIRECTIONS (Question 161 through 165): For each of the items in this section, ONE or MORE of the numbered options is correct. Choose answer

    (A) if only (1), (2), and (3) are correct,
    (B) if only (1) and (3) are correct,
    (C) if only (2) and (4) are correct,
    (D) if only (4) is correct,
    (E) if all are correct.

Questions 161 through 165

161. Diminution or absence of femoral pulses combined with absence of popliteal and pedal pulses is most likely to occur in patients with

    (1) abdominal aortic aneurysm
    (2) diabetes mellitus as well as aortoiliac occlusion
    (3) Buerger's disease
    (4) aortoiliac occlusive disease

162. The rationale behind education of diabetics to the importance of proper foot care includes the following:

    (1) It is likely that diabetics will develop atherosclerosis in their lower extremities.
    (2) Diabetics may not notice minor trauma.
    (3) Diabetics have a propensity for developing infections.
    (4) The foot of the diabetic has distinct characteristics that can quickly progress to threaten life and limb.

163. Patients with aortoiliac occlusive disease may also have

    (1) coronary artery atherosclerosis
    (2) aneurysmal disease
    (3) cerebral atherosclerosis
    (4) hypercoagulability

164. What is usually responsible for the development of venous stasis ulcers at the ankle?

    (1) greater saphenous vein
    (2) perforator or communicating vein
    (3) lesser saphenous vein
    (4) venous valvular incompetence

165. Ischemic stroke

    (1) refers to cerebral infarction occurring as a result of impairment of regional blood flow
    (2) is secondary to cerebral embolization of thrombi that originate in the heart
    (3) is due to fibromuscular hyperplasia
    (4) is associated with obliterative arteritis of the great vessels

DIRECTIONS (Questions 166 through 168): Each set of items in this section consists of a list of lettered options followed by several numbered words or phrases. For each numbered word or phrase, select the ONE lettered option that is most closely associated with it. Each lettered option may be selected once, more than once, or not at all.

Questions 166 through 168

Select the study that will be helpful in establishing the diagnosis of the following diseases.

    (A) Adson's maneuver
    (B) Allen's test
    (C) submersion test
    (D) exercise stress test
    (E) valsalva maneuver

166. Raynaud's disease

167. Thoracic outlet syndrome

168. Femoropopliteal disease

DIRECTIONS (Question 169): Each of the numbered items or incomplete statements in this section is followed by answers or by completions of the statement. Select the ONE lettered answer or completion that is BEST in each case.

Question 169

169 The statements below are true EXCEPT:

    (A) Venous valves assure proximal flow and prevent distal reflux.
    (B) The number of venous valves increase the greater the distance from the heart.
    (C) Venous valves have little if any role in venous disease.
    (D) Venous valves may be weakened in patients with varicose veins.
    (E) Venous valves are absent from the vena cava and the common iliac veins.

DIRECTIONS (Question 170 through 172): For each of the items in this section, ONE or MORE of the numbered options is correct. Choose answer

    (A) if only (1), (2), and (3) are correct,
    (B) if only (1) and (3) are correct,
    (C) if only (2) and (4) are correct,
    (D) if only (4) is correct,
    (E) if all are correct.

Questions 170 through 172

170. The lymphedema associated with radiation following mastectomy may be

    (1) primary lymphedema
    (2) secondary lymphedema
    (3) unavoidable and treated with a compression stocking
    (4) due to infection caused by staphylococcus or beta hemolytic streptococcus

171. Which disease(s) has/have been known to cause heart disease in children?

    (1) varicella or chickenpox
    (2) rubella
    (3) diphtheria
    (4) rheumatic fever

172. The main physiologic disturbances resulting from congenital heart disease are

    (1) obstructive lesions
    (2) pulmonary congestion
    (3) left-to-right shunts
    (4) right-to-left shunts

DIRECTIONS (Questions 173 and 174): Each of the numbered items or incomplete statements in this section is followed by answers or by completions of the statement. Select the ONE lettered answer or completion that is BEST in each case.

Questions 173 and 174

173. The following statements about congenital heart disease are true EXCEPT:

(A) Congenital heart disease occurs as an isolated malformation resulting from defective embryonic development without known cause.

(B) Atrial or ventricular septal defects result from incomplete formation of the respective septa.

(C) Transposition and other abnormalities of the aorta result from abnormalities in the spiral division of the primitive bulbus cordis.

(D) Although a large number of congenital heart defects have been recognized, three malformations will comprise the majority of abnormalities seen in a large pediatric cardiac clinic.

(E) Cardiac development occurs early in uterine life, for virtually all fetal heart structures are formed between the third and eighth week of pregnancy.

174. All the following physical findings point to a severe congenital cardiac malformation EXCEPT

(A) hepatic enlargement
(B) clubbing of the fingers and toes
(C) delayed growth and development
(D) normal growth and development
(E) cyanotic lips

DIRECTIONS (Questions 175 through 178): Each set of matching questions in this section consists of a list of lettered options followed by a set of numbered words or phrases. For each numbered word or phrase, select the ONE lettered option that is most closely associated with it. Each lettered option may be selected once, more than once, or not at all.

Questions 175 through 178

(A) acyanotic
(B) cyanotic
(C) both
(D) neither

175. Tetralogy of Fallot

176. Ventricular septal defect

177. Atrial septal defect

178. Transposition of the great vessels

DIRECTIONS (Questions 179 through 185): For each of the items in this section, ONE or MORE of the numbered options is correct. Choose answer

(A) if only (1), (2), and (3) are correct,
(B) if only (1) and (3) are correct,
(C) if only (2) and (4) are correct,
(D) if only (4) is correct,
(E) if all are correct.

Questions 179 through 185

179. What are the most common forms of congenital heart disease?

(1) atrial septal defects
(2) ventricular septal defects
(3) patent ductus arteriosus
(4) tetralogy of Fallot

180. In obtaining the history of a 3-year-old patient who presents with signs and symptoms of recurrent pneumonia, what other questions should be asked of the mother?

(1) Did the mother have rubella in the first trimester?
(2) Does anyone in the family have congenital heart disease?
(3) Has she noticed the child's lips, fingertips, or lobes of the ears turning blue?
(4) Does the child squat frequently while walking or during outdoor play?

181. Which of the following is/are (a) late sign(s) of advanced cardiac disease?

(1) dyspnea
(2) edema
(3) syncope
(4) angina

182. Which symptom(s) is/are the hallmark(s) of coronary artery disease?

(1) dyspnea
(2) syncope
(3) arrhythmia
(4) angina

183. Extracorporeal circulation includes

(1) a roller pump to provide practically nonpulsatile flow of blood
(2) a disposable membrane or bubble oxygenator

(3) heparinization

(4) the use of protamine

184. Problems from perfusion include

    (1) derangement of normal clotting mechanisms

    (2) renal insufficiency

    (3) transient neurological abnormalities

    (4) multiple organ injury

185. Myocardial preservation may be accomplished by

    (1) topical hypothermia

    (2) arresting the heart with cold blood potassium technique

    (3) blood cardioplegia

    (4) crystalloid cardioplegia

DIRECTIONS (Questions 186 and 187): Each of the numbered items or incomplete statements in this section is followed by answers or by completions of the statement. Select the ONE lettered answer or completion that is BEST in each case.

Questions 186 and 187

186. The most serious complication following extracorporeal circulation is

    (A) postoperative bleeding

    (B) cardiac arrhythmias

    (C) stroke

    (D) renal failure

    (E) respiratory insufficiency

187. The cerebral anoxia following circulatory arrest produces brain damage within

    (A) 30 to 60 seconds

    (B) 1 to 2 minutes

    (C) 3 to 4 minutes

    (D) 5 to 7 minutes

    (E) 6 to 8 minutes

DIRECTIONS (Questions 188 and 189): Each set of matching questions in this section consists of a list of lettered options followed by a set of numbered words or phrases. For each numbered word or phrase, select the ONE lettered option that is most closely associated with it. Each lettered option may be selected once, more than once, or not at all.

Questions 188 and 189

    (A) syncope

    (B) dyspnea

    (C) both

    (D) neither

188. Mitral stenosis

189. Aortic stenosis

DIRECTIONS (Questions 190 through 195): For each of the items in this section, ONE or MORE of the numbered options is correct. Choose answer

    (A) if only (1), (2), and (3) are correct,

    (B) if only (1) and (3) are correct,

    (C) if only (2) and (4) are correct,

    (D) if only (4) is correct,

    (E) if all are correct.

Questions 190 through 195

190. The myocardial ischemia produced by coronary artery disease can cause one or more of the following events:

    (1) angina pectoris

    (2) sudden death

    (3) myocardial infarction

    (4) congestive heart failure

191. The best therapy for acute myocardial infarction includes

    (1) angioplasty

    (2) IV administration of a thrombolytic agent

    (3) intracoronary administration of a thrombolytic agent

    (4) immediate bypass preceded by intra-aortic balloon support

192. Occlusion of a vein graft within the first 5 years following coronary artery bypass grafting may be due to

    (1) anastomotic technique
    (2) trauma to the vein graft at the time of operation
    (3) postoperative adhesions
    (4) the use of dipyridamole and aspirin

193. Which is/are the best bypass grafting material(s)?

    (1) brachial vein
    (2) greater saphenous vein
    (3) lesser saphenous vein
    (4) internal mammary artery

194. Chronic constrictive pericarditis may be due to

    (1) viral pericarditis
    (2) *Haemophilus influenzae*
    (3) intensive radiation
    (4) *Staphylococcus*

195. Which pacemaker(s) has/have the ability to cause ventricular fibrillation?

    (1) demand pacemaker
    (2) atrioventricular pacemaker
    (3) programmable pacemaker
    (4) fixed-rate asynchronous pacemaker

DIRECTIONS (Questions 196 and 197): Each of the numbered items or incomplete statements in this section is followed by answers or by completions of the statement. Select the ONE lettered answer or completion that is BEST in each case.

Questions 196 and 197

196. The findings listed below are typical of a mild pericardiotomy syndrome EXCEPT

    (A) fever
    (B) pericardial friction rub
    (C) pleural effusion

    (D) elevated white blood cell count
    (E) normal white blood cell count

197. The statements about left ventricular aneurysms are true EXCEPT:

    (A) The aneurysm usually enlarges a moderate degree and then becomes stationary.
    (B) They are due to a severe transmural myocardial infarction.
    (C) The aneurysm undergoes progressive enlargement and rupture.
    (D) More than 80% of aneurysms are in the anterolateral portion of the left ventricle.
    (E) Lateral or posterior aneurysms are uncommon.

DIRECTIONS (Questions 198 through 200): Each set of items in this section consists of a list of lettered options followed by several numbered words or phrases. For each numbered word or phrase, select the ONE lettered option that is most closely associated with it. Each lettered option may be selected once, more than once, or not at all.

Questions 198 through 200

    (A) penetrating cardiac trauma
    (B) blunt cardiac trauma
    (C) both
    (D) neither

198. Steering wheel injury

199. Tamponade and hemorrhage

200. Pericardial effusion and chest pain

Answers and Explanations

1. **(A)** Thrombocytopenia is by far the most common bleeding disorder seen in the postoperative patient. This results from platelet consumption in the control of bleeding or may be the result of drug interaction or massive blood transfusion. The most common cause of bleeding in a surgical patient is poor local control. This should be suspected in patients who are bleeding from a single site, not multiple sites. *(Schwartz, pp. 115–120)*

   Shock is a clinical entity in which the cardiovascular system cannot adequately perfuse the vital organs and can be caused by trauma, metabolic derangement, infection, or cardiac injury.

2. **(A)** Lower extremity paresthesia is most commonly associated with neurogenic shock, as the symptom of paresthesias is associated with a neurologic injury. This causes interruption of the sympathetic innervation responsible for vasoconstriction and results in hypotension.

3. **(E)** Cardiogenic shock. Muffled heart sounds, especially in the hypotensive patient with distended neck veins, should suggest the presence of cardiac tamponade.

4. **(D)** Hypovolemic shock. The fracture of a femur is associated with a large loss of blood into the surrounding tissue and depletes the intravascular space. This in turn causes the reduction in the volume the heart can pump and decreases the systemic blood pressure.

5. **(B)** Septic shock. The individual with an overwhelming infection becomes hyperdynamic, meaning his/her heart is working very hard; however, the toxins produced by the bacteria, notably gram-negative, will cause a vasodilation. This vasodilation is responsible for the decrease in blood pressure and also the warmth of skin, because there is more blood flowing there. *(Shires et al, pp. 139–140)*

6. **(D)** Pain is not a symptom associated with carcinoma of the breast. This is more commonly seen in mastitis, pregnancy, or in fat necrosis following trauma. The remainder of the symptoms are all suspicious of carcinoma and should be thoroughly evaluated. *(Rush, pp. 556–559)*

7. **(C)** Mammography is indicated initially at the age of 40. All women should be encouraged to have annual or biannual examinations up to the age of 50, at which point the indication is an annual examination. This examination should consist of a physician or physician's assistant breast examination as well as mammography. Studies have documented that the early findings on mammogram have led to earlier detection of malignant lesions. *(American Cancer Society Guidelines; Rush, p. 556)*

8. **(E)** All of these are important historical points ascertained in the evaluation of the patient with a breast mass. There are associated risks of breast carcinoma in females who have had no children or their first child after the age of 30. In addition, there is an increased risk of breast cancer in those patients with family history of carcinoma and in those people with benign breast lesions. *(Rush, pp. 556–558; Wilson, p. 533)*

9. **(D)** Diffuse abdominal pain that is "wave-like" and associated with vomiting is most likely the result of a luminal-type obstruction. Generally, this is a bowel obstruction, either small or large. Pancreatitis, which is also associated with diffuse abdominal pain, is generally a constant pain that often radiates into the back. The remaining choices are occasionally colicky or "wave-like," although they are generally not diffuse in nature. *(Schwartz, pp. 1065,1074–1079; Cope, pp. 20–27)*

10. **(C)** Biliary colic is often an insidious pain that is postprandial in its onset. Perforation of viscus, ureteral colic, the rupturing of an abdominal aneurysm, or severe pancreatitis can be severe in onset and, in fact, can cause a patient to collapse. *(Schwartz, p. 1065; Cope, pp. 21–23)*

11. **(D)** When evaluating a patient with abdominal pain that you suspect to be an intestinal obstruction, a flat and upright radiograph of the abdomen

will provide sufficient information to differentiate a simple obstruction or a dynamic ileus from a perforation of a viscus by the demonstration of free air. Further radiographic investigation would involve the use of a barium enema that would outline the inferior margins of an obstructing lesion. (Schwartz, pp. 1078–1079)

12. **(C)** "Pain out of proportion" to physical findings is a clue to an underlying vascular etiology. The ischemic pain resulting from either a venous or arterial occlusive process is significant with minimal signs; eg, peritonitis or localized tenderness. This unfortunately is often a diagnosis of exclusion that is only made via arteriography. (Adams, pp. 1504–1505)

13. **(B)** The recurrent laryngeal nerve lies in the tracheoesophageal groove bilaterally and is responsible for innervation of the vocal cord on the ipsilateral side. It must be identified during thyroidectomy to avoid iatrogenic injury. The cervical sympathetic chain and vagus nerve lie along the path of the carotid artery and jugular vein and are not usually encountered during thyroid surgery. The laryngeal nerves lie adjacent to the superior and inferior thyroid arteries and are identified during ligation of those vessels. (Kaplan, p. 1614; Zollinger et al, pp. 346–347)

14. **(E)** The most useful diagnostic test in the preoperative evaluation of a solid thyroid mass is a needle biopsy. Ultrasound and needle aspiration are useful in the determination of cystic lesions. The radioactive scan is important in the differentiation of a cold or nonfunctioning nodule; however, the majority of benign lesions are also cold and this is not in any way diagnostic of carcinoma. In addition, thyroid function tests have no role, because the majority of patients with thyroid carcinoma are found to be euthyroid. (Kaplan, p. 1632)

15. **(B)** Papillary carcinoma of the thyroid has an excellent prognosis following surgical excision. In recent studies, 10-year survival rates were approximately 89%. Follicular carcinoma has a propensity for a mulicentric focus of carcinoma. Studies have shown this to have a 10-year survival of between 44% and 86% based upon the apparent invasiveness of the original tumor. (Kaplan, pp. 1634–1635)

16. **(E)** Findings associated with thyroid carcinoma include those of pressure within the neck such as dysphagia, which may be the result of pressure on the esophagus. In addition, tumor invasion may result in injury to the recurrent laryngeal nerve with resultant vocal cord paralysis and hoarseness. Palpable mass is associated with both benign and malignant processes within the thyroid but should certainly be suspect for a malignant

process. A Delphian node is usually palpable on the trachea just above the thyroid isthmus and is usually associated with malignant disease or thyroiditis. (Kaplan, pp. 1633–1638)

17. **(B)** The historical information that places an individual at high risk for cancer involves previous irradiation to the head and neck. In addition, there have been increased instances of carcinoma of the thyroid demonstrated in individuals who have family members with histories of medullary thyroid carcinoma. This is most likely a result of the familial medullary carcinoma syndrome that is a genetic inheritance in 50% of their offspring. Changes in thyroid function, either hyperfunctioning or hypofunctioning glands, have not been proven to increase the risks of carcinoma. (Kaplan, p. 1631)

18. **(D)** Vitamin D deficiency is not a cause of primary hyperparathyroidism. Parathyroid adenomas, hyperplasia of the parathyroid gland, as well as carcinoma of the parathyroid gland are all cited in the etiology of primary hyperparathyroidism. In addition, nonparathyroid tumors can secrete a parathormone-like substance that can mimic primary hyperparathyroidism. (Kaplan, pp. 1649–1654)

19. **(D)** The most common causes of hypoparathyroidism are related to surgery. This is the result of either surgical removal, trauma, or devascularization during thyroid surgery. Metastatic carcinoma and renal failure are generally associated with elevation of the serum calcium level. Idiopathic hypoparathyroidism is an exceedingly rare condition and would present prior to the age of 16. (Kaplan, p. 1677)

20. **(B)** The superior mesenteric artery gives rise to the right colic, middle colic, and ileocolic vessels. The inferior mesenteric artery gives rise to the left colic, sigmoid, and hemorrhoidal vessels. Collateral circulation is provided by the marginal artery of Drummond which traverses the mesenteric border of the colon. (Zollinger et al, p. 13; Schrock, pp. 633–634)

21. **(B)** The taenia coli, which are longitudinal muscles of the colon, and the haustra, which are outpouchings between the taenia, give the colon its classic appearance. Valvulae conniventes are semicircular valves seen in the small intestine. The ligament of Treitz is a landmark denoting the end of the duodenum and the start of jejunum. (Schrock, p. 633; Goldberg et al, p. 1225)

22–26. **22. (A); 23. (A); 24. (B); 25. (A); 26. (A)** Crohn's colitis is associated with a number of anorectal complications including anal fistulae and fissures. It is a disease of the entire alimentary tract that can be seen in different sections with normal tissue between the involved areas. Crohn's is almost always a full-thickness disease in contrast to ulcerative colitis, which generally involves the mucosa and submucosa only. Because of Crohn's transmural involvement, it can cause localized perforation and inflammatory masses in the abdomen. *(Goldberg et al, pp. 1246–1247)*

27. **(D)** Overgrowth of *Clostridium difficile* and the increased production of exotoxin are responsible for the colitis seen after antibiotic use. This can result from the use of most antibiotics. However, ampicillin and clindamycin are most frequently associated. *(Goldberg et al, pp. 1251–1252)*

28. **(D)** Treatment of pseudomembranous colitis involves the cessation of all present antibiotics, the replacement of fluid and electrolytes, and the use of vancomycin 500 mg PO qid. Steroids, sulfasalizine, and colectomy are not used for treatment of this type of colitis. *(Goldberg et al, p. 1252)*

29. **(A)** Cobblestoning results from the changes in mucosal pattern and loss of haustra seen in colitis. In addition, Crohn's frequently causes perforation and fistulization with adjacent structures, that is, bladder and rectum. Stenosis and stricture result from long-standing inflammatory reaction. *(Goldberg et al, p. 1246)*

30. **(E)** There are a number of complications associated with ulcerative colitis including all those listed. Each of them is, in and of itself, serious, and justify surgical intervention. The prognosis for cancer in patients with colitis is poor. A 20% 5-year survival is seen in this group compared to 40% in the general population. *(Goldberg et al, pp. 1239–1242)*

31. **(A)** An initial management of colitis includes the use of sulfasalizine (azulfidine), ACTH, corticosteroids, and occasionally azathioprine. Surgery is indicated for the management of specific complications, that is, perforation or hemorrhage. *(Schrock, pp. 669–673)*

32. **(B)** Surgical management of ulcerative colitis involves total colectomy and creation of an ileostomy, as the disease is confined to the colon. This is often a curative approach. A number of procedures have been devised to provide continence of the fecal stream via ileal pouches or anastomosis of the ileum to the rectal musculature. *(Goldberg et al, pp. 1242–1243)*

33. **(C)** Bleeding from diverticulosis represents about two thirds of all massive lower gastrointestinal bleeds. It is usually the only symptom and can be sudden in onset and profuse, requiring emergent surgical repair. *(Goldberg et al, pp. 1255–1259)*

34. **(D)** Angiography is the most beneficial study in massive lower GI bleeding that is greater than 2.0 mL/min. It accurately localizes the bleeding site and allows the use of selective intra-arterial vasoconstrictive agents. Technetium-labeled RBC is helpful in bleeding as slow as 0.5 mL/min. The remaining studies have limited value in brisk bleeding. *(Schwartz, p. 1091)*

35. **(D)** Carcinoma is not a complication of diverticulitis, although they may present with similar symptoms. The remaining are all associated with diverticulitis and can necessitate surgical resection. *(Goldberg et al, pp. 1257–1260)*

36. **(E)** Juvenile polyposis has no malignant potential and the usual symptoms includes bleeding. Polyposes coli is seen in Gardner's syndrome and, along with villous adenoma and familial polyposis, all have significant malignant potential. Tubular adenomas generally remain carcinoma in situ, since they rarely extend beyond the muscularis. *(Goldberg et al, pp. 1264–1270)*

37. **(D)** Diabetes is not associated with anal fissure, although the inability to heal wounds is associated with diabetes. Conservative management to include anal hygiene, laxatives, and lubricants should precede surgery unless the fissure is associated with perirectal abscess, which should be incised and drained. *(Goldberg et al, p. 1303)*

38. **(E)** All these are indications for surgical relief of hemorrhoidal symptoms. Failure of dietary manipulation, topical medications, and/or rubber band ligation often lead to surgery. *(Goldberg et al, pp. 1302–1303)*

39. **(A)** Diverticulitis results from inflammation of a diverticulum and presents with pain, fever, anorexia, and change in bowel habits. Nausea is frequent; however, vomiting is infrequent unless there is obstruction. *(Goldberg et al, p. 1256)*

40. **(B)** Screening for colon carcinoma involves hemoccult study and colonoscopy. The hemoccult study or stool for blood is a very sensitive and inexpensive test that can be done by the patient at home. Colonoscopy should be done once in the fourth or fifth decade and then biannually. CEA is a useful blood test for determining recurrence of tumor. *(American Cancer Society Guidelines; Goldberg et al, pp. 1277–1278)*

41. **(C)** Characteristically, esophageal achalasia has unsynchronized contractions of the esophagus that gives it the absence of peristalsis. Failure of the lower esophageal sphincter to relax makes it impossible for food to pass into the stomach. Gastroesophageal reflux is not seen in this condition un-

less it results from mechanical dilation of the lower esophageal sphincter. *(Pairolero et al, pp 1109–1111)*

42. **(B)** There is at present no cure for esophageal achalasia. A number of procedures have been proposed with regard to therapy for this condition. Of late, esophagomyotomy has proven to be the most successful in relieving the diffuse esophageal spasm. This procedure involves dissection of the muscular layer of the esophagus through a thoracic approach down onto the gastric wall. This is offered to all but the worst of surgical risk patients, in which case esophageal dilation would be performed. Vagal denervation is avoided in these patients, as this would relax the lower esophageal sphincter but is associated with a high incidence of esophageal reflux. The Nissan fundoplication, which is an antireflux procedure, is of no benefit in esophageal achalasia. *(Pairolero et al, pp. 1112–1113)*

43. **(B)** The evaluation of esophageal motility is most often done through manometric means. There are several devices that, through the use of balloon-covered transformers, will measure the upper and lower esophageal sphincters as well as the pressures generated within the esophageal mucosa. In addition, the use of contrast radiography, specifically cineradiography or the barium swallow, is also an important adjunct in the diagnosis of motility disorders. Endoscopy, although critical for the evaluation of esophageal disease per se, is not of significant value in the evaluation of esophageal function. *(Pairolero et al, pp. 1106–1110)*

44. **(A)** Complications associated with herniation of the abdominal viscera through the diaphragm are volvulus and obstruction. Should this condition persist, an ischemic injury will occur to the abdominal viscera. There is, however, no increased incidence of carcinoma either within the hernia itself or within the abdominal viscera. This condition is usually amenable to simple reduction and surgical repair. *(Pairolero et al, pp. 1118–1123)*

45. **(B)** Acute pancreatitis is often a clinical diagnosis, although elevation of the serum amylase is helpful. A more reliable indicator is total urinary amylase in 2 hours. Care must be taken not to ascribe an elevated serum amylase alone to pancreatitis, as this can occur with cholecystitis, perforated ulcer, infarcted bowel, renal failure, and mumps. *(Silen and Steer, pp. 1420–1421)*

46. **(A)** The mainstay of therapy for acute and chronic pancreatitis is supportive; repletion of fluids and electrolytes is paramount, because these patients are frequently dehydrated secondary to nausea, vomiting, and thirdspacing of fluid. In addition, the GI tract is put at rest with nasogastric suctioning to avoid stimulus of the exocrine function, and analgesics are used for the pain. Surgery is not indicated unless a complication ensues such as pseudocyst, abscess, necrosis, or hemorrhage. *(Silen and Steer, pp. 1421–1422)*

47. **(E)** Mallory–Weiss syndrome is not a complication of gastroesophageal reflux. This is a condition seen after repeated forceful vomiting and is associated with bleeding and pain. The remainder are all associated complications of gastroesophageal reflux. As a result of the distal esophagus being persistently exposed to the low PHs from the stomach, esophageal ulceration with bleeding occurs and, following prolonged exposure, muscle contractures and mucosal changes such as Barrett's esophagus. *(Pairolero et al, p. 1151)*

48. **(D)** The earliest and almost constant feature associated with carcinoma of the esophagus is dysphagia. This is initially seen with the swallowing of solid foods but, if undetected, will eventually progress to involve liquids and even saliva. Advanced stage malignancies will be associated with painful swallowing and, to some extent, bleeding, although massive bleeding is not associated with esophageal malignancies. *(Pairolero et al, pp. 1138–1139)*

49. **(C)** The main duct emptying the pancreas is the duct of Wirsung. The minor duct is the duct of Santorini. These enter into the second part of the duodenum at the ampulla of Vater. *(Silen and Steer, pp. 1413–1414)*

50. **(A)** The development of a pancreatic pseudocyst is the most common complication of pancreatitis. It should be suspected in those patients with anorexia, weight loss, and upper abdominal pain after an episode of pancreatitis. *(Silen and Steer, p. 1421)*

51. **(D)** The advent of ERCP has made it possible to document the status of the pancreatic ducts and the presence of intraductal calcification. In the patient with chronic pancreatitis, such repeated episodes lead to deposition of calcium and eventual ductal obstruction. This is frequently the cause of the pain in these patients. CT and ultrasound are helpful in evaluating the pancreas for pseudocyst or abscess. *(Silen and Steer, pp. 1427–1428)*

52. **(D)** Drainage of a pancreatic pseudocyst is recommended to avoid the complications of infection or hemorrhage into the cyst. This would ideally

involve total excision of the cyst; however, this is rarely possible. Hence, these are incised and internally drained by anastomosis to the stomach or duodenum. *(Silen and Steer, pp. 1428–1429)*

53. (A) The classic triad of weight loss, diabetes, and steatorrhea should indicate severe pancreatic disease. The presence of fever would be associated with complications such as an infected pseudocyst. *(Silen and Steer, pp. 1422–1424; Reber and Way, pp. 572–575)*

54. (E) All these symptoms may be seen in a patient with carcinoma of the pancreas. Pruritis is related to increasing bilirubin and often precedes the onset of jaundice. It is often thought that pain is not associated with carcinoma of the pancreas; however, retrospectively, about 75% of patients complain of dull epigastric aching that radiates to the back or lower quadrants. *(Silen and Steer, p. 1430)*

55. (A) The Whipple procedure consists of a resection involving the distal stomach, pylorus, duodenum, proximal pancreas and gallbladder. The remaining jejunum is anastamosed to the biliary and pancreatic duct as well as to the stomach. The spleen is not involved in this resection. *(Zollinger et al, p. 212; Silen and Steer, pp. 1432–1433)*

56. (D) The primary function of the spleen is the sequestration of aging erythrocytes. It is not involved in the production of erythrocytes nor in the formation of products for the clotting cascade. *(Schwartz, pp. 1442–1443)*

57. (C) An unreducible hernia in which the content of the hernia develops ischemia is said to be strangulated. *(Morton, p. 1525)*

58. (B) A hernia through which bowel or omentum extend and then becomes edematous, usually secondary to venous congestion, is unreducible. The contents are then incarcerated. *(Morton, p. 1525)*

59. (E) A direct hernia occurs as the result of weakened muscles in the floor of the inguinal canal. This occurs in Hesselbach's triangle, the boundaries of which are medial to the inferior epigastric artery, lateral to the rectus sheath, and superior to the inguinal ligament. *(Morton, pp. 1526–1527)*

60. (D) The indirect hernia in males extends through the internal ring and is found within the spermatic cord and cremasteric fibers. The path of herniation is along the tunica vaginalis. This has not completely closed since descent of the testicle. These are also referred to as congenital hernias. *(Gray's Anatomy, p. 1051; Morton, pp. 1527–1528)*

61. (A) A sliding hernia is the situation in which one wall of the hernia sac is composed of an intraperitoneal organ such as cecum or sigmoid colon. This may coexist with other forms of hernia, that is, indirect hernia. Care must be taken in resection of the hernia sac to rule out this possibility. *(Morton, p. 1525)*

62. (C) The most common type of hernia in a female is the femoral hernia. This starts off with a defect in the transversalis fascia; however, it extends under the inguinal ligament and can often grow quite large prior to its diagnosis. *(Morton, p. 1528)*

63. (A) Brain tumors occur in five patients per 100,000 in the United States and account for about 2.7% of all cancer deaths. Glioblastomas comprise about 40% of the brain tumors. Meningiomas occur in about 15% to 20% and metastatic lesions represent 5% to 10% of intracranial lesions. *(Youman's, pp. 2682–2685; Spencer et al, pp. 1847–1848)*

64. (B) This patient most likely has a ruptured disc between the L5 and S1 vertebrae, which has caused weakness in the gastrocnemius muscles and elimination of the ankle jerk, which are both controlled by the first sacral nerve root. This can also involve hypalgesia of the lateral aspect of the foot. The L5 nerve root classically causes pain along the posterolateral leg to the dorsum of the foot along with dorsiflexion weakness. *(Youman's, pp. 2540–2543; Spencer et al, pp. 1871–1872)*

65. (E) All these are complications associated with herniorrhaphy. Hemorrhage, severing of the vas deferens or of the ilioinguinal, iliohypogastric, or genitofemoral nerves are potential complications. Testicular swelling may result from a tight closure of the inguinal ring. Recurrence is a complication that may occur in 20% to 30% of patients, according to varying sources. Underlying problems such as diabetes, obesity, and infection all increase the risk of recurrence. *(Morton, pp. 1543–1544; SCNA [1983], pp. 1363–1371)*

66. (E) All these can be seen with brain tumors. Signs and symptoms will vary according to the location of the tumor. Increased intracranial pressure will generally cause headache and, because of its long course, the sixth cranial nerve is also sensitive to pressure, which can cause double vision. Seizures, weakness, and visual change arise according to tumor location. Any of these symptoms should raise suspicion of brain tumor. *(Youman's, pp. 2874–2875; Spencer et al, pp. 1848–1849)*

67. (A) Melena is generally produced from upper gastrointestinal tract bleeding. Red or currant-jelly stools, however, may be produced if the bleeding is massive. The stimulatory effect of intraluminal blood increases gastrointestinal motility and will produce a rapid transit time. Melena results from the interaction of gastric acid and hemoglobin, and as little as 50 mL of blood may be enough to produce melena. Other substances, especially iron, have been known to cause black stools. Black stools can persist for up to 5 days after a significant upper gastrointestinal hemorrhage. (Schwartz, p. 1085)

68. **(C)** The incidence of gastric ulcer increases with age. In Western countries, duodenal ulcers are much more prevalent than are gastric ulcers. Increased acid production and stress are associated with duodenal, NOT gastric, ulcers. (Moody, et al, pp. 1168–1175)

69. **(A)** There are several surgical procedures designed to decrease gastric acid production. Parietal cell vagotomy would denervate parietal cells, or the acid-producing cells of the stomach. Antrectomy would lead to decreased gastrin production, and proximal gastrectomy removes the acid-producing cells. A procedure such as pyloroplasty will increase gastric emptying but should not significantly affect gastric acid secretion. (Moody et al, pp. 1172–1173)

70. **(A)** The pathophysiology of duodenal ulcer formation has a multifaceted etiology. Forty percent of patients have gastric acid hypersecretion secondary to an increase in the parietal cell mass. Fasting gastrin levels are usually normal. Increased pepsinogen production, rapid gastric emptying, and an absence of sufficient duodenal buffers have all been implicated in the role of duodenal ulcers, but as yet the role has not been proven. (Moody et al, pp. 1168–1169)

71. **(D)** Radionucleotide imaging is emerging as an effective, minimally invasive, and safe method for determining gastrointestinal bleeding. Because most gastrointestinal bleeding is not a continuous process and radionucleotide imaging can be continued for up to 24 hours, it is a useful method for determining the source of such bleeding. The accuracy and sensitivity of this imaging is as good as selective angiography, although the imaging cannot pinpoint the site of bleeding as well as does angiography. Colonoscopy is of little use in detecting the cause of massive gastrointestinal bleeding because the amount of bleeding obscures the bleeding site. Barium enema should not be performed as an early procedure because the contrast material involved will obscure subsequent angiograms. (Schwartz, pp. 1088–1089)

72. **(D)** For those patients in whom medical therapy has not been successful, surgical treatment of bleeding peptic ulcer is necessary. All the options listed in this question are capable of controlling upper gastrointestinal hemorrhage caused by peptic ulcer. However, the procedure that offers the lowest mortality and morbidity rates, reasonable long-term protection from recurrence, and control of the bleeding is oversewing the ulcer, bilateral truncal vagotomy, and a pyloroplasty. (Moody et al, pp. 1174–1175)

73. **(E)** Of all the gastric malignancies, lymphoma accounts for approximately 2%. The treatment of choice for those with gastric lymphoma is radiotherapy. This accounts for a 5-year survival rate of approximately 40%. If outlet obstruction is present, the treatment of choice would be subtotal gastrectomy with postoperative radiotherapy. (Moody et al, p. 1178)

74. **(A)** Gallstones are usually composed of a combination of calcium, bile pigments, and cholesterol. Cholesterol stones, which are the most predominate type of gallstone in the United States, are formed when the proportion of bile salts and lecithin in the bile are inadequate to form micelles to dissolve cholesterol. It is possible to have pure cholesterol stones; however, this is rare. Approximately 30% of patients diagnosed with gallstones in the United States will have pigmented stones. Pigmented stones are of two types: black pigmented stones are associated with hemolysis, cirrhosis, and old age; brown pigmented stones (or earthy stones) are usually associated with infection. (Schwartz, pp. 1390–1391)

75. **(E)** Cholelithiasis may be present whenever conditions occur that alter the concentrations of the major elements involved in gallstone formation. Pigmented stones may occur in patients who have hematological diseases associated with increased hemolysis. Also, hemolysis caused by mechanical trauma such as that found in a patient with aortic valve replacement results in the formation of pigmented stones. Increases in the concentration of cholesterol in the blood and bile and suppression of gallbladder emptying may be found with prolonged administration of estrogen, such as that found in the use of birth control pills. People who have undergone ileal resection of the distal third of their small intestine have an interruption in their enterohepatic circulation and a decrease of the secretion of bile salts and phospholipids, both necessary for the solubility of cholesterol. It is likely that such patients will develop cholelithiasis. (Schwartz, pp. 1390–1391)

76. **(B)** The HIDA scan or technetium 99-labeled N substituted iminodiacetic acid scan uses a gamma-emitting isotope with a 6-hour half-life. These isotopes are selectively extracted by the liver and se-

creted into the bile. In patients with acute chole-cystitis secondary to cystic duct obstruction, the isotope will fail to enter the gallbladder. This makes it the diagnostic choice for such a condition. This technique can also define obstruction of ex-trahepatic bile ducts, in which case the radionu-clides fail to enter the intestine. These scans are associated with less toxicity than the contrast me-dia involved in IV cholangiography. They provide adequate visualization even when bilirubin levels are as high as 10 to 20 mg per 100 mL. *(Schwartz, p. 1388)*

77. **(A)** Sclerosing cholangitis appears to occur more frequently in males than in females, which is in contrast to acute cholecystitis. There have been a significant number of sclerosing cholangitis cases found to be associated with ulcerative colitis. Be-cause it has been found that most individuals who have sclerosing cholangitis do not have stones in their gallbladder or common bile duct, this disease does not appear to be caused by irritation of the common duct due to the passage of gallstones. The cause of the disease is unknown, although it has been suggested that it may be related to viral in-fection. The entire extrahepatic and intrahepatic bile duct system may be involved, or the hepatic duct may be spared and the disease restricted to the common duct. The gallbladder is usually not involved. The clinical and laboratory presentation is usually that of extrahepatic jaundice. It is usu-ally noted that the serum alkaline phosphatase level is elevated out of proportion to that of the serum bilirubin level. *(Schwartz, pp. 1400–1401)*

78. **(E)** The solubility of cholesterol depends on the relative concentrations of conjugated bile salts, cholesterol, and phospholipids (lecithin being pre-dominant). Cholesterol is insoluble in aqueous so-lution, but becomes soluble when incorporated into lecithin bile salt micelles. The ratio of the sum of the molar concentrations of bile salts plus lecithin to the molar concentration of cholesterol is termed the lithogenous ratio. A lowering of this ratio by either a decrease in the concentration of bile salts or lecithin, or an increase in the concentration of cholesterol, makes the cholesterol less soluble and results in a more lithogenic bile. Bilirubinate, a major constituent of pigmented stones, has no ef-fect on the solubility on other bile constituents. *(Schwartz, pp. 1390–1391)*

79. **(B)** Cholecystokinin, which is released from the intestinal mucosa in response to food (particularly fat) and enters into the duodenum, is the primary stimulus for gallbladder emptying. Cholecys-tokinin also relaxes the terminal bile duct, the sphincter of Oddi, and the duodenal musculature. Vagal stimulation causes the gallbladder to con-tract, but the rate of gallbladder emptying is un-changed following vagotomy. Sympathetic stimu-lation is inhibitory to the motor activity of the gallbladder, whereas secretin and hydrochloric acid have little effect on motor activity. *(Schwartz, p. 1385)*

80. **(B)** Chenodeoxycholic acid replenishes the bile acid pool and so tends to return super-saturated bile to a more normal composition. It has also been found to decrease hepatic cholesterol synthesis. Chenodeoxycholic acid is less effective in dissolv-ing large (1.5 cm) than small stones, and ra-diopaque rather than radiolucent stones. When treatment is terminated, cholelithiasis is likely to return. Side effects of this type of treatment in-clude clinically significant hepatotoxicity. *(Schwartz et al, p. 1391)*

81. **(E)** In several large series of asymptomatic pa-tients with gallstones who were followed and who did not receive surgical treatment, symptoms de-veloped in 50% and serious complications devel-oped in 20%. An operative mortality of 0.7% has been reported for asymptomatic patients in con-trast to a 5% mortality rate for patients with acute cholecystitis. Based on a high incidence of ulti-mate development of symptoms or complications and the small risk of operative mortality, it is gen-erally felt that, unless there is a strong contrain-dication, the presence of cholelithiasis with or without symptoms is an indication for a chole-cystectomy. *(Schwartz, p. 1391)*

82. **(B)** In patients with chronic cholecystitis, ultra-sonography is approximately 95% accurate for the detection of gallstones and has, for the most part, replaced oral cholecystography as the initial method of diagnosis. Oral cholecystography is still useful, however, in the evaluation of patients with typical symptoms of chronic cholecystitis who have equivocal and negative ultrasounds. HIDA scan-ning is most useful in the diagnosis of acute chole-cystitis. CT scans can demonstrate gallstones, but this method is not appropriate for initial screening evaluations. Direct visualization of the bile duct by percutaneous transhepatic cholangiography is im-portant in the evaluation of common duct obstruc-tion. *(Schwartz, pp. 1386–1388,1398)*

83. **(A)** Charcot's triad, consisting of fever, jaundice, and abdominal pain, is the clinical hallmark of acute cholangitis. Initial treatment consists of fluid resuscitation and antibiotics to cover gram-negative organisms, aerobes, and enterococci. If the patient improves with these measures, cholan-giographic assessment of the biliary tract is car-ried out in order to plan definitive therapy. Most cases of acute cholangitis are caused by calculous disease, although benign strictures and malignan-cies must be excluded. If the patient does not re-

spond to initial nonoperative therapy, decompression of the biliary tract must be carried out. This may be done either surgically, or through percutaneous techniques. (Schwartz, p. 1399)

84–87. 84. (C); 85. (A); 86. (D); 87. (A) Cholecystitis is considered to be acute or chronic, dependent on the clinical presentation. The pathophysiology of both implies that the cystic duct is obstructed, usually by gallstones. In acute cholecystitis, persistent obstruction of the cystic duct leads to a chemical and bacterial inflammation of the gallbladder wall itself and potential complications are empyema, gangrene, perforation, and fistula formation. HIDA scan is considered a specific test for acute cholecystitis because of the low rate of false-positive studies. Acute cholecystitis requires cholecystectomy but the timing of the operation is controversial. Early cholecystectomy prevents complications and recurrent symptoms and has been shown to be as safe in terms of morbidity and mortality as the delayed operation when symptoms resolve. Proponents of the delayed cholecystectomy have suggested that because most episodes of acute cholecystitis resolve, and because the operation may be more difficult in the case of acute inflammatory process, the operation is more appropriately carried out later. In chronic cholecystitis, intermittent cystic duct obstruction produces biliary colic. The diagnosis is usually made on the basis of symptoms and an ultrasound demonstrating cholelithiases. Chronic cholecystitis is treated by elective cholecystectomy. (Schwartz, pp. 1395–1398)

88. (A) Anatomically, the liver is divided into right and left lobes by a plane between the gallbladder fossa and inferior vena cava. The left lobe is divided into medial and lateral segments by the falciform ligament. The right lobe is divided into the anterior and posterior segments that do not have external landmarks. (Way, p. 497)

89. (A) The liver performs a wide range of synthetic and metabolic functions and is an important component of the reticuloendothelial systems. Albumin and other plasma proteins such as urea, fibrinogen, and most coagulation factors are principally synthesized in the liver. The liver also has a central role in lipid and glucose metabolism. In the well-fed state, the liver is a site of glycogen synthesis and during periods of fasting it provides energy substrate by glycogenolysis and gluconeogenesis as well as by the formation of ketone bodies. In addition, the liver is also the primary site of cholesterol synthesis and has a controlling function in the enterohepatic circulation. Primary bile acids are synthesized, conjugated, actively secreted, and then effectively retrieved during this process. Furthermore, the liver is critical in the role of metabolism of fat and water-soluble vita-

mins, and is the site of the initial 25 hydroxylation of vitamin D. The liver is responsible for the metabolism of many drugs and toxins by the oxidative reactions of the cytochrome P450 system. (Schwartz, pp. 1329–1331)

90. (B) The hepatic arterial supply is normally derived from the celiac axis by way of the proper hepatic artery, which becomes the common hepatic artery after giving off the gastroduodenal branch. The common hepatic artery subsequently bifurcates into the right and left hepatic branches. In approximately 15% to 20% of persons, the right hepatic artery can arise from the superior mesenteric artery. The left hepatic artery may originate from the left gastric artery in 15% of persons. These variations must be kept in mind when considering surgical approaches. The hepatic arterial blood supply accounts for approximately 25% of the hepatic blood flow with the remainder supplied by the portal vein. (Schwartz, pp. 1327–1328)

91. (E) The most common primary tumor associated with metastases to the liver is bronchogenic carcinoma. However, considering patients with primary cancers, those with gastrointestinal primaries will develop liver metastases in a greater percentage than those with lung cancers. When colorectal cancers metastasize, they do so commonly to the liver. The diagnosis of hepatic metastases is confirmed by CT scan, ultrasound, or biopsy. (Schwartz, pp. 1349–1350; Way, p. 504)

92. (D) Surgical excision is the only definitive treatment for primary hepatocellular carcinoma. Three criteria should be met before attempts are made for surgical resection. (1) The cancer should be solitary. (2) There should be no involvement of the lymph nodes, vasculature, or bile ducts. (3) There should be no distant metastases. Even with the advances of improved surgical techniques, anesthesia, and blood replacement, hepatic resection has only reached an acceptable level of less than 5%. Overall, only 20% to 30% of patients can undergo resection, and 5-year survival rates approach 30%. In the face of extensive cirrhosis, and with its associated morbidity and mortality, resection is contraindicated. Orthotopic liver transplantation results have not been encouraging. Radiation and/or chemotherapy have not been shown to prolong survival. (Schwartz, pp. 1347–1349)

93. (B) The protein alpha-fetoprotein (AFP) is normally present in the fetus at birth, but disappears after a few weeks. In patients in the United States with primary hepatic neoplasms, 30% will be found to have AFP in their serum. If present, AFP may be used as a marker because resection of the tumor converts the test to negative. Recurrence of the same tumor would be evident by a return of

AFP to the serum. The AFP may also be elevated in embryonic tumors of the ovary and testes, giving a false-positive test result. In metastatic tumors of the liver, the AFP is usually negative. *(Schwartz, p. 1348)*

94. **(E)** The etiology of portal hypertension arises from four categories of pathology: (1) increased hepatopedal flow without obstruction, such as that seen with hepatic arterial-portal venous fistulas (an infrequent cause); (2) extrahepatic outflow obstruction, as in Budd–Chiari syndrome or endophlebitis of the hepatic veins; (3) obstruction of the extrahepatic portal venous system, as in cavernomatous transformation of the portal vein (the most common etiologic factor in this category in childhood is some form of infection carried by a patent umbilical vein [neonatal omphalitis]); (4) the overwhelming majority of cases of portal hypertension are caused by intrahepatic obstruction. This category accounts for 90% of all cases. Cirrhosis (nutritional, postnecrotic, or biliary) is the most common reason for this type of postsinusoidal obstruction to portal blood flow. *(Schwartz, pp. 1352–1355)*

95. **(E)** In a patient with alcoholic cirrhosis, abstinence from alcohol is the most important factor in determining survival postshunting. A low-salt diet, control of ascites, a low-protein diet, and the use of lactulose are various therapies that are used depending on the severity of the disease. *(Schwartz, pp. 1352–1360)*

96. **(B)** Bleeding from varices that have not responded to endoscopic sclerosis in an alcoholic cirrhotic patient is the most accepted indication for surgery. Because only 30% of cirrhotic patients with varices, regardless of size, will ever bleed, choice (A) is incorrect. Emergency shunting results in an operative survival of 50% to 71% and a 7-year survival in 42% of patients. If possible, emergency shunting should be avoided. Prophylactic shunts, such as for choice (E) do not increase survival, and may produce encephalopathy. If at all possible, patients with encephalopathy should not be shunted. *(Schwartz, pp. 1362–1374)*

97–101. **97. (A); 98. (C); 99. (A); 100. (A); 101. (B)** Hepatic abcesses are related to two distinct types of pathogens: *Entamoeba histolytica* and pyogenic bacteria. With pyogenic abscesses, *Escherichia coli* or other gram-negative bacteria are the most commonly isolated organism. The most common source of these bacteria is a contiguous infection in the biliary system. Amebic abscesses are caused by *Histolytica* and no bacteria are typically isolated from these abscesses. However, in 22% of patients, secondary infection is a complication. Pyogenic abscesses may be solitary, multiple, and

multilocular. Amebic abscesses are usually single. The right lobe of the liver is commonly involved in any abscesses of the liver because of the so-called streaming effect in the portal vein. Treatment of pyogenic abscesses consists of appropriate antibiotics plus surgical drainage. The mortality rate with a solitary pyogenic abscess is 24%, whereas multiple abscesses carry a 70% mortality. Undrained pyogenic abscesses have a mortality rate approaching 100%. With amebic abscesses, the treatment is conservative, consisting of the use of amebicidal drugs. Aspiration is indicated if the patient fails to respond to medication or if signs of secondary infection develop. With amebic abscesses, the mortality rate is only 7% in uncomplicated cases and 43% in cases where complications such as secondary infection develop. *(Schwartz et al, pp. 1334–1340)*

102. **(E)** Approximately 60% of benign tumors of the small bowel occur in the ileum, 25% occur in the jejunum, and 15% in the duodenum. Often, these tumors are discovered at autopsy and are asymptomatic during life. Unless obstruction is present, the physical diagnosis is rarely helpful and radiologic examination may fail to show an existing tumor, even if suspected clinically. The two most common clinical manifestations are bleeding and obstruction. Bleeding occurs in roughly 30% of patients and is rarely gross hemorrhage. The bleeding is usually occult. Obstruction is either from encroachment, in which case the obstruction is chronic and partial, or by intussusception. *(Townsend and Thompson, pp. 1205–1206)*

103. **(C)** Malignant tumors of the small bowel are relatively infrequent, accounting for about 2% of all gastrointestinal malignancies. Histologically, adenocarcinoma is the most frequent, followed by carcinoid, lymphoma, and leiomyosarcoma. Survival is lowest with adenocarcinoma (20%) and higher with the other cell types (40%). Treatment of malignant small bowel tumors is wide resection, including regional lymph nodes. This requires pancreaticoduodenectomy in duodenal lesions. With lymphomas, postoperative radiation and/or chemotherapy is indicated but has no effect with the other cell types. *(Townsend and Thompson, pp. 1207–1209)*

104. **(B)** Carcinoid tumors were histologically first described in 1808, although their potential for malignancy was not recognized until 1911. The cell of origin is the Kultschitzsky cell, and carcinoid tumors may arise anywhere in the gastrointestinal tract that these cells occur, that is, from stomach to anus. The appendix is, however, the most frequently involved, followed by the ileum, and rectum. Carcinoid tumors may also be found outside the gastrointestinal tract, including the bronchus

and ovary. Carcinoid tumor has a tendency for multicentricity that exceeds any other neoplasm of the gastrointestinal tract. The prognosis is a function of tumor size and its site of origin, along with its histological type. *(Townsend and Thompson, pp. 1208–1209)*

105. **(C)** Meckel's diverticulum is the most frequently encountered diverticulum of the small intestine. It occurs in 2% of the population. It is a true diverticulum and is found on the antimesenteric border of the ileum about 2 feet from the ileocecal valve. Complications of Meckel's diverticulum include intestinal obstruction, which is the most common, followed by bleeding and, finally, Meckel's diverticulitis. Occasionally, Meckel's diverticulum contains ectopic gastric mucosa and can be seen with a technetium pertechnetate scan. *(Townsend and Thompson, p. 1212)*

106. **(A)** Abdominal pain is the prime symptom of appendicitis. Classically, the pain is initially diffuse, but centered in the periumbilical region. The pain is characterized as a steady, moderately severe, occasionally crampy, type of pain. Usually within 4 to 6 hours, the pain localizes in the right lower quadrant. There is, however, a high degree of variability to this classic sequence. Anorexia is so closely associated with acute appendicitis that the diagnosis should be questioned if the patient is not anorectic. Vomiting occurs in about 75% of patients but is not prolonged. Changes in bowel function, particularly obstipation or constipation, frequently occur but are of little diagnostic value. In more than 95% of patients with acute appendicitis, anorexia is the first symptom, followed by abdominal pain and then vomiting, if vomiting occurs. The diagnosis should be questioned if vomiting precedes the onset of abdominal pain. *(Schwartz, p. 1317)*

107. **(A)** Acute appendicitis in the elderly is a very serious disease. Less than 10% of patients operated on for appendicitis are more than 60, but greater than 50% of all deaths from appendicitis are in this age group. Classic symptoms and physical findings may be present but are generally much milder or difficult to elicit. Fever and/or leukocytosis are less than expected and in some patients, normal. Because of these conditions, 67% to 90% of elderly patients will have a ruptured appendix at the time of operation. This often results in a diffuse peritonitis. Mortality rates of ruptured appendicitis in the elderly is about 15%, a fivefold increase from the overall rate. *(Schwartz, p. 1321)*

108. **(C)** Obstruction of the lumen of the appendix is the principle factor in the pathogenesis of acute appendicitis. Fecaliths are the most common cause of appendiceal obstruction. Other less common causes of appendiceal obstruction are vegetable and fruit seeds, intestinal worms, and inspissated barium from x-ray studies. Fecaliths are found in simple appendicitis in about 40% of cases. In gangrenous appendicitis without rupture, they are found in approximately 65%; if the appendix is gangrenous and ruptured, a fecalith is found approximately 90% of the time. *(Schwartz, pp. 1316–1317)*

109. **(B)** At birth, the appendix arises from the inferior tip of the cecum. Through growth and differentiation, the appendix in the adult comes to lie on the posteromedial aspect of the cecum, below the ileocecal valve. The base of the appendix and its relationship to the cecum is relatively constant. The distal end may, however, be found in a variety of places, such as the pelvis, retrocecal, or even on the left side. The three taeniae coli are a useful surgical landmark in that they converge at the junction of the cecum and the appendix. Here, they form the outer longitudinal muscle layer of the appendix. *(Schwartz, p. 1315)*

110. **(E)** With acute appendicitis, the differential diagnosis is essentially that of the acute abdomen. A diverse number of pathologies can present with a seemingly identical picture of appendicitis. In general, about 85% of the cases diagnosed preoperatively as appendicitis are positive, accounting for an acceptable 15% false-negative rate. The most common inaccurate preoperative diagnoses include mesenteric lymphadenitis, no pathology found; acute pelvic inflammatory disease; twisted ovarian cyst; and epiploic appendicitis. Diverticulitis of the sigmoid colon, particularly that portion that lies on the right side, is also included in the differential. The diagnosis of appendicitis depends on three factors: (1) the location of the inflamed appendix, (2) the sex and age of the patient, and (3) the type of appendicitis, that is, ruptured or simple. *(Schwartz, pp. 1319–1321)*

111. **(E)** Although acute appendicitis is a diagnosis of clinical findings, radiography may be used to narrow the list of the differential diagnosis or to demonstrate complications of appendicitis. Radiographic findings consistent with, but not diagnostic of, appendicitis include distended loop(s) of small bowel in the right lower quadrant, visualization of a gas-filled appendix, and a partially filled appendix on barium enema examination. Some studies show that, with barium enema examination, the findings of a partially filled appendix, a mass effect on the medial and inferior borders of the cecum, and a mass effect or mucosal changes of terminal ileum, are pathognomonic for acute appendicitis. *(Schwartz, p. 1318)*

112. (B) Acute appendicitis is a surgical disease. Delaying surgery places the patient at greater risk for increased morbidity and mortality. In pregnancy, there is a fourfold increase in fetal mortality associated with appendiceal rupture. In the elderly, nonoperative treatment increases the chance of rupture and death. In patients with periappendiceal abscess formation, the treatment is controversial. Nonoperative treatment initially, in combination with antibiotic therapy, and close monitoring of the patient's clinical and laboratory course is an acceptable option in a patient with subsiding symptoms and a palpable right lower quadrant mass. An elective appendectomy should be performed 6 weeks to 3 months later, if the patient remains stable. The interval appendectomy is needed because of the high rate of recurrence. *(Schwartz, p. 1322)*

113. (A) Carcinoma of the prostate is the most frequent malignant tumor in males over the age of 65. It should be noted, however, that many men die with carcinoma of the prostate and not because of it. Elevations in the serum acid phosphatase occurs from many sources, including multiple myeloma, bony tumors, benign prostatic disease, and acute urinary retention. The portion of the total serum acid phosphatase that comes from the prostate may be detected by the addition of tartate to the serum, making it a more specific test. An elevation of the prostatic serum acid phosphatase is not specific for carcinoma. The normal prostate contains acid phosphatase and minor serum elevations may be seen following rectal examinations. These elevations may persist for up to 36 hours. The presence of an elevated serum acid phosphatase in cases of prostatic cancer usually indicates metastatic disease or extensive local disease, precluding surgical cure. It is useful as a tumor marker to gauge effectiveness of treatment. It is not generally elevated in early disease and so it is not useful as a screening method. Digital examination of the prostate and serum prostate specific antigen is the most important method of detecting asymptomatic prostate cancer. *(Williams and Donovan, pp. 932–934)*

114. (C) Detection of the asymptomatic prostate nodule is essential in order to find prostate cancer in its potentially curable form. The vast majority are found on routine physical examination. Greater than 50% of prostatic nodules palpated on rectal examination are found to be positive for carcinoma on biopsy. The objective of treatment for asymptomatic prostate cancers should be to cure. Only surgical excision, namely, radical prostatectomy, or radical radiation therapy can offer a cure for this disease. The 5-year survival rate in selected cases can be greater than 50%. *(Frank, p. 1766)*

115. (B) Benign tumors of the testis are very rare. Whenever a testicular mass is found, it should be considered malignant until proven otherwise. Testicular malignancies account for 1% of all cancers in the male. The average age at diagnosis is 32 years. Patients typically present with a nonpainful lump in the testis, which is hard, nontender, and solid. The mass does not transilluminate. If a testicular tumor is suspected, surgical exploration is indicated. Serum alpha-fetoprotein and human chorionic gonadotropin should be obtained, as these are useful tumor markers in many testicular tumors. Exploration via an inguinal incision, so as to control the spermatic vessel at the inguinal ring, is the preferred method. Palpation of induration of the testis is the indication for orchiectomy. Because these tumors are heterogeneous, incisional biopsy has no role. *(Frank, pp. 1768–1770)*

116. (D) The differential in this patient is that of acute epididymitis versus testicular torsion. Because prompt treatment of testicular torsion is necessary to prevent testicular infarction, it may occasionally be required that the patient with acute epididymitis be explored in order to prevent the loss of a testis from torsion. Four hours appears to be the maximal amount of time that a testis can undergo torsion, after which irreversible damage is done. If time allows, isotopic scanning of the testis may show the characteristic absence of testicular blood flow. However, time should not be wasted in order to confirm the diagnosis. *(Frank, p. 1735)*

117. (B) Testicular masses are malignant until proven otherwise. Testicular masses are most often found in the 20- to 35-year-old age group. Benign tumors, usually fibromas of the tunica vaginalis, are in the differential diagnosis but are rare. Of malignant tumors, germinal cell tumors are the most common. This cell type includes seminoma (40%), embryonal cell carcinoma (25%), teratocarcinoma (25%), and choriocarcinoma (1%). *(Frank, pp. 1768–1769)*

118. (C) The composition of urinary calculi is significant, in that therapy aimed at prevention of recurrence and the etiological abnormality may both be determined by knowing the make-up of the calculi. Calcium oxalate stones are the most common urinary calculi. They account for approximately 75% of all urinary stones. Ammonium-magnesium phosphate stones make up 15% of stones and are typically found in infected urine. Uric acid stones constitute about 8% of all calculi. Finally, cystine stones represent only 1% of urinary calculi. *(Frank, p. 1748)*

119–121. 119. (B); 120. (C); 121. (A) Joints are either fibrous or cartilaginous based on the nature of the tissue joining the bones together. A fibrous joint, such as the sutures of the skull, is made up of bones united by fibrous tissue. When bones are joined by either hyaline cartilage or fibrocartilage, they are called cartilaginous joints. The pubic symphysis and the intervertebral discs are examples of this type of joint. Synovial joints, also known as diarthrodial joints, are movable joints united by a capsule. This capsule is lined with synovium. Most joints of the extremities are synovial joints. *(Duthie and Hoaglund, p. 1981)*

122–125. 122. (B); 123. (A); 124. (C); 125. (D) After the age of 35, pain after minor strains of the shoulder or spontaneous pain is common. Before attaching the diagnosis to a local condition of the shoulder, one must be certain to rule out diseases that may cause referred pain to the shoulder. Cardiac, pulmonary, and gastrointestinal pathologies may all cause referred pain to the shoulder. Pathology in the neck including cervical arthritis and brachial plexus irritation, Pancoast's tumors, and central nervous system disease need to be considered. Once the pathology has been located at the shoulder, knowledge of the anatomy of the shoulder makes the diagnosis easier. Disorders of the rotator cuff, bicipital tendonitis, and subacromial bursitis are the three most common causes of primary painful shoulder disorders. The rotator cuff is made up of the common tendinous insertions of the supraspinatus, infraspinatus, teres minor, and the subscapularis muscle tendons (SITS). The rotator cuff is intimately adherent to the shoulder capsule that lies just beneath it. The rotator cuff comes in contact with the undersurface of the coracoacromial ligament when the arm is abducted past 90° or is fully elevated. This may lead to mechanical irritation and subsequent degeneration. The subacromial bursa lies between the coracoacromial ligament, the acromion, and the rotator cuff. Inflammation may occur here as a result of the mechanical irritation, causing bursitis. This typically causes unrelenting pain that is unaffected by position changes. With supraspinatus tendonitis, the patient usually complains of low-grade shoulder pain with sudden motion or with full internal rotation and the extremes of abduction. Bicipital tendonitis presents with similar symptoms but differentiation may be made on the basis of the anatomical location of the biceps tendon. Pain and tenderness are found over the bicipital groove. A rotator cuff tear is a physical disruption of the rotator cuff and is usually partial. Partial tears can be treated with shoulder immobilization in a sling. Complete tears may be treated conservatively but surgical repair is often required. *(Duthie and Hoaglund, pp. 2001–2002)*

126. (B) Injury to the peripheral nerves may accompany soft tissue injuries with or without fractures.

The clinical manifestations of these injuries are dependent on the severity of the injury. Neurapraxia is the least severe type of nerve injury and is characterized by a transient loss of nerve conduction. With more severe injuries, Wallerian degeneration of the axon may take place. The Schwann sheath may remain intact. The combination is termed *axonotmesis*. If the nerve is completely divided, the term used is *neurotmesis*. *(Spencer et al, p. 1845)*

127. (C) As with any pathology, the history and physical examination are important. In internal derangements of the knee, however, the practitioner is rarely able to make an accurate diagnosis. Arthroscopy, especially of the lateral compartment, is more accurate than arthrography, and permits visualization of portions of the knee that are not viewed at arthrotomy. *(Duthie and Hoaglund, pp. 1966–1967)*

128. (B) Chondromalacia of the patella represents degeneration of the cartilage surface of the patella and the earliest changes occur on its medial facet. X-rays are negative early in the disease but are used to rule out other forms of pathology. The cause of chondromalacia is unknown, but repetitive trauma may play a role. The patient will typically complain of discomfort in the knee with acute flexion or when kneeling or walking down stairs. Most patients may be treated conservatively with good results. In those patients who do not respond to conservative management, surgical treatment is needed. Realignment of the quadriceps patellar mechanism, or patellectomy are the surgical treatments of choice. *(Duthie and Hoaglund, pp. 1995–1996)*

129. (A) Peripheral nerves are most sensitive to anoxia. Paralysis and anesthesia quickly develop when arterial blood flow is severely decreased. Striated muscle is almost equally sensitive and will usually become necrotic if arterial blood flow is decreased to such a degree that anesthesia and paralysis are present. Skin, bone, and tendon may survive an ischemic injury that produces irreversible, extensive muscle necrosis. *(Imparato and Riles, p. 936)*

130–131. 130. (B); 131. (A) In acute arterial occlusion, the level of arterial obstruction may be diagnosed from the history because the exertional muscle pain occurs one joint distal to the site of occlusion. Superficial femoral artery occlusion results in calf pain. An occlusion in the external iliac artery can produce thigh pain, and aortic occlusion may be diagnosed by buttock pain. The level of occlusion can often be estimated from the color and temperature level as well as the pulse findings. The arterial pulse is absent at the site of occlusion, frequently with accentuation of the pulse immediately proximal to this point. Sensory impairment varies from hypesthesia to anesthesia, and motor disturbances from weakness to paralysis. (Imparato and Riles, p. 951)

132–133.   132. (C); 133. (A) The gangrenous digits represent occlusion of a critical digital artery. Diabetics may have a type of arterial occlusive disease that typically involves the popliteal artery and its branches down to the pedal arches. Minor trauma, unnoticed by diabetics because of their diabetic neuropathy, may progress to gangrene of the toes. Trophic ulcers, which are usually sharply demarcated, punched-out areas on the sole of the foot overlying a pressure point, are frequently found in diabetics. Palpable pedal pulses may be present. Buerger's disease is a form of chronic arterial insufficiency in which tobacco plays a major role. With its progression, superficial ulceration and gangrene will develop if arterial circulation is not improved. (Imparato and Riles, pp. 971–972,995)

134.   (E) Signs of chronic tissue ischemia include loss of hair from the digits, atrophy of the skin, brittle opaque nails, and rubor on dependency. Muscle atrophy in the feet with increasing prominence of the interosseous spaces may be present. The importance of the examination of the foot is emphasized by the fact that gangrene seldom appears in an extremity with chronic vascular disease until these stigmata of chronic ischemia are present. (Imparato and Riles, p. 949)

135.   (B) The classic five abnormal findings associated with acute ischemia are pain, paralysis, paresthesia or anesthesia, absent pulses, and pallor. Paralysis and paresthesia are most important because loss of neurologic function indicates a degree of tissue ischemia that will progress to gangrene unless arterial blood flow is improved. (Imparato and Riles, pp. 936–939)

136.   (A) Congenital arteriovenous fistulas constitute one manifestation of a number of more commonly related abnormalities of the vascular system. The appearance may vary from a simple port wine stain to the massively hypertrophied extremity that has multiple arteries, capillaries, and veins dilated and visible in and through the skin with or without abnormal arteriovenous communications. The hallmark of the complex congenital arteriovenous fistula is the palpation of a thrill and the auscultation of a bruit. The key note of treatment is conservativism. The decision to treat malformations on the surface of the body need only to be based upon whether a lesion threatens to ulcerate or bleed, whether the hemihypertrophy of the extremity may lead to serious orthopedic prob-

lems, or whether the deformity is so cosmetically repulsive that the patient must have help. (Imparato and Riles, p. 934)

137.   (C) The most important consideration following operation is to detect peripheral pulses, which indicate satisfactory restoration of arterial flow. If pulses cannot be detected or if previously palpable pulses disappear, an arteriogram should be performed or the site of anastomosis should be reexplored. The important principle to emphasize is that, with modern vascular techniques, traumatic injury of a normal artery can almost always be successfully repaired. Anticoagulant therapy is not recommended routinely after arterial repair, for it provides little protection from thrombus but does increase the risk of bleeding into the wound. (Imparato and Riles, p. 938)

138.   (E) Control of bleeding is the most urgent immediate problem and can usually be accomplished by direct digital pressure on the bleeding site or by tightly packing the wound with gauze and applying a pressure dressing. Tourniquets are best avoided for most injuries. If they are used, they must be carefully padded to avoid the risk of permanent injury to peripheral nerves. (Imparato and Riles, p. 937)

139.   (C) Anterior compartment syndrome should be treated by decompression fasciotomy early to avoid anoxic necrosis of the muscle mass. The dorsalis pedis pulse may be normal, diminished, or absent. Its absence is a late sign and occasionally follows the loss of motor power of the muscles of the anterior compartment. (Imparato and Riles, p. 940)

140.   (E) Diabetics may have high ankle brachial indices due to calcification of the arterial wall. Claudicators range from 0.50 to 1.00. Patients with more advanced degrees of ischemia will generally have an index less than 0.50. The ankle brachial index is a ratio between the pressure of the affected extremity and the normal systolic blood pressure. (Imparato and Riles, p. 949)

141.   (A) Noninvasive studies using ultrasound, plethysmography, x-ray, and magnetic resonance imaging have been useful in confirming the diagnosis and differentiating arterial disease from other syndromes. Arteriography continues to be the most important laboratory technique. A high-quality study is essential in planning the surgical approach to reconstruction. (Imparato and Riles, p. 949)

142–143.   142. (D); 143. (C) Emboli arising from the heart, constituting the majority of emboli seen, are referred to as cardioarterial embolization. In about 90% of patients with lower extremity emboli, the embolus originates in the heart from one of three causes: mitral stenosis, atrial fibrillation, or myocardial infarction. In some patients, it is the first sign of unrecognized heart disease. Emboli and thrombi are terms that are not interchangeable. A thrombus is a blood clot obstructing a blood vessel. A thrombosis is inferred when there are signs of diffuse vascular disease. An embolism may occur during atrial fibrillation when there is a dislodgement of a thrombus from the left ventricle. *(Imparato and Riles, p. 950; DeGowin and DeGowin, p. 427)*

144. **(A)**   Incompetent valves of the deep veins enable a long column of blood to transmit pressures of over 100 mm Hg to venules. This promotes fluid and protein loss into tissues. The perivascular fibrinous deposits interfere with normal oxygenation and metabolism of tissues. This causes the thickening and liposclerosis of the subcutaneous tissues to produce the characteristic nonpitting edema. In patients with long-standing chronic venous insufficiency, hemosiderin deposits from the red cells are responsible for the brown pigment. *(Greenfield, p. 1029)*

145. **(A)**   Abdominal aortic aneursyms are the most common of the atherosclerotic aneurysms. Men are affected more frequently than women in a ratio approximating 10:1. Except for traumatic and congenital malformations, almost all peripheral aneurysms result from arteriosclerosis. The majority of the peripheral aneurysms are in the popliteal artery. Infrequent sites include the femoral, carotid, and subclavian arteries. *(Schwartz, p. 988)*

146. **(E)**   The prompt IV administration of heparin to inhibit the development of thrombi distal to the embolus is the most important therapeutic measure in the treatment of an arterial embolus. For operations on the lower extremity, local anesthesia may be used. The emboli can be removed by the insertion of a Fogarty balloon catheter through a short incision placed directly over the uppermost level of the arterial occlusion. If the embolus is localized to the incision site, the balloon catheter should be used to clear out the entire artery. An operative arteriogram should be performed to confirm the patency of the artery. A fasciotomy may help preserve limb viability if embolectomy has been delayed beyond 4 to 6 hours and increased muscle turgor was palpated before operation. *(Imparato and Riles, p. 954)*

147–148.   **147. (B); 148. (A)**   The majority of abdominal aneurysms are arteriosclerotic in nature and their pathogenesis is probably different from occlusive disease. Aneurysms result from degenerative changes in the media. Atherosclerotic occlusion results from a proliferative reaction in the media causing narrowing of the lumen. The distri-

bution of the two processes is also different. The atherosclerotic occlusive process involves the aorta at sites of bifurcations, attachments, tapers, and curvatures. Aneurysmal disease occurs at the abdominal aorta, popliteal, carotid, femoral, iliac, and subclavian arteries. *(Imparato and Riles, p. 981)*

149–150.   **149. (D); 150. (C)**   In the 1940s, Leriche described the clinical characteristics of occlusion of the abdominal aorta. These are claudication, sexual impotence in the male, and absence of gangrene. The luminal narrowing may be due to fibrointimal thickening, ulceration of atherosclerotic plaques, and superimposed thrombus or embolization of portions of atherosclerotic plaques. The progress of aortoiliac occlusive disease is slow. Symptoms of claudication appear with exercise. Sexual impotence is frequent because of decreased blood flow through the hypogastric arteries. Patients with abdominal aortic aneurysms are usually asymptomatic. They may have associated lesions but for the most part do not complain of claudication or impotence. Occasionally, low back pain caused by tension on the retroperitoneum by the aneurysm may be a patient's complaint. *(Imparato and Riles, pp. 957,982)*

151–153.   **151. (C); 152. (B); 153. (A)**   Livedo reticularis, an unusual vasomotor condition, is characterized by a persistent mottled reddish-blue discoloration of the skin of the extremities. It is most prominent in the legs and, although it never disappears, it does worsen on exposure to the cold. The pathologic feature apparently is a stenosis of the arterioles that pierce the cutis at right angles and arborize into peripheral capillaries of the skin, which accounts for the nature of the discolorization. Peripheral pulses are normal. Acrocyanosis is a disorder characterized by persistent but painless cold and cyanosis of the hands and feet. The basic pathologic condition is a slow rate of blood flow through the skin, the result of chronic arteriolar constriction, that results in a high percentage of reduced hemoglobin in the blood in the capillaries and production of the cyanotic color. This disorder is usually found in young women who note persistent coldness and blueness of the fingers or hands for many years, worsening on exposure to the cold. Peripheral pulses are normal. In erythromelalgia, the basic abnormality is an unusual sensitivity to warmth. Skin temperatures of 32° to 36° C, which produce no effects in normal individuals, will regularly induce a painful burning sensation. The increase in temperature is usually a result of vasodilatation with increased blood flow. The exact basis for the spontaneous vasodilatation with rise in temperature and the burning sensation is not known. *(Imparato and Riles, pp. 998–1000)*

154–156. **154. (C); 155. (A); 156. (D)** Raynaud's phenomenon and Raynaud's disease have the same recurrent episodes of vasocontriction in the upper extremities initiated by exposure to cold or emotional stress. In 10% to 15% of patients, the legs may be involved as well as the arms. Three sequential phases classically occur—pallor, cyanosis, and rubor. Raynaud's phenomenon may exist as a primary disorder, termed Raynaud's disease, or it may be a secondary manifestation of a more serious vascular disease. The disorders associated with Raynaud's phenomenon include Buerger's disease, scleroderma, thoracic outlet syndrome, atherosclerosis, periarteritis nodosa, and disseminated lupus erythematosus.

A critical point in the evaluation of Raynaud's disease is to determine the existence of a more severe disorder. Buerger's disease or thromboangiitis obliterans is an inflammatory process involving the walls of arteries with involvement of neighboring nerve and vein that may terminate into thrombosis of the artery. Both upper and lower extremities may be affected. Heavy tobacco smoking has been almost universally associated with Buerger's disease. *(Imparato and Riles, pp. 994, 996,997)*

157–158. **157. (A); 158. (B)** The degrees of severity of a frostbite injury have been grouped into four different types analogous to the classification of burn injury. First degree injury consists of edema and redness of the affected part without necrosis of the skin. Formation of blisters occurs in a second degree injury. There is necrosis of the skin in a third degree injury. In a fourth degree injury, gangrene of the extremity develops that requires amputation. *(Imparato and Riles, p. 1000)*

159. (C) Rapid rewarming of injured tissue, using water with a temperature in the range of 40° to 44° for 20 minutes is the most important aspect of treatment of frostbite. Higher temperatures are more injurious than beneficial. A frostbitten part should never be exposed to hot water, an open fire, or an oven, for the loss of sensitivity can result in a thermal injury. *(Imparato and Riles, p. 1000)*

160. (A) Buerger's disease, or thromboangiitis obliterans, is most often seen in men who smoke greater than 20 cigarettes per day, and are between 20 and 40 years of age. The distribution of the arterial involvement is not the same as in atherosclerotic disease. Smaller, more peripheral arteries, usually in a segmental distribution are involved, similar to the diabetic. *(Imparato and Riles, pp. 994–995)*

161. (D) The principle finding in aortoiliac occlusive disease is diminution or absence of femoral pulses, combined with absence of popliteal and pedal pulses. Diabetics most often have occlusive disease of the tibial arteries, although some do also have aortoiliac disease. Patients with Buerger's disease may also have tibial occlusive disease. The femoral and popliteal arteries in these patients should not be affected. Unless patients with abdominal aneurysm have concomitant aortoiliac occlusive disease or arterioemboli from their aneurysm, their peripheral pulses should be intact. *(Imparato and Riles, pp. 958,967)*

162. (E) In the diabetic, arterial occlusive disease typically involves the popliteal artery and its branches down to the pedal arches. Because of diabetic neuropathy, the patient may not be aware of minor trauma to the foot. Within hours or days of a trivial injury, a virulent necrotizing infection can appear, rapidly spreading along musculofascial planes because of the diabetic's extraordinary susceptibility to infection. *(Imparato and Riles, p. 971)*

163. (E) In patients with aortoiliac disease, concomitant coronary artery or cerebral atherosclerosis occurs frequently. It has been found that 10% of persons with aortoiliac disease have small aneurysms as well. A younger group of patients in their fifth or sixth decades who have hypercoagulability and thrombose their abdominal aortas while only having mild atherosclerosis of the common iliac arteries has been identified. *(Imparato and Riles, p. 957)*

164. (C) The perforators adjacent to the medial malleolus are often responsible for the development of stasis ulcers at that level. When they become incompetent, the findings of perforator or deep venous disease are more serious than disease of the superficial system, which is composed of the greater and lesser saphenous veins. Primary varicosities due to valvular weakness or weakness of vein walls are associated with the superficial system, whereas secondary varicosities are present in those patients with other symptoms of deep venous disease (stasis ulcers, brawny edema, dermatitis). *(Greenfield, pp. 1012,1028)*

165. (E) The term ischemic stroke refers to cerebral infarction occurring as a result of impaired blood flow. Atherosclerosis is the basis of this in the vast majority of patients but it can also occur when the lumen is occluded by emboli, hematoma, fibromuscular hyperplasia, or arteritis. Injury, trauma, or thoracic aneurysms involving the carotid artery can result in dissection and tearing of the intima. *(Imparato and Riles, p. 974)*

166–168. **166. (C); 167. (A); 168. (D)** The Adson's maneuver that demonstrates the obstruction of the subclavian artery by the scalenus anticus muscle is the most useful test to indicate thoracic outlet syndrome. The Allen's test will show the integrity of the palmar arches. In patients with thoracic outlet syndrome, the radial pulse will decrease or obliterate during the Adson's maneuver, but the radial pulse should be present during the Allen's test. The submersion test is performed for patients who complain of cold-related color and temperature changes to their upper extremities. If the submersion test is positive, patients will show classic color changes of Raynaud's phenomenon, pallor, cyanosis, and rubor. The exercise stress test is most helpful in documenting exercise-induced claudication in patients with femoropopliteal disease. At rest, these patients may show only slightly decreased Doppler pressures and pulses. However, following exercise that produces the symptoms, the drop in pressure and recovery time are proportional to the extent of arterial occlusive disease. The Valsalva maneuver can be used to assess venous, not peripheral, arterial disease. *(Imparato and Riles, pp. 944,997)*

169. **(C)** Venous valves are the focal point of most of the pathology of venous thrombosis. The sinus in which the valve lies is where the initial thrombus forms. In addition, the loss of valvular function after recannulization of a vein produces venous insufficiency. *(Greenfield, p. 1011)*

170. **(C)** The most common cause of secondary lymphedema in the United States is malignant disease metastatic to lymph nodes. Surgical removal of lymph nodes, particularly when combined with radiation therapy that produces lymphatic fibrosis, is another common cause. Lymphangitis is most often caused by staphylococcus or beta-hemolytic streptococcus. Compression stockings or gloves may help to reduce the edema. *(Greenfield, pp. 1036,1038)*

171. **(C)** Varicella and diphtheria are not known to cause heart disease. However, rubella, occurring in the first trimester of pregnancy, is one of the few infectious diseases known to cause congenital heart disease, usually patent ductus arteriosus. All evidence indicates that mitral stenosis is almost always due to rheumatic fever. Since it is now rare, the most common heart disease in children is congenital heart disease. *(Spencer, p. 771; Spencer and Culliford, p. 855)*

172. **(E)** Obstructive lesions, which occur in pulmonic valvular stenosis, aortic valvular stenosis, and coarctation of the aorta, impede emptying of the involved ventricular chamber. This results in systolic overloading and corresponding hypertrophy of the ventricle. As pressures in the left atrium and left ventricle are normally greater than those in the right atrium and ventricle, a defect in either atrial or ventricular septum results in a shunt of oxygenated blood from the left to the right side of the heart. This causes pulmonary congestion from an increase of pulmonary blood flow and a corresponding decrease in systemic blood flow. Right-to-left shunting produces cyanosis and is seen in tetralogy of Fallot and other types of cyanotic heart disease due to the emptying of venous blood into the systemic circulation. *(Spencer, p. 774)*

173. **(D)** Seven malformations will comprise the majority of abnormalities seen in a large pediatric cardiology clinic. Ventricular septal defect with or without pulmonic stenosis is the most common, representing 20% or more of all patients. The other six malformations, each occurring in 10% to 15% of patients are atrial septal defect, pulmonic valvular stenosis, patent ductus arteriosus, aortic valvular stenosis, coarctation of the aorta, and transposition of the great vessels. The frequency of the different defects varies with the age of the group evaluated. *(Spencer, pp. 771–772)*

174. **(D)** Abnormalities in growth and development are among the most common signs of cardiac disease. Cyanosis may be obvious, and results simply from a decrease in cardiac output with sluggish regional blood flow through the capillary circulation. More oxygen is extracted and a greater amount of reduced hemoglobin is present. Cyanosis and clubbing, a consequence of chronic cyanosis, and polycythemia are often seen in congenital heart disease. Hepatic enlargement is the hallmark of congestive failure in children. *(Spencer, pp. 774–776)*

175–178. **175. (B); 176. (A); 177. (A); 178. (B)** Cyanosis does not occur in isolated atrial and ventricular septal defects. In atrial and ventricular septal defects, the pressure in the left atrium and ventricle are greater than those in the right atrium and ventricle. The blood that is shunted is oxygenated. Pulmonary congestion occurs from an increase in pulmonary blood flow, and often a corresponding decrease in systemic blood flow occurs. With the increase in blood flow, pulmonary hypertension occurs. Patent ductus arteriosus also produces this same left-to-right shunt. Cyanotic heart diseases produce a right-to-left shunt of blood. Unoxygenated blood is in the systemic circulation producing arterial hypoxemia and cyanosis. This is due to the combination of an intracardiac septal defect with obstruction to the normal flow of blood into the pulmonary artery. The classic example of this is the tetralogy of Fallot, a combination of ventricular septal defect and pulmonic stenosis. Venous blood entering the right ventricle is then shunted directly into the aorta to produce cyanosis. In addition to the cyanosis, the malformation decreases the pulmonary blood flow and hence limits the capacity of the lungs to absorb oxygen. With transposition of the great vessels, the aorta originates from the right ventricle and the pulmonary artery from the left ventricle. As a result, venous blood returning through the vena cavae to the right atrium enters the right ventricle and is then ejected directly into the aorta. Oxygenated blood returning from the lungs through the pulmonary veins to the left ventricle is then expelled through the pulmonary artery to the lungs. Cyanosis and dyspnea in the newborn are the most prominent symptoms. *(Spencer, pp. 772,774,812,820)*

179. **(E)** Atrial septal defects are among the most common cardiac malformations. Ventricular septal defects occur in 20% to 30% of congenital defects. Patent ductus arteriosus occurs once in every 2000 births and constitutes 10% of all cases of congenital heart disease. Tetralogy of Fallot is one of the most common cyanotic malformations, occurring in more than 50% of all cases of cyanotic heart disease. *(Spencer, pp. 796,802,807,812)*

180. **(E)** Pulmonary congestion in the child with congenital heart disease produces a susceptibility to bacterial infections. Recurrent episodes of pneumonia may occur in the first few years of life. Rubella in the first trimester has been emphasized because of the high incidence of cardiac defects. In the majority of patients with congenital heart disease, there is about a 2% associated occurrence of congenital heart defects in other members of the same family. Whether it occurred at birth or in-fancy, cyanosis, its variations in appearance as well as its location, is important in these patients. A decrease in exercise tolerance, exhibited by squatting, may be a sign of exertional dyspnea. *(Spencer, pp. 772,775)*

181. **(A)** The frequent symptoms of cardiac disease include dyspnea, edema, hepatomegaly, ascites, arrhythmia, angina, syncope, and fatigue. With the exception of angina, these symptoms are usually a late sign of advanced cardiac disease. The initial change in most cardiac disease is a rise in intracardiac pressure in the involved chamber followed by cardiac hypertrophy, a manifestation of Starling's law of the heart. Symptoms develop as compensatory mechanisms fail. *(Spencer and Culliford, p. 843)*

182. **(D)** Angina is the hallmark of coronary artery disease, a symptom of myocardial anoxia with subsequent anaerobic metabolism. Classic angina is described as precordial discomfort appearing with exercise, emotion, or eating, relieved by rest or nitroglycerin. Dyspnea is one of the cardinal symptoms of left heart failure, and it is a late sign of heart disease. Syncope occurs with aortic stenosis from the transient decrease in cerebral blood flow. Arrhythmias are usually found in patients with mitral stenosis, in older patients with intrinsic disease in the atrioventricular conducting mecha-

nism, and in severe cardiac failure. *(Schwartz et al, p. 844)*

183. **(E)** The majority of heart–lung machines use a simple roller pump that produces an almost non-pulsatile flow of blood. Disposable membrane and bubble oxygenators are used to oxygenate venous blood prior to return to the patient. The blood must be anticoagulated by heparin just prior to bypass. At the end of the bypass procedure, protamine is given to neutralize the heparin. *(Spencer and Culliford, p. 846)*

184. **(A)** Extracorporeal circulation does produce some trauma. Derangement of normal clotting mechanisms may occur, producing an increased tendency towards bleeding for 18 to 24 hours. A slight degree of renal insufficiency may occur, manifested by a rise in blood urea nitrogen, returning to normal in 2 to 3 days. Reports from Scandinavia and England found a high frequency of transient neurologic abnormalities following perfusion. Multiple organ injury was common in the first two decades of extracorporeal perfusion so that pump times longer than 1 to 3 hours were regularly associated with signs of multiple organ injury. *(Spencer and Culliford, p. 848)*

185. **(E)** Myocardial preservation can be accomplished by arresting the heart with hyperkalemic hypothermic cardiac arrest. Both crystalloid and blood cardioplegia are widely used, with little difference in the two techniques for cardiac arrest periods of 60 to 90 minutes. Continuous topical hypothermia, constantly irrigating the pericardium with a 4° electrolyte solution, is an important part of the procedure to keep the heart from being rewarmed as the temperature of the perfusate in the pump oxygenator is usually 25° to 30° C. With the combination of periodic infusion of cold blood and hypothermia, the myocardial temperature can easily be kept below 15° C. *(Spencer and Culliford, p. 848)*

186. **(C)** Stroke is perhaps the most serious complication following extracorporeal circulation, occurring with a frequency of 1% to 2% following open-heart operations. Possible causes of stroke include carotid disease, emboli from the heart, or air emboli from incomplete evacuation of air from cardiac chambers. In the majority of patients who suffer stroke, the cause remains unknown, so stroke remains a distressing and serious cause of morbidity following open-heart surgery. Postoperative bleeding, cardiac arrhythmias, renal failure, and respiratory insufficiency are all complications, but they can be monitored, followed, and controlled. *(Spencer and Culliford, pp. 849–851)*

187. (C) When the diagnosis of cardiac arrest is considered, it should be either excluded within 30 to 60 seconds, or treatment should be initiated. Depending on the temperature, cerebral anoxia following circulatory arrest produces brain injury within 3 to 4 minutes. Periods of anoxia for 6 to 8 minutes may produce extensive but reversible brain injury, whereas longer periods regularly cause irreversible injury. *(Spencer and Culliford, p. 852)*

188–189. 188. (B); 189. (C) Dyspnea is the most important symptom in patients with mitral stenosis. This appears whenever mean left atrial pressure exceeds 30 mm Hg long enough to produce significant transudation of fluid into the pulmonary capillaries. At first, it appears with extreme exertion, but it subsequently occurs with lesser degrees of exertion as the stenosis progresses. Other symptoms of advanced disease include chronic cough, orthopnea, paroxysmal nocturnal dypsnea, hemoptysis, and pulmonary edema. Aortic stenosis may present early on as slight dyspnea on exertion. The turning point in the illness is heralded by the appearance of one or more of three symptoms: angina pectorus, syncope, or left ventricular failure. Syncope develops in about one third of patients with aortic stenosis and does not occur in patients with mitral stenosis. *(Spencer and Culliford, pp. 856,870)*

190. (E) Angina pectoris, occurring most frequently, is a periodic discomfort usually substernal, appearing typically with exertion, after eating, or with extreme emotion. The symptoms subside with sublingual nitroglycerin. There is a constant risk of sudden death with angina pectoris, probably due to an acute disturbance of rhythm with terminal vertricular fibrillation. Myocardial infarction, with or without thrombosis of a diseased coronary artery, is another frequent and fatal complication. In some patients, congestive heart failure develops and may become the principal disability causing death. *(Spencer and Culliford, p. 885)*

191. (E) Although the best therapy for acute myocardial infarction is rapidly changing, the results from immediate administration of thrombolytic agents, both through IV and intracoronary route, has demonstrated a decrease in mortality. Angioplasty may be used in combination with intracoronary thrombolytics to reduce residual stenosis in the once-thrombosed vessel. Patients with triple vessel disease who suffer a massive infarction should probably undergo immediate bypass, with insertion of an intraaortic balloon pump prior to their operation. *(Spencer and Culliford, p. 888)*

192. (A) With proper technique, combined with the preoperative use of dipyridamole and aspirin, pa-

tency 1 month following operation should be in the range of 90% to 95%. In the first 5 years after operation, patency decreases slowly, about 2% to 3% each year, so the five-year patency rate is in the range of 75% to 80%. Occlusion of the graft during this time is probably due to anastomotic technique, trauma to the vein graft during harvesting, or, rarely, postoperative adhesions. *(Spencer and Culliford, p. 890)*

193. (D) In the period 5 to 10 years after operation, there is an increase of atherosclerotic disease in vein grafts and the patency rate is probably no better than 50%. For this reason, the use of the internal mammary artery has increased markedly. The 10-year patency rate is near 95%, and the internal mammary artery seems to be relatively immune to atherosclerosis. *(Spencer and Culliford, pp. 890,891)*

194. (B) The most common organisms that cause acute pyogenic pericarditis are *Haemophilus influenzae* and *Staphylococcus*. In the majority of patients with chronic constrictive pericarditis, the cause is unknown, probably the end-stage viral pericarditis. In recent years, intensive radiation has become a significant cause in some series. *(Spencer and Culliford, pp. 894,895)*

195. (D) Unfortunately, the fixed-rate asynchronous units, the initial pacemakers, stimulated the ventricle at a fixed rate that could possibly compete with the patient's own rhythm and produce ventricular fibrillation. The fixed-rate pacemakers have been supplanted by demand pacemakers, usually triggered from a ventricular electrode. A more complex type is the atrioventricular pacemaker, requiring an electrode in the right atrium as well as the right ventricle. All these have the advantage of coordinating with the patient's own cardiac rhythm and supplying an "atrial kick" when the atrioventricular sequential pacing is employed. Programmable pacemakers permit adjustment of rate, pulse, amplitude, and duration. *(Spencer and Culliford, p. 897)*

196. (D) Pericardiotomy syndrome is fairly common and usually responds to therapy with ibuprofen. A mild postoperative pericardiotomy syndrome consists of fever, a pericardial friction rub, pleural effusion, and a normal white blood count. Although many postoperative patients experience a transient elevated white blood cell count, it is not a part of the pericardiotomy syndrome. *(Spencer and Culliford, p. 889)*

197. (C) A left ventricular aneurysm results when a severe transmural infarction destroys virtually all muscular fibers in the area of the infarction and are subsequently replaced by fibrous tissue. The aneurysm usually enlarges to a moderate degree and then becomes stationary; progressive enlargement and rupture, as usually occurs with atherosclerotic aneurysms, is rare. More than 80% of aneurysms develop in the anterolateral portion of the left ventricle. Lateral or posterior aneurysms are rare. *(Spencer and Culliford, pp. 891–893)*

198–200. 198. (B); 199. (A); 200. (B) The two life-threatening problems for patients with penetrating cardiac trauma are tamponade and hemorrhage. Tamponade develops rapidly as the normal pericardium can accommodate only 100 to 250 mL of blood. Small wounds, such as those from an icepick or knife, often produce tamponade because the laceration in the pericardium is small. Bullets or large knives threaten immediate death from exsanguination as blood can be expelled through the pericardial laceration into the pleural cavity. The treatment should be control of the hemorrhage through emergency thoracotomy. The key to tamponade is considering the diagnosis in any patient with hypotension and a penetrating thoracic wound and performing a pericardial aspiration. Blunt cardiac trauma usually results from automobile accidents when the steering wheel impacts against the chest. The direct injury may be a cardiac contusion. The contusion varies from simple subepicardial hemorrhage to a full-thickness myocardial contusion. The clinical picture is that of pericarditis with a pericardial effusion and chest pain. *(Spencer and Culliford, pp. 880–881)*

REFERENCES

Adams JT. Abdominal wall, omentum, mesentery, and retroperitoneum. In Schwartz SI, et al (eds). *Principles of Surgery,* 5th ed. New York: McGraw-Hill; 1989: 1491.

Degowin EL, Degowin RL. *Bedside Diagnostic Examination,* 5th ed. New York: Macmillan; 1989.

Duthie RB, Hoaglund FT. Orthopaedics. In Schwartz SI, et al (eds). *Principles of Surgery,* 5th ed. New York: McGraw-Hill; 1989: 1879.

Frank IN. Urology. In Schwartz SI, et al (eds) *Principles of Surgery,* 5th ed. New York: McGraw-Hill; 1989: 1729.

Greenfield LJ. Venous and lymphatic disease. In Schwartz SI, et al (eds). *Principles of Surgery,* 5th ed. New York: McGraw-Hill; 1989: 1011.

Goldberg SM, Nivatvongs S, Rothenberger DA. Colon, rectum, and anus. In Schwartz SI, et al (eds). *Principles of Surgery,* 5th ed. New York: McGraw-Hill; 1989: 1225.

Imparato AM, Riles TS. Peripheral arterial disease. In Schwartz SI, et al (eds). *Principles of Surgery,* 5th ed. New York: McGraw-Hill; 1989: 933.

Kaplan EL. Thyroid and parathyroid. In Schwartz SI, et al (eds). *Principles of Surgery,* 5th ed. New York: McGraw-Hill; 1989: 1613.

Moody FG, McGreevy JM, Miller TA. Stomach. In Schwartz SI, et al (eds). *Principles of Surgery,* 5th ed. New York: McGraw-Hill; 1989: 1157.

Morton JH. Abdominal wall hernias. In Schwartz SI, et al (eds). *Principles of Surgery,* 5th ed. New York: McGraw-Hill; 1989: 1525.

Pairolero PC, Trastek VF, Payne WS. Esophagus and diaphragmatic hernias. In Schwartz SI, et al (eds). *Principles of Surgery,* 5th ed. New York: McGraw-Hill; 1989: 1103.

Rush BF Jr. Breast. In Schwartz SI, et al (eds). *Principles of Surgery,* 5th ed. New York: McGraw-Hill; 1989: 549.

Schrock TR. Large Intestine. In Way LW (ed). *Current Surgical Diagnosis & Treatment,* 9th ed. Norwalk, CT: Appleton & Lange, 1991: 633.

Schwartz SI. Appendix. In Schwartz SI, et al (eds). *Principles of Surgery,* 5th ed. New York: McGraw-Hill; 1989: 1315.

Schwartz SI. Gallbladder and extrahepatic biliary system. In Schwartz SI, et al (eds). *Principles of Surgery,* 5th ed. New York: McGraw-Hill; 1989: 1381.

Schwartz SI. Hemostasis, surgical bleeding and transfusion. In Schwartz SI, et al (eds). *Principles of Surgery,* 5th ed. New York: McGraw-Hill; 1989: 115.

Schwartz SI. Liver. In Schwartz SI, et al (eds). *Principles of Surgery,* 5th ed. New York: McGraw-Hill; 1989: 1327.

Schwartz SI. Manifestations of gastrointestinal disease. In Schwartz SI, et al (eds). *Principles of Surgery,* 5th ed. New York: McGraw-Hill; 1989: 1061.

Schwartz SI. Spleen. In Schwartz SI, et al (eds). *Principles of Surgery,* 5th ed. New York: McGraw-Hill; 1989: 1441.

Shires GT III, Canizaro PC, Carrico CJ. Shock. In Schwartz SI, et al (eds). *Principles of Surgery,* 5th ed. New York: McGraw-Hill; 1989: 137.

Silen W, Steer M. Pancreas. In Schwartz SI, et al (eds). *Principles of Surgery,* 5th ed. New York: McGraw-Hill; 1989: 1413.

Spencer DC, Chyatt D, Collins WF, et al. Neurologic surgery. In Schwartz SI, et al (eds). *Principles of Surgery,* 5th ed. New York: McGraw-Hill; 1989: 1831.

Spencer FC. Congenital heart disease. In Schwartz SI, et al (eds). *Principles of Surgery,* 5th ed. New York: McGraw-Hill; 1989: 771.

Spencer FC, Culliford AT. Acquired heart disease. In Schwart SI, et al (eds). *Principles of Surgery,* 5th ed. New York: McGraw-Hill; 1989: 843.

Townsend CM Jr, Thompson JC. Small intestine. In Schwartz SI, et al (eds). *Principles of Surgery,* 5th ed. New York: McGraw-Hill; 1989: 1189.

Way, LW. Liver. In Way LW (ed). *Current Surgical Diagnosis & Treatment,* 9th ed. Norwalk, CT: Appleton & Lange; 1991: 497.

Williams RD, Donovan JF. Urology. In Way LW (ed). *Current Surgical Diagnosis & Treatment,* 9th ed. Norwalk, CT: Appleton & Lange; 1991: 886.

Subspecialty List: Surgery

QUESTION NUMBER AND SUBSPECIALTY

1. Hemostasis
2. Neurogenic shock—characteristics
3. Cardiogenic shock—characteristics
4. Hypovolemic shock—characteristics
5. Septic shock—characteristics
6. Breast carcinoma—characteristics
7. Mammography—indications
8. Breast mass—history
9. Bowel obstruction—physical findings
10. Biliary colic—characteristics
11. Intestinal obstruction—laboratory evaluation
12. Mesenteric occlusion—characteristics
13. Thyroid surgery—risks
14. Thyroid cancer—evaluation
15. Thyroid cancer—prognosis
16. Thyroid mass—characteristics
17. Thyroid cancer—characteristics
18. Primary hyperparathyroidism—characteristics
19. Hypothyroidism—characteristics
20. Surgical anatomy
21. Colon anatomy
22. Crohn's disease—characteristics
23. Crohn's disease—characteristics
24. Ulcerative colitis—characteristics
25. Crohn's disease—characteristics
26. Crohn's disease—characteristics
27. Colitis—causes
28. Pseudomembranous colitis—treatment
29. Crohn's disease—x-ray findings
30. Ulcerative colitis—complications
31. Colitis—treatment
32. Ulcerative colitis—surgical management
33. Diverticulosis—characteristics
34. Lower gastrointestinal bleeding—evaluation
35. Diverticulitis—complications
36. Polyps—malignant potential
37. Anal fissure—characteristics
38. Hemorrhoidectomy—indications
39. Diverticulitis—complications
40. Colon cancer—screening
41. Esophageal achalasia—characteristics
42. Esophageal achalasia—treatment
43. Esophageal motility—evaluation
44. Diaphragmatic hernias—complications
45. Pancreatitis—diagnosis
46. Pancreatitis—treatment
47. Gastroesophageal reflux—complications
48. Esophageal cancer—characteristics
49. Pancreas—anatomy
50. Pancreatitis—complications
51. Pancreatitis—evaluation
52. Pancreatic pseudocyst—treatment
53. Pancreatitis—characteristics
54. Pancreatic cancer—characteristics
55. Whipple procedure—characteristics
56. Spleen—physiology
57. Strangulated hernia—characteristics
58. Incarcerated hernia—characteristics
59. Direct hernia—characteristics
60. Indirect hernia—characteristics
61. Sliding hernia—characteristics
62. Femoral hernia—characteristics
63. Brain tumors—characteristics
64. Lumbar radiculopathy—characteristics
65. Hernia repair—complications
66. Brain tumors—characteristics
67. Melena—characteristics
68. Gastric ulcers—characteristics
69. Stomach—physiology
70. Duodenal ulcers—characteristics
71. Gastrointestinal bleeding—evaluation
72. Duodenal ulcers—treatment
73. Gastric lymphoma—treatment
74. Cholelithiasis—physiology
75. Cholelithiasis—characteristics
76. Gallbladder—laboratory evaluation
77. Sclerosing cholangitis—characteristics
78. Bile—physiology
79. Gallbladder—physiology
80. Cholelithiasis—treatment
81. Cholelithiasis—characteristics
82. Chronic cholecystitis—evaluation
83. Acute cholangitis—treatment
84. Cholecystitis—characteristics
85. Cholecystitis—characteristics
86. Cholecystitis—characteristics
87. Cholecystitis—characteristics
88. Liver—anatomy
89. Liver—physiology
90. Liver—anatomy

91. Hepatic metastases—characteristics
92. Hepatocellular carcinoma—characteristics
93. Tumor markers
94. Portal hypertension—causes
95. Cirrhosis—prognosis postshunting
96. Cirrhosis—indications for shunting
97. Liver abcess—characteristics
98. Liver abcess—characteristics
99. Liver abcess—characteristics
100. Liver abcess—characteristics
101. Liver abcess—characteristics
102. Small bowel tumors—characteristics
103. Small bowel tumors—characteristics
104. Carcinoid—characteristics
105. Meckel's diverticulum—characteristics
106. Appendicitis—characteristics
107. Appendicitis—characteristics
108. Appendicitis—pathogenesis
109. Appendix—anatomy
110. Right lower quadrant pain—differential diagnosis
111. Appendicitis—x-ray findings
112. Appendicitis—management
113. Prostatic disease—laboratory evaluation
114. Prostate cancer—treatment
115. Testicular mass—management
116. Scrotal swelling—management
117. Testicular mass—differential diagnosis
118. Urinary tract calculi—pathology
119. Joints—characteristics
120. Joints—characteristics
121. Joints—characteristics
122. Subacromial bursitis—characteristics
123. Bicipital tendonitis—characteristics
124. Supraspinatus tendonitis—characteristics
125. Rotator cuff tear—characteristics
126. Neuropraxia—characteristics
127. Meniscal tears—diagnosis
128. Chondromalacia patella—characteristics
129. Anoxia—complications
130. Aortic occlusion—characteristics
131. Superficial artery occlusion—characteristics
132. Diabetes mellitus—skin changes
133. Buerger's disease—skin changes
134. Chronic tissue ischemia—characteristics
135. Arterial injury—clinical findings
136. Congenital arteriovenous fistula—characteristics
137. Arterial reconstruction—management
138. Bleeding—management
139. Anterior compartment syndrome—characteristics
140. Stocking neuropathy—diagnosis
141. Arterial occlusive disease—laboratory evaluation
142. Thrombi—characteristics
143. Emboli—characteristics
144. Chronic venous insufficiency—characteristics
145. Aneurysms—characteristics

146. Embolic disease—treatment
147. Abdominal aortic aneurysm—characteristics
148. Atherosclerotic occlusive disease—characteristics
149. Abdominal aortic aneurysms—characteristics
150. Aortoiliac occlusive disease—characteristics
151. Livedo reticularis—symptoms
152. Erythromelalgia—symptoms
153. Acrocyanosis—symptoms
154. Raynaud's phenomenon—characteristics
155. Raynaud's disease—characteristics
156. Buerger's disease—characteristics
157. Frostbite—characteristics
158. Frostbite—characteristics
159. Cold exposure—management
160. Buerger's disease—characteristics
161. Aortoiliac disease—characteristics
162. Diabetes—foot care
163. Aortoiliac disease—characteristics
164. Venous stasis ulcers—pathogenesis
165. Ischemic stroke—characteristics
166. Raynaud's disease—diagnosis
167. Thoracic outlet syndrome—diagnosis
168. Femoropopliteal disease—diagnosis
169. Venous valves—characteristics
170. Secondary lymphedema—causes
171. Heart disease in children—causes
172. Congenital heart disease—pathophysiology
173. Congenital heart disease—characteristics
174. Congenital heart disease—physical findings
175. Tetralogy of Fallot—characteristics
176. Ventricular septal defect—characteristics
177. Atrial septal defect—characteristics
178. Transposition of the great vessels—characteristics
179. Congenital heart disease—characteristics
180. Congenital heart disease—history
181. Cardiac disease—symptoms
182. Coronary artery disease—symptoms
183. Extracorporeal circulation—characteristics
184. Extracorporeal circulation—complications
185. Myocardial preservation—characteristics
186. Extracorporeal circulation—complications
187. Cerebral anoxia—characteristics
188. Mitral stenosis—characteristics
189. Aortic stenosis—characteristics
190. Coronary artery disease—characteristics
191. Myocardial infarction—management
192. Coronary artery bypass grafting—complications
193. Coronary artery bypass grafting—characteristics
194. Chronic constrictive pericarditis—characteristics
195. Pacemakers—characteristics
196. Pericardiotomy syndrome—characteristics
197. Ventricular aneurysms—characteristics
198. Blunt cardiac trauma—characteristics
199. Penetrating cardiac trauma—characteristics
200. Blunt cardiac trauma—characteristics

CHAPTER 2

Pediatrics
Questions

DIRECTIONS (Questions 1 through 3): For each of the items in this section, ONE or MORE of the numbered options is correct. Choose answer

- (A) if only (1), (2), and (3) are correct,
- (B) if only (1) and (3) are correct,
- (C) if only (2) and (4) are correct,
- (D) if only (4) is correct,
- (E) if all are correct.

Questions 1 through 3

1. Which of the following would be included in the differential diagnosis of a child with chronic diarrhea (more than 14 days)?

   (1) milk protein allergy

   (2) celiac disease

   (3) lymphangiectasia

   (4) AIDS

2. The most common malignancy of childhood is acute lymphoblastic leukemia (ALL). Which of the following is/are true in relationship to this disease?

   (1) it occurs more frequently in patients with chromosomal abnormalities

   (2) anemia, thrombocytopenia, and neutropenia are common at presentation

   (3) the disease is heterogenous, requiring different treatment regimens

   (4) prognosis is worse for patients with onset greater than 2 years old

3. Transient tachypnea of the newborn is characterized by which of the following?

   (1) chest x-ray shows hyperaeration with milk cardiomegaly, prominent vascular markings, and streaky lung field

   (2) most require more than 40% oxygen

   (3) there is a history of heavy maternal sedation, maternal diabetes, or delivery by elective cesarean section

   (4) blood gases are normal

DIRECTIONS (Questions 4 through 17): Each set of items in this section consists of a list of lettered options followed by several numbered words or phrases. For each numbered word or phrase, select the ONE lettered option that is most closely associated with it. Each lettered option may be selected once, more than once, or not at all.

Questions 4 through 7

For each cardiac lesion select the physical findings with which it is commonly associated.

- (A) decreased and delayed or absent femoral pulses
- (B) bounding pulses with hyperdynamic precordium, in premature infants with murmur, if any
- (C) loud first heart sound with widely split second heart sound
- (D) evidence of gross congestive failure without a systolic murmur
- (E) holosystolic murmur along the lower left/sternal border not heard in the first days of life

4. Secundum atrial septal defect

5. Ventricular septal defect

6. Persistent ductus arteriosus

7. Coarctation of aorta

Questions 8 through 11

Dermatological diseases are common in pediatric patients. Match the diagnosis with the most appropriate statement.

    (A) the pattern of inheritance can be autosomal dominant or recessive

    (B) subsides after the first few months of life

    (C) slow, but spontaneous involution

    (D) a staphylococcal infection

    (E) may involve the diaper area

  8. Neonatal pustular melanosis

  9. Strawberry hemangiomas

10. Seborrheic dermatitis

11. Epidermolysis bullosa

Questions 12 through 15

For each age group select the orthopedic problem with which it is commonly associated.

    (A) subluxation of radial head

    (B) scoliosis

    (C) fracture of clavicle

    (D) Legg-Calvé-Perthes disease

    (E) slipped capital femoral epiphysis

12. Adolescent female

13. Newborn

14. 5 to 9 years, male

15. 1 to 4 years

Questions 16 and 17

    (A) involves the dorsa of the toes and distal aspect of the foot

    (B) seen in prepubertal children

    (C) both

    (D) neither

16. Allergic contact dermatitis

17. Tinea pedis

DIRECTIONS (Questions 18 through 23): Each of the numbered items or incomplete statements in this section is followed by answers or by completions of the statement. Select the ONE lettered answer or completion that is BEST in each case.

Questions 18 through 23

18. An 8-year-old female presents with evidence of polyarthritis. The chart shows that she had a documented beta-streptococcus infection 20 days previously. The differential diagnosis includes rheumatic fever. What additional finding would permit you to make the diagnosis of rheumatic fever based on clinical examination? (Modified Jones Criteria)

    (A) fever

    (B) arthralgia

    (C) acute pharyngitis

    (D) carditis

    (E) erythema multiforme

19. Which of the following is true regarding adolescent gynecomastia?

    (A) Gynecomastia begins in Tanner Stage II–III and disappears in 1 to 2 years.

    (B) The underlying mass may be fixed and there may be skin dimpling.

    (C) Gynecomastia is due to excess fatty tissue in an obese patient.

    (D) Gynecomastia is not a painful condition.

    (E) Surgical intervention is not a consideration in treatment of gynecomastia.

20. The most common vasculitis in childhood is Henoch–Schonlein purpura (HSP). All the following are true about this condition EXCEPT

    (A) colicky abdominal pain may be present

    (B) a protein-losing enteropathy secondary to intestinal involvement is part of the spectrum of disease

    (C) most children with HSP have renal involvement

    (D) platelet counts are abnormal, as are coagulation studies

    (E) joint, ankle, and knee pain are associated with HSP

21. The most common thrombocytopenia of childhood is ITP. To substantiate the diagnosis, what laboratory test would you order?

    (A) clot retraction

    (B) bleeding time

    (C) platelet count

(D) CBC

(E) ANA antibody test

22. The nevus is a common skin lesion in childhood. Which one of the following types of nevi should be excised?

(A) acquired pigmented nevi

(B) lentigines (macular nevi)

(C) halo nevus

(D) nevus sebaceous

(E) achromic nevi (nevus depigmentosus)

23. A patient is brought into the emergency room after an automobile accident. His skin is cold, clammy, and pale and his neck veins are flat. You notice signs of trauma at the right upper quadrant of the abdomen. What type of shock is this patient likely to have?

(A) cardiogenic shock

(B) hypovolemic shock

(C) simple shock

(D) distributive or vasogenic shock

(E) terminal shock

DIRECTIONS (Questions 24 through 31): For each of the items in this section, ONE or MORE of the numbered options is correct. Choose answer

(A) **if only (1), (2), and (3) are correct,**

(B) **if only (1) and (3) are correct,**

(C) **if only (2) and (4) are correct,**

(D) **if only (4) is correct,**

(E) **if all are correct.**

Questions 24 through 31

24. A child presents with a history of viral gastroenteritis and has mildly dry mucous membranes. The child's vital signs are normal and the child clinically appears to be less than 5% dehydrated. Which of the following is/are true about the treatment of this child?

(1) If the child is able to tolerate oral fluids, oral rehydration may be instituted instead of parenteral fluid administration.

(2) Commercially available oral electrolyte products are usually recommended, although flat soda, Gatorade, or Jell-O water may be used as well.

(3) If the child has a history of vomiting, clear fluids should be given in small amounts and administered slowly (1 teaspoon every 20 minutes), and amounts of fluid may be increased slowly as tolerated. After 8 hours without vomiting, the child may be gradually returned to a normal diet.

(4) Rice water, juice, boiled milk, and tea are acceptable fluids to use in oral rehydration.

25. Fever is a common chief complaint in pediatrics. Which of the following is/are true regarding fever(s) in children?

(1) A child is considered to have a fever if his or her rectal temperature is $\geq 38.0°C$.

(2) Laboratory tests for a child 3 months of age or younger who has been febrile for 24 hours or greater, who looks clinically well, and has no focal physical findings, may be delayed after 6 to 12 hours of close follow-up.

(3) Children who are less than 2 years old, have a fever of $39.4°C$ or above, have a WBC count of $15,000$ mm^3 or above, and have an ESR of 30 mm/hr or above are likely to be bacteremic and may have an underlying disease such as pneumonia or meningitis.

(4) Effective treatment for children with fevers include use of acetaminophen or aspirin, alcohol baths, drinking clear liquids, and reduction in the amount of clothes the child wears.

26. Animal bites, particularly dog bites, are common in pediatric patients. Which of the following characteristics are true about animal bites?

(1) The most common organism found in animal bites is *Yersinia pestis*.

(2) Hand injuries and bites older than 24 hours should be sutured.

(3) Animal bites that are sutured are less likely to become infected; puncture wounds are more likely to become infected.

(4) Other treatment considerations include administration of tetanus toxoid, wound irrigation, and debridement of devitalized tissue.

27. Which of the following is/are true about the treatment of burns?

(1) Electrical burns should be followed up in 7 days to assure proper healing.

(2) Intact blisters should be opened, cleaned, and debrided.

(3) Initial treatment of minor burns should include packing the area in ice to retard heat damage to the skin.

(4) Partial thickness burns may be cleaned and dressed with 1% silver sulfadiazine cream or fine mesh impregnated with petrolatum jelly.

28. Which of the following should be initiated when treating a patient with a severe head injury?

(1) Establish an airway, remembering to rule out cervical spine injury.

(2) Hyperventilate, keeping the P_{CO_2} at 20 to 25 mm Hg, and P_{aO_2} of 90 mm Hg.

(3) Elevate the head if shock is not present.

(4) Observe for signs of shock but do not introduce IV fluids for treatment as this might increase intracranial pressure.

29. Which of the following is/are true about acute asthma attacks?

(1) Asthma is a common pediatric entity and has the physical finding of wheezing, which is found in the majority of children with acute asthma attacks.

(2) Inhaled beta-agonist therapy is very helpful in the initial management of an acute asthma attack. Humidified oxygen is a must when dealing with the acute asthmatic.

(3) Rectal theophylline suppositories are a helpful way to give a loading dose of theophylline to a vomiting patient with an acute asthma attack. An acceptable serum theophylline level is between 15 and 25 µg/mL

(4) Status asthmaticus is present when a patient fails to have a significant response to initial attempts at bronchodilator therapy.

30. Which of the following growth patterns for children is/are correct?

(1) A newborn may lose up to 15% of birthweight in the first few days of life.

(2) An infant should double his or her birthweight by 5 months of age.

(3) For the first 2 months of life, the infant should gain 30 g (1 ounce) per day.

(4) An infant should triple his or her birthweight by 15 months.

31. Failure to thrive is a common pediatric condition that occurs in about 8% of this population. Which of the following statement(s) is/are also true regarding FTT?

(1) FTT is most commonly seen in children under 2 years of age.

(2) Children with FTT always need hospitalization to determine the cause of their growth delay.

(3) FTT may be defined as height and/or weight below the 3rd percentile.

(4) Laboratory studies are very helpful in the diagnosis of failure to thrive.

DIRECTIONS (Questions 32 through 35): Each set of items in this section consists of a list of lettered options followed by several numbered words or phrases. For each numbered word or phrase, select the ONE lettered option that is most closely associated with it. Each lettered option may be selected once, more than once, or not at all.

Questions 32 through 35

Match the following types of poisonings with their antidote.

(A) methylene blue
(B) oxygen
(C) atropine sulfate
(D) naloxone
(E) syrup of ipecac

32. Carbon monoxide

33. Methemoglobin (nitrates)

34. Narcotics

35. Organophosphates

DIRECTIONS (Questions 36 through 38): Each of the numbered items or incomplete statements in this section is followed by answers or by completions of the statement. Select the ONE lettered answer or completion that is BEST in each case.

Questions 36 through 38

36. The most dangerous inflicted injury in terms of morbidity and mortality is

(A) a skull fracture
(B) an intra-abdominal injury
(C) a subdural hematoma
(D) a subgaleal hematoma
(E) multiple fractures of the extremities

37. Radiologic characteristics of inflicted injuries include all of the following EXCEPT

(A) spiral fractures
(B) multiple fractures in different stages of healing
(C) symmetrical fractures
(D) fractures of the scapula or sternum
(E) evidence of subperiosteal bleeding

38. The diagnosis of childhood sexual molestation is most frequently made by

(A) the child's emotional distress and fearfulness of a physical examination

(B) the child's detailed explicit account of his/her experience

(C) physical evidence of perineal trauma; that is, redness, swelling, discharge, abrasions

(D) laboratory evidence of gonorrhea in cultures of the mouth, anal area, or vaginal discharge

(E) parental complaints of recent onset of sexualized behaviors, including masturbation, and explicit sexual vocabulary

DIRECTIONS (Question 39): For each of the items in this section, ONE or MORE of the numbered options is correct. Choose answer

(A) if only (1), (2), and (3) are correct,

(B) if only (1) and (3) are correct,

(C) if only (2) and (4) are correct,

(D) if only (4) is correct,

(E) if all are correct.

Question 39

39. In the United States, placing children in foster care can be life saving for abused, neglected, or abandoned children. However, studies indicate there are also certain identifiable difficulties with foster care. These include

(1) foster care rarely provides comprehensive integrated services for children

(2) foster parents rarely receive support or guidance

(3) natural parents who retain custody can change a child's placement

(4) frequent placement changes affect how a child forms attachments, learns to trust, and relates to adults and peers

DIRECTIONS (Questions 40 and 41): Each of the numbered items or incomplete statements in this section is followed by answers or by completions of the statement. Select the ONE lettered answer or completion that is BEST in each case.

Questions 40 and 41

40. Clinical experience indicates that most infants with polycythemia

(A) are in respiratory distress

(B) develop convulsions

(C) exhibit priapism

(D) are asymptomatic

(E) develop necrotizing enterocolitis

41. All the following are true with regard to hyaline membrane disease (HMD) EXCEPT

(A) symptoms usually develop within minutes of birth

(B) the infant with HMD is almost always premature

(C) the unventilated infant may require an increasing oxygen requirement over 24 to 48 hours

(D) chest x-rays show bilateral lung infiltrates

(E) current prevention includes surfactant replacement before 1–2 hours

DIRECTIONS (Questions 42 through 45): Each set of items in this section consists of a list of lettered options followed by several numbered words or phrases. For each numbered word or phrase, select the ONE lettered option that is most closely associated with it. Each lettered option may be selected once, more than once, or not at all.

Questions 42 through 45

From statistical reviews of reported cases of childhood maltreatment, the abuser is

(A) in 1% of the cases

(B) in 4% of the cases

(C) in 5% of the cases

(D) in 25% of the cases

(E) in 90% of the cases

42. A caretaker related to the child

43. A sibling of the victim

44. An unrelated babysitter

45. A male friend of the mother's

DIRECTIONS (Questions 46 through 60): For each of the items in this section, ONE or MORE of the numbered options is correct. Choose answer

(A) **if only (1), (2), and (3) are correct,**
(B) **if only (1) and (3) are correct,**
(C) **if only (2) and (4) are correct,**
(D) **if only (4) is correct,**
(E) **if all are correct.**

Questions 46 through 60

46. The health care providers' main responsibilities to abused and neglected children is/are

    (1) detection (diagnosis)
    (2) prevention
    (3) reporting
    (4) treatment

47. If a 6-year-old female child presents within 72 hours of an alleged sexual attack, laboratory data should include

    (1) a wet mount preparation for sperm
    (2) acid phosphatase
    (3) vaginal, rectal, and throat cultures for gonorrhea
    (4) pregnancy testing

48. In the case of adoptions, most authorities agree that

    (1) adoptions should be accomplished through approved agencies
    (2) adoptions of older children, or those of different religious or ethnic heritage than the adoptive parents, should be discouraged
    (3) the adopted child should be told of his or her adoption as soon as he or she is able to comprehend the situation
    (4) adoption should be accomplished as soon after birth as possible, in order to ensure success

49. In unilateral sensorineural hearing loss

    (1) the Weber test lateralizes to the unaffected ear
    (2) the Weber test follows the pattern found in normal patients
    (3) the Rinne test follows the pattern found in normal patients
    (4) the Rinne test reveals that bone conduction is greater than air conduction

50. Physical examinations in the newborn

    (1) need only be done at designated times
    (2) should always be timed and dated on the chart note
    (3) should be performed after adequate handwashing; jewelry need not be removed before the examination.
    (4) can be stressful in sick infants or if done by an unskilled examiner

51. Which of the following is/are true concerning children born to substance abusing parents?

    (1) They are at increased risk for physical, sexual, and emotional abuse.
    (2) Opiate withdrawal peaks during the first week of life.
    (3) Signs and symptoms of neonatal withdrawal include high-pitched cry, sweating, tremulousness, excoriation of extremities, and GI disturbance.
    (4) Urine toxicology screens will be positive if drugs have been ingested by mothers within 48 hours of the delivery.

52. True polycythemia in children can be caused by

    (1) cyanotic congenital heart disease
    (2) placental dysfunction
    (3) hemoglobinopathies
    (4) tumors

53. Factors known to affect neonatal bilirubin levels include

    (1) genetics
    (2) perinatal events
    (3) infant feeding practices
    (4) ethnic factors

54. Absolute contraindications to the administration of DPT vaccine include

    (1) viral respiratory infection without fever
    (2) convulsion 24 hours after previous DPT
    (3) family history of epilepsy
    (4) temperature of 105.1°F following previous DPT

55. Which of the following are true of hepatitis A?

    (1) Transmission is via the oral fecal route.
    (2) There is a 10% to 15% incidence of chronic infection.
    (3) Incubation period is 15–50 days (avg. 25–30 days).
    (4) Young children and infants are more likely to have fulminant disease.

56. An 18-month-old unimmunized infant who is infected with human immunodeficiency virus (HIV) should receive which of the following vaccines?

    (1) IPV
    (2) MMR

(3) DPT

(4) OPV

57. A 4-month-old infant born to a mother infected with human immunodeficiency virus (HIV)

    (1) may be infected but asymptomatic

    (2) has a 90% to 95% chance of developing AIDS

    (3) may be ELISA-positive for HIV due to a transplacental antibody

    (4) cannot be definitely diagnosed with AIDS until 15 months of age

58. Patients at an increased risk of acquiring infection with cytomegalovirus (CMV) include the following:

    (1) toddlers in daycare

    (2) neonatal ICU nurses

    (3) parents of toddlers in daycare

    (4) renal transplant nurses

59. Which of the following regimens is accepted for therapy of group A streptococcal pharyngitis in a 9-year-old who weighs 75 pounds?

    (1) PenVK 250 mg PO tid for 10 days

    (2) PenVK 500 mg PO bid for 10 days

    (3) benzathine penicillin 1.2 million U intramuscularly

    (4) PenVK 750 mg PO qd for 10 days

60. Which of the following infants should be given varicella-zoster immune globulin (VZIG)?

    (1) an infant whose mother develops varicella one day after delivery

    (2) a 1-day-old infant whose 2-year-old brother develops varicella

    (3) an infant whose mother developed varicella 2 days prior to delivery

    (4) a 1-month-old infant with varicella

DIRECTIONS (Questions 61 through 65): Each set of items in this section consists of a list of lettered options followed by several numbered words or phrases. For each numbered word or phrase, select the ONE lettered option that is most closely associated with it. Each lettered option may be selected once, more than once, or not at all.

Questions 61 through 65

For each of the following vaccines, select the best description of the biological components.

    (A) live virus vaccine

    (B) killed bacteria

    (C) bacterial toxoid

    (D) purified bacterial capsule

    (E) killed virus vaccine

61. Diphtheria vaccine

62. MMR vaccine

63. Oral polio virus (OPV) vaccine

64. Pertussis vaccine

65. *Haemophilus influenzae* type b

DIRECTIONS (Questions 66 through 76): For each of the items in this section, ONE or MORE of the numbered options is correct. Choose answer

    (A) if only (1), (2), and (3) are correct,

    (B) if only (1) and (3) are correct,

    (C) if only (2) and (4) are correct,

    (D) if only (4) is correct,

    (E) if all are correct.

Questions 66 through 76

66. Diagnostic criteria for the mucocutaneous lymph node syndrome (Kawasaki syndrome) include which of the following?

    (1) fever greater than 5 days

    (2) generalized lymphadenopathy

    (3) swelling of the hands and feet

    (4) diarrhea and vomiting

67. Risk factors for acute otitis media in the first year of life include

    (1) parental history of acute otitis media

    (2) male gender

    (3) parental or sibling with history of atopy

    (4) exposure to cigarette smoke

68. Which of the following is/are true regarding mortality in adolescence?

(1) Neoplasms are the most common natural cause of death.

(2) Over 75% of adolescent deaths are due to accidents, homicide, and suicide.

(3) Males outnumber females 5:1 in completed suicides.

(4) Males outnumber females in attempted suicides.

69. Normal pubertal growth and development is demonstrated by which of the following?

(1) Menarche always occurs after the peak height velocity has been attained.

(2) Axillary hair precedes pubic hair by about 2 years in both males and females.

(3) For males, pubertal development usually begins with testicular enlargement followed by the appearance of pubic hair.

(4) For females, appearance of pubic hair usually precedes breast budding.

70. The following statement(s) is/are true when speaking of jaundice in the newborn.

(1) It normally begins on the extremities and spreads caudally.

(2) It becomes visible at 6 to 8 mg/dL.

(3) An infant with polycythemia is at no greater risk for jaundice.

(4) A small percentage of ABO-incompatible infants have hemolytic disease.

71. Criteria that rule out physiologic jaundice of the newborn are

(1) jaundice in the first 24 hours of life

(2) total serum bilirubin concentrations greater than 12.9 mg/dL in a full-term infant, or 15 mg/dL in a premature infant

(3) direct serum bilirubin concentration greater than 1.5 to 2 mg/dL

(4) clinical jaundice persisting longer than 1 week in a full-term infant or 2 weeks in a premature infant

72. Juvenile rheumatoid arthritis is characterized by which of the following?

(1) migratory arthritis

(2) chronic nonsuppurative inflammation of the synovium

(3) conjunctivitis

(4) morning stiffness

73. Which of the following is/are true regarding adolescent suicide?

(1) It is higher for boys than girls.

(2) Victims are often intoxicated with alcohol at the time of death.

(3) Firearms are the most common method for suicide.

(4) The majority of adolescents had previously been referred to a mental health professional.

74. Which of the following is/are true about sinusitis in childhood?

(1) Common organisms causing infection include *Streptococcus pneumoniae*, Branhamella catarrhalis, and nontypable *Haemophilus influenzae.*

(2) Frontal sinuses are a frequent site of infection in preschool children.

(3) Sinus headache is an infrequent complaint in children under 5 years of age.

(4) The incidence of acute and chronic sinusitis decreases in latter childhood.

75. Which of the following is/are true about bacterial meningitis in childhood?

(1) *H. influenzae* type B, *S. pneumoniae,* and *Neisseria meningitidis* are responsible for most cases of meningitis in the 2-month to 12-year age group.

(2) Parents of children in daycare who are exposed to a child with *H. influenzae* meningitis should be alerted to the potential of *H. influenzae* infection in their child.

(3) Both *N. meningitidis* and *H. influenzae* type B meningitis have the potential sequelae of hearing loss.

(4) The peak incidence of *S. pneumoniae* meningitis is in the school-aged child.

76. Which of the following is/are true about cystic fibrosis (CF)?

(1) It is probably inherited as an autosomal dominant trait.

(2) The gene for CF resides in the middle of the long arm of chromosome 7.

(3) Diagnosis can be attained via the sweat chloride test, quantitative stool trypsin, and immunoreactive trypsin.

(4) Recurrent pulmonary infections caused by group A beta hemolytic strep and *H. influenzae* are common.

DIRECTIONS (Questions 77 through 82): Each of the numbered items or incomplete statements in this section is followed by answers or by completions of the statement. Select the ONE lettered answer or completion that is BEST in each case.

Questions 77 through 82

77. The Jones criteria for diagnosis of rheumatic fever includes all of the following as *major* criteria EXCEPT

    (A) carditis
    (B) polyarthritis
    (C) Sydenham's chorea
    (D) erythema chronicum migrans
    (E) subcutaneous nodules

78. All of the following are true of infant colic EXCEPT

    (A) colicky crying can occur at any time of the day
    (B) colic is more common in males than females
    (C) colic begins in the first month of life, usually the first week
    (D) colic is sometimes believed to be related to swallowed air
    (E) colic is not felt to be related to gas pains

79. All of the following are true regarding cryptorchidism EXCEPT

    (A) it is more common in premature than normal-term infants
    (B) it is more commonly unilateral than bilateral
    (C) it is frequently associated with Fragile X syndrome
    (D) it may be easily confused with retractile testes in childhood
    (E) cryptorchid testes have an increased rate of testicular cancer

80. All the following are true regarding sports participation by teens EXCEPT

    (A) epiphyseal injuries, although uncommon, can cause variation in growth
    (B) the cardiac abnormality most associated with sudden death is hypertrophic cardiomyopathy
    (C) children with Down syndrome should not be allowed to participate in contact sports until an x-ray evaluation is done of the neck
    (D) isometric exercise should be encouraged for teens with mildly elevated blood pressure
    (E) swimming is an activity with low likelihood of inducing bronchospasm in an asthmatic

81. Suicide is the third leading cause of death among 15- to 19-year-olds in the United States. All the following statements about adolescent suicide are true EXCEPT

    (A) the method of suicide most commonly used by teenagers is ingestion of medication
    (B) leaving a suicide note suggests premeditation and should be considered a sign of serious intent
    (C) male adolescents lead female adolescents in the incidence of suicide attempts, but females outnumber males in completed suicides
    (D) it is difficult to assess the seriousness of intent by the actual potency or medical lethality of the method

82. The incidence of anorexia nervosa and bulimia has increased in the past two decades; 1 in every 100 16- to 18-year-old females has such an eating disorder. Anorexia is characterized by all of the following EXCEPT

    (A) they were "model" children before the illness
    (B) they exhibit excessive physical activity
    (C) they are preoccupied with food preparation
    (D) their academic performance is poor

DIRECTIONS (Questions 83 through 87): Each set of items in this section consists of a list of lettered options followed by several numbered words or phrases. For each numbered word or phrase, select the ONE lettered option that is most closely associated with it. Each lettered option may be selected once, more than once, or not at all.

Questions 83 through 87

For each age group, select the developmental milestone in personal–social behavior one would look for in an assessment of the child.

    (A) 28 weeks
    (B) 12 months
    (C) 18 months
    (D) 3 years
    (E) 5 years

83. Plays with feet and toys; expectant in feeding situations

84. Uses spoon with moderate spilling; toilet regulated

85. Cooperates in dressing; gives toy; finger feeds

86. Dresses without assistance; asks meaning of words

87. Uses spoon well; puts on shoes; takes turns

DIRECTIONS (Questions 88 and 89): For each of the items in this section, ONE or MORE of the numbered options is correct. Choose answer

(A) if only (1), (2), and (3) are correct,
(B) if only (1) and (3) are correct,
(C) if only (2) and (4) are correct,
(D) if only (4) is correct,
(E) if all are correct.

Questions 88 and 89

88. A normal 18-month-old's language development includes

    (1) using plurals and pronouns
    (2) pointing to three body parts when asked
    (3) repeating three digits
    (4) jargon and ten-plus words

89. A normal 4-year-old's language development includes

    (1) asks questions: why? how?
    (2) knows four-plus colors
    (3) beginning concepts of time: past, future
    (4) knows opposites

DIRECTIONS (Question 90): Each of the numbered items or incomplete statements in this section is followed by answers or by completions of the statement. Select the ONE lettered answer or completion that is BEST in each case.

Question 90

90. The average 3-year-old can

    (A) catch a ball
    (B) copy a triangle
    (C) knows the days of the week
    (D) climb stairs with alternating feet
    (E) skips smoothly

DIRECTIONS (Questions 91 and 92): For each of the items in this section, ONE or MORE of the numbered options is correct. Choose answer

(A) if only (1), (2), and (3) are correct,
(B) if only (1) and (3) are correct,
(C) if only (2) and (4) are correct,
(D) if only (4) is correct,
(E) if all are correct.

Questions 91 and 92

91. Traditionally, a child's development is divided into the following categories:

    (1) gross motor
    (2) fine motor/adaptive
    (3) speech and language
    (4) personal–social behavior

92. Concerning childhood neoplasms

    (1) the leukemias are the most common form of childhood cancer
    (2) the occurrence of osteosarcoma and accelerated bone growth seem to be correlated
    (3) the EB virus is increasingly being implicated in Hodgkin's lymphoma
    (4) males have a higher incidence of Wilms' tumor

DIRECTIONS (Questions 93 through 98): Each set of items in this section consists of a list of lettered options followed by several numbered words or phrases. For each numbered word or phrase, select the ONE lettered option that is most closely associated with it. Each lettered option may be selected once, more than once, or not at all.

Questions 93 through 96

(A) tender, swollen tibial tuberosity in an adolescent
(B) obese child with progressive pain and limp
(C) pain and crepitus
(D) incomplete tearing of a muscle or tendon
(E) incomplete tearing of a ligament with associated pain and swelling

93. Osteoarthritis

94. Mild or moderate sprain

95. Osgood–Schlatter disease

96. Slipped capital femoral epiphysis

Questions 97 and 98

(A) stretching of tendon or muscle
(B) stretching of ligament
(C) both
(D) neither

97. Sprain

98. Strain

DIRECTIONS (Question 99): For each of the items in this section, ONE or MORE of the numbered options is correct. Choose answer

(A) if only (1), (2), and (3) are correct,
(B) if only (1) and (3) are correct,
(C) if only (2) and (4) are correct,
(D) if only (4) is correct,
(E) if all are correct.

Question 99

99. There are several types of dehydration. Which of the following is/are true regarding the effect of the type on physical signs?

(1) In hyponatremic dehydration, intracellular fluid (ICF) volume is increased.
(2) In isonatremic dehydration, the mucous membranes are dry.
(3) In hypernatremic dehydration, the extracellular fluid (ECF) volume is decreased.
(4) In hyponatremic dehydration, the blood pressure is high.

DIRECTIONS (Question 100): Each of the numbered items or incomplete statements in this section is followed by answers or by completions of the statement. Select the ONE lettered answer or completion that is BEST in each case.

Question 100

100. Down syndrome involves all the following EXCEPT

(A) the incidence in the general population is 1 in 600 to 800 live births
(B) the presence of an extra number 18 chromosome
(C) increased frequency of congenital heart disease
(D) an association with advanced maternal age
(E) varying degrees of mental retardation

Answers and Explanations

1. **(E)** The differential diagnosis includes *G. lamblia*, milk protein allergy, AIDS, ulcerative colitis, pseudomembranous colitis, acrodermatitis enteropathica, primary immunodeficiency syndromes, secondary or primary disaccharidase deficiencies, celiac disease, Schwachman syndrome, ganglioneuroma or other vasoactive-secreting tumors, intestinal lymphangiectasia, immunoproliferative small intestinal disease, and congenital chloride or sodium-losing diarrhea. Many of these can be distinguished on the basis of history, physical, or screening laboratory examinations. *(Behrman et al, pp. 979–980)*

2. **(A)** Lymphoid leukemias occur more often than expected in patients with immunodeficiencies, chromosomal abnormalities, and ataxia-telangiectasia. On initial examination most patients have anemia and thrombocytopenia, although as many as 25% may have platelet counts greater than 100,000/mm³. A significant percentage will have white blood counts less than 3,000/mm³ and about 20% will have counts less than 50,000/mm³. The treatment of ALL varies with the clinical risk features. Unfavorable prognostic features include onset at age less than 2 years or greater than 10 years of age, with a white cell count over 100,000/mm³, or with a mediastinal mass. *(Behian et al, pp. 1297–1299)*

3. **(B)** All of these findings are typical of the chest x-ray with transient tachypnea of the newborn with the radiographic abnormalities resolving over the first 2 to 3 days after birth. Infants seldom require more than 40% oxygen. Arterial blood gas tensions often reveal a respiratory acidosis which resolves within 8 to 24 hours, and mild to moderate hypoxia. Heavy maternal sedation, maternal diabetes, or delivery by cesarean section are all commonly seen in the history. *(Taeusch et al, pp. 504–505)*

4. **(C)** With ASDs the first heart sound is often split and the second component is of increased intensity. The characteristic finding is wide, fixed splitting of the second heart sound. *(Oski et al, pp. 1418–1423)*

5. **(E)** The murmur of a VSD is not present in the immediate newborn period until pulmonary vascular resistance falls. It is a high-pitched harsh nolosystolic murmur well localized along the left sternal border. *(Oski et al, pp. 1426–1428)*

6. **(B)** The classical auscultatory finding of a patent ductus arteriosus is a continuous machine-like murmur localized under the left clavicle. It should be suspected in any premature infant with hyperdynamic precordium and bounding pulses even in the absence of significant murmur. *(Oski et al, p. 358)*

7. **(A)** Below the coarct there is a narrowed pulse pressure with decreased systolic and diastolic pressure. There may be a tactile sensation of delay between radial and femoral pulses, though the pulse discrepancy may not be apparent in the infant because the widely patent ductus serves as a route of flow to the descending aorta. *(Oski et al, pp. 1438–1442)*

8. **(B)** This is a recently described condition that presents with clusters of easily ruptured vesicopustules on the forehead, neck, and lower back. The lesions have a rim of scale after they rupture and the base may be hyperpigmented. The melanosis gradually subsides over the first few months of life. *(Crapo et al, p. 501; Hoekelman, p. 468)*

9. **(C)** Strawberry hemangiomas are raised from the skin. At birth they may be identified as macular areas of erythema. These hemangiomas grow during the first months of life and eventually involute spontaneously without scarring. Therapy is not advised in the great majority of cases. Occasionally, the location will necessitate therapy. Prednisone for 6 to 12 weeks is the initial therapy. Radiation and laser therapy are used if the lesion does not respond to steroids, but the cosmetic result is poorer. *(Avery et al, p. 1149; Crapo et al, p. 502; Hoekelman, p. 469)*

10. **(E)** Seborrheic dermatitis may be identified in the axillae, neck folds, scalp, and diaper area. The presence of greasy-appearing plaques that are adherent suggests the diagnosis. It is an inflammatory disorder of the sebaceous glands. For severe and persistent lesions, and particularly for lesions in the diaper area, 1% hydrocortisone cream is helpful. *(Crapo et al, pp. 503–504)*

11. **(A)** Epidermolysis bullosa can be either autosomal dominant or autosomal recessive in inheritance. The recessive form is the most severe and can be lethal. The dominant form can range from being a nuisance to a moderate medical problem. Emollients to decrease friction and the prevention of bacterial infection of the blisters are important steps in management of this disease. *(Crapo et al, p. 503)*

12. **(B)** Idiopathic scoliosis is more common in adolescent females than in males. There appears to be a pattern of inheritance that is multifactorial and an autosomal dominant genetic pattern with variable penetrance. *(Behrman et al, pp. 1713–1714)*

13. **(C)** The most common fracture in the newborn is that of the clavicle, which occurs during labor and delivery. In treating this lesion, immobilization is unnecessary. Pinning the total sleeve to the shirt and gentle handling will reduce the discomfort. *(Behrman et al, p. 457)*

14. **(D)** Legg-Calvé-Perthes disease (avascular necrosis of the femoral head) is more common in males. It occurs in children from 3 to 11 with the most common age range being 5 to 9. *(Behrman et al, pp. 1706–1709)*

15. **(A)** Subluxation of the radial head (nursemaid elbow) is a very common injury that occurs in children between 1 and 4 years of age. The child presents with refusal to move the arm and holds it slightly flexed at the elbow and pronated at the forearm. The lesion is a tear in the annular ligament at its attachment on the radius. *(Behrman et al, p. 1724)*

Slipped capital femoral epiphysis (not a correct answer) is most frequently seen in obese adolescents, usually males from 10 to 16 years of age. *(Behrman et al, pp. 1710–1711)*

16. **(C)** Allergic contact dermatitis in children, often caused by a reaction to shoe dyes, rubber, and other chemicals, involves the dorsum of the toes and the distal foot. The lesions are erythematous, scaly, and vesicular and are seen in prepubertal children. *(Polin et al, p. 38; Crapo, pp. 490–491)*

17. **(D)** Tinea pedis presents as interdigital maceration, scaling, and fissures. The scaling occurs primarily on the instep or weightbearing surface. Pruritus is a common symptom. Secondary bacterial infection is common. It is rare before puberty. *(Polin et al, p. 38; Crapo, pp. 490–491)*

18. **(D)** The diagnosis of rheumatic fever is based on clinical grounds. The modified Jones' criteria are the classic for diagnosis. Two major manifestations or one major and two minor manifestations strongly suggest rheumatic fever. The major criteria are polyarthritis, carditis, erythema marginatum, subcutaneous nodules, Sydenham's chorea. The minor manifestations are fever, arthralgia, previous rheumatic fever or rheumatic heart disease, an elevated sedimentation rate or C-reactive protein, and a prolonged P-R interval. *(Behrman, pp. 642–643)*

19. **(A)** Gynecomastia begins in Tanner Stage II–III and disappears in 1 to 2 years. The underlying mass is mobile and there is no skin dimpling that would suggest a cancerous mass. The tissue is breast tissue, not fatty tissue secondary to obesity. Tenderness is a common symptom, as is irritation by clothing, which is relieved by wearing undershirts. Surgical intervention is not a common consideration; however, there are those males who have persistent breast tissue beyond the usual time for resolution and who are having significant psychologic problems with this disorder. Hence, surgery is considered, recommended, and successful. *(Kempe et al, p. 245)*

20. **(D)** Colicky abdominal pain is a common presenting symptom but not invariably present. The edema experienced by these patients is thought to be related to a protein-losing enteropathy secondary to the intestinal involvement in the disease. Most children have renal involvement in HSP. Not all patients have hematuria, but renal biopsy confirms the presence of renal disease in all patients. Platelet counts and coagulation studies are normal. Joint, ankle, and knee pain may be the presenting complaint. *(Hoekelman, pp. 276–277)*

21. **(C)** In idiopathic thrombocytopenic purpura, the platelet count is reduced below 20,000/mm³ (some authors say less than 50,000/mm³). Clot retraction, bleeding time, and the tourniquet test are dependent upon platelet function and are abnormal in ITP. The WBC is normal and anemia is usually not present. Although the differential smear may show decreased platelets, the working diagnosis is made by a platelet count and confirmed by bone marrow examination. In adolescents, systemic lupus erythematosus is a consideration in the differential diagnosis of thrombocytopenic purpura. This would make the ANA test appropriate for ruling out that disease, but would not substantiate the diagnosis of ITP. *(Behrman et al, pp. 1281–1283)*

22. **(D)** Nevus sebaceous (Jadassohn) usually occurs on the head and is present at birth as a yellowish placque without hair. At puberty, there are changes that histologically reveal hyperplasia of the epidermis. In adulthood, there are frequently malignant changes. The usual recommendation is for removal in early adolescence. Acquired pigmented nevi are benign lesions and need be removed only for cosmetic purposes or because their location causes chronic irritation. A very small number of these nevi become malignant. Lentigines are small round dark macules that appear anywhere on the body. The lesions are benign and may be viewed as normal when the number is small. Halo nevus reflects the disappearance of melanocytes in a common pigmented nevus. These lesions are seen frequently in adolescents and children. Eventually, the lesions disappear. Excision would only be considered if there is something unusual about the nature of the central lesion. Achromic nevi are present at birth. They are areas of macular hypopigmented patches with irregular borders. They represent a focal defect in melanin production. *(Behrman et al, pp. 1631–1635)*

23. **(B)** Hypovolemic shock occurs after a reduction in blood volume caused by factors that include hemorrhage (internal or external), plasma loss via burns, sepsis, nephrotic syndrome, fluid shift due to third spacing, fluid and electrolyte loss, or fluid shift due to endocrine conditions such as diabetes mellitus, diabetes insipidus, hypothyroidism, and adrenal insufficiency. Cardiogenic shock stems from a dysfunction of the heart that may result from myocardial insufficiency or mechanical obstruction to the flow of blood into and out of the heart. Distributive or vasogenic shock is due to decreased intravascular volume secondary to leaky capillaries resulting from conditions such as septic shock, anaphylaxis, or barbiturate intoxication. Clinically, the patient's skin is warm, dry, and flushed initially. Terminal shock is irreversible damage to the heart and brain due to altered metabolism and tissue perfusion. This results in death. *(Barkin, pp. 20–32)*

24. **(A)** Many juices are hyposmolar and may draw water into the intestinal lumen. Rice water and tea lack carbohydrates and are not acceptable fluids for oral rehydration. Because it contains large amounts of sodium, boiled milk is also not acceptable. *(Barkin, pp. 50–51; Schmitt, pp. 591–596,608–611)*

25. **(B)** Rectal temperatures are more accurate than axillary temperatures. Antipyretics may be used with children who are uncomfortable due to fever, or have a temperature of 38.6°C. Antipyretics may be held off until that time. Aspirin should not be used in children who have chickenpox or influenza-like illnesses because of the link with

Reye's syndrome. Most providers use no aspirin with children at all. Children under the age of 3 months should have laboratory tests drawn because of the danger of severe underlying disease. Common organisms in bacteremic children include: *Staphylococcus aureus, Streptococcus pneumoniae, Haemophilus influenzae,* and *Neisseria meningitides.* Sponging, not alcohol baths, is useful in treating fevers, along with antipyretics and limiting the amount of clothes worn. *(Barkin, pp. 178–183)*

26. **(D)** *Pasteurella multocida* is the most common organism with *S. aureus*, a secondary organism. Animal bites should be vigorously cleaned, irrigated, and debrided of devitalized tissue. Suturing is determined by functional or cosmetic reasons. Hand injuries, those involving extensive tissue damage, or wounds older than 24 hours' duration should not be sutured. Along with puncture wounds, sutured wounds are more likely to become infected. Tetanus prophylaxis is indicated along with antibiotic prophylaxis for those bites considered high risk for infection. *(Barkin, pp. 230–231)*

27. **(D)** Initial treatment of burns includes immersing the burn in cold water or applying cold compresses to the area. Ice may damage tissue or cause hypothermia in severe burns. Treatment of partial-thickness burns is conducted by cleaning; blisters should remain intact and 1% silver sulfadiazine or petrolatum gauze should be applied. The dressings should be changed every 24 hours initially and every 2 to 3 days thereafter. Electrical burns commonly show little tissue damage at first but increased tissue damage with time is common. These burns should be followed daily. *(Barkin, pp. 237–241)*

28. **(A)** Injury to the cervical spine must always be ruled out. Airway management including intubation and oxygen should be initiated, particularly for the acutely unconscious patient. Hyperventilation and elevation of the head of the bed are crucial in the treatment of severe head injury. Shock is another important consideration. It should be managed aggressively because cerebral perfusion pressure depends on an adequate blood pressure. Shock must be treated first and fluids are generally administered at two-thirds maintenance. *(Barkin, pp. 315–323)*

29. **(C)** Asthma is a common pediatric problem, but children having an acute asthma attack do not always wheeze. Clinicians must conduct a complete history and physical for all children to establish the diagnosis of asthma, but some children may need chest x-rays and a CBC to rule out other causes of wheezing and respiratory difficulty. It is important to establish their respiratory status, but pulmonary function tests may not be helpful in

children because of their difficulty inspiring and expiring into a machine. Humidified oxygen is a necessity and inhaled and/or injected beta agonists are important initial therapy. Rectal theophylline suppositories have erratic absorption and should not be used. Liquid rectal theophylline preparations may be used in the same dose as oral preparations, but only for a short time. The therapeutic serum theophylline level is 10 to 20 µg/mL. Status asthmaticus is present when a patient fails to respond to epinephrine or beta agonists administered as initial therapy. *(Barkin, pp. 581–588)*

30. (C) Infants should gain between 15 and 30 g per day during the first 2 months of life. In the newborn period, they may initially lose up to 10% of their body weight. Infants should double their birthweight at 5 months and triple their birthweight at 12 months. *(Barkin, p. 655)*

31. (B) Failure to thrive is a label applied to children who are below the third percentile in height, weight, or both, or whose growth velocity has slowed and the growth chart reflects a significant decrease in the growth percentiles. The term is usually applied to children under age two, but older children may also be affected. While hospitalization may be necessary in the initial treatment of severely malnourished children, mild to moderate failure to thrive may be managed on an outpatient basis. Laboratory studies may be useful in ruling out organic etiologies for growth failure, but as many as 90% of these children are growing poorly because of inadequate intake. The causes of inadequate intake include economic, educational, and psychosocial factors. *(Hoekelman et al, pp. 704–707)*

32–35. 32. (B); 33. (A); 34. (D); 35. (C) Causes of methemoglobinemia include nitrates, nitrites, and sulfonamides. Organophosphates in pesticides include malathion and parathion. Ipecac is an emetic, not an antidote. *(Barkin, p. 274)*

36. (C) Subdural hematoma is the most dangerous inflicted injury, often causing death or serious neurologic sequelae (ie, seizures, blindness, and/or mental retardation). Subdurals may be associated with skull fractures, but fractures will heal. Intra-abdominal injuries are the second most common cause of death in battered children. Because the abdominal wall is flexible, the force of a blow to the abdomen is usually absorbed by the internal organs, thus causing a ruptured liver or spleen, tears of the small intestine, or intramural hematomas. Subgaleal hematomas, although unsightly, usually resolve within a month, leaving no residual. Extremity fractures, if properly treated, heal without deformity or residual deficit in function. *(Behrman et al, p. 80)*

37. (C) Bone trauma is found in 10% to 20% of physically abused children. Inflicted fractures of the shaft of bones are usually spiral rather than transverse, and spiral fractures of the femur prior to the age of walking are usually inflicted. Multiple bony injuries at different stages of healing imply repeated assaults and are diagnostic of nonaccidental trauma. Fractures of the scapula or sternum are so unusual that they should arouse suspicion of inflicted injury. Many inflicted injuries result from pulling on an extremity. This force tears the periosteum from the bone, thus causing subperiosteal bleeding. By 4 to 6 weeks after the injury, calcification occurs. Rare bone diseases such as scurvy and syphilis may radiologically resemble nonaccidental bone trauma, but the bony changes are symmetrical. *(Behrman et al, p. 80)*

38. (B) Most frequently, children do not disclose sexual molestation for long periods of time. Therefore, at the time they present to the health care provider they are not having acute emotional distress. Also, because of the delay in disclosure, physical findings are usually absent. Positive cultures for gonorrhea are confirmatory evidence of sexual activity, but in and of themselves do not make the diagnosis. Parental assessments of a child's emotional state and behavioral changes are also supportive of the diagnosis but do not make it. The diagnosis most often rests on the graphic history offered by the victim. This can include descriptions of sexual behaviors not commensurate with a child's development or experience level. *(Behrman et al, p. 82)*

39. (E) Foster care is typically provided by local welfare authorities for children who have been neglected and abused. For many children this gives them an environment for physical and emotional safety. However, for others it becomes another episode of deprivation. The United States does not have a comprehensive and well-integrated system for foster care. Foster care is usually managed by individual counties, rather than by state or national authorities, allowing for wide variations in policies. Understaffed and underbudgeted welfare departments do not have the means to develop well-integrated, child-oriented foster care programs to offer support and guidance for foster parents, nor to screen foster parents and children adequately to anticipate problems that may result in another change of placement. The legal system also has been slow to respond to permanent planning for children, making it possible for repeated placement changes. *(Behrman et al, p. 51)*

40. (D) Most polycythemic infants are asymptomatic. Common early symptoms include plethora, cyanosis, lethargy, hypotonia, poor suck and feeding, and tremulousness. Serious complications include cardiorespiratory disease, seizures, peripheral gangrene, necrotizing enterocolitis, renal failure and priapism. *(Taeusch et al, pp. 822–823)*

41. **(D)** Symptoms of hyaline membrane disease (HMD) occur after the onset of breathing. The incidence is 60% at 29 weeks' gestation and declines with maturation to near 0 by 39 weeks. The unventilated infant frequently requires 40% to 50% oxygen after birth but then develops an increasing oxygen requirement over 24 to 48 hours reaching as high as 100%. Chest x-rays show diffuse, fine granular densities. The appearance may be more marked at the lung bases than at the apices, and lung volume is ultimately decreased.

Current prevention includes prevention of premature birth, antenatal treatment of women with premature labor with glucocorticoid hormones and surfactant replacement, either prophylactically for small premature infants at risk for HMD or treatment of infants with established HMD. *(Taeusch et al, pp. 498–504)*

42–45. **42. (E); 43. (A); 44. (B); 45. (C)** The abuser is a related caretaker in 90% of cases, a male friend of the mother in 5%, an unrelated babysitter in 4%, and a sibling in 1%. These statistics are apt to change as do social conditions; that is, currently, women are more likely to be involved in abuse, but this difference disappears in families in which the mothers work and fathers are the primary caretakers. Presently there is also a trend for increased reporting of abuse in daycare settings. *(Behrman et al, p. 79)*

46. **(A)** Physicians, physician assistants, and all health care providers must be able to recognize abused children and confirm the diagnosis. Recognition during the first 6 months of life is extremely important because the risk of a fatal outcome is highest in this age group. Prevention should be provided at all contacts with the parents by offering support, anticipatory guidance, and asking questions that allow parents to express any difficulties they are experiencing. All 50 states have laws requiring that health care providers report suspected cases of child abuse and neglect to a local child protective agency. Physician assistants, without specific training in psychiatry or mental health, rarely provide direct treatment for abused children and their families. *(Behrman et al, p. 79)*

47. **(A)** In the vagina, sperm are motile for 6 hours and nonmotile for 72 hours or longer. The presence of sperm substantiates the victim's story. Acid phosphatase is present for 24 hours and confirms ejaculation. Gonorrhea cultures are positive less than 5% of the time, but are evidence that confirm the victim's history. When the cultures are positive, the alleged perpetrator will also need to be cultured. Pregnancy testing is not contributory (therefore, not indicated) in a child of this age, but in a postmenarcheal child, medication to prevent pregnancy should be given. *(Behrman et al, p. 82)*

48. **(B)** Adoptions accomplished through approved agencies are preferred to independent adoptions, as they tend to have more adequate assessment of the psychosocial setting of the prospective adoptive family. Although, in general, adoptive placement should be made as soon after birth as possible, adoptions of older children, or across religious or ethnic lines, are appropriate and reasonable alternatives to having adoptable children languish in institutions or temporary homes. The adopted child should be told of his/her adoption as soon as reasonably good verbal faculty and comprehension have been achieved, usually about ages 3 to 4. *(Behrman et al, p. 50)*

49. **(B)** In sensorineural hearing loss, the Weber test lateralizes to the healthy ear. The affected inner ear or nerve is less able to receive vibrations arriving by any route, including bone. The sound is therefore heard in the better ear. On the Rinne test, air conduction lasts longer than bone conduction because the affected inner ear or nerve is less able to perceive vibrations arriving by either route. Therefore, the normal pattern prevails. *(Bates, p. 188)*

50. **(C)** A one-time physical examination of the newborn is useless, except for identifying gross congenital conditions or malformations. Observations and physical examinations of newborns need to be a "running appraisal" of findings over time. This is to assess the baby's condition and adaptation to extrauterine life, rather than assessments just at previously designated times, namely, admission and discharge. In the newborn, physical examinations are highly time dependent; that is, what is normal at 5 minutes of age is not normal at 3 hours, especially in regard to respiration and color. For this reason, all chart notes need to be specifically timed and dated. Particularly when performed by the unskilled on a premature sick infant, the physical examination can have adverse results, such as decreased body temperature, decreased skin perfusion, and decreased oxygenation. Handwashing to the elbows after removal of rings, bracelets, and watches should be performed immediately before and after touching the infant with no handling of fomites in the period during which the infant is handled. Nosocomial infections are one of the results of casual "baby-to-baby" examinations. *(Avery and Taeusch, p. 55)*

51. **(C)** Infants born to substance-abusing parents are at increased risk for physical, sexual, and emotional abuse, as well as neglect and developmental delays. Opiate withdrawal may not reach a peak

until 10–14 days after birth and evidence of withdrawal from narcotics can persist in a subacute form for 4–6 months after birth. Significant signs and symptoms of neonatal abstinence include all of these symptoms. Neonates who are withdrawing from non-narcotic substances may exhibit irritability, restlessness, poor feeding, crying, and impaired neurobehavioral activity also seen in neonatal narcotic abstinence syndrome. Universal neonatal screening for illicit drugs is not recommended. Screening will be negative when drugs were used early in the pregnancy and can be negative even when a woman has taken drugs during the 48 hours before delivery. *(Freeman et al, pp. 224–227)*

52. **(E)** Polycythemia beyond the immediate neonatal period is seen with arterial hypoxia due to cyanotic heart disease or pulmonary disorders. It can be caused by renal, hepatic, or cellular tumors, or by hemoglobinopathies with increased oxygen affinity. *(Taeusch et al, pp. 822–823)*

53. **(E)** Genetic (parents' and infant's blood types) and ethnic factors are known to affect neonatal bilirubin levels. With Rh and ABO incompatibility, hemolysis of infant blood cells and subsequent release of bilirubin occurs. Serum bilirubin values appear to be significantly higher in apparently normal Chinese, Japanese, Korean, and American Indian babies. Some perinatal events associated with increased bilirubin include delayed cord clamping and traumatic delivery. Surveys indicate that somewhere between one in 50 and one in 200 breastfed infants will develop hyperbilirubinemia. This is usually of late onset (after the third day). Kernicterus has never been reported with breastfeeding jaundice. Temporary cessation of breast feeding should be performed only if bilirubin levels have approached 20 mg/dL or when such interruption is crucial in establishing an etiology. *(Taeusch et al, pp. 754–757)*

54. **(C)** The contraindications to DPT are previous severe reactions to DPT, including encephalopathy within 7 days, convulsion within 3 days, persistent high-pitched crying for 3 or more hours within 48 hours, collapse or shock-like state within 48 hours, temperature of 40.5°C or greater unexplained by another cause, and an immediate severe or anaphylactic reaction. Although some practitioners elect to defer immunization, a nonfebrile respiratory illness is not a contraindication to DPT. A family history of seizure is not a contraindication to vaccination. *(Red Book, pp. 28,363–366)*

55. **(B)** Hepatitis A is a viral illness. Symptoms include jaundice, anorexia, nausea, and malaise. Infants and preschool children are often asymptomatic. Chronic infection does not occur; fulminant disease is rare. Transmission is person to person via the fecal–oral route. The incubation period is 15–50 days, average 25–30 days. Treatment is supportive only. Immune globulin is used for contacts of infected people. *(Red Book, pp. 234–237)*

56. **(A)** An unimmunized child should be caught up as rapidly as possible, and DPT, OPV, and MMR may be given at one visit. However, a patient infected with HIV should receive inactivated polio virus (IPV) instead of oral polio vaccine (OPV). MMR, a live viral vaccine, is indicated because complications have not occurred in HIV-infected children, no killed-virus vaccine is available, and because measles is devastating in children with HIV. *(Red Book, p. 51)*

57. **(B)** In children younger than 15 months of age, HIV-seropositivity may be due to the passive transmission of maternal antibody in the perinatal period. Diagnosis of AIDS disease in younger children must be confirmed by a positive viral culture, a positive antigen or indirect abnormalities, or a decreased T/T ratio. Of infants born to HIV infected mothers, 30% to 50% will acquire HIV infection. *(Hoekelman et al, pp. 1115–1117)*

58. **(E)** A newborn without congenital CMV infection can be infected by his or her mother at the time of delivery, through breast milk, by acquisition from the nursery or home environment, or by transfusion of blood from a donor who is antibody positive. Acquisition from blood transfusion often results in severe, sometimes fatal, disease when maternal antibody is lacking. Perinatal or postnatal acquisition from the mother or the environment appears to be benign, although lower respiratory illness may occur. *(Taeusch et al, p. 335)*

59. **(A)** Streptococcal pharyngitis may be successfully treated with penicillin given intramuscularly or orally, two, three, or four times per day. Failure rates are unacceptably high (more than 20%) when dosed only once per day. *(Red Book, pp. 442–444; Gerber et al, pp. 153–155)*

60. **(B)** Varicella zoster immune globulin (VZIG) should be given to a newborn infant of a mother who had chickenpox within 5 days before delivery or within 48 hours after delivery. VZIG does not modify established varicella. A newborn exposed to a sibling with varicella is not considered to be at high risk for complicated varicella because transplacental maternal antibody will usually protect the infant. *(Red Book, pp. 521–523)*

61–65. **61. (C); 62. (A); 63. (A); 64. (B); 65. (D)** MMR and OPV are attenuated live virus vaccines. Diphtheria and tetanus toxoids are together with formalin-treated killed whole *B. pertussis* organisms in DPT vaccine. Purified polysaccharide from the capsule of *H. influenzae* type B is given alone in PRP vaccine, or covalently linked to a bacterial toxoid as in PRP-D vaccine. *(Red Book, p. 11)*

66. **(B)** Diagnostic criteria for Kawasaki syndrome are *fever for 5 days or longer;* and four of the five following: *conjunctival infection, rash, mucus membrane changes* such as cracked dry lips, injected pharynx or strawberry tongue, *extremity changes* such as redness and swelling of palms and soles, or desquamation, and cervical lymphadenopathy. Other illnesses that may mimic Kawasaki syndrome, for example, streptococcal infection, must be excluded. Diarrhea and vomiting and generalized lymphadenopathy, although occasionally seen in children with Kawasaki syndrome, are not diagnostic criteria. *(Bell, pp. 20–26)*

67. **(C)** Approximately 75% of children will have at least one episode of otitis media, with the peak incidence occurring between 6 and 24 months of age. Risk factors include race (with white children affected more commonly than blacks), craniofacial malformations, Down syndrome, bottle feeding instead of breast feeding, and exposure to cigarette smoke. *(Hoekelman et al, pp. 1417–1419)*

68. **(A)** In the 15- to 24-year age group, the main causes of death are accidents, homicide, suicide, and neoplasms, in that order. Males outnumber females 5:1 in completed suicide, but adolescent females attempt suicide four times more often than males. *(Hoekelman, pp. 22–23,788–791)*

69. **(B)** In females, onset of puberty is usually heralded by breast bud development. The growth spurt follows, with menarche occurring after peak height is attained. In males, growth of the testes is the first sign of puberty, followed by pigmentation and thinning of the scrotum and growth of the penis. Pubic hair then appears. The male growth spurt generally occurs after puberty is well under way. There are considerable variations in sequence of changes and age of onset in both sexes. *(Behrman et al, p. 1047)*

70. **(C)** Jaundice progresses in a cephalocaudal manner, with the extremities the last to be affected. Jaundice is visible clinically usually at 6 or 7 mg/dL. Cephalohematomas are reservoirs of RBCs that can act as an increased source of bilirubin. Jaundice is associated with all these syndromes (hypothyroidism, galactosemia, and PKU) and they should be included in the differential diagnosis. *(Merenstein et al, pp. 325,327–328)*

71. **(C)** Scleral and facial jaundice become visible at 6–8 mg/dL, jaundice of the shoulders and trunk at 8 to 10 mg/dL and jaundice of the lower body at 10–12 mg/dL as rough guidelines. Neonatal poly-

cythemia, when combined with shortened red blood cell survival time, may result in the accumulation of an increased bilirubin load. Although 25% of all pregnancies are potentially ABO incompatible, only 10% to 15% of these have hemolytic disease as documented by a positive Coombs' test. *(Oski, pp. 399–404)*

72. **(C)** Migratory arthritis is associated with rheumatic fever. Conjunctivitis occurs with Reiter's syndrome. Juvenile rheumatoid arthritis is characterized by mono-, pauci-, or polyarticular joint swelling constantly and daily for at least 6 weeks. It is almost always possible to elicit a history of morning stiffness. *(Tausch et al, p. 754)*

73. **(A)** Choices (1), (2), and (3) are correct. Unfortunately, only a minority (30% to 45%) of teens who are suicide victims had ever been referred for mental health evaluation. In one series, only 2 of 27 were in treatment at the time of suicide. *(Brent, pp. 269–270)*

74. **(B)** These organisms are usually recovered from sinus aspirates. Frontal sinuses are rarely a site of infection until age 6 to 10. Sinus headaches are infrequent in children 5 years or younger. Acute and chronic sinusitis increases in later childhood. *(Behrman et al, p. 1059)*

75. **(A)** These are the most common organisms in this age group. Children in daycare settings are at a higher risk for secondary cases of meningitis. Hearing loss does occur as a sequelae with both *H. influenzae* and *N. meningitidis*. The peak incidence of *S. pneumoniae* meningitis occurs in infants 3 to 5 months of age. *(Behrman et al, pp. 683–684)*

76. **(A)** Pulmonary infections are more common with *S. aureus* and *P. aeruginosa*. *P. aeruginosa* is responsible for a chronic low-grade infection that progresses. The patients colonized with *P. aeruginosa* may require recurrent hospitalizations for intensive inhalation therapy and antibiotics. *(Behrman et al, pp. 1106–1116)*

77. **(D)** Erythema chronicum migrans is the cutaneous manifestation of Lyme disease. This rash develops at the site of the tick bite and develops into an expanding erythematous annular lesion with central clearing of approximately 16 cm. The rash of rheumatic fever is erythema marginatum that occurs over the trunk and inner surfaces of arms and legs. The rash is barely red, slightly raised, nonpruritic, and spreads in wavy lines or rings with sharp margins. *(Behrman et al, p. 541)*

78. **(B)** Colic does not have any sexual predilection. It is important to realize that colicky crying can occur at any time of the day, although it frequently

occurs at the same time each day. The cause of colic is not known, but is felt to be associated with hunger and with swallowed air that has passed into the intestines. *(Behrman et al, pp. 128–129)*

79. (C) In Fragile X syndrome the testes are large. Fragile X syndrome is also associated with mental retardation. Cryptorchid testes are associated with many congenital and chromosomal abnormalities. *(Behrman et al, pp. 295,1378)*

80. (D) Isometric exercises such as weight lifting should be discouraged in adolescents with hypertension, because this form of exercise produces a marked increase in both systolic and diastolic pressures. Severe (Type IV or V) fractures involving the epiphysis may result in growth disturbance if not properly treated. Hypertrophic cardiomyopathy is characterized by massive ventricular hypertrophy with involvement of the ventricular septum. It can occur at any age and in some instances is transmitted in an autosomal dominant pattern. Many children are asymptomatic and are evaluated only because of heart murmur, but even those children are at risk for sudden death. As many as 10% to 20% of children with Down syndrome have atlantoaxial instability and children with this diagnosis should have cervical roentgenograms prior to their participation in sports. Activities such as swimming, which generally does not induce bronchospasm, should be encouraged for asthmatics. *(Behrman et al, pp. 587–592,1210–1211,1721–1725)*

81. (C) Female adolescents lead male adolescents in the incidence of suicide attempts. Males outnumber females in completed suicides. *(Behrman et al, p. 526)*

82. (D) Anorexic patients show excessive physical activity, deny hunger, and yet are preoccupied with food preparation and academic success. Most parents will describe their anorexic daughters as a "model" child before the onset of the illness. *(Behrman et al, p. 533)*

83–87. 83. (A); 84. (C); 85. (B); 86. (E); 87. (D) At 28 weeks, the toddler usually plays with feet and toys and is expectant in feeding situations. By 18 months, the infant uses a spoon with moderate spilling and is toilet regulated. By 12 months, the infant cooperates in dressing, gives toy, and finger feeds. By 5 years, the child dresses without assistance and asks the meaning of words. By 3 years, the child uses a spoon well, puts on shoes, and takes turns. *(Lewis, p. 163)*

88. (C) There are age-related norms established for articulation of speech and development of language and concepts. The correct response to this "K" question is (C) because (2) and (4) are correct

answers. An 18-month-old child has attained sufficient maturation in his/her language development to be able to point to three body parts (2), and to have jargon and ten-plus words (4). Choices (1) and (3) are incorrect responses because using plurals and pronouns (1) and repeating three digits (3) are 3-year-old skills. *(Kaye et al, pp. 35–36)*

89. (B) Using the established age-related norms for development of language and concepts, the correct response to this "K" question is (B). Choices (1) and (3) are correct responses because a 4-year-old has attained the language skills necessary to ask questions such as why and how and is beginning to understand concepts of time: past, future. Choices (2) and (4) are incorrect responses because knowing four-plus colors and opposites are 5-year-old skills. *(Kaye et al, p. 36)*

90. (D) A 3-year-old has attained the skill of climbing stairs with alternating feet, making (D) the correct choice. Knowing the days of the week is a 4- to 5-year-old skill; catching a ball and skipping smoothly are 5- to 6-year-old skills; copying a triangle is a 6- to 7-year-old skill. *(Kempe et al, p. 32)*

91. (E) Development follows a dynamic sequential pattern with the timetable varying not only in normal versus abnormal persons, but also reflecting individual differences among children. It is helpful to divide development into categories as above, making (E) the correct response. In the infant, assessment of development is dependent primarily on motor and reflex parameters. Later, language and visual motor perception assume greater relative importance. *(Kaye et al, pp. 24–26)*

92. (A) Leukemias are the most common cancer in childhood—one-third of all diagnosed cancers. Bone marrow dysfunction is the major pathologic finding. The mean age of the diagnosis of osteosarcoma is 15 years. Osteoma occurs most frequently at the metaphyseal ends of long bones. One study found that children at the time of diagnosis are taller than children with other kinds of cancer. There is recent evidence the EB virus is invoked in the pathogenesis of Hodgkin's disease, one type of lymphoma. With current treatment of Hodgkin's disease (radiation/chemotherapy), 90% will have an initial clinical remission. Wilms' tumor accounts for almost all kidney cancers in childhood. The median age of diagnosis is 3 years. It occurs equally in males and females. Treatment is surgical removal. Neuroblastomas may present with the same sign (abdominal mass) but these patients are older and appear less ill. *(Behrman, pp. 1297–1312)*

93–96. 93. (C); 94. (E); 95. (A); 96. (B) Osteoarthritis is manifested when the physical examination of the patellofemoral compartment of the knee joint yields pain and crepitus (C). A mild or moderate sprain is diagnosed by incomplete tearing of a ligament (E) as opposed to a strain, which involves the tendon. Complete tearing can result in instability of the joint. Osgood–Schlatter disease is suspected in an adolescent with knee pain and is demonstrated on physical exam by a tender, swollen tibial tuberosity (A). Slipped capital femoral epiphysis should be suspected in an obese child with pain and/or limp; greater than 40% of the children so affected are indeed obese. Additionally, it is important to always examine the hip joint in any child complaining of knee pain as pain can be referred. The (D) choice does not relate to any of the numbered items and is, therefore, an incorrect response. *(Bates, pp. 450–451; Kempe et al, pp. 639–642)*

97–98. 97. (B); 98. (A) Soft tissue trauma may be divided into several categories according to the anatomical area that has been injured. A sprain is the stretching of a ligament. A strain is defined as stretching of a tendon or muscle. In either of these injuries there may be some degree of tissue tearing. *(Kempe et al, p. 642)*

99. (A) The correct response to this "K" question is (A) as (1), (2), and (3) are true statements. Choice (1), hyponatremic dehydration or loss of sodium in excess of water, produces an increase in intracellular fluid (ICF) volume. Choice (2), an isonatremic dehydration, where there is a proportionate loss of water and sodium, mucous membranes are dry on physical examination. Choice (3), hypernatremic dehydration, loss of water in excess of sodium, produces a decrease in extracellular volume. Choice (4) is a false statement because in hyponatremic dehydration, the blood pressure is very low. *(Behrman et al, p. 200)*

100. (B) The appropriate answer is (B), which is the only incorrect choice given. Down syndrome involves the presence of an extra number 21 chromosome and has been the best recognized and most frequent human chromosomal syndrome. (A) applies to Down syndrome in that the incidence is indeed 1 in 600 to 800 live births. Actually, among all conceptuses, greater than twice this frequency occurs but more than one half of these are spontaneously aborted during early pregnancy. (C), frequency of congenital heart disease, is associated with Down syndrome, primarily septal defects, especially of the endocardial cushion. (D), associated with advanced maternal age, is correct with the reason for the correlation unknown. The major thought has to do with some aspect of aging of the oocyte. (E) is a correct statement, as all children with Down syndrome exhibit some degree of mental retardation, albeit there is a wide variability of severity. *(Behrman et al, pp. 282–283)*

REFERENCES

Avery ME, First LR (eds). *Pediatric Medicine,* 1st ed. Baltimore, MD: Williams & Wilkins; 1989.

Avery ME, Taeusch HW. *Scaffer's Diseases of the Newborn,* 5th ed. Philadelphia, PA: WB Saunders; 1984.

Barkin RM. *Emergency Pediatrics,* 3rd ed. St. Louis, MO: CV Mosby; 1990.

Bates B. *A Guide to Physical Examination and History Taking,* 5th ed. Philadelphia, PA: JB Lippincott; 1991.

Behrman RE. *Nelson Textbook of Pediatrics,* 14th ed. Philadelphia, PA: WB Saunders; 1992.

Bell DM. Kawasaki update: More answers, fewer questions. *Contemp Pediatr.* 1985;2:2–36.

Crapo JD, Hamilton MA, Edgman S (eds). *Medicine & Pediatrics in One Book.* Philadelphia, PA: Hanley & Belfus; St. Louis, MO: CV Mosby; 1988.

Dajani AS, Asmar BI, Thirumoorthi MC. Systemic *Haemophilus influenzae* disease: An overview. *J Pediatr.* 1979;94:355–364.

Freeman RK, Poland RL (eds). *Guidelines for Perinatal Care.* American Academy of Pediatrics, and American College of Obstetrics and Gynecology; 1992.

Gerber MA, Randolph MD, DeMae K, et al. Failure of once-daily penicillin V therapy for streptococcal pharyngitis. *Am J Dis Child.* 1989;143:153–155.

Hoekelman RA, et al. *Primary Pediatric Care,* 2nd ed. Mosby Year Book, Inc.; 1992.

Hathaway WE, et al. *Current Pediatric Diagnosis & Treatment,* 9th ed. CT: Appleton & Lange; 1991.

Lewis M. *Clinical Aspects of Child Development.* Philadelphia, PA: Lea & Febiger; 1982.

Markowitz LE, Preblud SR, Orenstein WA, et al. Patterns of transmission in measles outbreaks in the United States, 1985–1986. *N Engl J Med.* 1989;320: 75–81.

Merenstein GB, Gardner SL. *Handbook of Neonatal Intensive Care,* 2nd ed. St. Louis, MO: CV Mosby Company; 1989.

Neinstein L. *Adolescent Health Care. A Practical Guide.* Baltimore–Munich: Urban & Schwarzenberg; 1991.

Oski A (ed). Principles and practice of pediatrics. Lippincott; 1990.

Polin RA, Ditmar MF. *Pediatric Secrets.* Philadelphia, PA: Hanley & Belfus; St. Louis, MO: CV Mosby; 1989.

Report of the Committee of Infectious Diseases (*The Red Book*), 21st ed. Elk Grove Village, IL: American Academy of Pediatrics; 1991.

Rosenstein BJ, Fosarelli PD. *Pediatric Pearls: The Handbook of Practical Pediatrics.* Chicago, London, Boca Raton: Year Book Medical Publishers; 1989.

Schmitt BD. Colic: Excessive crying in newborns. *Clin Perinatol.* 1985;12:441–450.

Schmitt BD. *Your Child's Health.* Toronto: Bantam Books; 1991.

Taeusch HW, Ballard RA, Avery ME. *Schaffer and Avery's Diseases of the Newborn.* 6th ed. Philadelphia, PA: WB Saunders; 1992.

Subspecialty List: Pediatrics

QUESTION NUMBER AND SUBSPECIALTY

1. GI
2. Oncology
3. Neonatology
4. Cardiology
5. Cardiology
6. Cardiology
7. Cardiology
8. Dermatology
9. Dermatology
10. Dermatology
11. Dermatology
12. Orthopedics
13. Orthopedics
14. Orthopedics
15. Orthopedics
16. Dermatology
17. Dermatology
18. Rheumatology
19. Adolescent medicine
20. Renal
21. Hematology
22. Dermatology
23. Pediatric emergency medicine
24. Gastrointestinal
25. General pediatrics
26. Pediatric emergency medicine
27. Pediatric emergency medicine
28. Pediatric emergency medicine
29. Pediatric emergency medicine
30. Growth and development
31. Growth and development
32. Pediatric emergency medicine
33. Pediatric emergency medicine
34. Pediatric emergency medicine
35. Pediatric emergency medicine
36. Child abuse
37. Child abuse
38. Child abuse
39. Child abuse
40. Neonatology
41. Neonatology
42. Child abuse
43. Child abuse
44. Child abuse
45. Child abuse
46. Child abuse
47. Child abuse
48. General pediatrics
49. Ear, nose, and throat
50. Neonatology
51. Neonatology
52. Neonatology
53. Neonatology
54. Immunization
55. Immunization
56. Immunization
57. Infectious disease
58. Infectious disease
59. Infectious disease
60. Infectious disease
61. Infectious disease
62. Infectious disease
63. Infectious disease
64. Infectious disease
65. Infectious disease
66. Infectious disease
67. Ear, nose, and throat
68. Adolescent medicine
69. Adolescent medicine
70. Neonatology
71. Neonatology
72. Rheumatology
73. Adolescent medicine
74. Ear, nose, and throat
75. Infectious disease
76. Pulmonary
77. Rheumatology
78. General pediatrics
79. General pediatrics
80. Adolescent medicine
81. Adolescent medicine
82. Adolescent medicine
83. Child development
84. Child development
85. Child development
86. Child development
87. Child development
88. Child development
89. Child development
90. Child development

91. Child development
92. Orthopedics
93. Orthopedics
94. Orthopedics
95. Orthopedics

96. Orthopedics
97. Orthopedics
98. Orthopedics
99. Emergency medicine
100. Genetics

CHAPTER 3

Emergency Medicine
Questions

Questions

DIRECTIONS (Questions 1 through 3): Each of the numbered items or incomplete statements in this section is followed by answers or by completions of the statement. Select the ONE lettered answer or completion that is BEST in each case.

Questions 1 through 3

1. The most common form of shock in the initial phase of multisystem trauma is

   (A) hypovolemic shock
   (B) septic shock
   (C) neurogenic shock
   (D) cardiogenic shock
   (E) burn shock

2. Using the rule-of-nines, calculate the body surface area (BSA) involvement of an adult with a circumferential burn injury involving the left leg and right arm.

   (A) 9%
   (B) 18%
   (C) 27%
   (D) 36%
   (E) 70%

3. Alcohol is involved in what percent of fatal single vehicle accidents?

   (A) 10%
   (B) 20%
   (C) 40%
   (D) 60%
   (E) 100%

DIRECTIONS (Questions 4 through 7): Each set of items in this section consists of a list of lettered options followed by several numbered words or phrases. For each numbered word or phrase, select the ONE lettered option that is most closely associated with it. Each lettered option may be selected once, more than once, or not at all.

Questions 4 through 7

Match the type of shock with its characteristic physical findings.

   (A) hypotension without tachycardia, peripheral vasodilatation
   (B) hypotension, tachycardia, distended neck veins
   (C) near normal blood pressure, tachycardia, wide pulse pressure
   (D) tachycardia, peripheral vasoconstriction, narrow pulse pressure
   (E) tachycardia, edema due to loss of plasma volume

4. Hypovolemic shock

5. Septic shock

6. Cardiogenic shock

7. Neurogenic shock

DIRECTIONS (Questions 8 through 17): For each of the items in this section, ONE or MORE of the numbered options is correct. Choose answer

    (A) if only (1), (2), and (3) are correct,
    (B) if only (1) and (3) are correct,
    (C) if only (2) and (4) are correct,
    (D) if only (4) is correct,
    (E) if all are correct.

Questions 8 through 17

8. Potentially lethal chest trauma includes

    (1) hemothorax
    (2) open chest wounds
    (3) cardiac tamponade
    (4) pneumothorax

9. Characteristics of Boerhaave syndrome include

    (1) sudden onset of severe chest pain
    (2) esophageal reflux associated with postural changes
    (3) often precipitated by forceful vomiting
    (4) gradual onset of dull epigastric pain

10. Common causes of hypovolemic shock in the trauma patient include

    (1) femur fractures
    (2) pelvic fractures
    (3) hemothorax
    (4) closed head injury

11. Compartment syndromes often result from crush injuries or fractures of an extremity. Early signs and symptoms include

    (1) pulselessness
    (2) decreased sensation
    (3) poor capillary refill
    (4) pain

12. Emergency care of the major burn patient includes

    (1) administration of prophylactic IV antibiotics
    (2) vigorous administration of IV fluids
    (3) application of ice to affected areas
    (4) fiberoptic bronchoscopy to diagnose inhalation injury

13. Radiographic findings suggestive of aortic transection include

    (1) widened mediastinum
    (2) abnormal aortic contour
    (3) depression of left mainstem bronchus
    (4) left hemothorax

14. Treatment of flail chest injuries include

    (1) positioning patient on the affected side
    (2) positioning patient away from affected side
    (3) placement of sandbags on flail segment
    (4) intubation and positive pressure ventilation in patients with respiratory distress

15. Signs and symptoms of acute pancreatitis include

    (1) severe epigastric pain
    (2) rapid onset of pain
    (3) radiation of pain to the back
    (4) nausea and vomiting

16. Cardinal signs of a felon (infection of the finger tuft) include

    (1) fingers held in flexion
    (2) intense pain upon passive extension of the finger
    (3) sensitivity upon palpation along the course of the tendon sheaths
    (4) uniform swelling of the finger

17. A boutonniere deformity is characterized by

    (1) avulsion of the extensor digitorum communis tendon from its insertion on the middle phalanx
    (2) avulsion of the extensor digitorum communis tendon from its insertion on the distal phalanx
    (3) the proximal interphalangeal joint becomes markedly flexed and the distal interphalangeal joint extended
    (4) loss of extension in the distal phalangeal joint

DIRECTIONS (Questions 18 and 19): Each of the numbered items or incomplete statements in this section is followed by answers or by completions of the statement. Select the ONE lettered answer or completion that is BEST in each case.

Questions 18 and 19

18. Which spinal nerve supplies sensation to only the middle finger?

    (A) C5
    (B) C6
    (C) C7
    (D) C8
    (E) T1

19. Sensation to the skin of the legs and feet is derived from lumbar and sacral nerves. Which spinal nerve supplies sensation to the lateral aspect of the foot?

 (A) L3
 (B) L4
 (C) L5
 (D) S1
 (E) S2

DIRECTIONS (Questions 20 and 21): For each of the items in this section, ONE or MORE of the numbered options is correct. Choose answer

 (A) if only (1), (2), and (3) are correct,
 (B) if only (1) and (3) are correct,
 (C) if only (2) and (4) are correct,
 (D) if only (4) is correct,
 (E) if all are correct.

Questions 20 and 21

20. Clinical features of acute diverticulitis often include

 (1) crampy abdominal pain
 (2) persistent vomiting
 (3) left lower quadrant pain
 (4) left flank pain

21. Radiographic findings suggestive of small bowel obstruction include

 (1) free intraperitoneal air seen best under the diaphragm on the upright KUB
 (2) air fluid levels within the bowel loops
 (3) a large amount of gas within the large bowel
 (4) distended loops of small bowel, proximal to the point of obstruction

DIRECTIONS (Question 22): Each of the numbered items or incomplete statements in this section is followed by answers or by completions of the statement. Select the ONE lettered answer or completion that is BEST in each case.

Question 22

22. A 35-year-old male presents to the ER with a 2-hour history of severe epigastric pain. He reports the sudden onset of this discomfort. The patient denies vomiting. He reports a long history of intermittent abdominal pain relieved by antacids. The patient is lying on the stretcher, avoiding all movement. The abdomen is diffusely tender with muscular rigidity and guarding. The most likely diagnosis is

 (A) acute cholecystitis
 (B) perforated duodenal ulcer
 (C) acute appendicitis
 (D) acute diverticulitis
 (E) cholelithiasis

DIRECTIONS (Questions 23 through 25): For each of the items in this section, ONE or MORE of the numbered options is correct. Choose answer

 (A) if only (1), (2), and (3) are correct,
 (B) if only (1) and (3) are correct,
 (C) if only (2) and (4) are correct,
 (D) if only (4) is correct,
 (E) if all are correct.

Questions 23 through 25

23. Common causes of small bowel obstruction include

 (1) adhesions from previous abdominal surgery
 (2) abdominal wall or internal hernias
 (3) intussusception
 (4) mesenteric lymphadenopathy

24. Common features of ruptured ectopic pregnancy include

 (1) sudden onset of abdominal and pelvic pain
 (2) history of scant or missed menstrual period
 (3) evidence of intraabdominal bleeding
 (4) unilateral, tender adnexal mass

25. Proper care of the patient with acute abdominal pain includes

 (1) nasogastric suctioning
 (2) serial physical examinations
 (3) careful attention to intravascular volume replacement
 (4) adequate anesthesia

DIRECTIONS (Question 26): Each of the numbered items or incomplete statements in this section is followed by answers or by completions of the statement. Select the ONE lettered answer or completion that is BEST in each case.

Question 26

26. Murphy's sign is best described as

   (A) referred pain from the abdomen to the shoulder or scapula
   (B) rebound tenderness often seen in peritonitis
   (C) pain with palpation of the RUQ upon deep inspiration, pain causes patient to halt inspiratory effort
   (D) abdominal pain elicited by gently rocking the pelvis
   (E) a fetal position assumed by the patient with abdominal pain

DIRECTIONS (Questions 27 through 30): Each set of items in this section consists of a list of lettered options followed by several numbered words or phrases. For each numbered word or phrase, select the ONE lettered option that is most closely associated with it. Each lettered option may be selected once, more than once, or not at all.

Questions 27 through 30

Match the following pain patterns and location with the most likely diagnosis.

   (A) sudden, severe midepigastric pain that progresses to diffuse abdominal discomfort
   (B) sudden, severe right upper quadrant pain with radiation to the right scapular and shoulder region
   (C) severe epigastric pain with radiation to the back
   (D) vague midabdominal pain that localizes to the right lower quadrant

27. Perforated duodenal ulcer

28. Acute cholecystitis

29. Appendicitis

30. Acute pancreatitis

DIRECTIONS (Question 31): For each of the items in this section, ONE or MORE of the numbered options is correct. Choose answer

   (A) if only (1), (2), and (3) are correct,
   (B) if only (1) and (3) are correct,
   (C) if only (2) and (4) are correct,
   (D) if only (4) is correct,
   (E) if all are correct.

Question 31

31. Sources of emboli causing acute arterial occlusions can include

   (1) endocardium secondary to myocardial infarction
   (2) embolized atheromatous material from abdominal aortic aneurysms
   (3) left atrium secondary to atrial fibrillation
   (4) arterial arteriosclerotic stenosis with secondary thrombosis

DIRECTIONS (Questions 32 and 33): Each of the numbered items or incomplete statements in this section is followed by answers or by completions of the statement. Select the ONE lettered answer or completion that is BEST in each case.

Questions 32 and 33

32. A 60-year-old male presents to the ER with hematemesis. Past medical history is significant for cirrhosis. Physical examination is significant for disorientation, ascites, and splenomegaly. The most likely diagnosis is

   (A) UGI bleeding secondary to perforated duodenal ulcer
   (B) UGI bleeding secondary to erosive gastritis
   (C) UG bleeding secondary to Mallory–Weiss tears
   (D) UGI bleeding secondary to gastroesophageal varices
   (E) UGI bleeding secondary to Boerhaave syndrome

33. Proper treatment of soft tissue abscesses in an otherwise healthy individual consists of which of the following?

   (A) application of hot packs
   (B) observation and close follow-up
   (C) administration of broad spectrum antibiotics
   (D) incision, drainage, and local wound care
   (E) application of topical antibiotics

DIRECTIONS (Questions 34 through 37): For each of the items in this section, ONE or MORE of the numbered options is correct. Choose answer

    (A) if only (1), (2), and (3) are correct,

    (B) if only (1) and (3) are correct,

    (C) if only (2) and (4) are correct,

    (D) if only (4) is correct,

    (E) if all are correct.

Questions 34 through 37

34. Which of the following statements are true regarding pilonidal abscesses?

    (1) They commonly have a chronic waxing and waning course.

    (2) They arise from fistulous communications with the rectosigmoid colon.

    (3) They require wide excision for definitive treatment.

    (4) During acute episodes frank abscess formation can be readily appreciated over the presacral area.

35. Which of the following statements regarding infected sebaceous cysts are true?

    (1) They result from obstructed secretory glands.

    (2) They result from infected hair follicles within the dermis.

    (3) They require excision of the cyst capsule to prevent recurrence.

    (4) They respond well to oral antibiotics.

36. A paronychia is characterized by

    (1) an infection localized around the nail base

    (2) often tracks proximally along the tendon sheath

    (3) often accompanied by subungual abscess

    (4) an infection localized to the finger tuft

37. Proper care following venomous snake bite includes

    (1) application of a tourniquet proximal to wound

    (2) application of ice to affected part

    (3) immobilization of the affected part

    (4) performing a cruciate incision above the bite, followed by suctioning of the subcutaneous tissues

DIRECTIONS (Questions 38 through 41): Each set of items in this section consists of a list of lettered options followed by several numbered words or phrases. For each numbered word or phrase, select the ONE lettered option that is most closely associated with it. Each lettered option may be selected once, more than once, or not at all.

Questions 38 through 41

Match the following KUB findings with the most likely corresponding abdominal process.

    (A) free air beneath the diaphragm

    (B) loss of psoas shadow

    (C) dilated loops of small bowel with air fluid level

    (D) lower rib fractures

    (E) essentially normal KUB

38. Small bowel obstruction

39. Retroperitoneal abscess

40. Duodenal ulcer perforation

41. Hemoperitoneum

DIRECTIONS (Question 42): Each of the numbered items or incomplete statements in this section is followed by answers or by completions of the statement. Select the ONE lettered answer or completion that is BEST in each case.

Question 42

42. The most common cause of large bowel obstruction in the adult is which of the following?

    (A) diverticulitis

    (B) abdominal wall hernias

    (C) carcinoma

    (D) sigmoid volvulus

    (E) adhesions

DIRECTIONS (Questions 43 through 46): For each of the items in this section, ONE or MORE of the numbered options is correct. Choose answer

    (A) if only (1), (2), and (3) are correct,
    (B) if only (1) and (3) are correct,
    (C) if only (2) and (4) are correct,
    (D) if only (4) is correct,
    (E) if all are correct.

Questions 43 through 46

43. Epistaxis from the anterior inferior septal plexus of blood vessels is usually adequately controlled by

    (1) compression of the mobile portion of the nose for 5 to 10 minutes
    (2) compression of the bleeding site with a pledget impregnated with a topical vasoconstrictor
    (3) cauterization with silver nitrate
    (4) packing the anterior nasal cavity with 1/4-inch petroleum gauge

44. Clinical findings in orbital blowout fractures include

    (1) history of direct orbital injury
    (2) impaired extraocular movement
    (3) dysplasia
    (4) numbness of the upper lip

45. Factors that mediate wound infection in the acute setting include the

    (1) degree of bacterial contamination
    (2) body part involved
    (3) amount of devitalized tissue in the wound
    (4) past medical history

46. Early signs and symptoms suggestive of inhalation injury in the burn victim include

    (1) singed nasal hair
    (2) carbonaceous sputum
    (3) darkened oral or nasal mucosa
    (4) patchy infiltrates on chest radiograph

DIRECTIONS (Question 47): Each of the numbered items or incomplete statements in this section is followed by answers or by completions of the statement. Select the ONE lettered answer or completion that is BEST in each case.

Question 47

47. Burn shock is best described as

    (A) hypovolemia due to loss of plasma volume into the extravascular spaces
    (B) hypovolemia due to widespread thermal lysis of blood vessels
    (C) cardiogenic shock due to myocardial depression
    (D) hypovolemia due to bleeding from the burn wound
    (E) heart failure due to renal failure and volume overload

DIRECTIONS (Questions 48 and 49): For each of the items in this section, ONE or MORE of the numbered options is correct. Choose answer

    (A) if only (1), (2), and (3) are correct,
    (B) if only (1) and (3) are correct,
    (C) if only (2) and (4) are correct,
    (D) if only (4) is correct,
    (E) if all are correct.

Questions 48 and 49

48. Which of the following statements regarding chemical burns is true?

    (1) Burned areas should be copiously lavaged with tap water.
    (2) Dry chemical agents should be brushed from the skin prior to lavage.
    (3) All clothing should be removed from the patient as it may retain caustic agents.
    (4) Acid and alkaline burns are best treated by application of a neutralizing agent to the surface of the burn wound.

49. Which of the following statements regarding escharotomy is true?

    (1) It is used to prevent compartment syndromes in circumferential burn wounds.
    (2) It is associated with significant blood loss.
    (3) It is used to relieve respiratory distress.
    (4) It requires general anesthesia.

DIRECTIONS (Question 50): Each of the numbered items or incomplete statements in this section is followed by answers or by completions of the statement. Select the ONE lettered answer or completion that is BEST in each case.

Question 50

50. The most effective method of providing anesthesia for repair of finger lacerations, fractured phalanx, or abscess drainage is

(A) topical anesthetics
(B) bier block
(C) digital block
(D) intramuscular analysis
(E) ice packs

DIRECTIONS (Question 51): For each of the items in this section, ONE or MORE of the numbered options is correct. Choose answer

(A) if only (1), (2), and (3) are correct,
(B) if only (1) and (3) are correct,
(C) if only (2) and (4) are correct,
(D) if only (4) is correct,
(E) if all are correct.

Question 51

51. Without epinephrine, lidocaine is toxic in doses exceeding 4.5 mg/kg. Symptoms of lidocaine toxicity include

(1) apprehension
(2) disorientation
(3) nausea
(4) excitement

DIRECTIONS (Questions 52 and 53): Each of the numbered items or incomplete statements in this section is followed by answers or by completions of the statement. Select the ONE lettered answer or completion that is BEST in each case.

Questions 52 and 53

52. The most commonly fractured bone is the

(A) distal tibia
(B) clavicle
(C) distal radius
(D) rib
(E) mandible

53. The best method of restoring adequate intravascular volume in the hypovolemic patient is

(A) central venous lines, namely, subclavian or jugular lines

(B) saphenous vein cutdowns
(C) large peripheral IVs
(D) fluid boluses via the infusion part of pulmonary artery catheters
(E) administration of antidiuretic hormone

DIRECTIONS (Questions 54 and 55): For each of the items in this section, ONE or MORE of the numbered options is correct. Choose answer

(A) if only (1), (2), and (3) are correct,
(B) if only (1) and (3) are correct,
(C) if only (2) and (4) are correct,
(D) if only (4) is correct,
(E) if all are correct.

Questions 54 and 55

54. Chest tubes are indicated in a variety of emergency conditions including hemothorax, tension pneumothorax, open thoracic wounds, etc. General principles of chest tube insertion include

(1) inserting chest tube no lower than the 5th intercostal space
(2) placing the tube over the superior aspect of the rib
(3) inserting chest tube between the anterior to midaxillary line
(4) placing a gloved finger through the pleura to check for adhesed lung after puncturing the pleura

55. Signs and symptoms of airway compression include

(1) altered mental status
(2) hoarseness
(3) gurgling, snoring
(4) abnormal chest wall motion

DIRECTIONS (Questions 56 through 63): Each set of items in this section consists of a list of lettered options followed by several numbered words or phrases. For each numbered word or phrase, select the ONE lettered option that is most closely associated with it. Each lettered option may be selected once, more than once, or not at all.

Questions 56 through 59

Match the following types of fractures with their common complications.

    (A) femoral shaft fractures
    (B) femoral neck fractures
    (C) open tibial fractures
    (D) supracondylar humeral fracture
    (E) scapular fractures

56. Osteomyelitis

57. Volkmann's ischemic contracture

58. Avascular necrosis

59. Fat emboli syndrome

Questions 60 through 63

Spinal cord lesions can produce a variety of clinical manifestations. Match the following cord syndromes with their clinical characteristics.

    (A) anterior cord syndrome
    (B) Brown–Sequard syndrome
    (C) nerve root syndrome
    (D) complete cord syndrome
    (E) disc herniations

60. Flaccid paralysis below cord lesion

61. Complete paralysis, loss of pain perception with preservation of light touch, proprioception, and temperature sensation

62. Hemisection of the cord resulting in loss of proprioception, vibration, and light touch on the side of the lesion, loss of pain and temperature on the contralateral side

63. Typically occurs as a cervical injury with motor deficits that are more severe than sensory deficit

DIRECTIONS (Question 64): For each of the items in this section, ONE or MORE of the numbered options is correct. Choose answer

    (A) if only (1), (2), and (3) are correct,
    (B) if only (1) and (3) are correct,
    (C) if only (2) and (4) are correct,
    (D) if only (4) is correct,
    (E) if all are correct.

Question 64

64. Clinical signs of lumbar disc herniation include
    (1) reduction of deep tendon reflex
    (2) sciatic pain with straight leg raising
    (3) muscle weakness
    (4) low back pain made worse by valsalva

DIRECTIONS (Question 65): Each of the numbered items or incomplete statements in this section is followed by answers or by completions of the statement. Select the ONE lettered answer or completion that is BEST in each case.

Question 65

65. A 65-year-old male presents to the ER with anorexia, malaise, shaking, chills, and watery diarrhea. Chest x-ray demonstrates small alveolar infiltrates. Sputum samples are somewhat watery with Gram stains demonstrating a few polymorphonuclear leukocytes and no predominant bacterial species. Temperature is 103°F. The most likely diagnosis is

    (A) *Klebsiella pneumoniae*
    (B) Lyme disease
    (C) Legionnaire's disease
    (D) mycoplasma pneumonia
    (E) viral meningitis

DIRECTIONS (Questions 66 through 68): For each of the items in this section, ONE or MORE of the numbered options is correct. Choose answer

    (A) if only (1), (2), and (3) are correct,
    (B) if only (1) and (3) are correct,
    (C) if only (2) and (4) are correct,
    (D) if only (4) is correct,
    (E) if all are correct.

Questions 66 through 68

66. Phenytoin is often used intravenously for the treatment of status epilepticus. Side effects include
    (1) hypotension
    (2) tachycardia

(3) bradycardia

(4) tachypnea

67. Proper treatment of the adult with acute asthma includes

(1) β-adrenergic agonists (epinephrine, terbutaline)

(2) sedation

(3) supplemental O_2

(4) mucolytic agents

68. Clinical manifestation of diabetic ketoacidosis include

(1) hypotension

(2) a "fruity" odor to the patient's breath

(3) tachycardia

(4) nausea

DIRECTIONS (Question 69): Each of the numbered items or incomplete statements in this section is followed by answers or by completions of the statement. Select the ONE lettered answer or completion that is BEST in each case.

Question 69

69. The most common precipitating factor in the development of diabetic ketoacidosis is

(A) omission of daily insulin

(B) misuse of oral hyperglycemia medications

(C) pancreatitis

(D) infection

(E) inappropriately high doses of insulin

DIRECTIONS (Question 70): For each of the items in this section, ONE or MORE of the numbered options is correct. Choose answer

(A) if only (1), (2), and (3) are correct,

(B) if only (1) and (3) are correct,

(C) if only (2) and (4) are correct,

(D) if only (4) is correct,

(E) if all are correct.

Question 70

70. Symptoms of cocaine toxicity include

(1) seizures

(2) hallucinations

(3) dysrhythmias

(4) vertical nystagmus

DIRECTIONS (Questions 71 and 72): Each of the numbered items or incomplete statements in this section is followed by answers or by completions of the statement. Select the ONE lettered answer or completion that is BEST in each case.

Questions 71 and 72

71. A male multisystem trauma patient is found to have a "free-floating" prostate on rectal exam and blood is noted at the urinary meatus. The initial step in evaluating these findings is

(A) intravenous pyelogram

(B) pelvic CT scan

(C) retrograde urethrogram

(D) insertion of a Foley catheter to obtain a urine sample

(E) insertion of suprapubic catheter

72. The proper rate and sequence of ventilation and chest compression in one-person CPR is

(A) one ventilation per 15 compressions at a rate of 80 to 100 compressions per minute

(B) two ventilations per 7 compressions at a rate of 80 to 100 compressions per minute

(C) one ventilation per 7 compressions at a rate of 80 to 100 compressions per minute

(D) two ventilations per 15 compressions at a rate of 80 to 100 compressions per minute

(E) three ventilations per 15 compressions at a rate of 80 to 100 compressions per minute

DIRECTIONS (Questions 73 and 74): For each of the items in this section, ONE or MORE of the numbered options is correct. Choose answer

(A) if only (1), (2), and (3) are correct,

(B) if only (1) and (3) are correct,

(C) if only (2) and (4) are correct,

(D) if only (4) is correct,

(E) if all are correct.

Questions 73 and 74

73. True statements regarding the Heimlich maneuver include

(1) airway obstruction can be relieved by subdiaphragmatic compression forcing an artificial cough

(2) proper hand position is in the midline abdomen below the xiphoid process and above the umbilicus

(3) each thrust should be separate and distinct

(4) proper hand position is in the midline atop the xiphoid process

74. Characteristics of a ruptured Achilles tendon include

  (1) the acute onset of severe lower calf pain

  (2) loss of plantar flexion of the foot

  (3) common in males aged 40 to 50

  (4) loss of dorsiflexion

DIRECTIONS (Question 75): Each of the numbered items or incomplete statements in this section is followed by answers or by completions of the statement. Select the ONE lettered answer or completion that is BEST in each case.

Question 75

75. A young athlete comes to the Emergency Department with complaints of a dull ache in the upper third of the calf. The pain was mild at first but over the last week has increased, with pain present at rest. Initial radiography is negative. This history suggests

  (A) ruptured Achilles tendon

  (B) lower extremity fascial hernia

  (C) shin splints

  (D) Osgood–Schlatter disease

  (E) fibular stress fracture

DIRECTIONS (Question 76): For each of the items in this section, ONE or MORE of the numbered options is correct. Choose answer

  (A) if only (1), (2), and (3) are correct,

  (B) if only (1) and (3) are correct,

  (C) if only (2) and (4) are correct,

  (D) if only (4) is correct,

  (E) if all are correct.

Question 76

76. Which of the following statement(s) regarding pediatric fractures is/are correct?

  (1) The most common site of fractures in children is at the epiphyseal plate.

  (2) Metaphyseal fracture alignment is, as a rule, less important in children than in adults.

  (3) The strongest element of a child's bone is the periosteum.

  (4) Salter type II fractures, which involve a metaphysis fracture and epiphyseal plate slip, usually require open reduction and are at risk for bone growth arrest.

DIRECTIONS (Questions 77 through 80): Each set of items in this section consists of a list of lettered options followed by several numbered words or phrases. For each numbered word or phrase, select the ONE lettered option that is most closely associated with it. Each lettered option may be selected once, more than once, or not at all.

Questions 77 through 80

Match the following fractures and dislocations with their anatomical description.

  (A) comminuted

  (B) subluxation

  (C) compression

  (D) diastasis

  (E) avulsion

77. Disruption of the interosseous membrane connecting two joints

78. Caused by impaction of one bone upon another

79. Disruption of a joint with partial contact remaining between the two bones that make up the joint

80. Any fracture where there are more than two segments

Answers and Explanations

1. **(A)** The most common form of shock in the initial stages of multisystem trauma is hypovolemic shock from hemorrhage. Neurogenic shock can occur from spinal injuries that result in a loss of peripheral vascular sympathetic tone. Cardiogenic shock can occur with severe chest trauma and is characterized by shock that is unresponsive to fluid resuscitation accompanied by high central venous pressures. Septic shock occurs as a result of bacterial infection, usually late in the trauma patient's hospital course. *(Committee on Trauma, ACS, pp. 62–64)*

2. **(C)** The "rule-of-nines" is a method for calculating the BSA involvement of burn injuries. The system divides various parts of the body into multiples of nine (Fig. 3–1). Bear in mind that the full BSA value for an extremity is assigned only for circumferential injuries. For example, if only the anterior surface of the arm were involved, this would constitute 4.5% BSA. BSA for various body parts varies in adults and children. *(Moylan, p. 448)*

3. **(D)** Alcohol is involved in greater than half of all drownings, fires, falls, pedestrian injuries, assaults, and suicides. The use of alcohol is one of the major predisposing factors to an individual sustaining a traumatic injury. *(Waller, pp. 307–347)*

4. **(D)** *Hypovolemic shock* produces peripheral vasoconstriction as central organ systems are preferentially perfused. Tachycardia results from an effort to maintain adequate perfusion. A narrow pulse pressure is often noted. *(Committee on Trauma, ACS, pp. 62–64)*

5. **(C)** *Septic shock* produces a hyperdynamic cardiac output with a wide pulse pressure, near-normal blood pressure, and tachycardia. This frequently results from gram-negative septicemia secondary to exotoxin release. *(Committee on Trauma, ACS, pp. 62–64)*

6. **(B)** *Cardiogenic shock* results from cardiac failure; distention of the neck veins is a classic characteristic. Hypotension and tachycardia are com-

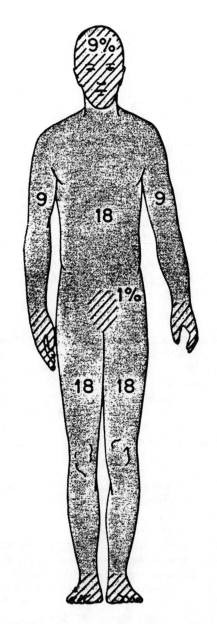

Fig. 3–1. The percentage of body area is calculated by the rule-of-nines.

mon findings. Cardiogenic shock can arise from infarctions occurring at the time of the traumatic event, cardiac contusions, and direct cardiac injury. *(Committee on Trauma, ACS, pp. 62–64)*

7. (A) *Neurogenic shock* occurs when spinal trauma causes a loss of peripheral vascular sympathetic tone, resulting in vasodilatation with hypotension and bradycardia. Isolated head injuries do not cause shock in the adult. Infants and small children can lose sufficient intravascular volume with a head injury for hypovolemic shock to occur. *(Committee on Trauma, ACS, pp. 62–64)*

8. (A) Hemothorax can result in significant blood loss and hypoxemia. Open chest wounds can cause equilibration between atmospheric and intrathoracic pressure, thus resulting in impaired gas exchange. Cardiac tamponade commonly results from penetrating chest injuries. Even small amounts of blood trapped within the pericardium can restrict cardiac filling. Pneumothorax is usually well tolerated by the healthy adult. *(Committee on Trauma, ACS, pp. 94–95)*

9. (B) Boerhaave syndrome is rupture of the esophagus, which can occur from instrumentation, trauma, or spontaneously. Pain at the site of perforation is often sudden and severe. This condition is often precipitated by forceful vomiting. Esophageal reflux associated with postural changes is most characteristic of hiatal hernia. *(Skinner, pp. 701–704)*

10. (A) Isolated head injury does not cause hypovolemic shock. For symptomatic hypovolemia to occur, an adult must lose up to 35% of total blood volume. The cranial vault cannot accommodate this amount of volume. Pelvic and femur fractures are often associated with significant bleeding that can often be unappreciated due to the expandibility of surrounding soft tissues. Hemothorax can cause significant blood volume loss. *(Committee on Trauma, ACS, p. 136)*

11. (C) Compartment syndromes develop from an increase in pressure within fascial planes, causing local ischemia. Decreased sensation from nerve compression and local pain as well as tense swelling and weakness are early signs and symptoms. Pulselessness and decreased capillary refill are late signs associated with compartment syndromes. *(Committee on Trauma, ACS, pp. 189–190)*

12. (C) Major burn victims require vigorous volume resuscitation to combat burn shock. Fiberoptic bronchoscopy is the key to definitive diagnosis of inhalation injury. Prophylactic IV antibiotics are contradicted, as this will merely encourage the development of resistant organisms. Ice to the

burn wound further damages compromised skin tissue. *(Moylan, p. 445)*

13. (E) Aortic rupture results from stresses caused by unequal rates of horizontal deceleration. These stresses are greatest at fixation points of the arch, such as the great vessels. Most aortic tears occur at the isthmus. Definitive diagnosis is achieved by aortography. The clinician must have a high index of suspicion for this entity, as the radiographic findings listed are suggestive, not diagnostic. *(Peyton and Wolfe, pp. 184–185)*

14. (D) Flail chest occurs when multiple contiguous ribs are fractured, resulting in a free-floating segment of chest wall. Normal respiratory motion of the chest is impaired. The main pathophysiological event is contusion of the lung beneath the bony injury. Sandbags do nothing to address this problem. Positioning the patient onto the affected side is impractical in the multiple-injury patient. In patients with respiratory distress secondary to flail chest and contusion of the underlying lung, intubation and positive pressure ventilation are indicated. *(Committee on Trauma, ACS, p. 15)*

15. (E) The majority of patients suffering from acute pancreatitis have associated gallstone disease or alcohol abuse. The pain of this condition has a rapid onset and quickly becomes severe, deep, and unremitting. The pain often radiates toward the back or around the costal margins *(Diethelm, pp. 736–755)*

16. (E) A felon is a localized infection of the finger tuft (Fig. 3–2). These infections have no way to spontaneously decompress as they are trapped between the septa that attach the skin to bone. As the infection spreads, it travels along the tendon sheath. The patient is forced to assume a flexed position for comfort. This tendon sheath involvement causes discomfort upon passive extension. *(Hoppenfeld, p. 88)*

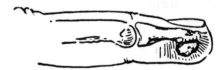

Fig. 3–2. An infection (a felon) of the finger tufts.

17. (B) A boutonniere deformity (Fig. 3–3) results from separation of the extensor tendon from its insertion on the middle phalanx. Pain is demonstrated by palpation of the middle phalanx. Avulsion of the extensor tendon from the distal phalanx (2) results in inability to extend the tip of the finger and is characteristic of a mallet finger deformity. *(Hoppenfeld, p. 87)*

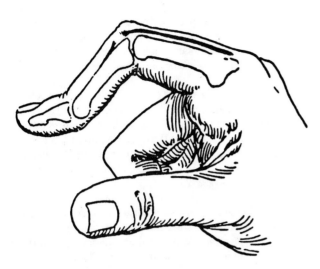

Fig. 3–3. A boutonniere deformity.

18. (C) C5 supplies sensation to the lateral aspect of the arm. C6 supplies sensation to the lateral forearm, thumb, and index finger. C7 supplies the middle finger (Fig. 3–4). C8 supplies ring and little finger, medial palm. *(Galli et al, p. 73)*

19. (D) (See Fig. 3–5). The L3 dermatome covers the anterior thigh. The L4 dermatome covers the medial aspect of the leg. The L5 dermatome covers the lateral leg and dorsum of the foot while the S1 dermatome involves the lateral aspect of the foot. *(Hoppenfeld, p. 230)*

20. (B) Diverticulitis is an inflammatory process within diverticula, most commonly affecting the sigmoid colon in older adults. Sigmoid involvement accounts for the characteristic left lower quadrant pain. Persistent vomiting is not a common feature. Flank pain would be more indicative of renal disease. *(Diethelm, pp. 736–755)*

21. (C) The abdominal radiograph of a small bowel obstruction will often reveal air fluid vessels within distended loops of small bowel, proximal to the point of obstruction. Free air denotes perforation of the stomach, or small or large bowel. Minimal gas will be found in the large bowel, or beyond the point of obstruction. *(Diethelm, pp. 736–755)*

22. (B) The sudden onset of abdominal pain and signs of peritonitis occurring in a patient with a history of dyspepsia are keys to the differential di-

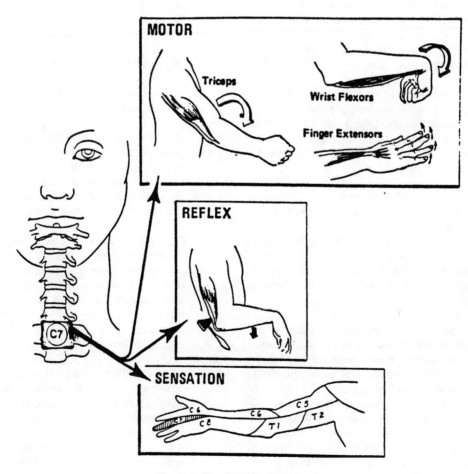

Fig. 3–4. The C7 neurologic level.

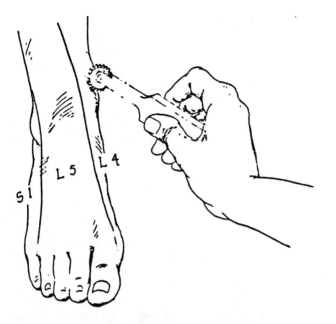

Fig. 3–5. Sensation of the foot.

agnosis. Acute cholecystitis is often accompanied by nausea and vomiting; patients are also quite restless in the early stages. Appendicitis begins with rather dull pain that gradually worsens. Patients with acute diverticulitis often give a history of episodic left lower quadrant pain. The pain occurs rather suddenly but is usually localized to the left lower quadrant. *(Diethelm, pp. 736–755)*

23. **(A)** Intra-abdominal adhesions and abdominal hernias are the most common causes of small bowel obstruction. In children, intussusception is frequently encountered. Mesenteric lymphadenopathy would not, in and of itself, cause the bowel to obstruct. *(Diethelm, pp. 736–755)*

24. **(E)** A ruptured ectopic pregnancy requires prompt diagnosis and rapid surgical intervention. Sudden sharp pain occurs at the time of rupture. Vital signs will change in relationship to the degree of intra-abdominal bleeding. Rupture commonly occurs 6 to 12 weeks following conception. Nausea and vomiting are often present. *(Diethelm, pp. 736–755)*

25. **(A)** Nasogastric suctioning acts as both a treatment and diagnostic maneuver in the patient with acute abdominal pain. Nasogastric suctioning relieves gastric dilatation and helps lessen the likelihood of aspiration. Suctioned material can be examined for occult blood. Serial abdominal exams provide a wealth of data regarding the progression or regression of an abdominal process. Many abdominal diseases cause significant third-space volume losses, necessitating careful attention to intravascular volume status. Providing a patient

with analgesia prior to the establishment of a definitive diagnosis is extremely dangerous, as it renders further serial exams and patient reports meaningless. *(Diethelm, pp. 736–755)*

26. **(C)** Murphy's sign is caused by the descent of the liver and gallbladder during deep inspiration coming into contact with the examiner's fingers during right subcostal palpation. If the gallbladder is inflamed, pain will be produced, halting the inspiratory effort. This is pathognomonic for cholecystitis. *(Diethelm, pp. 736–755)*

27. **(A)** *Perforated duodenal ulcer.* Pain begins suddenly, located in the midepigastric region. As peritonitis progresses, generalized abdominal pain is noted. This can cause a rigid or "board-like" abdomen on exam. There may be "free air" noted on plain radiographs of the upright abdomen. *(Diethelm, pp. 736–755)*

28. **(B)** *Acute cholecystitis* often begins suddenly with rapidly increasing pain. Pain is referred to the right shoulder and scapular area as subdiaphragmatic irritation triggers the phenic nerve. Nonvisualization of radionucleotide in the gallbladder during HIDA scan is diagnostic. *(Diethelm, pp. 736–755)*

29. **(D)** *Appendicitis* has rather vague and variable initial symptoms. However, over time, pain usually localizes to the right lower quadrant. Anorexia or even aversion to food is frequently seen. Fever of greater than 101°F is uncommon. *(Diethelm, pp. 736–755)*

30. **(C)** In *acute pancreatitis,* patients usually complain of the rapid onset of deep unrelenting midepigastric pain with radiation to the back. Patients may often give a history of intermittent dull epigastric pain. Alcoholism and cholelithiasis are the most frequent causes. *(Diethelm, pp. 736–755)*

31. **(E)** Acute arterial occulsion can be either intrinsic or extrinsic. Intrinsic occlusion is more common, resulting from embolic or thrombotic events. Extrinsic occlusions are usually the result of trauma. Common sources for emboli in addition to those described include valvular vegetation and thrombosis secondary to congestive heart failure and cardiomyopathies. *(Quinones–Baldrich, pp. 578–598)*

32. **(D)** Bleeding from gastroesophageal varices is a result of portal hypertension due to a relative or absolute obstruction of splenic blood flow. Cirrhosis resulting from acute alcoholic hepatitis is a common cause of portal hypertension. Cirrhosis is commonly associated with variceal bleeding, encephalopathy, and ascites. Splenomegaly is a common finding. Emergency endoscopy should be per-

formed on all patients with UGI bleeding, as other causes of bleeding may be present. *(Olthoff et al, pp. 636–668)*

33. **(D)** Definitive care of soft tissue abscesses is achieved through incision and drainage. Antibiotics in the healthy individual are unnecessary. Packing gauze should be placed into the wound to permit drainage and prevent premature closure of the skin edges. *(Warren, pp. 591–609)*

34. **(B)** Pilonidal abscesses are presacral soft tissue infections, usually chronic in nature. These do not communicate with the rectosigmoid. It is often easy to overlook the subtle appearance of these abscesses in the perisacral area. As multiple septations occur within the abscess cavity, wide excision is required for resolution. *(Warren, pp. 591–609)*

35. **(B)** Sebaceous cysts arise from occluded secretory glands within the dermis. These require excision of the cyst capsule to prevent recurrence. Oral antibiotics are of little help in resolving infected sebaceous cysts, as the abscess cavity is avascular and does not permit antibiotic penetration. *(Warren, pp. 591–609)*

36. **(B)** A paronychia is commonly seen as a "run around" or "hangnail" infection. It does not localize, as the infectious process has room to spread around the base of the nail. Infection that involves the finger tuft or track along the tendon sheath is more indicative of a felon. *(Warren, pp. 591–609)*

37. **(B)** Management of snake bite involves lessening the absorption of venom. This is best accomplished by application of a tourniquet proximal to the wound. Care is taken that arterial inflow is not compromised; the tourniquet should *not* be taken down at intervals. The limb should be immobilized. Ice should *not* be applied. Cruciate incisions heal poorly; a single, linear incision is sufficient to allow for adequate drainage. *(Rammings, pp. 249–258)*

38. **(C)** Dilated small bowel with air-fluid levels is indicative of small bowel obstruction. The dilation is seen proximal to the point of obstruction with decompressed bowel distal to the lesion. *(Diethelm, pp. 736–755)*

39. **(B)** The psoas muscle is a posterior retroperitoneal structure. This paired set of muscles is usually easily discerned on plain abdominal radiographs. Loss of this shadow may be indicative of a mass effect obscuring the psoas outline. *(Diethelm, pp. 736–755)*

40. **(A)** Free intra-abdominal air is indicative of perforation of a hollow viscus, that is, the small or large bowel or stomach. It is best seen in an upright film where air will accumulate under the diaphragm. *(Diethelm, pp. 736–755)*

41. **(D)** Hemoperitoneum is a difficult diagnosis to make based on a plain x-ray alone. Associated injuries such as lower rib fractures indicate that the patient's abdomen has been subjected to great force. Such findings would lead the clinician to strongly suspect liver or spleen injuries. *(Diethelm, pp. 736–755)*

42. **(C)** Carcinoma of the colon is the most common cause of large bowel obstruction in the adult. Diverticulitis can also cause large bowel obstruction, and patients often give a history of intermittent left lower quadrant pain. Sigmoid volvulus is a less common cause of large bowel obstruction. It is seen most often in elderly persons with poor bowel habits and chronic constipation. *(Diethelm, pp. 736–755)*

43. **(E)** All the methods are acceptable and will control the majority of cases with anterior nasoseptal bleeding. Posterior nasal bleeding, as seen in patients with hypertension or atherosclerosis, is much more difficult to control and may require extensive packing and the use of occlusive balloons. These are managed in step-wise fashion from compression to cauterization and, finally, packing. *(Snow, pp. 1187–1209)*

44. **(E)** Orbital blowout fractures occur when external forces increase intraorbital pressure, fracturing the orbital floor and entrapping extraocular musculature. Inspection of the orbital rim may reveal a stepoff. Numbness of the upper lip suggests compression of the infraorbital nerve. Diplopia is a common finding. Orbital x-rays will often show clouding of the maxillary sinus. *(Georgiade and Manstein, pp. 14.1–14.16)*

45. **(E)** The blood supply and ability of certain areas of the body to resist bacteria will greatly affect the propensity for wound infection. Past medical history that is significant for immunosuppressive disorders will also affect wound outcome. Foreign bodies and devitalized tissue within the wound will predispose the development of infection. *(Lammers, pp. 515–564)*

46. **(A)** Singed nasal hair, carbonaceous sputum, darkened oral or nasal mucous membranes, and history of burns in an enclosed space are highly suggestive for the presence of an inhalation injury. Bronchoscopy is used for definitive diagnosis. Even with the most severe inhalation injury, early chest x-rays appear normal. *(Herndon et al, p. 157)*

47. **(A)** Burn shock results from increased capillary permeability that permits the loss of plasma volume and macromolecules from the intravascular

to the extravascular spaces. This transmigration of fluid leads to extensive edema formation and hypovolemia. Formulas for aggressive fluid resuscitation are designed to combat this phenomenon. All burn patients with injuries to greater than 20% BSA are at risk for significant plasma volume loss. (*Demling, p. 189*)

48. **(A)** Prolonged lavage with tap water is the most effective treatment of liquid chemical burns. Application of neutralizing agents produces an exothermic reaction, thus worsening tissue damage. Clothing that may retain noxious agents should be removed. (*Luteman and Curreri, p. 233*)

49. **(B)** Eschar is the thick, nonelastic material that forms on the surface of a full-thickness burn wound. In patients with circumferential chest or extremity burns, compartment pressures can rise beneath the eschar. This process compromises breathing and/or arterial inflow. The treatment is to make a longitudinal incision through the eschar to relieve compartment pressures. This procedure is accompanied by little blood loss and is relatively painless. (*Monafo and Freedman, pp. 247–248*)

50. **(C)** Digital blocks are accomplished by the injection of local anesthesia (without epinephrine) into nerves on the lateral and medial aspects of the digit. Bier block is the IV introduction of anesthesia into the limb that is occluded by an inflated BP cuff. This method is useful in soft tissue procedures on the hand and forearm. Topical anesthetics and intramuscular analgesia are ineffective in providing proper patient comfort. (*Simmon and Brenner, p. 108*)

51. **(E)** All these symptoms, which can be easily overlooked, can be prodromes to the onset of convulsions due to lidocaine toxicity. The severity of toxic reactions is dependent on the rapidity of drug absorption and the susceptibility of the patient. The use of lidocaine with epinephrine will allow for less rapid absorption and the use of higher doses. (*Simmon and Brenner, p. 87*)

52. **(B)** The most commonly fractured bone is the clavicle. Overall clavicular fractures account for 5% of all fractures in all age groups. These fractures are usually treated with a figure-of-eight clavicular wrap. (*Simmon and Brenner, p. 218*)

53. **(C)** Flow through a catheter is adversely affected by its length. Long indwelling central venous lines such as subclavian, jugular, or pulmonary artery catheters do not have the flow characteristics necessary for volume resuscitation. These types of lines are time-consuming to place and carry with them significant morbidity. The proper method of volume replacement is via two or more short-length, large-bore peripheral IVs. (*Committee on Trauma, ACS, p. 16*)

54. **(E)** Chest tubes should be placed no lower than the 5th intercostal space to avoid injury to the diaphragm. Placement of the tube medial to the anterior axillary line increases the risk of lacerating the internal mammary vessels. The tube should be placed over the rib to avoid the intercostal neurovascular bundle. (*Committee on Trauma, ACS, p. 108*)

55. **(E)** It is important to recognize the somewhat subtle signs that may indicate airway obstruction. Agitation can often be attributed to intoxication when in actuality it heralds impending respiratory obstruction. A good test of airway patency is the patient's ability to converse with the examiner. A conversant patient indicates that the airway is patent and brain perfusion is adequate. (*Committee on Trauma, ACS, p. 33*)

56. **(C)** *Osteomyelitis* is infection of the bone, which often becomes chronic. Destruction of bone is often the consequence of this condition. This is most often the result of an open or "compound" fracture. This complication can be prevented by meticulous wound care designed to remove all foreign and devitalized material. (*Adams, p. 54*)

57. **(D)** Volkmann's ischemic contracture results from brachial artery injury in the setting of supracondylar humeral fracture. Ischemic damage to the flexor muscles of the forearm result in a flexion contraction of the hand and wrist. Other injuries that result in compartment syndromes may yield the same ischemic injury. (*Adams, p. 143*)

58. **(B)** Avascular necrosis is bony necrosis secondary to insufficient blood supply. It usually occurs in a fracture near the articular surface of a bone, especially if the terminal fragment is devoid of soft tissue attachments. This may occur following fracture of the femoral neck. Other common sites include navicular, scaphoid, and talar fractures. (*Adams, p. 60*)

59. **(A)** Fat emboli syndrome is an uncommon but serious complication of long bone fractures, mainly at the femur or tibia. It usually occurs 2 days following injury and is characterized by alterations in mental status and/or respiratory insufficiency. Patients will often demonstrate a petechial rash. The etiology remains unclear; however, it is postulated that fat globules or released fatty acids play a role. (*Adams, p. 54*)

60. **(D)** Complete cord syndrome is characterized by complete flaccid paralysis and loss of all sensation below the level of injury. Deep tendon reflexes are absent. Injuries to the C1–C4 level result in respi-

ratory arrest due to the respiratory muscle paralysis. *(Galli et al, pp. 12–19)*

61. **(A)** Anterior cord syndromes occur most commonly in hyperflexion injuries of the cervical spine. Clinically, there is immediate, complete paralysis and loss of sensation below the lesion. Light touch, proprioception, and vibratory sense are spared, as they are controlled through the intact dorsal columns. These patients have a much better prognosis for recovery then do those with complete cord lesions. *(Galli et al, pp. 12–19)*

62. **(B)** Brown–Sequard syndrome results from functional or anatomic hemisection of the spinal cord. The consequence is loss of proprioception, vibration, and light touch on the ipsilateral side of the injury and loss of pain and proprioception on the contralateral side. *(Galli et al, pp. 12–19)*

63. **(C)** Nerve root syndrome commonly occurs in the cervical region and results from isolated nerve root injuries. Unilateral facet dislocations and disc herniations are the most common causes. *(Galli et al, pp. 12–19)*

64. **(E)** Lumbar disc herniation results from herniation of the central nucleus pulposus causing nerve root compression with sciatica and lower extremity symptoms. The pain of lumbar disc herniation is worsened by coughing, sneezing, and the valsalva maneuver. It is associated with flattening of the lumbar curve and muscle spasm. Nerve root compression, most commonly L4–L5 or L5–S1, often results in muscle weakness and neurologic deficits. *(Galli et al, p. 256)*

65. **(C)** Legionnaire's disease is suggested by the presence of a constellation of symptoms including fever, respiratory symptoms, toxemia, constitutional symptoms, diarrhea, and a typically nonproductive cough.

    Mycoplasma pneumonia accounts for 25% of all community-acquired pneumonia. Symptoms include upper and lower respiratory tract complaints, fever, cough, and headaches. The treatment of choice is erythromycin.

    Klebsiella pneumoniae is seen most commonly in immunosuppressed individuals as a necrotizing lobar pneumonia. The entity is frequently associated with lung abscess and empyema. *Klebsiella* often has a rapid onset associated with pleuritic chest pain, shortness of breath, and rigors.

    Lyme disease is a tick-borne illness characterized by malaise, fatigue, fever, myalgia, lymphadenopathy, and malar rash. *(Zwanger, p. 257; Pavikrishnan, p. 253)*

66. **(B)** Phenytoin should always be given intravenously when intervening in acute neurologic

emergencies. Intramuscular injection leads to uncertain absorption and pain. Phenytoin slows conduction through the AV node leading to bradycardia and hypotension. All patients receiving IV phenytoin should be closely followed by EKG monitoring. *(Sacks, p. 567)*

67. **(B)** Beta-adrenergic agonists are the preferred medications for the treatment of asthmatics. Theophylline should be withheld for the more refractory case. Mucolytic agents are contraindicated as they may further bronchospasm. Sedation is contraindicated as it may lead to further respiratory compromise. *(Sherman, p. 278)*

68. **(E)** The osmotic diuresis and loss of intracellular water seen in diabetic ketoacidosis produces total body fluid depletion resulting in hypotension and reflex tachycardia. Ketone bodies are oxidized to acetone, causing the characteristic sweet or fruity odor to the breath. Nausea, vomiting, and abdominal pain are common occurrences, due in part to gastric dilatation and paralytic ileus. *(Ragland, pp. 490–491)*

69. **(D)** The most common precipitating factor in diabetic ketoacidosis is infection. All ketoacidotic patients must be thoroughly screened for the presence of an occult infectious process. Stressors, such as infection, cause the production of counterregulatory hormones such as glucagon, catecholamines, and cortisol. Stress hormone production, and their resultant anti-insulin effect, in conjunction with a relatively insufficient supply of insulin, set the stage for the development of ketoacidosis. *(Ragland, pp. 490–491)*

70. **(E)** Neurologic findings in cocaine toxicity range from apprehension and restlessness to twitching and generalized seizures, coma, and areflexia. Cardiac toxicity can lead to a wide range of dysrhythmias. It has been postulated that coronary artery vasospasm causes the myocardial infarctions seen in cocaine abusers. *(Gerkin, p. 121)*

71. **(C)** A "high-riding" or "free-floating" prostate on rectal exam, or blood at the urinary meatus is indicative of urethral injury. IVPs or pelvic CT scans are less then optimal imaging modalities to assess this entity. Insertion of a Foley catheter is contraindicated, as a partial urethral tear may be completed. Retrograde urethrograms should be performed to assess the integrity of the urethra prior to catheterization. *(Ahlering, p. 663)*

72. **(D)** The proper sequence of one-person CPR as proposed by the American Heart Association is 15 compressions alternating with 2 ventilations. Two-person CPR is performed using five compressions to one ventilation. *(Albarran-Sotelo et al, p. 47)*

73. (A) The Heimlich maneuver is performed with the rescuer either kneeling astride the recumbent victim or standing behind the upright victim. Sharp, abdominal thrusts designed to quickly raise intra-abdominal pressures are applied. Care is taken to maintain hand placement below the xiphoid process to lessen the risk of rib fracture. *(Albarran-Sotelo et al, p. 58)*

74. (A) The most common site of Achilles tendon rupture is approximately 2 inches above the point of calcaneal attachment. This injury is common among sedentary men aged 40 to 50 years, but is also seen in athletes. Patients will often complain of agonizing lower calf pain and demonstrate an inability to plantar flex the foot. Partial tears are often misdiagnosed as some plantar flexion is preserved. *(Simon, p. 407)*

75. (E) The fibula is the most common site of stress fractures. It is commonly seen in young athletes, military recruits, and dancers. Early radiographs are often negative, but in 10 to 14 days a fine transverse line will often be seen, tracing the fracture site. The entity is commonly misdiagnosed as shin splints, which are more often characterized by pain on the anteriomedial surface of the distal leg. Fascial hernias are easily diagnosed by the presence of a reducible mass when the muscle is relaxed. Osgood–Schlatter disease is a painful condition of the tibial tuberosity seen in adolescents. *(Simon, p. 392)*

76. (A) Children's bones are more porous than adults. The periosteum is the strongest element, with the epiphyseal plate the weakest. The epiphysis is the "growth plate" of young bones. Salter classification III and IV fractures have a high risk of growth arrest. As a general rule metaphyseal fractures in children require less alignment than those in adults (Fig. 3–6). *(Simon, p. 19)*

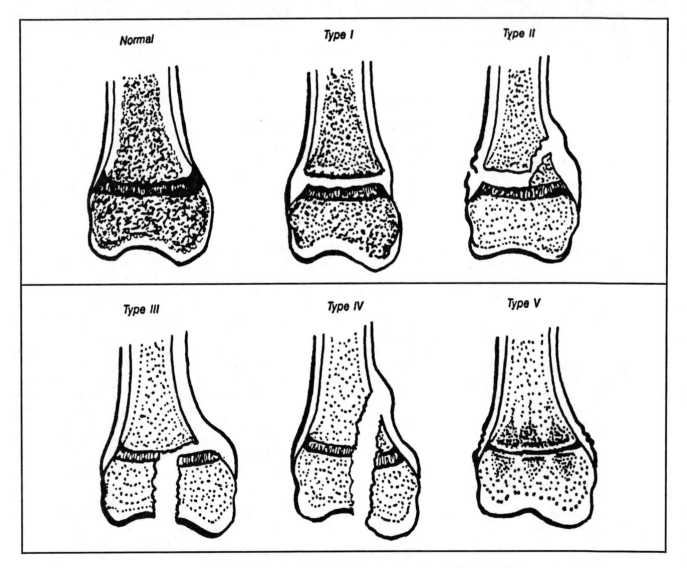

Fig. 3–6. The Salter–Harris classification system used in epiphyseal injuries.

77. (D) Diastasis is a disruption of the interosseus membrane of a joint. This presents as a joint injury with edema and tenderness, as in a superior ankle dislocation. *(Simon, pp. 4–5,402)*

78. (C) Compression fractures occur as a result of axial loading of one bone upon another. Most commonly seen in the spinal vertebrae of the elderly with complaints of pain and occasionally radicular nerve pain. *(Simon, pp. 4–5)*

79. (B) Subluxation involves a partial dislocation of a joint in that there is continued contact of the bones. The clinical presentation is similar to a dislocation. *(Simon, pp. 4–5)*

80. (A) Comminuted fracture by definition implies more than two bone fragments. Variation of this is the butterfly fracture where a v-shaped fragment is seen, or a segmented fracture where there are two transverse fractures with a piece or segment of bone between. *(Simon, pp. 2–3)*

REFERENCES

Adams JC. Complications of fractures. In Adams JC. *Outline of Fractures*. Churchill Livingston; Edinburgh: 1992.

Ahlering T, Weintraub P, Weinburg A, Skinner D. Urologic surgery and trauma. In Civetta E (ed). *Critical Care*. London: JB Lippincott; 1992.

Albarran-Sotelo R, Flint L, Kelly K, eds. *Instructor's Manual for Basic Life Support*. Washington, D.C.: American Heart Association; 1987.

Committee on Trauma. *Advanced Trauma Life Support Program of the American College of Surgeons*. Chicago, IL: ACS; 1989.

Demling R. Fluid resuscitation. In Bostwick JA (ed). *The Art and Science of Burn Care*. Rockville, MD: Aspen Publishers; 1987.

Diethelm AG, Stanley RJ. The acute abdomen. In Sabiston DS (ed). *Textbook in Surgery*. Philadelphia, PA: WB Saunders; 1991: 736–755.

Galli RL, Spraite DW, Simon RR. *Emergency Orthopedics of the Spine*. Norwalk, CT: Appleton & Lange; 1989.

Georgiade DG, Manstein ME. Maxillofacial trauma. In Moylan JA (ed). *Trauma Surgery*. Philadelphia, PA: JB Lippincott; 1992: 14.1–14.16.

Gerkin RD. Cocaine. In Tintinalli JE (ed). *Emergency Medicine: A Comprehensive Study Guide*. New York: McGraw-Hill; 1992.

Herndon DJ, Thompson PB, Brown M, Traber DL. Diagnosis, pathophysiology and treatment of inhalation injury. In Boswick JA (ed). *The Art and Science of Burn Care*. Rockville, MD: Aspen Publishers; 1987.

Hoppenfeld S. *Physical Examination of the Spine and Extremities*. New York: Appleton-Century-Crofts; 1976.

Lammers RL. Principles of wound management. In Roberts JR, Hedges JR (eds). *Clinical Procedures in Emergency Medicine*. Philadelphia, PA: WB Saunders; 1991: 515–564.

Luteman A, Curreri P. Chemical burn injury. In Boswick JA (ed). *The Art and Science of Burn Care*. Rockville, MD: Aspen Publishers; 1987.

Monafo WW, Freedman BM. Electrical and lightning injury. In Boswick JA (ed). *The Art and Science of Burn Care*. Rockville, MD: Aspen Publishers; 1987.

Moylan JA. Burn injury. In Moylan JA (ed). *Trauma Surgery*. Philadelphia, PA: JB Lippincott; 1992: 17.2–17.16.

Olthoff KM, Brown SL, Busuttil RW. Portal hypertension. In Moore W (ed). *Vascular Surgery: A Comprehensive Review*. New York: Grune & Stratton; 1991: 636–668.

Pavikrishnan KP. Viral and mycoplasma pneumonias in adults. In Crome JE, Ruiz RL (eds). *Emergency Medicine, A Comprehensive Study Guide*. New York: McGraw-Hill; 1988.

Peyton RB, Wolfe WG. Traumatic thoracic aneurysm. In Moylan JA (ed). *Trauma Surgery*. Philadelphia, PA: JB Lippincott; 1988.

Quinones-Baldrich, WJ. Acute arterial occlusions. In Moore W (ed). *Vascular Surgery: A Comprehensive Review*. New York: Grune & Stratton; 1991: 578–598.

Ragland G. Diabetic ketoacidosis in adults. In Krome JE, Ruiz RL (eds). *Emergency Medicine. A Comprehensive Study Guide*. New York: McGraw-Hill; 1988.

Rammings KP. Bites and stings. In Sabiston DC (ed). *Textbook of Surgery*. Philadelphia, PA: WB Saunders, 1991: 249–258.

Sacks C. Seizures and status epilepticus in adults. In Krome JE, Ruiz RL (eds). *Emergency Medicine. A Comprehensive Study Guide*. New York: McGraw-Hill; 1988.

Sherman S. Acute asthma in adults. In Krome JE, Ruiz RL (eds). *Emergency Medicine. A Comprehensive Study Guide*. New York: McGraw-Hill; 1988.

Simmon RR, Brenner BE. Anesthesia and regional blocks. In Simmon RR, Brenner BE (eds). *Emergency Procedures and Techniques*. Baltimore, MD: Williams & Wilkins; 1987.

Simmon RR, Brenner BE. Orthopedic procedures. In Simmon RR, Brenner BE (eds). *Emergency Procedures and Techniques*. Baltimore, MD: Williams & Wilkins; 1987.

Simon R, Koenigknecht SJ. *Emergency Orthopedics, The Extremities*. Norwalk, CT: Appleton & Lange; 1987.

Skinner DB. Perforation of the esophagus: Spontaneous (Boerhaave syndrome), traumatic and following esophagoscopy. In Sabiston DC (ed). *Textbook of Surgery*. Philadelphia, PA: WB Saunders; 1991: 701–704

Snow JB. Surgical disorders of the ears, nose, paranasal sinuses, pharynx, and larynx. In Sabiston DC (ed).

Textbook of Surgery. Philadelphia, PA: WB Saunders; 1991: 1187–1209.

Urbaniak JR. Replantation of amputated digits and hands. In Sabiston DC (ed). *Textbook of Surgery.* Philadelphia, PA: WB Saunders; 1991: 1377–1382.

Waller JA. Alcohol and unintentional injury. In Kissin B, Begleiter H (eds). *The Biology of Alcoholism,* vol. 4. New York: Plenum; 1976.

Warren T. Incision and drainage of cutaneous abscesses and soft tissue infections. In Roberts JR (ed). *Clinical Procedures in Emergency Medicine.* Philadelphia, PA: WB Saunders; 1991: 591–609.

Zwanger M. Legionnaire's disease. In Krome JE, Ruiz RL (eds). *Emergency Medicine. A Comprehensive Study Guide.* New York: McGraw-Hill; 1988.

Subspecialty List: Emergency Medicine

QUESTION NUMBER AND SUBSPECIALTY

1. Shock
2. Burns
3. Trauma
4. Hypovolemic shock
5. Septic shock
6. Cardiogenic shock
7. Neurogenic shock
8. Chest trauma
9. Boerhaave syndrome
10. Shock
11. Compartment syndromes
12. Burn care
13. Chest trauma
14. Chest trauma
15. Abdominal pain
16. Infections
17. Orthopedics
18. Neurology
19. Neurology
20. Abdominal pain
21. Radiographic findings
22. Abdominal pain
22. Abdominal pain
23. Abdominal pain
24. Abdominal pain
25. Abdominal pain
26. Abdominal pain
27. Abdominal pain
28. Abdominal pain
29. Abdominal pain
30. Abdominal pain
31. Arterial occlusive disease
32. Upper GI bleeding
33. Soft tissue infections
34. Soft tissue infections
35. Soft tissue infections
36. Soft tissue infections
37. Wound care
38. Radiographic findings
39. Radiographic findings
40. Radiographic findings
41. Radiographic findings
42. Bowel obstruction
43. Epistaxis
44. Facial trauma
45. Wound care
46. Inhalation injury
47. Burn care
48. Burn care
49. Burn care
50. Regional anesthesia
51. Regional anesthesia
52. Orthopedics
53. Trauma management
54. Trauma management
55. Trauma management
56. Orthopedics
57. Orthopedics
58. Orthopedics
59. Orthopedics
60. Neurology
61. Neurology
62. Neurology
63. Neurology
64. Neurology
65. Infectious disease
66. Neurology
67. Pulmonary
68. Diabetic management
69. Diabetic management
70. Toxicology
71. Trauma management
72. CPR
73. CPR
74. Orthopedics
75. Orthopedics
76. Orthopedics
77. Orthopedics
78. Orthopedics
79. Orthopedics
80. Orthopedics

CHAPTER 4

Internal Medicine: Acquired Immunodeficiency Syndrome
Questions

DIRECTIONS (Questions 1 through 8): Each set of items in this section consists of a list of lettered options followed by several numbered words or phrases. For each numbered word or phrase, select the ONE lettered option that is most closely associated with it. Each lettered option may be selected once, more than once, or not at all.

Questions 1 through 4

For each disease process, select the drug of choice with which it is treated.

    (A) amphotericin B
    (B) ganciclovir
    (C) trimethoprim-sulfamethoxazole (Bactrim/Septra)
    (D) acyclovir
    (E) pyrimethamine and sulfadiazine

1. *Pneumocystis carinii* pneumonia (PCP) C

2. Toxoplasmic encephalitis

3. Cryptococcal meningitis A

4. Cytomegalovirus (CMV) chorioretinitis B

Questions 5 through 8

    (A) cryptococcal meningitis
    (B) toxoplasmic encephalitis
    (C) both
    (D) neither

5. Computerized tomography (CT) of the head is usually normal A

6. Presenting symptoms of headache, fever, and altered sensorium C

7. Cerebrospinal fluid (CSF) may show normal protein and glucose as well as absence of pleocytosis A

8. Chronic suppressive therapy is required to prevent recurrences

DIRECTIONS (Questions 9 through 13): Each of the numbered items or incomplete statements in this section is followed by answers or by completions of the statement. Select the ONE lettered answer or completion that is BEST in each case.

Questions 9 through 13

9. All the following statements about patterns of HIV infection in the United States are true EXCEPT

    (A) the cumulative incidence of AIDS cases is disproportionately higher in African-Americans and Hispanics than in whites
    (B) the percentage of reported AIDS cases in New York and San Francisco compared to the total United States population has gradually decreased over time
    (C) the percentage of reported AIDS cases in women has gradually decreased over time
    (D) the highest risk of HIV infection in pediatric patients occurs in children born to women who themselves are at risk of HIV infection

10. Which one of the following tests is used initially to evaluate the presence of HIV infection in a patient?

    (A) HIV antibody status by ELISA
    (B) HIV serum p24 antigen status
    (C) HIV antibody status by western blot
    (D) T-lymphocyte subset studies
    (E) in vitro culture of HIV from patient's blood

11. HIV-infected patients are at increased risk for all the following CNS diseases EXCEPT

   (A) progressive multifocal leukoencephalopathy (PML)
   (B) primary CNS lymphoma
   (C) cryptococcoma
   (D) bacterial meningitis
   (E) TB meningitis

12. Which one of the following statements is true about pediatric HIV infection?

   (A) A positive HIV antibody status in a neonate reflects the presence of HIV infection.
   (B) Symptoms of HIV infection are often seen in the first 6 weeks of life.
   (C) Chronic lymphocytic infiltrative pneumonia (LIP) and chronic parotid enlargement are commonly seen in children.
   (D) Kaposi's sarcoma is frequently diagnosed in children but is difficult to treat.
   (E) Neurologic involvement, principally progressive encephalopathy, has been described in 10% to 20% of pediatric AIDS cases.

13. Which of the following would be LEAST appropriate in the evaluation of an HIV-infected patient with profuse diarrhea?

   (A) routine stool evaluations
   (B) sigmoidoscopy/colonoscopy with biopsy
   (C) stool for acid-fast bacteria (AFB)
   (D) barium enema
   (E) blood cultures for CMV (cytomegalovirus) and MAC (mycobacterium avium complex)

DIRECTIONS (Questions 14 through 25): For each of the items in this section, ONE or MORE of the numbered options is correct. Choose answer

   (A) if only (1), (2), and (3) are correct,
   (B) if only (1) and (3) are correct,
   (C) if only (2) and (4) are correct,
   (D) if only (4) is correct,
   (E) if all are correct.

Questions 14 through 25

14. Which of the following do didanosine (ddI) and zalcitabine (ddC) have in common?

   (1) Both are nucleoside analog reverse transcriptase inhibitors.
   (2) Peripheral neuropathy is a common adverse effect.

   (3) Both are alternative antiretroviral agents to zidovudine in the event of development of intolerance or disease progression.
   (4) Dosing for both medications is twice a day.

15. Retrosternal pain or burning on swallowing in an HIV infected patient may be due to

   (1) candidiasis
   (2) cytomegalovirus (CMV)
   (3) herpes simplex virus (HSV)
   (4) oral hairy leukoplakia

16. Administration of zidovudine in HIV-infected patients is often associated with

   (1) anemia and neutropenia
   (2) myopathy
   (3) headache and nausea
   (4) peripheral neuropathy

17. The incidence of new HIV infection in groups at recognized risk between 1985 and the present has shown

   (1) a decline in the percent of men who have sex with men
   (2) an increase in the percent of hemophiliacs
   (3) an increase in the percent of IV-drug users
   (4) elimination of the category of persons with no known risk factor

18. Which of the following clinical conditions were included in the expanded CDCP surveillance case definition effective January 1, 1993?

   (1) pulmonary tuberculosis (TB)
   (2) recurrent pneumonia
   (3) invasive cervical cancer
   (4) HIV-infected people with CD4+ T-lymphocyte count of less than 200 cells/mm or a CD4+ percentage of less than 14.

19. *Mycobacterium avium* complex (MAC)

   (1) often infects the bone marrow causing pancytopenia
   (2) can be present in any organ in the body
   (3) often produces symptoms of chronic fever, diaphoresis, and weight loss
   (4) is a multiresistant organism whose therapy typically involves a multidrug regimen

20. Which of the following medications are acceptable treatment for prophylaxis of *Pneumocystis carinii* pneumonia (PCP)?

   (1) trimethoprim-sulfamethoxazole (TMP-SMX)
   (2) aerosolized pentamidine

(3) Dapsone

(4) ciprofloxacin

21. Neurologic syndromes seen in HIV-infected patients include which of the following disorders?

    (1) aseptic meningitis

    (2) myelopathy

    (3) dementia

    (4) peripheral neuropathy

22. The risk of HIV transmission

    (1) for homosexual men increases when practicing receptive anal intercourse

    (2) for blood recipients decreased dramatically in 1985 when routine screening of blood for HIV antibodies became available

    (3) by sexual contact increases in the presence of genital ulcers

    (4) for blood recipients decreases if blood is donated by a family member

23. The risk of HIV transmission to health-care workers

    (1) is greatly reduced when universal precautions are implemented

    (2) is lower than the risk of hepatitis B virus (HBV) transmission

    (3) is approximately 0.33% following a single needlestick exposure to blood from an HIV-infected patient

    (4) has been documented from exposure to body fluids other than blood, such as feces, sputum, urine, or vomitus

24. Which of the following statements regarding herpes virus infections in AIDS patients are true?

    (1) Isolation of CMV from the lung is uncommon and warrants initiation of antiviral treatment.

    (2) Prompt administration of antiviral treatment for active HSV infection reduces morbidity and risk of serious complications.

    (3) In treatment of mucocutaneous HSV, topical acyclovir reduces the formation of new lesions as well as the risk of dissemination.

    (4) Disseminated varicella zoster virus (VZV) infection warrants hospitalization and treatment with high-dose IV acyclovir.

25. AIDS-associated Kaposi's sarcoma

    (1) may present in the lung as nodular infiltrates

    (2) is seen primarily in IV-drug users

    (3) may respond to alpha-interferon administration

    (4) when treated with radiotherapy is associated with a high-response rate and an improved prognosis

Answers and Explanations

1. **(C)** Trimethoprim/sulfamethoxazole is the drug of choice in treating *P. carinii* pneumonia (PCP); dosing is based on the trimethoprim component at 15 to 20 mg/kg/day intravenously in divided doses for 21 days. Trimethoprim/sulfamethoxazole is associated with a high frequency of adverse reactions that include rash, leukopenia, thrombocytopenia, nausea, vomiting, or nephritis. If patients have a history of intolerance to sulfonamides or trimethoprim, pentamidine is the second-line drug for PCP treatment at a once daily dose of 4 mg/kg intravenously. Adverse effects of pentamidine include renal dysfunction (elevation of blood urea nitrogen and serum creatinine); hypoglycemia, which may be followed by hyperglycemia, orthostatic hypotension; leukopenia; thrombocytopenia; nausea; and metallic taste. Most of these side effects are reversible after the medication is discontinued; however, the hyperglycemia may be permanent and necessitate insulin. In severe cases of PCP where the patient is acutely ill with a PO_2 < 70 mm Hg, early treatment with prednisone has been demonstrated to decrease respiratory failure and death. Prednisone should be started orally at a dose of 40 mg twice a day for 5 days, then 40 mg daily for 5 days, then 20 mg daily for the remainder of the anti-PCP treatment. In mild cases of PCP where the patient is not acutely ill and is able to take oral medications, TMP/SMX can be given orally or Dapsone 100 mg daily and TMP 15-20 mg/kg in divided doses, both orally, can be given to sulfonamide-allergic patients. Since Dapsone may cause hemolytic anemia, particularly in G6PD-deficient patients, this must be ruled out prior to its usage. *(Masur and Kovacs, pp. 419–424; Bozzette, Sattler, Chiu et al, pp. 1451–1457)*

2. **(E)** Standard treatment of an acute episode of toxoplasmic encephalitis is the combination of pyrimethamine at 200 mg loading dose, then 50 to 100 mg daily orally and sulfadiazine at 4 to 6 g daily in divided doses orally. This combination blocks folic acid metabolism of the proliferative form of *Toxoplasma gondii* and is synergistic against the organism. Corticosteroids are often indicated to manage increased intracranial pressure from mass effect. Associated with this treatment is a high frequency of toxic side effects, most commonly bone marrow suppression and rash. Folinic acid should be added to the therapy at doses of 10 to 30 mg daily in an effort to prevent bone marrow suppression. In the advent of severe toxicity, sulfadiazine should be discontinued, as it is more often responsible for the toxicity. Clindamycin has been recognized to be an effective drug for the treatment of toxoplasmosis and may be used as a second-line agent with pyrimethamine. The recommended dosage is 2400 to 4800 mg/d intravenously in divided doses depending on the patient's clinical status and tolerance to the medication. The toxic effects include nausea, vomiting, diarrhea, neutropenia, rash, and pseudomembranous colitis. Recently, three new macrolide/azolide antibiotics—clarithromycin, azithromycin, and roxithromycin—have been found to be effective alternative treatments for toxoplasmosis. *(Luft and Remington, pp. 211–222)*

3. **(A)** Standard treatment for cryptococcal meningitis is amphotericin B at 0.5 to 0.8 mg/kg per day IV. The side effects of amphotericin B commonly include high fever, rigors, nausea, vomiting, hypotension, and renal dysfunction. Cerebrospinal fluid (CSF) cultures should become sterile during initial therapy, and CSF cryptococcal antigen titers usually fall with therapy. Flucytosine, another antifungal agent may prove useful when added to amphotericin B in patients with severe cryptococcal disease at a dose of 150 mg/kg daily in divided doses. Fluconazole, an oral triazole antifungal agent has been shown to be an effective first-line treatment for mild to moderate cryptococcal disease, ie, patients with normal mental status and a CSF cryptococcal antigen titer of less than 1:1024, and a CSF white cell count above 20 cells/mm. The treatment dose should be 400 mg daily for 6 to 10 weeks. There are authorities who would continue to treat mild to moderate disease with amphotericin B as described above. *(Grant and Armstrong, pp. 459–462; Saag, Powderly, Cloud et al, pp. 83–94)*

4. **(B)** Ganciclovir is the recommended treatment of CMV chorioretinitis. Initial treatment consists of 5 mg/kg, intravenously, bid for 14 to 21 days with duration of "induction therapy" dependent on degree of response determined by follow-up ophthalmologic exams. Maintenance treatment 5 to 7 days a week at 6 mg/kg once daily is required in an effort to prevent recurrence of lesions, as it has been shown that with cessation of therapy, retinal lesions usually recur. The toxicity of ganciclovir includes bone marrow suppression (particularly neutropenia and thrombocytopenia), rash, headache, confusion, nausea, and vomiting, and may be the limiting factor in determining dose and duration of maintenance treatment. Because both ganciclovir and zidovudine (AZT) are myelosuppressive, patients treated with ganciclovir may not be able to tolerate the full recommended dose of zidovudine. Foscarnet, another antiviral agent, is an alternate drug used in the treatment of CMV chorioretinitis. The induction dose is 60 mg/kg intravenously every 8 hours for 14 to 21 days, with a maintenance dose of 90 to 120 mg/kg IV daily. The primary toxicity of foscarnet is renal with one third of patients experiencing decrease in renal function requiring adjustment in dose or interruption of therapy. However, full doses of zidovudine can be used with foscarnet. *(Drew, pp. 495–501; Studies of Ocular Complications of AIDS Research Group, in Collaboration with the AIDS Clinical Trials Group, pp. 213–220)*

5. **(A)** CT of the head is usually normal in cryptococcal meningitis, although in rare circumstances, a ring-enhancing lesion can be demonstrated if a cyptococcoma is present. Diagnosis of cryptococcal meningitis requires isolation of *Cryptococcus neoformans* from CSF. A head CT has become indispensable for diagnosis and management of patients with toxoplasmic encephalitis. The study most often reveals multiple hypodense, ring-enhancing lesions more frequently seen in the basal ganglia and corticomedullary junction. Double-dose contrast gives maximal enhancement of lesions and is, therefore, preferable to single-dose studies. Magnetic resonance imaging (MRI) is more sensitive and may demonstrate lesions not picked up by CT scan, but there are no findings pathognomonic for toxoplasmosis. Definitive diagnosis is made by demonstration of *T. gondii* cysts or tachyzoites in brain tissue obtained by biopsy. This procedure is recommended for patients with presumptive toxoplasmic encephalitis based on head CT or MRI who have not responded to empiric therapy within 3 to 4 weeks. *(Grant and Armstrong, pp. 457–459; Luft and Remington, pp. 211–222)*

6. **(C)** Clinical presentation of toxoplasmic encephalitis, the most common CNS infection in AIDS patients, includes fever and headache in more than one-half of patients, altered mental status, focal neurologic deficits and seizures. Hemiparesis is the most common focal finding, but patients may also present with ataxia, visual field loss, and cranial nerve palsies. Less commonly, toxoplasma may involve retina, lung, heart, abdomen, and testes. Cryptococcal meningitis, the second most common opportunistic infection of the CNS associated with AIDS, presents with fever (often low grade), headache, and altered mental status. Less frequently seen are focal neurologic deficits, seizures, meningismus, and photophobia. Extracranial disseminated disease occurs in up to 50% of patients. *(Grant and Armstrong, pp. 457–459; Luft and Remington, pp. 211–222)*

7. **(C)** In toxoplasmic encephalitis, CSF may be completely normal or may show mild pleocytosis and elevated protein. Although the presence of IgG toxoplasma antibodies in serum does not predict the development of toxoplasmic encephalitis in patients, its absence argues strongly against the presence of disease in a patient with intracerebral lesions. However, more sensitive assays are needed to improve diagnosis. Production of toxoplasma-specific antibodies in the CSF may be useful in diagnosing active CNS infection. The CSF of patients with cryptococcal meningitis may reveal normal glucose and protein with absence of pleocytosis. Latex agglutination detects cryptococcal polysaccharide antigen in serum and CSF, a positive titer indicating active disease. Less commonly, an India ink stain of CSF may reveal organisms with their typical large capsules. CSF cryptococcal antigen titers are serially followed to determine response to therapy; however, serum titers may remain high and cannot be correlated with clinical improvement. *(Grant and Armstrong, pp. 457–459; Luft and Remington, pp. 211–222)*

8. **(C)** Duration of initial treatment of toxoplasmic encephalitis is approximately 6 weeks, providing there is steady improvement of intracerebral lesions on neuroradiographic imaging. Chronic suppressive therapy is required indefinitely to prevent recurrence of lesions or development of new lesions. Although the combination of pyrimethamine with sulfadiazine or clindamycin is highly active against the proliferative form of *T. gondii*, it is not effective against the dormant cyst. Therefore, if therapy is withdrawn, relapse may occur in up to 80% of cases. Pyrimethamine at 25 to 50 mg daily and sulfadiazine at 2 to 4 g daily, both taken orally with folinic acid, appears to be an adequate suppressive regimen. In instances when sulfonamides cannot be continued, pyrimethamine at 75 mg daily with clindamycin 450 mg tid can be used orally. Recurrences may still present on suppressive treatment, requiring reinitiation of high-dose therapy. Initial management of cryptococcal

meningitis usually consists of daily amphotericin B until the patient is stable and becomes afebrile and free of nausea, vomiting and headache. Treatment can then be changed to oral fluconazole 400 mg daily to complete an 8 to 10 week course. Maintenance therapy with fluconazole 200 mg daily should begin immediately to prevent relapse. Adverse effects of fluconazole include skin rash, nausea, vomiting, abdominal pain, diarrhea, and elevated SGOT and SGPT. *(Grant and Armstrong, pp. 459–462; Luft and Remington, pp. 211–222; Saag, Powderly, Cloud et al, pp. 83–94)*

9. **(C)**   The cumulative incidence of reported AIDS cases in the United States is disproportionately higher in African-Americans and Hispanics. Although 80% of the population in the United States is composed of whites, 53% of all persons with AIDS are white. Conversely, whereas African-Americans and Hispanics compose 12% and 6% of the United States population, they make up 30% and 17% of all AIDS cases, respectively. The geographic distribution of AIDS cases throughout the United States has shifted with time. The percent of AIDS cases in New York and San Francisco, although disproportionately larger than other areas in the United States, has gradually decreased since 1983; other areas have, however, seen an increase in cases. The proportion of adult AIDS cases in women has increased over time. As of December 1992, the percentage of reported AIDS cases in women was 13%, and gradually increasing. Close to 90% of HIV infection in children occurs in those born to women who are at risk of HIV infection. Women at increased risk should be counseled, tested for HIV antibody status, and advised of the risk of HIV transmission to fetus should pregnancy arise. *(CDC, HIV/AIDS Surveillance, pp. 1–23)*

10. **(A)**   The first step in evaluating the presence of HIV infection is the HIV antibody status using the enzyme-linked immunosorbent assay (ELISA) technique. HIV antibodies may be detected by this screening method 1 to 2 months after the onset of acute illness. If this test is found to be positive, it is confirmed by the more specific western blot (WB) method of HIV antibody detection. HIV serum p24 antigen may be detected by ELISA in the period prior to antibody seroconversion but is less sensitive than antibody status and may be present in the serum for only a brief period of time. Persistent p24 antigenemia or the reappearance of antigenemia may be associated with poor clinical outcome. In-vitro culture of HIV is used in clinical trials and in research, but is rarely indicated in routine practice. T-lymphocyte subset studies are routinely used only in known HIV infected patients. Major subsets include CD4⁺ (T-helper) cells and CD8 (T-suppressor) cells. A de-

crease in absolute number of CD4 cells generally correlates with a decline in function of the immune system and an increase in risk of opportunistic infection. *(Tindall et al, pp. 329–338)*

11. **(D)**   Progressive multifocal leukoencephalopathy (PML) results from destruction of oligodendrocytes by the JC papovavirus, a DNA "slow" virus. Neurologic deterioration occurs with diminished mental acuity, visual impairment, cranial nerve and motor dysfunction and, in terminal stages, altered consciousness. Neuroradiographic imaging reveals hypodense white matter lesions with irregular borders without contrast enhancement or mass effect on CT and multifocal demyelination on MRI. Definitive diagnosis requires brain biopsy. There is no standard treatment available; however, experimental treatments include interferon, vidarabine, cytarabine, and zidovudine (AZT). To date, results have been disappointing. Primary CNS lymphoma commonly presents with symptoms of confusion and memory loss, as well as hemiparesis, seizures, headache, aphasia, or cranial nerve palsies. Single or multiple lesions that are frequently hypodense and contrast enhancing are seen on CT or MRI scanning of the head. These lesions may be indistinguishable from toxoplasmosis; therefore, brain biopsy may be necessary for confirmation. Treatment for primary CNS lymphoma involves whole brain irradiation sometimes combined with a short course of steroids; however, survival is not significantly improved. Combination chemotherapy is being studied. HIV-infected patients are at increased risk for all forms of tuberculosis, both pulmonary and extrapulmonary; the latter includes TB meningitis. To date, there are no studies documenting an increased risk of bacterial meningitis in HIV-infected patients. Cryptococcoma is discussed briefly in Question 6. *(Chaisson and Griffin, pp. 79–82)*

12. **(C)**   HIV may be transmitted from mother to neonate during intrauterine life as well as during delivery. HIV antibodies cross the placenta; thus, the positive HIV antibody status of the infant may reflect the presence of maternal antibodies. Symptoms of HIV infection, fever, chronic diarrhea, and thrush may appear as early as 5 months of age. There is often a decrease in weight gain and linear growth, and an increase in infections such as otitis media and pneumonia. Staphylococcal and gram-negative infections begin to occur. Chronic lymphocytic infiltrative pneumonia (LIP) and chronic parotid enlargement are common in children. LIP appears on chest x-ray as interstitial, usually bilateral, infiltrates. PCP is the most common opportunistic infection in children but others include *Mycobacterium avium* complex (MAC), toxoplasmosis, viral, cryptococcal, and other fungal infections. Kaposi's sarcoma occurs rarely in children,

but lymphomas are seen frequently. Neurologic involvement, primarily progressive encephalopathy, has been described in more than half of pediatric AIDS cases. *(Grossman, pp. 533–541)*

13. **(D)** Diarrhea accompanied by weight loss and abdominal cramps are common presenting symptoms in HIV-infected patients. Although AIDS-wasting syndrome (HIV infection without superimposed enteric infection) is frequently seen in AIDS patients, intestinal infection should first be excluded. Initial evaluation should include stool culture for routine bacterial pathogens including *Salmonella, Shigella, Campylobacter,* and *Yersinia.* Therapy is directed at each specific organism and should be of 1 to 2 weeks' duration. Stool examination for ova and parasites may reveal *Giardia lamblia* and *Entamoeba histolytica,* and assay for *Clostridium difficile* toxin should be obtained, all of which are associated with acute enteritis. *Cryptosporidium* and *Isospora belli,* two atypical parasitic infections common in patients with AIDS, are easily identified by examination of stool with acid-fast stain. In patients with cryptosporidiosis, symptoms develop insidiously and become more severe with deterioration of the immune system. Symptoms may include voluminous (1 to 25 L daily) diarrhea, weight loss of more than 10% total body weight, severe abdominal pain, and dehydration. The biliary tract may become involved causing nausea and vomiting. Nonspecific treatment of cryptosporidiosis is empiric and depends on the use of antidiarrheal agents (opiates, diphenoxylate, and loperamide), nutritional management, and fluids. Hyperimmune bovine colostrum (HBC), a promising treatment under investigation, has been shown to ameliorate symptoms. Other potentially effective treatments include three macrolide antibiotics (azithromycin, clarithromycin, and roxithromycin), paromycin, a nonabsorbable aminoglycoside, and octreotide, a synthetic cyclic octapeptide analog of somatostatin. Isosporiasis is diagnosed less frequently than cryptosporidiosis but the symptoms are indistinguishable. Other chronic causes of enteritis include *Mycobacterium avium* complex (also demonstrated on acid-fast stain), CMV, and Kaposi's sarcoma. Blood cultures for CMV and MAC would be useful in detecting those infections, and treatment would be aimed at the specific organism. If the above evaluation revealed no specific pathogen, sigmoidoscopy/colonoscopy with biopsy would be an appropriate last step. Barium enema would be least helpful in diagnosing the etiology of diarrhea in HIV-infected patients. *(Bartlett, Belitsos, and Sears, pp. 726–735; Petersen, pp. 903–909; Chaisson, pp. 480–481)*

14. **(A)** Didanosine (ddI) and zalcitabine (ddC) are both nucleoside analogs found to be inhibitors of HIV reverse transcriptase thereby inhibiting HIV replication. Peripheral neuropathy, characterized by distal numbness, tingling, or pain, occurs in 13% to 34% of patients on ddI and 17% to 31% of patients on ddC. Pancreatitis, ranging from mild abdominal pain and elevated serum amylase concentrations to fatal disease, occurs in 5% to 10% of patients on ddI and <1% of patients taking ddC. Other adverse effects for ddI include elevations in serum uric acid and triglyceride levels, headache, diarrhea, and retinal depigmentation; and for ddC include oral and esophageal ulcers, rash, cardiomyopathy, and congestive heart failure. Both ddI and ddC can be used as alternate antiretroviral therapy in patients who become intolerant of zidovudine or display disease progression (decline in CD4$^+$ cell count or development of constitutional symptoms or opportunistic infection). Clinical studies examining combination therapy (such as AZT combined with ddI or ddC) are encouraging. Because of problems with viral resistance, drug failure, and drug toxicity, emphasis is now being placed on combination drug regimens in HIV therapy. Dosing of ddI is 200 mg (two 100 mg tablets) twice daily in patients weighing >60 kg and 125 mg (one 100 mg and one 25 mg tablet) twice daily in patients weighing <60 kg. Administration should take place on an empty stomach and two tablets should be taken at each dose so that adequate buffering is provided to prevent gastric acid degradation of ddI. Dosing of ddC is 0.75 mg every 8 hours orally, with a dose reduction to 0.375 mg every 8 hours for mild drug toxicity or dose interruption for severe toxicity. *(Hirsch and D'Aquila, pp. 1686–1695; Sommadossi, pp. s7–s15)*

15. **(A)** Symptoms of dysphagia (difficulty swallowing), odynophagia (pain or burning on swallowing), and retrosternal pain are associated with esophagitis. The most common cause of esophagitis is *Candida albicans,* with most, but not all, patients having both oral thrush and esophageal candidiasis. An empiric trial of antifungal therapy, usually fluconazole at 200 mg orally for the first day, then 100 mg daily until improvement, is indicated in patients with oral thrush and esophageal complaints. Ketoconazole at 200 to 400 mg orally per day is an alternative treatment. If symptoms fail to improve on fluconazole, endoscopy is warranted to look for other etiologic agents. These include HSV and, less commonly, CMV. The clinical picture of esophagitis may be complicated by simultaneous presence of multiple infectious agents. Definitive diagnosis should be made by endoscopically directed biopsy of the esophageal mucosa. HSV esophagitis usually responds to a course of oral acyclovir at 200 mg 5 times daily, but may also require maintenance therapy at 400 mg 2 times daily to prevent recurrence. CMV esophagitis should be treated with IV ganciclovir and al-

though initial response is often favorable, relapses are common. Oral hairy leukoplakia caused by Epstein–Barr virus (EBV) produces a white thickening of the oral mucosa, particularly of the tongue. The lesions can range in size from a few millimeters to much of the dorsal surface of the tongue. Oral hairy leukoplakia does not extend into the esophagus or cause esophageal symptoms. (Drew, pp. 498–505; Greenspan et al, pp. 373–380; Laine et al, pp. 655–660)

16.   (A)   In early clinical trials, zidovudine (AZT) at a dose of 1600 mg per day was demonstrated to prolong survival and reduce the frequency of opportunistic infections in patients with advanced HIV infection. In subsequent trials conducted by the AIDS Clinical Trials Group (ACTG), lower doses of zidovudine were equivalent in efficacy to high doses in patients with advanced HIV infection and were associated with far less toxicity. The current recommended dose is 100 mg every 4 hours 5 times daily to be started when CD4⁺ lymphocyte count falls below 500. Current studies, however, have cast some doubt on the efficacy of zidovudine in patients whose CD4 cell count is above 300. Although the incidence of anemia and neutropenia has been reduced as zidovudine doses have decreased, they are still common with prolonged use. Blood transfusion, modification of dose, or a change to an alternate antiretroviral agent may be necessary. Hematopoietic hormones, erythropoietin (EPO) and granulocyte colony-stimulating factor (GCSF), are available for the treatment of zidovudine-induced anemia and neutropenia, respectively. Prolonged zidovudine use can cause a myopathy characterized by elevated serum creatine kinase concentrations. However, it is difficult to distinguish from myopathy caused by HIV itself unless it improves with the discontinuation of zidovudine therapy. Upon the initiation of zidovudine, there are patients who experience headache and nausea; however, in the majority of these patients the symptoms abate with continued use. (Hirsch and D'Aquila, pp. 1686–1695)

17.   (B)   Trends of newly diagnosed HIV infections in the United States in groups at recognized risk have changed over time. Evidence indicates a decrease in the incidence of new infections in men who have sex with men, reflecting reduced high-risk sexual behavior in this population. The risk of new infection in hemophiliacs has decreased dramatically with the development in 1984 of heat treatment of clotting factor concentrates. The incidence of new infection in IV-drug users and their heterosexual partners appears to be increasing. Seroprevalence in IV-drug users is strongly associated with the number of persons with whom needles are shared, and the use of shooting galleries. Effective interventions for behavior change are dif-

ficult but essential in an attempt to persuade IV-drug users to not share needles or to clean needles and drug paraphernalia with bleach. The incidence of new HIV infection in people with no known risk factors remains between 3% and 6%; however, 75% are reclassified into known-risk categories following additional questioning. (CDCP, HIV/AIDS Surveillance, pp. 1–23; Wofsy, pp. 307–319)

18.   (E)   The Centers for Disease Control and Prevention (CDCP), in collaboration with the Council of State and Territorial Epidemiologists (CTSE), expanded the AIDS surveillance case definition effective January 1, 1993. The expanded definition included pulmonary tuberculosis (TB), recurrent pneumonia, and invasive cervical cancer reflecting the importance of these diseases in the HIV epidemic. Pulmonary TB is the most common type of TB in HIV-infected patients. Patients co-infected with HIV and TB have a substantially increased risk of developing active TB compared with patients without HIV infection. With the exception of conditions included in the 1987 AIDS surveillance case definition, pneumonia is the leading cause of HIV-related morbidity and mortality. Two or more recurrent episodes of pneumonia in a one-year period are required for AIDS case reporting. Multiple episodes of pneumonia are more strongly associated with immunosuppression than are single episodes. Several studies have found an increased prevalence of cervical dysplasia, a precursor lesion for cervical cancer, among HIV-infected women. This finding is usually associated with greater immunosuppression, and HIV infection may adversely affect the clinical course and treatment of cervical dysplasia and cancer. Invasive cervical cancer is preventable by the proper recognition and treatment of cervical dysplasia. The inclusion of HIV-infected persons with CD4⁺ T-lymphocyte count of <200 cells/mm or a CD4⁺ percentage of <14 will enable AIDS surveillance to more accurately reflect the number of people with severe HIV-related immunosuppression and those at highest risk for severe HIV-related morbidity. (MMWR, No. RR-17, pp. 1–9)

19.   (E)   Mycobacterium avium complex (MAC) is the most common bacterial complication found in AIDS patients in the U.S. and causes widely disseminated infection. The patients at greatest risk for DMAC are those with CD4⁺ T-lymphocyte counts below 100/mm. DMAC frequently produces symptoms of chronic fever, diaphoresis, and weight loss; also associated are diarrhea and chronic abdominal pain with hepatosplenomegaly. It often infects bone marrow, causing pancytopenia. Anemia may be profound enough to require chronic transfusions. DMAC may be found in virtually any organ in the body including spleen, liver, lymph nodes, lungs, kidneys, adrenals, and

gastrointestinal tract. Patients with DMAC should be treated to reduce mycobacterial load and alleviate symptoms; however, it has not been proven that treatment elicits a durable response or extends survival. DMAC is a multiresistant organism and the initial treatment should include at least two to three antimycobacterial drugs depending on the patient's clinical status. Clarithromycin at a dose of 500 mg to 1 gm twice daily is the preferred first agent with azithromycin as an alternative first agent. Ethambutol at a dose of 15 mg/kg/d seems to be a rational second-choice agent. For third- or fourth-choice agents rifamycin derivatives, clofazimine, ciprofloxacin, or parental amikacin are all appropriate selections. *(Benson and Ellner, pp. 7–20)*

20. **(A)** One of the major advances in HIV treatment has been the development of prophylactic regimens to prevent *Pneumocystis carinii* pneumonia, prompting the U.S. Public Health Service task force to issue guidelines on PCP prophylaxis. Secondary prophylaxis should be started after a patient has been treated for a first episode of PCP. Primary prophylaxis should begin when an HIV-infected patient's CD4$^+$ cell count falls below 200 cells/mm or a CD4 cell percentage below 20, or an HIV-infected patient develops oral thrush or unexplained fevers over 100°F for longer than 2 weeks (even if the CD4$^+$ count is above 200 cells/mm). To monitor a patient's immune system more closely, CD4$^+$ cell counts should be measured every three months. The first-line agent for PCP prophylaxis is trimethoprim-sulfamethoxazole (TMP-SMX). Although optimal dose is unknown, the dose recommended in the new guidelines is one double-strength tablet (160 mg TMP plus 800 mg SMX) once a day. There is evidence that less frequent dosing (one double-strength tablet 3 times a week) is equally effective and less toxic, but this remains to be established. Approximately 25% of patients are unable to tolerate TMP-SMX secondary to bone marrow suppression, or skin and other allergic reactions. For patients experiencing myelosuppression secondary to zidovudine, TMP-SMX may not be an appropriate choice for PCP prophylaxis. The leading candidate for a second-line agent is Dapsone at a dose of 50 to 100 mg daily, although there have been reports that doses as low as 100 mg twice weekly may also be effective. Side effects include skin rash, nausea, vomiting, abdominal pain, and headache. Aerosolized pentamidine (AP), which in 1989 was the first drug approved by the FDA for PCP prophylaxis, has since been shown to be less effective than TMP-SMX. Studies showed that up to 20% of patients receiving AP had a recurrence of PCP within one year. In addition, uneven distribution of the medication in the lungs during treatment led to increased episodes of apical PCP, peripheral PCP, and extrapul-

monary PCP. AP at a dose of 300 mg once monthly is recommended for PCP in patients who are unable to tolerate either of the recommended oral agents. Ciprofloxacin is not a recommended treatment for PCP prophylaxis. *(MMWR, RR-4, p. 141)*

21. **(E)** Aseptic meningitis may occur acutely with seroconversion or later in the course of HIV infection in both symptomatic and asymptomatic patients. Progressive vacuolar myelopathy is a common complication of HIV infection that presents with progressive gait disturbance and ataxia, often followed by bowel and bladder dysfunction and paraplegia in advanced cases. It is often accompanied by dementia but may occur in relative isolation. Lab studies show multiple vacuoles of the white matter of the spinal cord. The etiology of vacuolar myelopathy is debated, but there is evidence for direct involvement of HIV. There is no standard treatment, but there are anecdotal reports that vacuolar myelopathy responds to antiretroviral therapy. AIDS dementia complex (ADC) is characterized by cognitive, motor, and behavioral abnormalities. This is the most common CNS disorder associated with HIV infection and is considered to eventually affect the majority of AIDS patients. Other disease processes must first be ruled out by history, physical examination, and laboratory studies. Radiologic imaging typically reveals atrophy and abnormalities in white matter by both CT and MRI. Zidovudine has been found to ameliorate symptoms of patients with ADC. Peripheral neuropathy can be seen at any stage of HIV infection and presents both sensory and motor dysfunction. The sensory symptoms are more common and include numbness, "burning," and pain, usually beginning in the toes and feet. It is believed that HIV is the causative agent, although neuropathy is also seen as an adverse effect of treatment with didanosine (ddI) and zalcitabine (ddC). Treatment is aimed at alleviating symptoms with tricyclic antidepressants, analgesics, and certain anticonvulsants. *(Clifford and Campbell, pp. 28–33)*

22. **(A)** In 1983, the self-deferral program of volunteer blood donors who thought they may be at risk for HIV infection was begun in an attempt to reduce HIV transmission through blood transfusions. However, it was not until April 1985 that HIV-antibody testing of donated blood was instituted. This dramatically decreased the risk of HIV transmission to blood recipients. Although blood recipients often wish to have blood donated by family members, this does not decrease the risk of HIV transmission, as risk factors for HIV infection in family members are usually not known or not admitted. Sexual transmission is responsible for the majority of AIDS cases; thus, safer sex practices have become essential. Receptive anal inter-

course carries the greatest risk of infection to homosexual men and female partners of bisexual men. The use of latex condoms with or without nonoxynol-9 (a spermicide displaying HIV viricidal activity) reduces the risk of HIV transmission. The presence of genital ulcers increases the risk of HIV transmission, likely on the basis of increased contact with blood at the ulcer site. *(CDCP, HIV/AIDS Surveillance, pp. 1–23; Jaffe and Lifson, pp. 299–306; Wolfsy, pp. 307–319)*

23. **(A)** The risk of HIV transmission to health care workers has been evaluated and demonstrated to be approximately 0.33% (1 in 300) following a single needlestick exposure to HIV-infected blood. Although the incidence of transmission is low, the magnitude of risk emphasizes the need for effective infection control procedures. Universal precautions—treating all blood and body fluids as though infected with HIV—reduce the risk of occupational exposure. Protective measures include handwashing before and after patient contact, proper disposal of sharp objects, no recapping of needles, use of gloves when handling blood or body fluids/tissues, and use of goggles and gowns when splatter of body fluids is anticipated. The use of masks is necessary only with procedures during which there is aerosolization of body fluids or with contagious airborne diseases. No cases of HIV transmission to health care workers from contact with body fluids other than blood have been documented. Zidovudine has been given prophylactically to people who have been inoculated with HIV-infected blood in an effort to prevent seroconversion. There has been no documentation to date to prove the effectiveness in such circumstances, and there have been anecdotal reports of the failure of zidovudine in preventing infection. The potential for HBV transmission to health care workers after accidental exposure is much greater than HIV transmission. Studies demonstrate that 10% to 30% of health care workers have serologic evidence of past or present HBV exposure. Twelve thousand health care workers become infected with HBV each year, of which 700 to 1200 become chronic carriers. *(Gerberding and Henderson, pp. 1179–1185; Henderson, Fahey, Willy et al, pp. 740–746)*

24. **(C)** CMV infection in AIDS patients is quite common and can cause several clinical illnesses, most frequently chorioretinitis, gastrointestinal disease, and pneumonia. Culture of CMV from pulmonary secretions or lung tissue is common, but its isolation does not always indicate active disease. Many patients with pulmonary disease and CMV isolation from the lung have concomitant infections, thereby raising doubt as to whether CMV is a true pulmonary pathogen. CMV is considered a possible pathogen when CMV-infected cells are seen histopathologically in tissue specimens. Therapy with ganciclovir or foscarnet should be considered when CMV is felt to be documented as a pulmonary pathogen and the patient's clinical course is deteriorating. HSV infection, common in HIV-infected patients, may cause oral, genital, and anorectal lesions, as well as esophagitis and other organ involvement. The severity of illness depends upon the degree of immunosuppression in the patient and site of infection. Prompt administration of therapy—acyclovir or foscarnet for acyclovir-resistant HSV—for active infection reduces morbidity and the risk of serious complications. Topical acyclovir, although reducing virus shedding, does not reduce formation of new lesions or risk of dissemination. Recurrent VZV infection manifesting as shingles occurs commonly in immunosuppressed HIV-infected patients. Dissemination of VZV to lung, liver, and CNS has been associated with a high mortality rate. This life-threatening disease process warrants hospitalization and treatment with high-dose IV acyclovir or foscarnet for acyclovir-resistant VZV. *(Drew, pp. 495–509; Studies of Ocular Complications of AIDS Research Group, in Collaboration with the AIDS Clinical Trials Group, pp. 213–220)*

25. **(B)** Kaposi's sarcoma (KS) is the most frequent AIDS-associated malignancy and is seen primarily in homosexual men. Unlike classic KS, which presents as relatively indolent cutaneous lesions, KS in AIDS patients is often aggressive and can be found as cutaneous lesions, visceral lesions, or both. Cutaneous KS can appear on any body surface but is commonly seen on the face and in the oral cavity. KS may cause pulmonary disease, gastrointestinal disease leading to gastric outlet obstruction, or GI bleeding, and cause lymphatic obliteration leading to severe lymphedema. Pulmonary KS may be seen on chest x-ray as nodular infiltrates, with or without pleural effusions, and patients often present with shortness of breath, hemoptysis, and dyspnea. Definitive diagnosis of Kaposi's sarcoma is readily made by biopsy. Radiotherapy is effective palliative treatment for KS lesions; however, progression and dissemination are not altered with treatment and prognosis is not improved. Multiple cytotoxic chemotherapeutic agents have been used in treatment of visceral KS with varying response rates. Most of these agents, including vincristine, vinblastine, doxorubicin, etoposide, and bleomycin, have been associated with severe toxicities. Alpha-interferon administered parenterally has proven effective against KS, particularly in patients with early disease who do not yet have marked depletion of CD4+ cells. *(Krown, pp. 24–29; Mitsuyasu, pp. 511–523)*

REFERENCES

Bartlett JG, Belitsus PC, Sears CL. AIDS enteropathy. *Clin Infect Dis.* October 1992;15:726–735.

Benson CA, Ellner JJ. *Mycobacterium avium* complex infection and AIDS: Advances in theory and practice. *Clin Infect Dis.* July 1993;17:7–20.

Bozzette SA, Sattler FR, Chiu J, et al. A controlled trial of early adjunctive treatment with corticosteroids for *Pneumocystis carinii* pneumonia in the acquired immunodeficiency syndrome. *NEJM.* December 1990;323:1451–1457.

Centers for Disease Control and Prevention. *HIV/AIDS Surveillance,* Year-End Edition. U.S. AIDS cases reported through December 1992. February 1993:1–23.

Centers for Disease Control and Prevention. 1993 revised classification system for HIV infection and expanded surveillance case definition for AIDS among teenagers and adults. *MMWR.* 1993;41:RR 17, 1–19.

Centers for Disease Control and Prevention. Recommendations for prophylaxis against PCP for adults and adolescents infected with HIV. *MMWR.* 1992;41:RR-4, 141.

Chaisson R, Griffin D. Progressive multifocal leukoencephalopathy in AIDS. *JAMA.* 1990;264:79–82.

Clifford DB, Campbell JW. Management of neurologic opportunistic disorders in human immunodeficiency virus infection. *Semin Neurol.* 1992;12(1):28–33.

Drew WL. Herpesvirus infections. How to use ganciclovir and acyclovir. *Infect Dis Clin North Am.* 1988;2(2):495–501.

Gerberding JL, Henderson DK. Management of occupational exposures to bloodborne pathogens: Hepatitis B virus, hepatitis C virus and HIV. *Clin Infect Dis.* June 1992;14:1179–1185.

Grant IH, Armstrong D. Fungal infections in AIDS. Cryptococcus. *Infect Dis Clin North Am.* 1988;2(2):457–464.

Greenspan JS, Greenspan D, Winkler JR. Diagnosis and management of the oral manifestations of HIV infection and AIDS. *Infect Dis Clin North Am.* 1988;2(2):373–385.

Grossman M. Children with AIDS. *Infect Dis Clin North Am.* 1988;2(2):419–428.

Henderson DK, Fahey BJ, Willy M, et al. Risk for occupational transmission of human immunodeficiency virus type 1 (HIV-1) associated with clinical exposures: A prospective evaluation. *Ann Intern Med.* 1990;113:740–746.

Hirsch MS, D'Aguila RT. Therapy for human immunodeficiency virus infection. *NEJM.* 1993;328:1686–1695.

Jaffe HW, Lifson AR. Acquisition and transmission of HIV. *Infect Dis Clin North Am.* 1988;2(2):299–306.

Krown SE. Evolving therapeutic options for Kaposi's sarcoma. *HIV Adv in Res and Ther.* October 1992;2(3):24–29.

Laine L, et al. Fluconazide compared with ketoconazole for the treatment of *Candida* esophagitis in AIDS. *Ann Intern Med.* 1992;117:655–660.

Luft BJ, Remington JS. Toxoplasmic encephalitis in AIDS. *Clin Infect Dis.* August 1992;18:211–222.

Masur H, Kovacs JA. Treatment and prophylaxis of *Pneumocystis carinii* pneumonia. *Infect Dis Clin North Am.* 1988;2(2):419–42.

Mitsuyasu RT. Kaposi's sarcoma. *Infect Dis Clin North Am.* 1988;2(2):511–523.

Petersen C. Cryptosporidiosis in patients infected with the human immunodeficiency virus. *Clin Infect Dis.* December 1992;15:903–909.

Saag MS, Powderly WG, Cloud GC, et al. Comparison of amphotericin B with fluconazole in the treatment of acute AIDS-associated cryptococcal meningitis. *NEJM.* January 1992;326:83–94.

Sommadossi JP. Nucleoside analogs: Similarities and differences. *Clin Infect Dis.* February 1993;16:s7–s15.

Studies of Ocular Complications of AIDS Research Group, in Collaboration with the AIDS Clinical Trial Group. Mortality in patients with the acquired immunodeficiency syndrome treated with either foscarnet or ganciclovir for cytomegalovirus retinitis. *NEJM.* January 1992;362:213–220.

Tindall B, Cooper DA, Donovan B, Pennt R. Primary human immunodeficiency virus infection. Clinical and serologic aspects. *Infect Dis Clin North Am.* 1988;2(2):329–341.

Wofsy CB. Prevention of HIV transmission. *Infect Dis Clin North Am.* 1988;2(2):307–319.

Subspecialty List:
Acquired Immunodeficiency Syndrome

QUESTION NUMBER AND SUBSPECIALTY

1. *P. carinii* pneumonia (PCP)—treatment and management
2. Toxoplasmic encephalitis—diagnosis, treatment, and management
3. Cryptococcal meningitis—diagnosis, treatment, and management
4. Cytomegalovirus (CMV) chorioretinitis
5. Cryptococcal meningitis—diagnosis, treatment, and management
6. Toxoplasmic encephalitis—clinical presentation
7. Toxoplasmic encephalitis—work-up
8. Toxoplasmic encephalitis—treatment
9. HIV—patterns of infection
10. HIV—testing
11. HIV—neurologic complications
12. Pediatric AIDS
13. HIV—gastrointestinal disorders
14. Didanosine (ddI) and zalcitabine (ddC)—comparisons
15. HIV—esophagitis
16. Zidovudine (AZT)—side effects
17. HIV—epidemiology
18. HIV—CDCP AIDS surveillance case definition
19. *Mycobacterium avium* complex (MAC)—characteristics
20. PCP—prophylaxis
21. HIV—neurologic syndromes
22. HIV—transmission and prevention
23. HIV—transmission and prevention
24. HIV—associated viral infections
25. AIDS—Kaposi's sarcoma

Internal Medicine: Dermatology
Questions

DIRECTIONS (Questions 1 through 11): Each of the numbered items or incomplete statements in this section is followed by answers or by completions of the statement. Select the ONE lettered answer or completion that is BEST in each case.

Questions 1 through 11

1. All the following are considered elevated lesions EXCEPT

   (A) plaques
   (B) macules
   (C) wheals
   (D) pustules
   (E) scales

2. Differential diagnosis of scaly feet must include all EXCEPT

   (A) pityriasis rubra pilaris
   (B) tinea pedis
   (C) dyshidrotic eczema
   (D) tinea versicolor
   (E) contact dermatitis

3. The differential diagnosis of papulosquamous lesions on the trunk includes

   (A) guttate psoriasis
   (B) secondary syphilis
   (C) erythema nodosum
   (D) A and B
   (E) all of the above

4. The most common skin cancer is

   (A) squamous cell carcinoma (SCC)
   (B) primary melanoma
   (C) actinic keratosis (AK)
   (D) keratoacanthoma
   (E) basal cell carcinoma (BCC)

5. Which of the following topical steroids should be used to treat a localized allergic contact dermatitis on the face?

   (A) Temovate (clobetasol propionate) 0.05% cream
   (B) Hytone (hydrocortisone) 2.5% cream
   (C) Cyclocort (amcinonide) 0.1% ointment
   (D) Lidex (fluocinonide) 0.05% cream
   (E) Halog (halcinonide) 0.1% ointment

6. Pityriasis rosea manifestations include all EXCEPT

   (A) prodromal symptoms such as malaise
   (B) a herald patch
   (C) pruritus
   (D) scaly oval papulosquamous lesions
   (E) resolution of rash within less than 2 weeks

7. The drug of choice in treating uncomplicated erysipelas is

   (A) tetracycline
   (B) cephalothin
   (C) vancomycin
   (D) penicillin
   (E) nafcillin

8. The most likely diagnosis for a severely pruritic, rough, erythematous, scaly lesion on the lateral aspect of the ankle which started from what was thought to be a mosquito bite three months ago is

   (A) allergic contact dermatitis
   (B) psoriasis
   (C) systemic lupus erythematosus
   (D) lichen simplex chronicus
   (E) pemphigus vulgaris

9. A necrotic skin ulcer is most commonly associated with the bite of a

    (A) gypsy moth
    (B) brown recluse spider
    (C) scabies
    (D) black widow spider
    (E) scorpion

10. Target lesions are characteristic of

    (A) erythema marginatum
    (B) erythema multiforme
    (C) erythema annulare
    (D) erythema nodosum
    (E) erythema gyratum repens

11. The factor NOT exacerbating acne vulgaris is

    (A) cosmetics
    (B) emotional stress
    (C) topical steroids
    (D) mechanical stress
    (E) food

DIRECTIONS (Questions 12 through 24): Each set of items in this section consists of a list of lettered options followed by several numbered words or phrases. For each numbered word or phrase, select the ONE lettered option that is most closely associated with it. Each lettered option may be selected once, more than once, or not at all.

Questions 12 through 15

Select the viral skin problem for each of the cutaneous lesions.

    (A) verruca vulgaris
    (B) herpes zoster
    (C) molluscum contagiosum
    (D) ecthyma contagiosum
    (E) erythema infectiosum

12. Grouped vesicles, unilateral along a dermatome

13. Slapped face appearance

14. 1.5 cm nontender, dome-shaped bulla with central crusting on the hand of a veterinarian

15. Dome-shaped papules with central umbilication

Questions 16 through 20

Match the appropriate diagnostic test with the listed diagnosis.

    (A) syphilis
    (B) erythrasma
    (C) herpes simplex
    (D) tinea versicolor
    (E) scabies
    (F) ecthyma

16. KOH (potassium hydroxide preparation)

17. Tzanck smear

18. Darkfield microscopy

19. Wood's light

20. Mineral oil scrape

Questions 21 through 24

For each characteristic nail change, select the most likely associated disease or disorder.

    (A) transverse depressions (Beau's lines)
    (B) chalk white nails
    (C) whitening (Terry's nails)
    (D) green
    (E) pitting

21. Cirrhosis

22. Psoriasis

23. Tinea unguium

24. Previous high fever or severe systemic disease

DIRECTIONS (Questions 25 through 27): Each group of items in this section consists of lettered headings followed by a set of numbered words or phrases. For each numbered word or phrase, select

    (A) if the item is associated with (A) only,
    (B) if the item is associated with (B) only,
    (C) if the item is associated with BOTH (A) and (B),
    (D) if the item is associated with NEITHER (A) NOR (B).

25. Therapy for severe Rhus dermatitis (poison ivy/oak) includes

    (A) systemic corticosteroids
    (B) desensitization

26. Curative Kaposi's sarcoma therapy may include

   (A) excisional surgery
   (B) chemotherapy

27. Eczematous dermatitis resulting from endogenous factors include

   (A) nummular dermatitis
   (B) dermatophytid

DIRECTIONS (Questions 28 through 36): For each of the items in this section, ONE or MORE of the numbered options is correct. Choose answer

   (A) if only (1), (2), and (3) are correct,
   (B) if only (1) and (3) are correct,
   (C) if only (2) and (4) are correct,
   (D) if only (4) is correct,
   (E) if all are correct.

Questions 28 through 36

28. Course and prognosis of toxic epidermal necrolysis (TEN) is highly dependent on

   (1) percentage of skin involvement
   (2) management of fluids and electrolytes
   (3) topical skin care
   (4) hospitalization

29. Which of the following cutaneous changes occur with renal insufficiency?

   (1) generalized pruritus
   (2) Muehroke's nails
   (3) Kyrle's disease
   (4) lichen planus-like dermatosis

30. Drugs most likely associated with erythema nodosum include

   (1) bromides
   (2) sulfonamides
   (3) oral contraceptives
   (4) salicylates

31. Skin manifestations suggestive of malignant disease are

   (1) dermatitis herpetiformis
   (2) Sweet's syndrome
   (3) purpura
   (4) leukocytoclastic vasculitis

32. Mongolian spots usually

   (1) disappear in childhood
   (2) are a malignancy indicator
   (3) occur in the lumbosacral area
   (4) are present in more than 30% of whites

33. Bullae on lower extremities include the following diagnosis:

   (1) pemphigus vulgaris
   (2) epidermolysis bullosa acquisita (EBA)
   (3) bullous diabeticorum
   (4) bullous pemphigoid

34. Atopic dermatitis is a chronic skin disorder associated with

   (1) elevated serum IgE
   (2) family history of atopic dermatitis
   (3) allergic rhinitis and/or asthma
   (4) geographic tongue

35. Varicella (chickenpox)

   (1) has an average incubation period of 14 days
   (2) cannot be transmitted through blood transfusions
   (3) is usually treated symptomatically
   (4) occurs only in children and young adults

36. Viral disease(s) occurring in children include

   (1) rubella
   (2) rubeola
   (3) Kawasaki
   (4) scarlet fever

Answers and Explanations

1. **(B)** Macules are flat, nonpalpable lesions marked by pigment alteration and vary in size and shape. Café au lait spots and vitiligo are examples of macules. Plaques are palpable, raised, plateau-like lesions of variable sizes and thickness. The scaly psoriatic plaques are an example of these. Wheals are inflamed, flat-topped papules or plaques formed by transient and superficial edema. They may appear as small papules or involve areas as large as the entire back; an example of these would be the wheals in urticaria (hives). Pustules are palpable vesicles filled with exudate that may contain bacteria, as in folliculitis, or they may be sterile, as in the lesions of pustular psoriasis. Scales are palpable results of abnormal shedding or the accumulation of the stratum corneum. An increased rate of cell production appearing as scaly plaques in psoriasis or the scaling with a dermatophyte infection, such as tinea versicolor, are examples. *(Fitzpatrick, pp. 32–44)*

2. **(D)** Tinea versicolor is a superficial fungal infection characterized by scaly hypopigmented and hyperpigmented macules involving the trunk and the proximal extremities. A positive KOH (potassium hydroxide) with the pathognomonic spaghetti and meatballs (very short hyphea and spores) is diagnostic for this. Pityriasis rubra pilaris is a chronic disorder, both familial and acquired. It manifests itself with reddish scaly plaques and keratotic follicular papules affecting the entire body, including the oral mucosa. Most commonly involved are the palms and soles. Tinea pedis may manifest itself with erythema, scaly plaques, and/or maceration on the feet. Pruritus may accompany the cutaneous symptoms. The diagnosis of tinea pedis can usually be confirmed by a positive KOH (long hyphea) and/or a dermatophyte culture. Scaling and fissuring may be present on the feet and hands with chronic dyshidrosis. It is often accompanied by secondary bacterial infection. Scaly feet secondary to shoe contact dermatitis can be very difficult to diagnose because of the insidious onset of the reaction. The lesions usually appear to be on the dorsal aspect of the feet. One method of establishing the diagnosis is to place a piece of the suspected shoe material as a patch test on the skin of the back. *(Epstein, p. 154; Fitzpatrick, pp. 544–546, 1525–1538,1574–1577,2437–2439,2462–2465)*

3. **(D)** Guttate psoriasis manifests with erythematous papulosquamous macules, papules, and plaques scattered over most of the body. Greater than 50% of all patients report a preceding streptococcal infection. These patients may go on to develop chronic psoriasis. Secondary syphilis skin lesions may include macules, papules, papulosquamous and follicular eruptions, with or without scaling, scattered over the body. The lesions represent a tissue reaction to the *Treponema pallidum* carried to the site by the blood and the lymphatics. The nontreponemal serologic test RPR should be done to rule out secondary syphilis. If positive, a fluorescent treponemal pallidum absorption test (FTA-ABS) should follow to confirm the diagnosis. Erythema nodosum usually presents with erythematous tender nodules on the anterior shins. They may also appear in areas containing subcutaneous fat. Spontaneous resolution usually occurs in 3 to 6 weeks. Bedrest, identification, and elimination of underlying causes are usually sufficient. *(Fitzpatrick, pp. 489–497,1338–1340,2710–2714)*

4. **(E)** Basal cell carcinoma (BCC) is the most common skin cancer in light-skinned people. The predominant occurrence is on sun-exposed areas. It rarely metastasizes. SCC is a skin cancer that develops mostly because of exposure to sunlight and chemical agents, that is, arsenic, coal tar, creosote oil. Exposure to x-rays and gamma rays with resulting SCC is experimentally and epidemiologically evident. Primary cutaneous malignant melanoma is the leading fatal illness arising in the skin. It is a highly visible tumor and occurs principally during the productive years except for the lentigo maligna melanoma, which is predominantly seen in the elderly. Sun exposure has been implicated in the etiology of primary melanoma. Actinic keratosis (AK), a precancerous lesion, presents on sun-exposed areas in almost 100% of the elderly white population. It may also be found on other fair-skinned people from teens to adults. AK

may progress into a SCC without therapy. A keratoacanthoma is a fast-growing benign skin tumor believed to arise from the hair follicles. It resembles the SCC during the active growth phase with sunlight, chemical carcinogens, trauma, and genetic predilection being factors in this. *(Fitzpatrick, pp. 804–807,821–847,848–855,1078–1114)*

5. **(B)** Hytone (hydrocortisone) 2.5% is the drug of choice of those listed for treatment of any lesion on the face because of its potency. Topical corticosteroids can be grouped in at least four separate groups, which include low-potency, mid-potency, high-potency, and ultra-high-potency, based on their strength of activity. The other four drugs listed are either in the high-potency or ultra-high-potency groups and should never be used on thin skin, such as faces, or in areas where they would be occluded, such as the groin or the intertriginous areas of the skin. High-potency steroids are useful primarily on very thick skin or on severely hyperkeratotic lesions, such as psoriasis. High-potency steroids used either on the face or in the intertriginous areas can cause severe atrophy. *(Sams and Lynch, pp. 51–52)*

6. **(E)** The duration of the secondary lesions in pityriasis rosea (PR) averages 2 to 10 weeks. PR is thought to be caused by an infectious agent but not to be contagious. Structures resembling mycoplasma have been detected on primary plaque. It is regarded as unusual to have recurrent PR. The disease is self-limiting and treatment is symptomatic. Prodromal symptoms of PR such as general malaise, headaches, and gastrointestinal distress appear to occur frequently. The herald patch is the primary lesion in 50% to 90% of cases. It is usually oval or round with fine scaling at the borders and can be found anywhere on the body. The secondary, symmetrical, papulosquamous lesions may appear over the following 7 to 10 days. Most patients will have oval lesions following the skin lines, particularly on the trunk, forming the classic "Christmas tree" pattern. These are usually limited from the neck down the trunk, ending at the wrists and midthighs. Pruritus (itching) may range from severe in 25% to moderate in 50% of patients. It appears to be absent in about 25%. Therapy is symptomatic, and ultraviolet radiation has been shown to be of benefit. *(Epstein, pp. 135–136; Fitzpatrick, pp. 1117–1123)*

7. **(D)** Penicillin is the drug of choice in the treatment of erysipelas, which is usually a group A streptococcal skin infection. Erysipelas, a superficial cellulitis, most often occurs in infants and older adults. The source is commonly the upper respiratory tract. As many as 40% of group A streptococci may be resistant to the tetracyclines. Cephalothin may be substituted in the very ill patient with a questionable penicillin allergy. In the case of an immediate type of reaction, the very ill patient may be treated with vancomycin. Nafcillin should be used in the patient with a suspected severe staphylococcal infection. *(Fitzpatrick, pp. 2323–2324)*

8. **(D)** Lichen simplex chronicus is a commonly seen chronic area of dermatitis, occurring in response to repeated scratching and/or rubbing. The most distinctive feature is lichenification, and the lesions are usually fairly well circumscribed. The most common sites are back of the neck, lower legs, ankles, wrists, and forearms. It frequently begins in a response to some small local irritation such as an insect bite. A scratch-itch cycle is initiated, which results in thickening of the skin and chronic irritation. The lesion sometimes takes on a nodular characteristic which is referred to as prurigo nodularis. Incorrect responses include contact dermatitis, which is usually of a much shorter duration and comes on much more suddenly. Psoriasis usually has a much more sharply demarcated border, is less pruritic, and occurs in multiple lesions. Systemic lupus erythematosus is usually an ill-defined lesion, mostly affecting the face, arms, shoulders, and upper trunk but can affect the hands. The lesions are more violaceous than those of lichen simplex chronicus. Pemphigus vulgaris is a blistering disease. *(Sams and Lynch, pp. 307–311, 381–383,419–420,563–565)*

9. **(B)** The brown recluse spider, often called the fiddleback spider because of the violin-shaped figure on its thorax, bites when humans accidentally disturb its habitat. The initial bite is often painless with the wound starting as a small erythematous papule over the first 6 to 12 hours, progressing to a blister and/or skin necrosis. The resultant necrotic skin ulcer heals slowly and may require a skin graft. The gypsy moth (*Lymantria dispar*), a caterpillar species, may cause irritation with its histamine-containing hairs. The lesions in this case may appear as grouped vesicles and/or bullae. Papules and vesicles are the most common lesions of scabies, but the burrow is the most characteristic and diagnostic feature. The black widow spider, also called the "hourglass" spider, has a neurotoxin venom. This produces minimal local reactions. Generalized pain may occur within 1 to 8 hours. Characteristically, the crampy abdominal pain may be associated with pain in the flanks or chest, or confused with acute appendicitis, renal colic, or acute myocardial infarction. Nausea and vomiting accompany most bites. Scorpions are of primary medical interest in tropical or desert areas, such as the southwestern United States, Mexico, and the Middle East. Their venom induces complex cardiac arrhythmias. It is not known whether the venom's effect on platelets or other

venom proteins induce ulcerative skin lesions. *(Fitzpatrick, pp. 2815–2818)*

10. **(B)** Erythema multiforme is an acute, self-limited eruption of the skin and the mucous membranes. The target or iris lesion, the most characteristic feature of this disease, develops abruptly and symmetrically on extensor surfaces, as well as on the palms and soles. Erythema marginatum is a specific skin manifestation of rheumatic fever. The lesion may begin as an erythematous papule or blotch, spreading peripherally. Lesions may appear on the trunk and the limbs with some pigmentary changes. Eruptions with erythema annulare centrifugum begin as erythematous or urticaria-like papules. These spread to form large rings with central clearing. Etiology appears to be related to underlying disease. Erythematous, tender nodules, usually on the anterior shins, are typical lesions of erythema nodosum. New lesions may be accompanied by fever, chills, and malaise. Numerous etiologies are attributed to this disease. Spontaneous resolution usually occurs. The lesions of erythema gyratum repens are rapidly growing, scaly, erythematous, concentric bands that may involve the entire body. Underlying malignancy appears to be etiology of this condition. *(Fitzpatrick, pp. 588–598,1183–1186,1338–1340)*

11. **(E)** Food does not appear to be an exacerbating factor with acne vulgaris. However, some patients cling to the belief that their flare-ups are associated with certain foods and, in particular, with the ingestion of chocolate. Although there is no scientific evidence for this, it is better to eliminate those dietary agents in these cases. Various cosmetics have been found to exacerbate acne, particularly thick, greasy ones such as actors' makeup. The use of water-based cosmetics may be of benefit. Just as emotional stress can worsen diseases such as hypertension, diabetes, and others, it can exacerbate acne as well. Topical corticosteroids, particularly fluorinated, may exacerbate acne and should not, therefore, be used as therapy. Repetitive trauma to the skin, such as rubbing, can exacerbate acne or produce acneiform lesions. Sports equipment, clothing, namely belts, etc., and excessive scrubbing of the skin are examples. *(Epstein, pp. 61–63; Fitzpatrick, pp. 709–724)*

12. **(B)** The most distinctive feature of herpes zoster is the localization of the rash. Its characteristic rash is nearly always unilateral, does not cross the midline, and is limited in most cases to the area of skin supplied by a single sensory dermatome. Lesions rarely occur below the elbows or knees. *(Fitzpatrick, p. 2552)*

13. **(E)** Erythema infectiosum, or Fifth disease, is a mild, febrile exanthematous disease of viral etiology. There is usually little or no prodrome. It has been determined that the human parvovirus B19 is the causative agent. Fifth disease begins as a low-grade fever, with or without conjunctivitis, upper respiratory infection, itching, and nausea and vomiting. In many cases, this vague early period is followed by a confluent erythema over the cheeks. This rash is the so-called "slapped face" appearance. It is typical for signs and symptoms to occur, then abate, only to reappear especially in times of stress. This may happen for a period of weeks. *(Harrison's, pp. 685–686)*

14. **(D)** Ecthyma contagiosum (ORF) is a contagious viral disorder caused by a poxvirus, which is usually contracted from infected sheep and goats and is seen in shepherds, slaughterhouse workers, shearers, veterinarians, and laboratory workers. The lesions closely resemble those of milker's nodules and are usually 1 to 2 cm in size and generally asymptomatic. The diagnosis is usually based on the clinical appearance of the lesion, the location of the lesion, and a history of exposure to sheep, goats, or cows. *(Sams and Lynch, pp. 109–110)*

15. **(C)** *Molluscum contagiosum* virus is a poxvirus. *M. contagiosum* is a benign viral disease of the mucous membranes and skin. It generally affects children. In adults, it may be transmitted by sexual contact. The lesions are individual, discrete, smooth, pearly to flesh-colored, dome-shaped papules. Often, these lesions have a central umbilication and a mildly erythematous base. Deep to the ulceration there is an easily expressible, white curd-like core. *(Fitzpatrick, p. 2609)*

16. **(D)** Tinea versicolor is a superficial recurring fungal infection of the stratum corneum. It is caused by pityrosporum orbiculare (*Malassezia furfur*). The fungus is readily identified in 10% KOH preparation. It typically shows a "spaghetti and meatball" appearance when viewed under a microscope. *(Fitzpatrick, pp. 2462–2464)*

17. **(C)** HSV infections may be rapidly diagnosed by obtaining cells from the base of the lesion and making a smear on a glass slide. This slide is then stained with Wright's stain or Giemsa's stain, and examined for multinucleated giant cells. This is a Tzanck preparation. In a number of studies there was only a 60% correlation between culture-documented HSV and the appearance of multinucleated giant cells. This stresses the importance of obtaining a positive culture result in order to confirm the diagnosis. *(Fitzpatrick, p. 2539)*

18. **(A)** Syphilis is a communicable disease caused by *Treponema pallidum*. The diagnosis of primary syphilis may be made by detecting the organism in early lesions. Serum from moist lesions or scrap-

ings of the base of dry lesions when viewed with a darkfield microscope may reveal characteristic movements of *T. pallidum*. These include corkscrew rotation, a gentle bending like a bamboo pole, and a spiral spring shortening and lengthening. *(Fitzpatrick, p. 52)*

19. (B) Erythrasma is a common superficial bacterial infection of the skin. It is caused by *Corynebacterium* species. It typically involves the skin of the intertriginous areas and is characterized by well-defined but irregular reddish-brown patches. Examination under a Wood's lamp shows a characteristic coral-red fluorescence, and confirms the diagnosis. *(Fitzpatrick, pp. 2331–2332)*

20. (E) The mineral oil technique of Muller and colleagues is excellent for isolating the mite that causes scabies. In this technique, a drop of sterile mineral oil is placed on a sterile scalpel blade. The oil is then applied to the surface of a burrow or papule. The burrow or papule is then scraped vigorously to remove the entire top of the papule. Tiny flecks of blood will appear in the oil, and when viewed under the microscope should reveal mites, ova, and/or feces. *(Fitzpatrick, p. 51)*

21–24. 21. (C); 22. (E); 23. (B); 24. (A) Close examination of the nails and nail beds can often be of great value in establishing a diagnosis. Terry's nails, which are a whiter color than normal, are often found in patients with cirrhosis. Patients with psoriasis often demonstrate pitting of the nails, although the nails themselves are not grossly involved. Tinea unguium is frequently associated with chalk white nails, which can otherwise also be grossly deformed. A clinical history of previous high fever or other systemic disease can be associated with transverse depressions in the nails known as Beau's lines, which correspond to a temporary slowing or cessation of nail growth during periods of severe stress on the body. *(Sams and Lynch, pp. 743–757)*

25. (A) A large-dose, short-term regimen of systemic corticosteroids, that is, 60 to 100 mg daily tapered over 2 to 3 weeks should be used for severe Rhus dermatitis mainly to suppress development of further lesions. Anecdotal experiences have also shown "rebound effects" such as a recurrence of the rash with low and short systemic therapy. Topical fluorinated steroids may be of benefit in patients with minimal cutaneous reaction but is not effective during the blistering stage. Desensitization to urushiol (the oil contained in the leaves of the plant) to increase tolerance has not been very successful. *(Epstein, pp. 138–139)*

26. (D) Neither surgery nor chemotherapy are considered curative with Kaposi's sarcoma. Although tumors may initially respond to therapy, the relapse rate is very disappointing; particularly with AIDS patients, it is almost 100%. Most clinicians agree treatment must be directed at the immunorestoration. *(Fitzpatrick, pp. 1250–1252)*

27. (B) Dermatophytid reactions are secondary, inflammatory responses of the skin at a side distant from the associated fungal infection. "Id" lesions are culture- and KOH-negative. It is suspected that the id response may involve a local immunologic reaction to systemically absorbed fungal antigens. Once the dermatophyte infection is treated, the dermatophytid disappears. Many factors are proposed as etiologic agents. The pathogenic role of bacteria has not been substantiated. Frequently, dry skin is associated with it, particularly during the winter months. This does not exclude exacerbation in the summer months. Frequent bathing, some topical medication, substances such as wool or soaps, and nutritional factors have been suggested as the cause without supporting evidence in nummular dermatitis. *(Fitzpatrick, p. 2427)*

28. (E) TEN is a severe reaction of the skin to multiple etiologies. Some of the precipitating factors are viral, bacterial, and/or fungal infections, neoplastic disease, and idiopathic and drug allergies, which are the most frequent. Some of the most common ones are nonsteroidal anti-inflammatories, antibiotics, phenolphthalein, barbiturates, and many others. Onset of TEN is acute, with symptoms of skin tenderness, malaise, and fever preceding a morbilliform rash concentrated on the face and extremities, within a few hours to a couple of days. The lesions may vesiculate before the rash becomes confluent. These vesicles become large, flaccid bullae that rupture easily and result in denuded areas. Mucous membranes, such as the lips, mouth, eyes, and genital areas, are usually severely involved. Among other complications are high fever, leukocytosis, electrolyte imbalance, pulmonary edema, and renal failure. Therapy consists of fluid, electrolyte therapy, and proper eye and skin care. The disease carries a greater than 30% mortality. *(Fitzpatrick, pp. 594–595)*

29. (B) 86% of uremic patients present with generalized pruritus. Because they are frequently on multiple medications, a drug reaction with generalized pruritus is not uncommon. Xerosis (dry skin) also contributes to pruritus and is usually relieved by topical emollients. Kyrle's disease, hyperkeratosis follicularis et parafollicularis in cutem penetrans, presents clinically with often pruritic papules and nodules with a central keratin plug. Topical tretinoin therapy may flatten the lesions and decrease pruritus.

Muehrcke's lines are paired, white, parallel

bands observed in patients with hypoalbumine-mia. Lichen planus lesions are tiny, flat-topped, polygonal papules with central umbilication and semitransparent scales known as Wickham's striae. Lichen planus-like dermatosis may develop as a result of drug therapy, namely, antimalarials. Treatment of lichen planus is complex. Systemic corticosteroids alleviate symptoms in most cases. *(Fitzpatrick, pp. 2058–2061)*

30. (A) Tender, erythematous subcutaneous nodules, usually located on the anterior shins in erythema nodosum, are most frequently caused by the use of oral contraceptives. Hypersensitivity to drugs other than bromides, sulfonamides, halogens, tetracycline, penicillin, and 13-cisretinoic acid. In severe or recurrent cases nonsteroidal anti-inflammatory drugs, such as acetylsalic acid, indomethacin, or naproxen, are commonly used as therapy. Systemic steroids are necessary for the more severe cases only. *(Fitzpatrick, pp. 1338–1339)*

31. (E) Dermatitis herpetiformis is associated with intestinal lymphoma. Cutaneous lesions are pruritic, grouped papules, vesicles, and crusts in a symmetric distribution, most commonly on the elbows, knees, buttocks, and shoulders. Sweet's syndrome consists of painful, red, raised plaques and nodules mostly on the face and extremities. It is most commonly associated with leukemia. The most common cause of idiopathic thrombocytopenic purpura (ITP) is lymphoma. The diagnosis of ITP may precede the most common associated lymphoma, Hodgkin's disease. Purpura may also be seen secondary to bone marrow infiltration by leukemia or carcinoma. Leukocytoclastic vasculitis can be a presenting sign in squamous cell carcinoma of the bronchus and malignant lymphoma. *(Fitzpatrick, pp. 2229–2245)*

32. (B) Mongolian spots are congenital and usually disappear, depending on the size, within a few years. Mongolian spots may persist into adulthood, with a 3% to 4% incidence in the Japanese. Mongolian spots are congenital and almost always located in the lumbosacral area and on the buttocks. When seen on the face it may be confused with the nevus of Ota. One point of difference in the pigmentation of the mongolian spot is a blue-black macule of varying sizes, whereas the nevus of Ota has a characteristic mottling with blue and brown spots. The nevus of Ota is not congenital and may persist through life. Laser therapy offers hope to decrease the color intensity with both.

Reference is made to the fact that one patient with mongolian spots on the nose was found to have metastatic melanoma of the liver and lymph nodes. Mongolian spots are observed in more than 90% of the Asiatic and Amerindian races, less fre-

quently in blacks, and in less than 10% of whites. *(Fitzpatrick, pp. 978–979)*

33. (E) Pemphigus vulgaris may present with flaccid bullae commonly involving the scalp, umbilicus, and other parts of the body including the mucous membranes. Delay of diagnosis may be life-threatening. EBA, a chronic blistering disease, is characterized by blister formation over joint surfaces. Extensor surfaces of the lower legs and the mucous membranes may also be involved. In general, these bullae are tense. Spontaneous bullae may appear in diabetics usually on the extremities, especially on the feet. In general, the bullae heal without scarring over several weeks. Large tense bullae in bullous pemphigoid are characteristic of this disease. The most common sites include the inner thighs, flexor surfaces of the forearms, axillae, abdomen, and other areas of the body, including the mucous membranes. This disease occurs predominantly in the sixth, seventh, and eighth decades of life. *(Fitzpatrick, pp. 608–610,615–619,632–633,2124)*

34. (E) During the course of atopic dermatitis there is an increased level of serum IgE. Eosinophilia is commonly associated with exfoliative dermatitis. To establish the diagnosis, a personal or family history of atopic dermatitis should be present. At least 50% of patients with atopic dermatitis develop allergic rhinitis or asthma. Hyperreactivity in the bronchi have been described by atopic dermatitis patients even without overt asthma. More than 60% of atopic dermatitis patients have a personal history of geographic tongue. This term describes the process of changing shapes on the surface of the tongue. *(Epstein, pp. 81–84; Fitzpatrick, pp. 1390–1393,1543–1560)*

35. (B) Varicella is an acute, highly contagious disease that occurs most often in childhood, but can occur at any age, worldwide. The average incubation period is 14 or 15 days with the main route of transmission through the respiratory tract. Presenting signs and symptoms may include a prodrome with a generalized pruritic rash following. Characteristic lesions progress from erythematous macules to papules. Vesicles and crusts at different stages throughout the disease may present. Constitutional symptoms are usually mild in normal children. Varicella may be associated with more extensive skin lesions, high fever, severe malaise, pneumonia and other life-threatening complications in adults, and immunologically compromised patients of any age. Treatment is usually symptomatic. *(Fitzpatrick, pp. 2543–2572)*

36. (A) Rubella (German measles) is a common viral infection in children and young adults. The rash appears first on the face, then generalizes with discrete erythematous macules and papules clearing within 2 to 4 days, followed by fine desquamation. This is in contrast to rubeola, which persists. Rubeola (measles) is also a highly contagious viral disease in children. Three distinct phases are present in measles: (1) an asymptomatic incubation period of about 10 to 12 days; (2) prodromal period with fever, chills, malaise, coryza, conjunctivitis, and cough; (3) onset of the rash, erythematous macules and papules starting on the face, then spreading downward. Koplik's spots usually appear in the mouth 24 to 48 hours prior to the rash. The average clinical course is about 10 days. Symptomatic therapy is usual unless complications such as encephalitis warrants antibiotic treatment. Kawasaki, a viral illness, has a list of six criteria to establish the diagnosis:

1. The disease begins with a high fever not responding to antipyretics. The fever must last for at least 5 days to be considered compatible with this disease. At the second stage, fever may fluctuate over the next week or two. Often myringitis and/or diarrhea may follow. A cough may be present as the third manifestation.
2. Conjunctival injection and uveitis may be present in 70% of the children.
3. Fissuring red lips and a hypertrophic tongue, as well as small mucosal ulcerations, may accompany the illness.
4. Palms and soles that turn bright red and peel as the fever declines.
5. A skin eruption; there are several kinds of eruptions—a red, confluent rash with papules or pustules in the diaper area, a scarlatiniform rash, and a third type presenting with large annular, brownish lesions such as those associated with erythema multiforme.
6. Cervical adenitis is the sixth manifestation.

There are many more signs and symptoms than those mentioned, such as abdominal pain as a most troublesome of all, cardiovascular disease. No specific form of treatment is available.

Scarlet fever presents with a diffuse erythematous eruption, having a sandpaper quality, as a sequela of a group A streptococci infection in the pharynx. Desquamation usually occurs within 4 to 6 days, lasting several weeks. Other clinical findings include enlarged tonsils, strawberry tongue, and generalized lymphadenopathy. It occurs usually in children—only rarely in adults. Early penicillin therapy prevents development of suppurative and nonsuppurative sequelae. *(Fitzpatrick, pp. 2318–2320,2513–2515,2516–2520,2693–2694)*

REFERENCES

Epstein E. *Common Skin Disorders,* 3rd ed. Oradell, NJ: Medical Economic Company Inc; 1988.

Fitzpatrick TB, Eisen AZ, Wolff K, Freedburg IM, Austen KF. *Dermatology in General Medicine,* 4th ed. New York: McGraw-Hill; 1993.

Isselbacher KJ, Adams RD, Braunwald E, Petersdorf RG, Wilson JD (eds). *Harrison's Principles of Internal Medicine,* 11th ed. New York: McGraw-Hill; 1987.

Sams WM, Lynch PJ. *Principals and Practice of Dermatology.* New York: Churchill Livingstone; 1990.

Subspecialty List: Dermatology

QUESTION NUMBER AND SUBSPECIALTY

1. Skin lesions—elevated
2. Scaly feet—differential
3. Papulosquamous lesions—differential
4. Skin cancer—frequency
5. Topical steroid use on the face
6. Pityriasis rosea—characteristics
7. Erysipelas—treatment
8. Lichen simplex chronicus—characteristics
9. Insect bites—characteristics
10. Erythema multiforme—characteristics
11. Acne vulgaris—exacerbating factors
12. Herpes zoster—characteristics
13. Erythema contagiosum—characteristics
14. Ecthyma contagiosum—characteristics
15. Molluscum contagiosum—characteristics
16. Tinea versicolor—laboratory evaluation
17. Herpes simplex—laboratory evaluation
18. Syphilis—laboratory evaluation
19. Erythrasma—laboratory evaluation
20. Scabies—laboratory evaluation
21. Cirrhosis—nail characteristics
22. Psoriasis—nail characteristics
23. Tinea unguium—nail characteristics
24. Previous severe systemic disease—nail characteristics
25. Rhus dermatitis (poison ivy/oak)—treatment
26. Kaposi's sarcoma—treatment
27. Eczematous dermatitis—characteristics
28. Toxic epidermal necrolysis—characteristics
29. Renal insufficiency—cutaneous changes
30. Erythema nodosum—causes
31. Malignancy—skin changes
32. Mongolian spots—characteristics
33. Bullae—differential diagnosis
34. Atopic dermatitis—characteristics
35. Varicella—characteristics
36. Viral disease in children—characteristics

Internal Medicine: Renal
Questions

DIRECTIONS (Questions 1 through 7): Each of the numbered items or incomplete statements in this section is followed by answers or by completions of the statement. Select the ONE lettered answer or completion that is BEST in each case.

Questions 1 through 7

1. Of the signs and symptoms listed below, which is LEAST likely to be associated with acute pyelonephritis?

   (A) nausea and vomiting with fever and chills
   (B) leukocytosis
   (C) CVA tenderness or pain on deep abdominal palpation
   (D) frequency and urgency
   (E) malaise

2. The filtrate that enters the proximal tubule immediately after the glomerulus should contain most all substances present in the plasma EXCEPT

   (A) sodium
   (B) potassium
   (C) protein
   (D) creatinine
   (E) water

3. Plasma creatinine concentration

   (A) is normally 0.6 to 1.3 mg/dl, with plasma levels in men being somewhat higher than women's
   (B) should remain constant in most individuals who are not undergoing muscle damage and have normally functioning kidneys
   (C) can be used to roughly estimate the number of functioning nephrons
   (D) is not immediately affected by sudden changes in glomerular filtration
   (E) all of the above

4. Hematuria

   (A) can arise from anywhere in the urinary tract
   (B) that is visible to the "naked eye" is of more concern than microscopic hematuria
   (C) is only significant when there is greater than 8 cells per HPF
   (D) is always due to tumor or stone in the collecting system
   (E) all of the above

5. White blood cell casts are most often seen with

   (A) urethral syndrome
   (B) acute pyelonephritis
   (C) cystitis
   (D) drug-induced tubulointerstitial nephritis
   (E) renal tuberculosis

6. Of the signs and symptoms listed below, which is the most ominous for a patient with symptomatic nephrolithiasis?

   (A) frequency
   (B) fever
   (C) intermittent flank pain
   (D) hematuria
   (E) nausea

7. In the absence of infection, approximately 90% of renal calculi are composed of

   (A) calcium compounds
   (B) uric acid compounds
   (C) cystine compounds
   (D) magnesium compounds
   (E) ammonium compounds

DIRECTIONS (Questions 8 through 12): Each set of items in this section consists of a list of lettered options followed by several numbered words or phrases. For each numbered word or phrase, select the ONE lettered option that is most closely associated with it. Each lettered option may be selected once, more than once, or not at all.

Questions 8 through 12

Of the causes of hematuria and proteinuria listed as (A)–(E) below, select a single best response to the following statements.

(A) nephrotic syndrome

(B) acute glomerulonephritis

(C) Berger's disease (IgA nephropathy)

(D) Goodpasture's syndrome

(E) systemic lupus erythematosus

8. These patients present with massive proteinuria but few formed elements (cells, casts, etc.) in their urine.

9. This disorder, caused by circulating immune complexes, presents in early adulthood and waxes and wanes between gross and microscopic hematuria. The disease progresses over a long period of time and is associated with slowly progressive renal impairment.

10. Patients with this complaint develop hemoptysis in association with rapid onset renal insufficiency.

11. The pathologic mechanism in this disease appears to be induced by antibodies to the glomerular basement membrane.

12. Renal involvement is a major cause of mortality in these patients.

DIRECTIONS (Questions 13 through 15): Each of the numbered items or incomplete statements in this section is followed by answers or by completions of the statement. Select the ONE lettered answer or completion that is BEST in each case.

Questions 13 through 15

13. A 72-year-old black male presents after several days of voiding difficulty complaining of complete loss of urine production, although he has the desire to void. He denies fever, chills, or recent illness. He admits to a 22-year history of diabetes mellitus and a 2-pack-per-day smoking habit. The most likely cause of his oliguria/anuria is

(A) prerenal anuria, due to CHF

(B) postrenal anuria, due to renal calculi

(C) intrinsic renal disease, due to bilateral renal cortical necrosis

(D) diabetic nephropathy

(E) postrenal anuria, due to bladder outlet obstruction

14. A 37-year-old white female presents with a history of right renal lithiasis diagnosed in the emergency room seven days ago. She is now hypotensive, nauseous, and has produced approximately one cup of smoky-colored urine in the past 24 hours. The most likely cause of her oliguria is

(A) acute glomerulonephritis

(B) renal calculus obstruction

(C) radiographic contrast media toxicity

(C) Alport syndrome

(E) Goodpasture's syndrome

15. A 32-year-old bank executive presents with a 24-hour history of fever, chills, perineal pain and frequency, urgency, and nocturia. He denies being at risk for sexually transmitted disease and has had no urethral discharge. On physical examination, he is noted to have an acutely inflamed prostate. The treatment of choice for his diagnosis is

(A) amoxicillin 500 mg qid for 30 days

(B) trimethoprim-sulfamethoxazole (160/800 mg) bid for 30 days

(C) trimethoprim-sulfamethoxazole (160/800 mg) bid for 10 days

(D) amoxicillin 500 mg qid for 10 days

(E) doxycycline 100 mg bid for 10 days

DIRECTIONS (Questions 16 through 23): Each set of items in this section consists of a list of lettered options followed by several numbered words or phrases. For each numbered word or phrase, select the ONE lettered option that is most closely associated with it. Each lettered option may be selected once, more than once, or not at all.

Questions 16 through 23

Match the list of disorders of the scrotum and its contents below to the single best response in the statements.

(A) cryptorchism

(B) testicular tumors

(C) testicular torsion

(D) acute epididymitis

(E) hydrocele

16. A life-threatening disorder in young men whose only sign may be a painless mass

17. Caused by rotation of the testicle and occlusion of its vascular supply

18. An effusion of fluid in the potential space in the tunica vaginalis

19. Is only serious if the testicle cannot be palpated

20. Increases chance of testicular malignancy

21. Leads to an extremely tender and swollen testicle with fever and chills; may require hospitalization

22. Is an indication for emergent surgical consultation in attempt to save testicle

23. May be associated with UTI or urethritis, especially chlamydia

DIRECTIONS (Questions 24 and 25): For each of the items in this section, ONE or MORE of the numbered options is correct. Choose answer

    (A) **if only (1), (2), and (3) are correct,**

    (B) **if only (1) and (3) are correct,**

    (C) **if only (2) and (4) are correct,**

    (D) **if only (4) is correct,**

    (E) **if all are correct.**

Questions 24 and 25

24. In the patient with hyperchloremic acidosis, you will find

    (1) decreased serum bicarbonate

    (2) sulfate and phosphate excreted normally

    (3) increased reabsorption of chloride ions

    (4) renal excretion of acid is reduced

25. Which has been converted by the kidney to its active form?

    (1) parathyroid hormone

    (2) antidiuretic hormone

    (3) aldosterone

    (4) 1,25-dihydroxycholecalciferol

Answers and Explanations

1. **(D)** Acute pyelonephritis is associated with nausea and vomiting, fever, chills, leukocytosis, costovertebral angle tenderness, or pain on deep abdominal palpation. The patient may or may not have symptoms of cystitis (ie, frequency, urgency, nocturia), and can be suffering from headache or malaise. *(Stams, pp. 1191–1192)*

2. **(C)** The glomerulus forms an essentially protein-free filtrate composed of all substances present in plasma at virtually the same concentration as in plasma. There is essentially no protein due to the glomerular membranes restricting movement of high molecular weight substance, the exception being some low molecular weight substance bound to proteins, such as fatty acids. In diseased kidneys, the glomerular membranes become increasingly permeable to protein and/or the tubules may lose their ability to remove protein. Traditionally, diseases of the kidney have been divided into four pathologic groups—glomerular, tubular, interstitial, and vascular. *(Walker, pp. 737–738)*

3. **(E)** Creatinine is freely filtered at the glomerulus and is not reabsorbed at the tubule and can be used to evaluate the percent of functioning nephrons. Normally the plasma creatinine concentration is 0.6 to 1.3 mg/dl, with men's levels being somewhat more elevated than women's. This value in most individuals, except for times of muscle damage, remains almost constant and is inversely proportional to the number of functioning nephrons, or the *glomerular filtration rate*. For example, if for some reason the number of functioning nephrons (glomerular filtration) drops, the excretion of creatinine in the urine (urine creatinine concentration) will decrease and the level of plasma creatinine will rise. Therefore, the level of plasma creatinine can be used to roughly estimate the number of functioning nephrons. Sudden changes in glomerular filtration (ie, renal artery thrombosis) will not cause immediate changes in the plasma creatinine. However, progressive retention will cause the plasma creatinine concentration to gradually rise. Two mechanisms aid in this attempt to maintain balance. First, compensation by remaining undamaged nephrons leads to increased filtration in functioning areas and, secondly, renal tubules can actively secrete creatinine and do so increasingly with rising levels of plasma creatinine. Plasma creatinine valves are best used to gauge GFR and to follow stable disease. *(Williams, p. 157)*

4. **(A)** Normally, there are no red blood cells present in a voided urine specimen. Anything greater than 3 to 4 RBCs per HPF is considered abnormal. Hematuria may be "gross" (visible to the naked eye) or microscopic, and the severity of hematuria may *not* be proportional to its clinical significance. Hematuria may be caused by glomerular bleeding, extraglomerular renal bleeding or extrarenal bleeding. *(Coe, p. 194)*

5. **(B)** Acute pyelonephritis often presents with fever, chills, flank pain, and dysuria. Urinalysis will reveal pyuria and often WBC casts. Cystitis and urethral infection do not affect the kidney and should not have casts. Renal tuberculosis should be considered when there is hematuria and "sterile" pyuria. Drug-induced tubulointerstitial nephritis will produce hematuria, pyuria, proteinuria and, at times, eosinophiluria. *(Walker, pp. 732–733)*

6. **(B)** Flank pain radiating to the groin, often crescendo and decrescendo in nature, and hematuria are the cardinal signs and symptoms of nephrolithiasis. The nature of the pain is intense and often associated with nausea. Patients may have nonspecific irritative symptoms of the urinary bladder. *Fever* should not be associated with nephrolithiasis and is a sign of impending sepsis. *(Walker, p. 778)*

7. **(A)** Calcium compounds are responsible for approximately 90% of all noninfected, non-struvite stones. The most common compounds are calcium oxalate and calcium phosphate. *(Walker, p. 775)*

8–12. 8. (A); 9. (C); 10. (D); 11. (D); 12. (E)

TABLE 1

	Nephrotic Syndrome	Acute Glomerulonephritis	Berger's Disease	Goodpasture's Syndrome	SLE
Presenting Signs and Symptoms	Massive loss of protein and associated lipiduria and edema. Variable renal function. If associated with systemic disease, those findings BUN and creatinine.	Usually follows pharyngitis, 3–12 incubation period, then decrease urine volume, edema and hematuria. Signs and symptoms of azotemia.	Mild to heavy gross hematuria that are episodic in nature and in association with proteinuria with slowly progressive renal failure.	Profuse and persistent hemoptysis with progressive renal insufficiency.	Fever, malaise, weight loss, joint symptoms & "butterfly" rash.
Labaratory Findings	Massive amounts of protein, but few formed elements. Some fatty casts, granular cast, no RBCs, RBC cast.	Urinalysis reveals hematuria, RBC cast and proteinuria. Positive ASO titers.	Varying disease of hematuria, RBC casts and proteinuria. Progressive azotemia, high serum IgA.	Anti-glomerular basement membrane antibodies in the serum. -	Positive ANA —occasional hematuria and mild proteinuria with or without RBC casts.
Pathologic Findings	Three types: (1) Nil disease—essentially normal findings. (2) Membranous glomerulonephritis—thickening of basement membrane and hypercellularity. (3) Focal sclerosing glomerulonephritis patchy involvement.	Epithelial deposits of IgG and hypercellularity.	Focal areas of hypercellularity (mostly endothelial and mesangical cells) and deposits of IgA and IgG.	Immunofluorescence of IgG deposits in the glomerular basement membrane on kidney biopsy.	Characterized by the presence of many different autoantibodies.
Treatment	Supportive	Penicillin, bedrest, salt restriction, antihypertensives as needed.	No treatment has demonstrated improvement or slows progression.	Corticosteroids and cyclophosphamide or azathioprine.	Corticosteroids and immunosuppressive agents such as cyclophosphamide or azathioprine.

(Walker, pp. 737–751)

13. **(E)** The complete absence of urine formation is relatively rare, even patients with very poor renal function usually void effectively. Anuria suggests a problem of outlet obstruction. One should consider two possibilities: obstruction above the bladder (rare unless there is a solitary kidney or periureteral metastasis) or bladder outlet obstruction. Bladder outlet obstruction is rare in women but is common in males, especially those who are prone to develop prostate hypertrophy, have a history of urethritis (especially gonorrhea) or have had previous instrumentation. Diagnosis and initial treatment can be made by insertion of a bladder catheter. *(Walker, p. 757)*

14. **(C)** When a patient presents with oliguria, historical information should be obtained and physical examination and laboratory data gathered to determine if the cause is prerenal, postrenal, or due to intrinsic renal disease. Prerenal causes of oliguria include any insult to the kidney that reduces cardiac output to the kidney, none is sug-

gested here. As mentioned earlier, postrenal or obstructive oliguria is rare in women, as long as the patient has two functioning kidneys. In this case, the patient's oliguria is most likely from an intrinsic renal problem. With a history of recent intravenous contrast media, a common toxic cause of acute renal failure, the most likely cause is radiographic contrast media toxicity. *(Walker, pp. 756–760)*

15. **(B)** Acute bacterial prostatitis is characterized by irritative bladder symptoms, fever, chills, and perineal discomfort. Pathogens in this disease are usually those associated with UTI, the gram-negative organisms. Patients usually respond dramatically to antibiotic therapy. Therapy should be continued for at least 30 days to prevent chronic prostatitis. Of the choices listed, trimethoprim-sulfamethoxazole 160/800 mg for 30 days is correct, due to its superior coverage of gram negative organisms and the duration of therapy. *(Meares, pp. 223–224)*

**16–23.   16. (B); 17. (C); 18. (E); 19. (A); 20. (A);
21. (D); 22. (C); 23. (D)**

TABLE 2

	Cryptorchism	Testicular Torsion	Testicular Tumors	Acute Epidydimitis	Hydrocele
Age	At birth	Adolescents	Early adolescence to mid-twenties	Most common in sexually active men and the elderly.	Can occur at any age, especially in infancy and in the elderly.
Pathophysiology	Testicle has failed to descend normally, cause is unclear.	Rotation of the testicle and spermatic cord on its axis leads to strangulation of its blood supply.	Neoplasms of the testicle are rare but the most common neoplasm in 15- to 25-year-old males; 90% are germ cell tumors.	Infection of epidy-dimis. Often an extension of infection elsewhere in urinary tract, such as with urethritis or UTI.	A collection of fluid in the potential space between tunica vaginalis and testicle. Can follow acute inflammatory processes, be in association with testicular tumors, or of unknown etiology.
Signs and Symptoms	On exam, testicle is not palpable in scrotum.	Sudden onset of severe pain in one testicle with an edema, erythema, retracted testicle on same side.	Small painless mass of the testicle, often with elevated tumor markers.	Acute onset of extremely painful, swollen testicle with fever, chills.	A rounded mass in scrotum anterior to the testicle, rarely painful; can be large; transluminates.
Treatment	Hormonal or surgical	Emergent surgical consultation to spare testicle.	Orchiectomy alpha-fetoprotein and human chorionic gonadotropin are used to follow for recurrence.	Treat likely organism (ie, GC, chlamydia or *E. coli*); scrotal support; may require admission if toxic.	Therapy is not required unless painful or when the testicle cannot be palpated to rule out carcinoma in at-risk populations.
Prognosis	Microscopic changes in undescended testicles noted in early childhood and leads to marked increase in neoplasms in untreated males.	If testicle can be detorsed before 12 hours, preservation is good.	Early diagnosis most always leads to complete cure; late disease does not respond well to therapy.	Can lead to chronic epididymitis, testicular atrophy.	Patients can have large hydroceles with no complaints often treated for cosmetics. Only serious if testicle cannot be palpated.

(McAnich, pp. 616–624)

24. (E) Hyperchloremic acidosis results from impaired renal excretion of acid and decreased serum bicarbonate. Sulfate and phosphate are excreted normally and increased reabsorption of chloride ions is also found. This form of metabolic acidosis is due to renal insufficiency and results in an increase in the normal ion gap. *(Coe, p. 1208)*

25. (D) Parathyroid hormone (PTH) arises in the parathyroid gland. Antidiuretic hormone (ADH) is made in the neurohypophysis and is active once it is released. Vitamin D (25-hydroxyvitamin D) is converted to its active form in the kidney. Its active metabolite, 1,25-dihydroxycholecalciferol, or another metabolite, 24,25-dihydroxycholecalciferol, are produced from the hydroxylation of 25-hydroxycholecalciferol. Vitamin D acts with PTH to maintain the level of ionized calcium in extracellular fluid. Vitamin D is best known for enhancing the intestinal absorption of calcium. Aldosterone is secreted in its active form from the adrenal cortex. *(Fitzgerald, pp. 876–877)*

REFERENCES

Coe FL. Alterations in urinary function. In Braunwald et al (eds). *Harrison's Principles of Internal Medicine,* 11th ed. New York: McGraw-Hill; 1987.

Fitzgerald PA. The parathyroids. In Tierney LM et al (eds). *Current Medical Diagnosis and Treatment.* Norwalk, CT: Appleton & Lange; 1993.

McAnich JW. Disorders of the testis, scrotum, and spermatic cord. In Tanagho EA, McAnich JW (eds). *Smith's General Urology,* 13th ed. Norwalk, CT: Appleton & Lange; 1988.

Meares EM. Nonspecific infections of the genitourinary tract. In Tanagho EA, McAnich JW (eds). *Smith's General Urology,* 13th ed. Norwalk, CT: Appleton & Lange; 1988.

Stam WE, Turck M. Urinary tract infection, pyelonephritis, and related conditions. In Braunwald et al (eds). *Harrison's Principles of Internal Medicine,* 11th ed. New York: McGraw-Hill; 1987.

Walker WG. Oliguria and acute renal failure. In Harvey AM et al (eds). *The Principles and Practice of Medicine,* 22nd ed. Norwalk, CT: Appleton & Lange; 1988.

Walker WG. Renal calculi. In Harvey AM et al (eds). *The Principles and Practice of Medicine,* 22nd ed. Norwalk, CT: Appleton & Lange; 1988.

Walker WG, Mitch WE. Pathophysiology of uremia and clinical evaluation of renal function. In Harvey AM et al (eds). *The Principles and Practice of Medicine,* 22nd ed. Norwalk, CT: Appleton & Lange; 1988.

Walker WG, Solez K. The proteinurias and hematurias. In Harvey AM et al (eds). *The Principles and Practice of Medicine,* 22nd ed. Norwalk, CT: Appleton & Lange; 1988.

Williams RD. Urologic laboratory examination. In Tanagho EA, McAninch JW (eds). *Smith's General Urology,* 13th ed. Norwalk, CT: Appleton & Lange; 1992.

Subspecialty List: Renal

Internal Medicine: Pulmonary
Questions

DIRECTIONS (Questions 1 through 5): Each set of items in this section consists of a list of lettered options followed by several numbered words or phrases. For each numbered word or phrase, select the ONE lettered option that is most closely associated with it. Each lettered option may be selected once, more than once, or not at all.

Questions 1 through 5

Select the most probable diagnosis given this initial presentation.

(A) *Streptococcus pneumoniae*
(B) mycoplasma pneumonia
(C) Legionnaire's disease (*L. pneumophilia*)
(D) *Pneumocystis carinii* pneumonia
(E) viral pneumonia

1. A 25-year-old white male with shortness of breath and a nonproductive cough. The patient's temperature is 103.5°F, respiration 40, and pulse 140. Physical exam reveals a thin dyspneic male in moderate respiratory distress, scattered rhonchi, and peripheral cyanosis. Chest x-ray reveals a diffuse interstitial infiltrate.

2. A 45-year-old black female with a one-week history of clear nasal drainage suddenly develops a single shaking chill followed by fever and cough productive of thick yellow mucous. Her temperature is 103°F. Rales are noted at the right base. Chest x-ray shows a right lower lobe pneumonia.

3. An 18-year-old female college co-ed complains of a three-day history of fever, headache, sore throat, left ear pain, and a productive cough of watery sputum. On exam, left bullous myringitis is noted. A chest x-ray reveals a left lower lobe segmental pneumonia.

4. A 58-year-old male smoker returns from vacation at the beach with anorexia, malaise, and a minimal cough that is nonproductive. The patient's wife states he has a continuous fever of 103.7°F,

respirations are 22, and the pulse rate is 55. Exam reveals dry oral membranes and rales over the right base with sharp stabbing pain upon inspiration. Chest x-ray shows a bilateral lower lobe pneumonia.

5. A 21-year-old Oriental male presents with diffuse myalgias, photophobia, and a nonproductive cough. His temperature is 100.8°F, and exam reveals slight nasal congestion, expiratory wheeze, and erythema multiforme. A chest x-ray shows scattered nodular interstitial infiltrate pattern.

DIRECTIONS (Questions 6 through 30): Each of the numbered items or incomplete statements in this section is followed by answers or by completions of the statement. Select the ONE lettered answer or completion that is BEST in each case.

Questions 6 through 30

6. A 50-year-old male presents with a history of persistent cough, hemoptysis, and weight loss. He states he has had "several lung infections" over the past 3 to 4 months. The patient is a 30-pack-per-year smoker, and also complains of right shoulder and chest pain. The patient is afebrile, pale, and dyspneic with exertion. The chest x-ray suggests mediastinal widening and perihilar adenopathy. Which of the following diagnoses is most consistent with the given history?

(A) bronchiectasis
(B) chronic obstructive pulmonary disease
(C) chronic bronchitis
(D) asthma
(E) bronchogenic carcinoma

7. A 62-year-old male patient presents with a history of exertional dyspnea and chronic cough that is worse in the morning. On exam, you notice decreased breath and heart sounds, an expiratory wheeze, and increased anterior-posterior chest diameter. The patient has a 42-pack-per-year history of smoking, and a chest x-ray shows hyperinflation of the lungs and flattened diaphragm. The FEV_1 and vital capacity are decreased. Which is the most likely diagnosis?

(A) emphysema
(B) congestive heart failure
(C) pulmonary embolism
(D) chronic bronchitis
(E) carcinoma of the lung

8. In the above patient, which of the following would improve pulmonary function and longevity?

(A) oxygen at 2 L/min by nasal cannula
(B) aminophylline intravenously; loading dose followed by oral theophylline
(C) antibiotics for suppressive therapy
(D) exercise reconditioning
(E) none of the above

9. Which of the following tests is the LEAST helpful in the diagnosis of bronchogenic carcinoma?

(A) sputum cytology
(B) bronchoscopy and biopsy
(C) ventilation–perfusion scan
(D) pulmonary function test
(E) CAT scan

10. Which of the following is the best screening exam for carcinoma of the lung?

(A) CAT scan
(B) bronchoscopy
(C) sputum cytology
(D) chest x-ray with previous comparison
(E) arterial blood gases

11. Which of the following is the most common cause for chronic obstructive pulmonary disease?

(A) air pollution
(B) recurrent infection
(C) smoking
(D) asthma
(E) trauma

12. Which is the most common cell type found in primary pulmonary neoplasm?

(A) small cell
(B) bronchioloalveolar cell
(C) large cell
(D) squamous cell
(E) hamartoma

13. A 19-year-old female is involved in an automobile accident; she is hospitalized with a fractured femur. Her past medical history is unremarkable. The patient suddenly develops dyspnea, cough, and anxiety, with retrosternal lateralized chest pain. Vital signs are pulse 120, respiration 32, blood pressure 120/80, and temperature 100.1°F. Chest x-ray shows mild bilateral atelectasis, and the ECG is normal. The most likely diagnosis is

(A) pneumonia
(B) myocardial infarction
(C) pulmonary embolism
(D) costochondritis with hyperventilation
(E) unrecognized pneumothorax

14. The most common cause of hemoptysis is

(A) tuberculosis
(B) trauma
(C) bronchogenic carcinoma
(D) bronchitis
(E) pulmonary embolism

15. Deep regular respirations with periods of apnea best describe

(A) Cheyne–Stokes respiration
(B) Biot's breathing
(C) Kussmaul's respiration
(D) stridulous breathing
(E) apnea

16. A 21-year-old thin male presents to your office with a sudden onset of vague chest pain radiating to the left shoulder, dyspnea, and cough. He states that his past medical history is unremarkable except for smoking. The onset of the above symptoms occurred while playing basketball. Vital signs are unremarkable except for a pulse of 110 and a respiratory rate of 28. You note decreased breath sounds, hyperresonance, and decreased vocal fremitus on the left thorax. At this time the most likely diagnosis is

(A) mycoplasmal pneumonia
(B) work-induced asthma
(C) spontaneous pneumothorax
(D) bronchial carcinoma
(E) aortic stenosis with angina

17. During your examination of the above patient, the x-ray returns to reveal air in the pleural space with visible retracted lung border; there is no pleural effusion. Treatment should consist of

    (A) nitroglycerin IV
    (B) epinephrine subcutaneously
    (C) further investigation with a CAT scan of the chest
    (D) aspiration of the air with a large needle or chest tube
    (E) endotracheal intubation

18. The most sensitive test for the diagnosis of a pulmonary embolism is

    (A) CAT scan of the chest
    (B) ECG
    (C) arterial blood gases
    (D) ventilation–perfusion scan
    (E) chest x-ray

19. A 22-year-old female presents to the emergency department with extreme shortness of breath after jogging. No past medical history is immediately available. Vital signs are pulse 120, respiration 32, temperature 98.7°F, and blood pressure 130/84. Exam reveals a lethargic and confused patient; there are diffuse expiratory wheezes and a prolonged expiratory phase. Hyperresonance to percussion is noted. The most likely diagnosis is

    (A) pneumothorax
    (B) bronchial asthma
    (C) bronchiolitis
    (D) pulmonary edema
    (E) pneumonia

20. Which of the following is not a clinical finding associated with adult respiratory distress syndrome (ARDS)?

    (A) tachypnea
    (B) air bronchogram
    (C) cardiomegaly
    (D) multiple organ failure
    (E) diffuse patchy infiltrate

21. Which of the following factors may precipitate an asthma attack?

    (A) anxiety
    (B) air pollution
    (C) exercise
    (D) beta-adrenergic blocking agents
    (E) all of the above

22. Which agent provides the most rapid effect and best therapeutic index in the treatment of asthma?

    (A) inhaled beta-adrenergic agonist medication
    (B) subcutaneous epinephrine
    (C) intravenous aminophylline
    (D) hydrocortisone
    (E) oral aminophylline

23. Which of the following is not an expected sign or symptom of pulmonary hypertension?

    (A) fatigue
    (B) dyspnea
    (C) right axis deviation
    (D) left atrial enlargement
    (E) cor pulmonale

24. During spontaneous ventilation, venous return to the heart is greatest

    (A) at end exhalation
    (B) during inhalation
    (C) during exhalation
    (D) at end inhalation
    (E) venous return to the heart is constant throughout spontaneous ventilation

25. Of the following, the best of all clinical respiratory measurements for assessing the progress of different types of pulmonary fibrotic diseases is

    (A) arterial blood gases
    (B) vital capacity
    (C) inspiratory reserve volume
    (D) total lung capacity
    (E) tidal volume

26. A child is brought to your office with high fever, difficulty swallowing, and drooling over the past several hours. On exam you notice an ill-appearing child with inspiratory stridor, breath sounds that are equal bilaterally, and symmetrical chest movement. The most likely diagnosis is

    (A) epiglottitis
    (B) bacterial pharyngitis
    (C) viral croup
    (D) foreign body aspiration
    (E) pneumonia

27. Of the following, the best and safest way to approach the child described in Question 26 would be

(A) direct visualization of the pharynx with a tongue blade

(B) obtaining a lateral soft tissue x-ray prior to exam

(C) direct visualization with the aid of a laryngoscope

(D) obtaining a bronchoscopy as soon as possible

(E) obtaining a rapid strep screen by blindly swabbing the oropharynx

28. A 2-year-old patient is brought to the emergency department by his mother with sudden onset of choking, gagging, coughing, and wheezing. The patient was last seen playing on the floor with several small toys. Vital signs are respiration 28, pulse 120, and temperature 98.6°F. Exam reveals decreased breath sounds over the right lower lobe with inspiratory rhonchi and a localized expiratory wheeze. Chest x-ray shows normal inspiratory views, but expiratory views show localized hyperinflation with mediastinal shift to the left. The most likely diagnosis is

(A) viral croup

(B) subglottic tumor

(C) foreign-body aspiration

(D) epiglottitis

(E) asthmatic bronchitis

29. In the above patient, the correct way to progress in the treatment of this case would be

(A) chest physiotherapy

(B) cool-mist therapy with racemic epinephrine

(C) bronchoscopy as soon as possible

(D) intubation as soon as possible

(E) antibiotics with antitussives

30. A 28-year-old female presents with sudden onset of shortness of breath, circumoral and carpopedal dysesthesia (tingling sensation), and carpopedal spasm. She complains of vague chest pain. Review of systems is unremarkable except for recent increase in stress at work. Vital signs are respiration 32, pulse 82, blood pressure 110/70, and temperature 98.6°F. ECG is normal. Exam reveals tachypnea, although the patient's breath sounds are normal, and the exam is otherwise normal. The most likely diagnosis is

(A) pneumonia

(B) primary pulmonary hypertension

(C) asthma

(D) hyperventilation

(E) myocardial infarction

DIRECTIONS (Questions 31 through 50): For each of the items in this section, ONE or MORE of the numbered options is correct. Choose answer

(A) if only (1), (2), and (3) are correct,

(B) if only (1) and (3) are correct,

(C) if only (2) and (4) are correct,

(D) if only (4) is correct,

(E) if all are correct.

Questions 31 through 50

31. The most commonly encountered endocrine syndromes found in lung cancer are

(1) inappropriate antidiuretic hormone secretion

(2) Cushing's syndrome

(3) gynecomastia

(4) hypothyroidism

32. Which of the following tests are best used to differentiate between restrictive and obstructive pulmonary disease?

(1) total lung capacity

(2) ventilation–perfusion scanning

(3) forced expiratory volume in 1 second divided by the forced vital capacity

(4) chest x-ray

33. Which of the following are physical findings consistent with a consolidated pneumonia?

(1) rales

(2) increased vocal fremitus

(3) dullness with percussion

(4) decreased whispered pectoriloquy

34. A patient newly diagnosed with pulmonary embolism should have which of the following treatment considerations?

(1) heparin therapy

(2) oxygen therapy

(3) thrombolitic therapy

(4) continued activities to prevent pneumonia

35. Which of the following might indicate that a trial of corticosteriods would be worthwhile in a patient with chronic obstructive pulmonary disease (COPD)?

(1) improved forced expiratory volume after 1 second greater than 20% after inhalation of a bronchodilator

(2) a history of fluctuation in the severity of pulmonary symptoms

(3) the finding of a prominent wheeze or "noisy" chest on physical examination

(4) finding of eosinophilia of the blood or sputum on microscopic examination

36. Which of the following clinical manifestations would you NOT expect to find in a patient with primary pulmonary hypertension?

(1) dyspnea

(2) chest pain resembling angina

(3) hoarseness

(4) clubbing

37. Which of the following could be used to determine if there is partial airway obstruction above or below the tracheal bifurcation?

(1) stridor

(2) pulmonary function tests

(3) chest x-ray

(4) ventilation–perfusion scanning

38. Initial treatment of COPD should include

(1) bronchodilators

(2) elimination of smoking

(3) instruction on bronchial hygiene

(4) corticosteroids

39. Findings consistent with a severe bronchial asthma attack would include which of the following?

(1) chest silent to auscultation

(2) $Paco_2 < 35$ mm Hg normal (35 to 45)

(3) $Paco_2 > 45$ mm Hg normal (35 to 45)

(4) loud generalized wheezes to auscultation

40. A 60-year-old male presents to your office with a history of asthma, new onset hypertension, and angina. The patient notes no change in his stable angina pattern. On exam you notice moderate expiratory wheezes and the patient states he has noted worsening of his asthma over the past week. There are no rales, jugular venous distention, or pedal edema noted on exam. His medications include Theodur (theophylline), 200 mg bid; Ventolin (albuterol) inhaler, 2 puffs qid; nitroglycerin patch, 10 cm^2 applied daily; and Inderal (propanolol), 40 mg bid recently added for control of hypertension. Vital signs are blood pressure 160/100, pulse 52, respiration +30; the patient is afebrile. Appropriate management of this patient should include

(1) epinephrine, 0.3 mL of 1:1000 solution subcutaneously

(2) obtain a theophylline level

(3) increase propanolol for better control of hypertension

(4) discontinue propanolol and start a calcium channel blocking agent

41. A 54-year-old male is brought to the emergency room by ambulance after a fall from 10 feet. The patient presents in acute respiratory distress. Vital signs are pulse 110, blood pressure 94/60, and respiration 38. Exam reveals marked decrease in breath sounds on the right, with dullness. Stat portable chest x-ray reveals a large air–fluid level on the right. Initial treatment of this patient should include

(1) establish two large-bore IVs with lactated Ringer's solution

(2) obtain blood for a CBC and type and cross-matching for possible blood transfusion

(3) placement of a right-sided chest tube

(4) perform an immediate thoracotomy in the emergency department

42. Which of the following will deliver oxygen in a concentration of 40% or above?

(1) face mask with oxygen reservoir

(2) nasal cannula at 2 L/min

(3) face mask without oxygen reservoir at 10 L/min

(4) mouth-to-mouth ventilation

43. Respiration is stimulated by which of the following?

(1) arterial pH

(2) exercise

(3) arterial Pco_2

(4) arterial Po_2

44. A term neonate is admitted to the neonatal intensive care unit after resuscitation with the diagnosis of meconium aspiration. Which of the following should be initiated in the management of this child?

(1) chest physiotherapy and suctioning of the oropharynx

(2) transcutaneous monitoring of the Po_2

(3) chest x-ray

(4) fluid restriction

45. Which of the following are risk factors for the development of hyaline membrane disease?

(1) female sex of child

(2) prematurity

(3) vaginal delivery

(4) maternal diabetes

46. The initial evaluation of hemoptysis should include

    (1) Gram stain of sputum
    (2) tuberculin skin test
    (3) chest x-ray
    (4) immediate bronchoscopy

47. A thoracentesis is performed on a patient with a pleural effusion on chest x-ray. The fluid obtained is cloudy with a protein greater than 3.5 g/dL and a specific gravity of 1.020. The differential diagnosis for this patient would include

    (1) bacterial infection
    (2) severe anemia
    (3) rheumatoid arthritis
    (4) liver disease

48. Which of the following statements are true concerning a pulmonary abscess?

    (1) They are frequently caused by aspiration related to altered consciousness.
    (2) Anaerobic bacteria are the primary organism recovered.
    (3) Cultures can reveal multiple bacterial organisms.
    (4) They are uncommon in edentulous patients.

49. Which of the following pneumonias is not likely to be complicated by the formation of a pulmonary abscess?

    (1) *Klebsiella pneumoniae*
    (2) *Staphylococcus aureus*
    (3) *Streptococcus pyogens*
    (4) pneumococcal pneumonia

50. Which of the following would you expect in a fresh water near-drowning patient?

    (1) hypoxia
    (2) pulmonary edema
    (3) acidosis
    (4) marked electrolyte abnormalities

Answers and Explanations

1. **(D)** *Pneumocystis carinii* pneumonia (PCP) is the most common opportunistic infection in AIDS. PCP is the initial infection in 60% of AIDS cases and occurs 80% at some time during the illness. The patient usually presents as acutely ill with an abrupt onset of tachypnea, mild cough, and cyanosis. Severe hypoxia is commonly present. Chest x-ray commonly shows diffuse interstitial infiltrates. *(Hardwood-Nuss et al, pp. 1048–1050)*

2. **(A)** Streptococcal pneumonia is still the most common community-acquired pneumonia, occurring between 40% and 80% of the time in this setting. The classical onset involves a single shaking chill, fever, and cough productive of yellow-green to rusty or bloody mucous. Gram stain reveals gram-positive diplococci, and chest x-ray most typically shows a single lobar pneumonia. *(Hardwood et al, pp. 910–912)*

3. **(B)** Mycoplasma pneumonia is a common cause of pneumonia in children and young adults, accounting for 10% to 50% of community-acquired pneumonias. Fever, headaches, and malaise precede the onset of pulmonary symptoms. Sputum is usually scant and sometimes blood-tinged. Bullous myringitis occurs in less than 25% of the cases. Tetracycline and erythromycin are drugs of choice. *(Hardwood et al, pp. 912–913; Wyngaarten and Smith, pp. 1561–1565)*

4. **(C)** Legionellosis most commonly occur in the summer. Other factors that are associated with risk of *L. pneumophilia* include male, middle or old age, smoking, and alcoholism. Sputum is usually scant along with influenza-type symptoms of fever, headache, and anorexia. Pleuritic chest pain, tachypnea, and lower than expected pulse rate often occurs. Chest x-ray shows patchy infiltrate, which progresses to lobar or segmented patterns and is commonly bilateral. *(Wyngaarden and Smith, pp. 1570–1572)*

5. **(E)** Influenza virus, adenovirus, and respiratory syncytial virus account for the majority of viral pneumonias. Coryza and sore throat, mild to moderate fever, myalgias, malaise, headache, and photophobia are common. Wheezing and dyspnea may develop as the disease progresses. Rash, conjuctivitis, and inflammation of the nasal mucosa may also be noted. Radiographs typically reveal a reticulonodular interstitial pattern. *(Hardwood-Nuss et al, pp. 912–913).*

6. **(E)** The clinical manifestations of bronchogenic carcinoma can vary, and many patients are asymptomatic when the pulmonary lesion is discovered. Cough, usually productive of scant sputum is a common symptom, hemoptysis frequently occurs secondary to ulceration in the pulmonary lesion. Frequently, because of a significant smoking history, patients with carcinoma also have obstructive pulmonary disease and dyspnea with exertion. Weight loss is also a common complaint of bronchogenic carcinoma but generally occurs with more extensive disease beyond the time frame that the neoplasm is limited to the lung. Chest pain may be due to pleural involvement but must also suggest metastatic disease. Pulmonary infections occur distal to the bronchial obstruction and can mask the tumor. Any atypical or recurrent pulmonary infection should suggest carcinoma. Chest x-ray may demonstrate hilar and mediastinal lymph node involvement, pleural effusion, rib metastasis, elevation of a diaphragm, tracheal compression or distortion, and pericardial effusion. Although pulmonary diseases, particularly at end stages, present with similar symptoms, the entire history, physical, laboratory, and roentgenographic findings must be correlated to form the correct diagnosis. Asthma and chronic obstructive pulmonary disease usually reveal hyperinflation of the lungs and flat diaphragms. Bronchiectasis shows coarse lung markings and even honeycombing due to the abnormal dilatation of the bronchial tree. Chronic bronchitis has been used in various ways, sometimes referring to a simple smoker's cough and at other times to severe COPD. It is usually described as a productive cough that is present on most days for at least 3 months of the year. *(Wyngaarden and Smith et al, pp. 457–460).*

7. **(A)** Emphysema is characterized by loss of elastic recoil of the lungs, resulting in abnormally enlarged air spaces with destructive changes in the alveolar walls. Pathogenesis is uncertain; there appears to be an inherited component. However, cigarette smoking is the major etiologic factor in developing emphysema. Diagnosis is usually inferred from clinical and lab findings. Dyspnea, chronic cough, and decreased pulmonary function occur with advanced disease. Radiograghic exam reveals an increase in the A-P diameter, with hyperinflation and depression of the diaphragms. *(Andreoli et al, p. 146)*

8. **(E)** All the answers may help the patient symptomatically, but there is no effective way, over the long term, to improve pulmonary function and longevity in emphysema. *(Tierney et al, pp. 197–200)*

9. **(D)** Pulmonary function tests are helpful in determining restrictive from obstructive pulmonary diseases but do not aid in the diagnosis of pulmonary carcinoma. Sputum cytology can yield a diagnosis in 40% to 60% of cases, and bronchoscopy with biopsy can give one a direct view of the lesion, as well as yield positive results in 75% to 80% of cases of pulmonary neoplasm. CAT scan is helpful in the visualization and location of a pulmonary lesion and is also helpful in the determination of metastases. Ventilation–perfusion scanning is a sensitive test for the examination for regional lung function and may be helpful in the diagnosis of pulmonary carcinoma. *(Andreoli et al, p. 167; Tierney et al, pp. 220–222)*

10. **(D)** All the examinations, except arterial blood gases, are helpful in the diagnosis of pulmonary carcinoma (see answer to Question 9). However, the chest x-ray, when compared to previous films, is the least expensive and least invasive examination. Therefore, it is the best screening exam for bronchogenic carcinoma. *(Tierney et al, pp. 220–221).*

11. **(C)** COPD results from some combination of chronic obstructive problems and pulmonary emphysema; both disorders are closely related to cigarette smoking. It is generally believed that emphysema results from the effect of proteolytic enzymes on lung tissue. When there is a very severe congenital deficiency of serum antiproteolytic activity, it is likely that emphysema will develop even if the subject does not smoke. This deficiency results in 0.5% to 2% of cases of COPD. The development of emphysema depends on prolonged exposure to noxious irritants, usually cigarette smoke. *(Wyngaarden and Smith, pp. 414–415)*

12. **(D)** Squamous cell and adenocarcinoma are the most common types of bronchogenic carcinoma accounting for about 30% to 35% each of primary tumors. Small-cell and large-cell tumors account for about 20% to 25% and 15%, respectively. Brochioloalveolar cell carcinoma represents about 2% of cases of bronchogenic carcinoma. Hamartoma is the most common type of benign lung tumor. *(Tierney et al, pp. 220–225).*

13. **(C)** People at risk for pulmonary embolism are those with hypercoagulable states, which may arise from the use of birth control pills, local stasis, immobilization that may be the result of an accident or illness, fractures, obesity, and congestive heart failure. Emboli that cause clinically significant pulmonary insult commonly arise in the ileofemoral and pelvic venous beds. Signs and symptoms often begin abruptly and include dyspnea, cough, anxiety, and chest pain (frequently pleuritic in nature). Hemoptysis may occur; tachycardia and tachypnea are common in this illness. A low-grade fever, hypotension, and cyanosis are also signs of pulmonary embolism. The presence of a deep venous thrombosis aids in the rapid clinical diagnosis. Radiographic evidence of consolidation may be present in cases of pulmonary embolism. *(Saunders and Ho, pp. 464,473–474)*

14. **(D)** Hemoptysis is the expectoration of blood or bloody sputum. Some of the important causes of hemoptysis include pneumonias, pulmonary emboli, bronchogenic carcinoma, mitral stenosis, COPD, tuberculosis, and other granulomatous diseases. However, the most common cause of hemoptysis is bronchitis. *(Sharts, pp. 215–216).*

15. **(A)** Cheyne–Stokes respiration is the most common form of periodic breathing. Periods of apnea alternate regularly with series of respiratory cycles. In each cycle, the rate and amplitude of successive respirations increase to a maximum, then decrease progressively until the series is terminated with an apneic period. Kussmaul respiration is applied to deep, regular, sighing respirations, regardless of rate. This pattern of breathing is seen in diabetic ketoacidosis, uremia, peritonitis, severe hemorrhage, and pneumonia. Biot's breathing is an uncommon variant of Cheyne–Stokes respiration, in which periods of apnea alternate irregularly with series of breaths of equal depth. This is most often seen in meningitis. Stridulous breathing is a high-pitched whistling or crowing sound with respirations when the air passes over a partially closed glottis. This occurs with edema of the vocal cords (ie, infection), neoplasm, abscess of the pharynx, and foreign body in the pharynx. Apnea is simply the absence of respiration. *(DeGowin and DeGowin, pp. 270–281)*

16. **(C)** Spontaneous pneumothorax is more likely to occur in young, thin, tall individuals. The patient usually complains of chest pain, dyspnea, or

cough, usually during exertion. Physical exam reveals decreased breath sounds, increased resonance, and decreased fremitus on the involved side. There may be deviation of the trachea and heart to the side opposite that of involvement. Distention of the neck veins may be visible if the pneumothorax is under tension and hypotension may occur. *(Saunders and Ho, pp. 271–272)*

17. **(D)** The description of the x-ray confirms the diagnosis of pneumothorax. Aspiration of the air to allow reexpansion of the lung must occur. This is most quickly achieved by aspiration with a large-bore needle but, frequently, chest tubes are required. Cough should be suppressed; pain control and bedrest are essential. Endotracheal intubation is not required in this patient. CAT scan delays the needed treatment, and the other choices are not beneficial in the treatment of a pneumothorax. *(Saunders and Ho, p. 272)*

18. **(D)** The ventilation–perfusion scan is the most sensitive screening procedure for embolization. The perfusion of the embolized area is profoundly impaired with minimal impairment of ventilation. A negative study of good technical quality excludes angiographically detectable pulmonary embolism. Chest x-rays are abnormal in most patients with pulmonary embolization with infarction; the abnormalities are, however, often nonspecific. ECGs are often normal or may show nonspecific changes. Clinically significant embolization is almost always associated with hypoxemia; however, this may be obscured by reflex hyperventilation and hypocapnia. Pulmonary angiography allows direct visualization of the vascular tree and is the procedure of choice for establishing the diagnosis. Nonetheless, this procedure has obvious limitations, and because of the controversy in this area, the choice of this procedure was not included in the answers. *(Mills et al, p. 535; Beeson et al, pp. 444–445)*

19. **(B)** With the history of acute onset of dyspnea during exertion and the findings of hyperresonance, expiratory wheezes, and prolonged expiratory phase, the obvious diagnosis is bronchial asthma. There are many aggravating activities and substances for the exacerbation of asthma, including infection, drugs, exertion, cold, inhaled irritants, and emotional stress. During an asthma attack, bronchospasm and hypersecretion of mucus results in airway obstruction and air trapping. Most patients with asthma are hypocapneic as a result of reflex hyperventilation. However, with progressive airway obstruction, fatigue, and increasing retention of carbon dioxide, mental status changes can occur and are evidence of a severe, possibly life-threatening episode. *(Saunders and Ho, pp. 457–459)*

20. **(C)** ARDS classically presents with rapid onset of tachypnea and dyspnea following the initiating event. Chest x-ray reveals diffuse patchy infiltrates that at first are interstitial and then become alveolar. Air bronchograms occur in 80% of patients. Most patients with ARDS demonstrate multiple organ failure commonly involving the kidneys, liver, gut, CNS, and cardiovascular systems. Heart size is normal and pleural effusions are small or nonexistent. *(Tierney et al, pp. 253–255)*

21. **(E)** All the choices may aggravate or stimulate an asthma attack. Inhaled allergens typically produce immediate "Type I," IgE-mediated allergic reaction in the airway, although "Type III," IgG-mediated reactions may also occur in some patients. The parasympathetic nervous system also plays a part in the asthmatic response. Cholinergic stimulation induces mediator production in the mast cell and causes contraction of bronchial smooth muscle. Vigorous exercise produces bronchoconstriction in some asthmatic patients. Furthermore, beta-adrenergic blockers as well as indomethacin, aspirin, and certain yellow coloring agents may induce asthma. Asthma-like reactions to inorganic chemicals and organic dusts are noted frequently. The role of emotional stress is difficult to assess, but clearly some subjects have exacerbations of their disease during stress. *(Beeson et al, pp. 403–408)*

22. **(A)** Therapy for asthma can include all the choices, but inhaled beta-adrenergic agonist provides the most rapid effect and, therefore, the best therapeutic index. Use of epinephrine is contraindicated in patients with known cardiac disease and is not recommended in patients over age 50. Aminophylline, IV and oral, has a slower onset of action, and therapeutic levels must be maintained and monitored. Hydrocortisone also has a delayed onset of action and its use should be limited if possible. *(Beeson et al, pp. 408–410)*

23. **(D)** Pulmonary hypertension is difficult to recognize clinically, and is present when pulmonary artery pressure rises to a high level inappropriate for a given level of cardiac output. Dyspnea, fatigue, and chest pain are usually present early in the disease with exertion and later may occur at rest. ECG changes are those of right axis deviation, right ventricular hypertrophy, right ventricular strain, or right atrial enlargement. In advanced cases cor pulmonale and right ventricular failure can occur. *(Beeson et al, pp. 298–300)*

24. **(D)** At end inhalation, blood flow to the heart is greatest because the pressure gradient between the thoracic vessels and vessels outside the thorax is greatest at that point. As we inspire, the intrathoracic pressure drops, and as the diaphragm

moves downward it increases intra-abdominal pressure and hence the pressure gradient. *(Dupuis, p. 11)*

25. **(B)** Vital capacity is the sum of the inspiratory reserve volume, the tidal volume, and the expiratory reserve volume. Any factors that reduce the ability of the lung to expand also reduce the vital capacity. Therefore, fibrotic lung diseases such as tuberculosis, emphysema, chronic asthma, lung cancer, chronic bronchitis, and fibrotic pleurisy can all reduce pulmonary compliance and reduce the vital capacity. For this reason, the vital capacity is the most important of clinical respiratory measurements in the assessment of the progression of these diseases. Arterial blood gases are helpful in the objective determination of the oxygenation of the blood, but are not reliable in the assessment of progression in fibrotic diseases. Changes in tidal volume may not become apparent until late in the disease process. *(Krupp et al, p. 126; Guyton, pp. 470–472)*

26. **(A)** Epiglottitis is an infection of the epiglottis and surrounding soft tissue. This is usually due to *Haemophilus influenzae* and is an immediate life-threatening illness. It most commonly occurs in children 3 to 6 years of age and usually has an abrupt onset presenting with high fever, stridor, difficulty swallowing, and severe sore throat, signaled by drooling. *(Saunders and Ho, pp. 445–446)*

27. **(B)** When epiglottitis is suspected, the mouth or neck should not be examined without first obtaining a soft tissue lateral neck x-ray, which would show edema and swelling of the epiglottis. The patient should be kept calm. If epiglottitis is noted on x-ray, orotracheal or nasotracheal intubation should be performed in the operating room, as an emergency tracheostomy may be needed. Visualization with a tongue blade or laryngoscope has been associated with abrupt laryngeal spasm, obstruction, and death. Chloramphenicol or cefuroxime IV are antibiotics appropriate for treatment of epiglottitis. *(Saunders and Ho, pp. 445–446)*

28. **(C)** Foreign-body aspiration presents in children usually from ages 4 months through 6 years; frequently, there is a history of playing with small objects. The aspiration of the foreign body classically precipitates an acute episode of choking, gagging, coughing, and wheezing. The chest x-ray results in this question are classic for foreign-body aspiration. *(Hathaway et al, pp. 479–480)*

29. **(C)** The treatment of foreign-body aspiration is hospitalization with immediate bronchoscopy to remove the foreign body. Chest physiotherapy should not be used for fear of completely obstructing the airway. Cool-mist therapy and antibiotics would not, of course, be helpful, and intubation in this patient is not required, as the foreign body is causing only local effects. *(Hathaway et al, pp. 479–480)*

30. **(D)** Hyperventilation usually occurs in young people without other evidence of cardiopulmonary disease, often in the presence of a recent emotional upset. Circumoral and carpopedal dysesthesias and spasm may occur. Frequently, anxiety exceeds the evidence for cardiopulmonary disease. Arterial blood gases are usually not needed but will show an increase in pH and a decrease in $PaCO_2$. Patients will usually improve rapidly, and reassurance is essential. *(Friedman, pp. 124–125)*

31. **(A)** In lung carcinoma, the most commonly encountered endocrine syndromes are inappropriate antidiuretic hormone secretion, Cushing's syndrome, and gynecomastia. Small-cell anaplastic carcinoma is especially associated with the development of these syndromes, suggestive of hormone overproduction. Small-cell anaplastic carcinoma cell may be of neural crest cell derivation and may have the potential for secreting many different chemical mediators. Hypothyroidism is not commonly encountered as a result of carcinoma of the lung. *(Beeson et al, pp. 459,1103)*

32. **(B)** The term *restrictive ventilatory disorder* denotes a pattern of abnormalities in lung function. The word *restrictive* is employed to indicate a restriction of, or limitation to, the amount of gas within the lungs. Thus, ventilatory disorders are characterized by reduction in lung volume. The hallmark of restriction is a decrease in the vital capacity. *Obstructive ventilatory disorder* denotes the constellation of abnormalities that resolves from airway obstruction, regardless of its cause. Obstructive disorders are detected principally by the tests of the behavior of the respiratory system under dynamic conditions. The FEV_1/FVC (forced expiratory volume in 1 second divided by the forced vital capacity) is the most widely used, although tests of maximal flow–volume relationships are increasingly being used. *(Beeson et al, pp. 416–417,427–428)*

33. **(A)** Patients with pneumonia may present in a variety of clinical presentations. However, findings disclosed by proper physical examination of the lungs should aid in the formulation of the differential diagnosis. Vocal fremitus is increased in consolidated pneumonias and by inflammation surrounding other pulmonary lesions by transmitting bronchotracheal air vibration with greater efficiency than do the air-filled pulmonary alveoli. Consolidated pulmonary tissue has increased density versus normal lung tissue, therefore yielding impaired resonance, dullness, and flatness to per-

cussion. This consolidated tissue also transmits whispered syllables distinctly, even when the pathological process is too small to produce bronchial breathing. Rales refer to sounds in the lungs from the movements of fluids or exudates in the airways. Although there are different types of rales, they sound like clicks or small bubbles and occur in bronchiectasis, pneumonia, consolidation, infarction, bronchitis, and TB. *(DeGowin and De-Gowin, pp. 296–319)*

34. (A) The treatment of a patient with a pulmonary embolism should include bed rest, analgesics, and oxygen, as indicated. Anticoagulation should begin as soon as possible if no contraindication exists. Anticoagulation is usually performed with heparin but in certain circumstances thrombolytics may be considered. *(Hardwood-Nuss, pp. 932–934)*

35. (E) The use of corticosteroids in COPD should be reserved for patients with potential reversibility of the disease. Some clues that a reversible component exist include: (1) improvement in the FEV_1, after inhalation of a bronchodilator, of greater than 20%; (2) history of considerable fluctuation in severity of symptoms or of acute attacks of wheezing dyspnea not brought on by exertion; (3) prominent wheeze or "noisy" chest on physical exam; (4) normal chest x-ray except for hyperinflation; (5) eosinophilia of the blood or sputum; (6) allergy skin test, or high serum IgE levels; (7) associated vasomotor rhinitis or nasal polyps; or (8) normal pulmonary diffusing capacity measurement. If no improvement of the FEV_1 is noted with a trial of a corticosteroid, the drug should be gradually tapered and discontinued. *(Beeson et al, pp. 416–417)*

36. (D) Because of the marked increase in pulmonary vascular resistance and pulmonary arterial pressure, there are a variety of clinical manifestations of primary pulmonary hypertension. Most frequently, dyspnea during exertion, fatigue, and weakness are noted. Substernal discomfort and even angina can be experienced during exertion; this is thought to be caused by right ventricular ischemia. Hoarseness may also be experienced due to compression of the left recurrent laryngeal nerve by the enlarged left pulmonary artery. Occasionally, cyanosis is noted, but clubbing is absent in this disease. If clubbing is present, it should prompt further investigation for the cause of pulmonary hypertension. Syncope in primary pulmonary hypertension is an ominous sign suggesting an abrupt fall in cardiac output and may result in sudden death. In almost every patient, an accentuated P_2 is noted with auscultation of the heart. *(Beeson et al, pp. 298–300; DeGowin and De-Gowin, p. 368)*

37. (E) The presence of partial airway obstruction below the tracheal bifurcation characteristically causes a localized wheeze over the site of obstruction and hyperinflation of the distal lung. Chest x-rays may be able to see the hyperinflation as well as the site of any foreign body or mass that is causing the obstruction. Inspiratory stridor is the hallmark of partial obstruction above the bifurcation. Pulmonary function testing reveals a relatively constant forced expiratory flow over a large portion of the FVC (forced vital capacity) in obstruction above the tracheal carina. Areas of localized decrease in airflow, as seen in obstruction below the carina, can be detected by ventilation–perfusion scanning. *(Beeson et al, pp. 418–419)*

38. (A) Because all patients with COPD should be regarded as having potentially reversible disease on initial exam, several measures should be instituted immediately. Bronchodilators should be given and drug levels monitored. Smoking and exposure to other pulmonary irritants should be avoided. A health care provider (MD, PA, RN, or RT) should provide the patient with instruction on bronchial hygiene and chest physical therapy. If it is found that the above measures do indeed improve pulmonary function by an appropriate amount, then at that time use of corticosteroids should be considered. *(Beeson et al, pp. 416–417)*

39. (B) Physical findings in a severe asthma attack with marked bronchospasm and dyspnea can be associated with a diminution of wheezing and breath sounds. This may lead to a silent chest, an especially serious finding that suggests impending respiratory failure. Arterial blood gas findings in mild to moderate asthma usually reveal normal to low $PaCO_2$ levels. As the bronchospasm worsens, hypoxia and CO_2 retention occur and, in severe episodes, the $PaCO_2$ rises to high levels. This elevation in $PaCO_2$ indicates a desperate situation and usually requires prompt and aggressive intervention. *(Hardwood-Nuss et al, pp. 726–727,922–923)*

40. (C) The patient presented has a somewhat complicated past medical history including asthma, which by the history and exam has worsened in the recent past. The patient appears, however, not to be in acute respiratory distress. The patient has recently been started on propanolol for treatment of hypertension. Because propanolol can accentuate bronchospasm and the patient appears to be at a therapeutic level (pulse rate 52) without normalization of the blood pressure, consideration should be given to discontinuing this medication and beginning another antihypertensive. The use of epinephrine is contraindicated in patients over age 50 and patients with a history of coronary artery disease. Any time a patient on theophylline presents with worsening of symptoms, a serum theophylline level should be obtained so that proper dosage is maintained. *(Beeson et al, pp. 408–410)*

41. (A) Blunt or penetrating trauma to the chest wall may result in intrapleural bleeding or hemothorax. The patient in question presents with a classical history and physical findings consistent with a hemothorax in the right chest. Hypotension, shock, or even cardiopulmonary arrest may be present, depending on blood loss and other injuries sustained. Emergency treatment should consist of the placement of at least two large-bore IVs; blood work should include CBC and the sending of clotted blood for type and crossmatching. A chest tube should be placed for the evacuation of the hemothorax and for treatment of a pneumothorax if present. The patient in question may indeed need surgery, but the above measures should be performed prior to thoracotomy. Every effort should be made to perform the thoracotomy in a well-prepared operating room by a trained cardiothoracic surgeon. *(Harwood-Nuss et al, pp. 310–314, 351–353)*

42. (B) All the choices are effective methods of oxygen delivery, and all health care providers should know the concentrations of O_2 delivered by each. A face mask with an oxygen reservoir at 6 L/min will provide an oxygen concentration at 60%. A nasal cannula at 2 L/min will provide O_2 at 28% to 30%. Mouth-to-mouth ventilation provides O_2 at 17%, and a face mask without an oxygen reservoir at 10 L/min will provide O_2 at a 60% concentration. *(Jaffe et al, pp. 35–36)*

43. (E) There are many factors involved in the control and stimulation of respiration. The most important factor in the control of ventilation under normal conditions is the Pco_2 of arterial blood. An increase in the Pco_2 is a strong stimulus to increase respiration and, similarly, a decrease in Pco_2 will cause a decrease in respiration. The role of hypoxia to stimulate respiration in the day-by-day control of respiration is small, as the PO_2 can be reduced by large amounts without stimulating an increase in respiration. However, patients with COPD have chronic CO_2 retention, and the pH of their cerebrospinal fluid has returned to normal, thus depressing the stimulation of respiration previously discussed. In these people, the hypoxic drive to ventilate becomes very important, and treatment of these patients with a high concentration of O_2 will act as a negative feedback and depress, and possibly stop, respiration. Reduction in the blood pH also stimulates respiration. Clinically, this response is difficult to differentiate from an accompanying rise in Pco_2, but animal models have demonstrated the response to pure acidosis convincingly. Exercise also increases respiration promptly for unclear reasons. During exercise the

arterial PO_2, Pco_2, and pH remain relatively constant, yet respiration increases at times to very high levels. *(West, pp. 124–125)*

44. (E) The management of infants with meconium aspiration must be closely observed for respiratory complication, and they must undergo treatment to prevent these complications. Chest physiotherapy and suctioning on a regular basis is suggested early and continued if signs of respiratory distress are encountered. Chest x-ray is important to help determine which child will develop respiratory distress and, because mechanical ventilation is often required, 10% to 20% of infants will develop pneumothorax or pneumomediastinum. Transcutaneous monitoring of the PO_2 early in the management of these infants aids in the assessment of the severity of the infant's condition. Fluid restriction is important to prevent cerebral and pulmonary edema during resuscitation. The response to asphyxiation may include the inappropriate secretion of antidiuretic hormone for 3 to 4 days after the insult. *(Cloherty and Stark, pp. 203–205, 319–320)*

45. (C) The advances in the prevention of hyaline membrane disease are closely related to the identification of risk factors for the development of the disease. Prenatal risk factors for hyaline membrane disease include prematurity, maternal diabetes, and a history of hyaline membrane disease in siblings. Also, male-sex children, second-born twins, and cesarean delivery without labor, are additional risk factors for hyaline membrane disease. *(Cloherty and Stark, p. 168)*

46. (A) The initial approach to evaluating hemoptysis involves several simple studies that can be instituted in almost any clinical setting. Studies should include determining if the sputum is blood-streaked or if gross blood is present, a Gram stain, a chest x-ray, a tuberculin skin test, and sputum cytology examination. These studies will aid in the determination for the direction of further studies or referrals. A bronchoscopy may be needed after the above tests are performed, but is not indicated as an initial study for the evaluation of hemoptysis. *(Harwood and Nuss, pp. 935–936)*

47. (B) The patient in this question has an exudative pleural effusion. An exudative effusion is defined as having a protein content of greater than 3 g/dL, is cloudy, and has a specific gravity greater than 1.016. The differential for an exudative pleural effusion includes bacterial and viral infections, TB, neoplasms, post-myocardial infarction, pulmonary infarction, rheumatoid arthritis, and SLE (lupus). Severe anemia and liver disease can cause a pleural effusion, but the effusion is a transudate that is clear, has a specific gravity less than 1.016, and has a protein content less than 2.5 g/dL. *(Harwood-Nuss et al, pp. 919–921)*

48. **(E)** By far the most important factor in the formation of a pulmonary abscess is aspiration, usually related to altered consciousness. Altered consciousness can be caused by a variety of conditions, such as alcoholism, stroke, drug use, seizure, or other serious illness. Lung abscess formation is rare in an edentulous person and, if present, suggests the possibility of bronchogenic carcinoma. In 60% of cases, only anaerobic bacteria are found, and there are generally an average of three organisms per case. *(Beeson et al, pp. 436–437)*

49. **(D)** Abscess formation may be a complication of pneumonias caused by *S. aureus, S. pyogenes,* and *K. pneumoniae.* Pneumococcal pneumonia is rarely associated with lung abscess formation unless other organisms are involved. *(Beeson et al, pp. 436–437)*

50. **(A)** As expected, there are many major complications in the near-drowning patient. Initially, the pulmonary effects must be evaluated and dealt with quickly. These include hypoxia, acidosis, and pulmonary edema that occurs in up to 75% of patients. Renal abnormalities have been reported, but significant electrolyte disturbances are usually not present. *(Harwood-Nuss et al, pp. 653–655)*

REFERENCES

Andreoli TE, Bennett JC, et al. *Cecil Essentials of Medicine,* 3rd ed. Philadelphia, PA: WB Saunders; 1993.

Cloherty JP, Stark AR. *Manual of Neonatal Care,* 2nd ed. Boston, MA: Little, Brown; 1986.

DeGowin EL, DeGowin RL. *Bedside Diagnostic Examination,* 5th ed. New York: Macmillan; 1982.

Guyton AC. *Textbook of Medical Physiology,* 7th ed. Philadelphia, PA: WB Saunders; 1986.

Hardwood-Nuss A, et al. *The Clinical Practice of Emergency Medicine.* Philadelphia, PA: JB Lippincott; 1991.

Hathaway WE, et al. *Current Pediatric Diagnosis and Treatment.* Norwalk, CT: Appleton & Lange; 1992.

Jeffe AS. *Textbook of Advanced Cardiac Life Support,* 2nd ed. Dallas, TX: American Heart Association; 1992.

Krupp MA, et al. *Current Medical Diagnosis and Treatment.* Norwalk, CT: Appleton & Lange; 1989.

Saunders CE, Ho MT. *Current Emergency Diagnosis and Treatment,* 4th ed. Norwalk, CT: Appleton & Lange; 1992.

Swartz MH. *Textbook of Physical Diagnosis, History and Examination.* Philadelphia, PA: WB Saunders; 1989.

Tierney LM, McPhee SJ, et al. *Current Medical Diagnosis and Treatment.* Norwalk, CT: Appleton & Lange; 1993.

West JB. *Respiratory Physiology,* 4th ed. Baltimore, MD: Williams & Wilkins; 1990.

Wyngaarden JP, Smith LH. *Cecil Textbook of Medicine,* 18th ed. Philadelphia, PA: WB Saunders; 1988.

Subspecialty List: Pulmonary

QUESTION NUMBER AND SUBSPECIALTY

1. *Pneumocystis carinii* pneumonia—characteristics
2. *Klebsiella pneumoniae*—characteristics
3. Mycoplasma pneumonia—characteristics
4. Legionnaire's disease—characteristics
5. Pneumococcal pneumonia—characteristics
6. Bronchogenic carcinoma—characteristics
7. Emphysema—characteristics
8. Emphysema—treatment
9. Bronchogenic carcinoma—laboratory evaluation
10. Lung carcinoma—laboratory evaluation
11. Chronic obstructive pulmonary disease—causes
12. Bronchogenic carcinoma—pathology
13. Pulmonary embolism—characteristics
14. Hemoptysis—causes
15. Cheyne–Stokes respiration—characteristics
16. Spontaneous pneumothorax—characteristics
17. Spontaneous pneumothorax—treatment
18. Pulmonary embolism—laboratory evaluation
19. Bronchial asthma—characteristics
20. Thoracentesis—procedure
21. Asthma—exacerbation
22. Asthma—treatment
23. Bronchitis—characteristics
24. Bronchitis—treatment
25. Pulmonary function tests
26. Epiglottitis—characteristics
27. Epiglottitis—evaluation
28. Foreign-body aspiration—characteristics
29. Foreign-body aspiration—treatment
30. Hyperventilation—characteristics
31. Lung cancer—associated endocrine syndromes
32. Restrictive vs. obstructive pulmonary disease
33. Pneumonia—physical findings
34. Pulmonary embolism—treatment
35. Chronic obstructive pulmonary disease—steroid indications
36. Pulmonary hypertension—characteristics
37. Airway obstruction—anatomic differential
38. Chronic obstructive pulmonary disease—treatment
39. Bronchial asthma—characteristics
40. Asthma—management
41. Hemopneumothorax—management
42. Oxygen therapy
43. Respiratory physiology
44. Meconium aspiration—management
45. Hyaline membrane disease—risk factors
46. Hemoptysis—evaluation
47. Thoracentesis—differential diagnosis
48. Pulmonary abscess—characteristics
49. Pulmonary abscess—differential diagnosis
50. Near drowning—characteristics

Internal Medicine: Infectious Diseases
Questions

DIRECTIONS (Questions 1 through 14): Each of the numbered items or incomplete statements in this section is followed by answers or by completions of the statement. Select the ONE lettered answer or completion that is BEST in each case.

Questions 1 through 14

1. A patient presents with symptoms consistent with infectious mononucleosis. During your work-up of this patient you would expect to find all the following EXCEPT

    (A) elevated liver function tests
    (B) hepatomegaly
    (C) lymphadenopathy
    (D) atypical lymphocytes on the differential
    (E) pharyngitis

2. All the following are true in cases of Lyme disease EXCEPT

    (A) there is an expanding erythematous annular lesion
    (B) the treatment of choice in early cases is trimethoprim-sulfamethoxazole
    (C) it is the most commonly reported tick-borne disease in the United States
    (D) it is a disease of stages if left untreated
    (E) if arthritis develops, it primarily affects the knee joint

3. You have taken a long-awaited 2-week vacation to Acapulco but have developed "turista" 3 days into your trip. Which of the following statements is true concerning your condition?

    (A) You probably became infected by drinking a bottle of local Mexican beer.
    (B) You can expect your symptoms to continue through your entire vacation.
    (C) Your symptoms may not have occurred if you had started your trip by taking amoxicillin 250 mg tid for 3 days.

    (D) Bismuth subsalicylate (Pepto-Bismol) may improve your symptoms.
    (E) The most common cause is one of the *Salmonella* serotypes.

4. The human papillomavirus (HPV) is the causative organism for the common wart as well as genital warts. Regarding genital warts, the following are true EXCEPT

    (A) in the U.S., the past ten years have seen HPV infections occur at five times the rate of genital herpes
    (B) no single treatment is effective in eradicating the virus and preventing recurrence
    (C) the treatment of choice is cryotherapy
    (D) the lesions can be confused with condylomata lata of secondary syphilis
    (E) of women with cervical dysplasia, more than 50% of male sexual contacts will have HPV

5. In the case of *Giardia lamblia,* stools can be characterized by all the following EXCEPT

    (A) they are mushy in recurrent cases
    (B) blood is not present
    (C) mucous is not present
    (D) there is little odor
    (E) they tend to be greasy and float

6. In a suspected case of food-borne botulism, you would expect to find all of the following EXCEPT

    (A) the patient had eaten home-canned vegetables two days prior
    (B) muscle twitching as the first neurological manifestation
    (C) impending respiratory failure if not treated promptly
    (D) the patient is afebrile
    (E) an alert, oriented individual, even in severe cases

7. Hepatitis D, also known as the delta agent, is a relatively new hepatic condition. All the following are true regarding this disease EXCEPT

   (A) it is an incomplete RNA virus
   (B) IV-drug users are at increased risk
   (C) it exists only as a co-infecting disease with hepatitis B
   (D) there is high infectivity rate among the homosexual population
   (E) its presence in chronic active hepatitis B can indicate a poor prognosis

8. In 1989 there was an outbreak of measles in the U.S. that had not been seen in recent years. As a result of this, the vaccination protocol has changed. Regarding measles prophylaxis, all of the following are true EXCEPT

   (A) in acute exposure, gamma globulin given within 6 days is preventative in most cases
   (B) a live, attenuated virus vaccine is used in routine immunization
   (C) an individual born before 1957 does not need to be revaccinated
   (D) in cases where gamma globulin has been used, a follow-up live, attenuated virus vaccination should be given at least 30 days later
   (E) in cases where outbreaks have occurred, a monovalent measles vaccine can be given as early as 6 months of age

9. Which of the following is incorrect when considering the treatment of genital herpes (HSV-2)?

   (A) For initial episodes use acyclovir 200 mg PO 5 times per day for 7 to 10 days.
   (B) For recurring episodes use acyclovir 200 mg PO 5 times per day for 5 days.
   (C) For those unable to tolerate oral medications, topical acyclovir q3 hours while awake for 5 days is as effective as oral acyclovir in recurrent cases.
   (D) For initial episode use acyclovir 400 mg PO tid for 7 to 10 days.
   (E) For suppression of recurrence, use acyclovir 400 mg PO bid, with treatment discontinued for 1 to 2 months per year to determine the frequency of recurrence.

10. Hepatitis B vaccine is recommended to all the following EXCEPT

   (A) infants born to a hepatitis B surface antigen (HBsAg) positive mother
   (B) established hepatitis B-infected individuals
   (C) promiscuous heterosexuals
   (D) persons receiving an accidental needlestick from HBsAg positive blood or body fluids
   (E) health care professionals exposed regularly to blood

11. A patient who has recently immigrated to the U.S. comes to your office with symptoms consistent with tuberculosis. After your work-up, you suspect this patient may have drug-resistant tuberculosis (DRTB). The following are true when considering DRTB EXCEPT

   (A) isoniazid and streptomycin are most frequently resistant to tuberculosis
   (B) risk for DRTB in this patient would be greater if they had immigrated from Haiti
   (C) suspected cases of DRTB could be treated properly with isoniazid, rifampin, ethambutol, and pyrazinamide until susceptibility testing is available
   (D) treatment should consist of two drugs that the patient has not taken previously
   (E) suspected cases of DRTB could be treated properly with isoniazid, rifampin, and streptomycin daily for 12 months

12. Nongonococcal urethritis (NGU) has become more prevalent than gonococcal urethritis (GU) in recent years. The following are true regarding NGU and GU EXCEPT

   (A) in the absence of gram-negative, intracellular diplococci on Gram stain, NGU can be diagnosed by seeing at least 5 PMNs/hpf
   (B) when treating GU, treatment should be aimed at eradicating causative organisms for GU, as well as NGU
   (C) the treatment of choice for GU is ceftriaxone 250 mg IM once
   (D) NGU occurs 20 times more frequently than GU in college students
   (E) nearly 50% of cases of NGU are caused by *Chlamydia trachomatis*

13. Of all hepatitis infections, hepatitis B (HBV) has the "alphabet soup" of lab values. All the following are true regarding these values EXCEPT

   (A) the presence of the surface antibody alone indicates past infection or immunization and is considered protective
   (B) the core antibody IgG can indicate infection even if the surface antigen is negative
   (C) the E antigen in the presence of the surface antigen can indicate a greater likelihood for chronic disease
   (D) the surface antigen is the first evidence of an acute infection
   (E) the core antigen is usually not detected in the serum by conventional lab methods

14. Childhood tuberculosis differs from adult tuberculosis in all the following EXCEPT

   (A) hilar lymphadenopathy is the hallmark of childhood tuberculosis

   (B) school-age children are particularly sensitive to becoming infected with tuberculosis

   (C) a child rarely develops progressive primary tuberculosis

   (D) the child has a recurrent nonproductive cough

   (E) caseation and cavity formation occur uncommonly in the child

DIRECTIONS (Questions 15 through 28): Each group of items in this section consists of lettered headings followed by a set of numbered words or phrases. For each numbered word or phrase, select

   (A) if the item is associated with (A) only,

   (B) if the item is associated with (B) only,

   (C) if the item is associated with BOTH (A) and (B),

   (D) if the item is associated with NEITHER (A) nor (B)

Questions 15 through 17

   (A) Kawasaki's disease

   (B) toxic shock syndrome

15. Bilateral, nonpurulent, conjunctival injection

16. Bacterial etiology believed to be the cause

17. Coronary artery involvement in some cases

Questions 18 through 20

   (A) Lyme disease

   (B) Rocky Mountain spotted fever

18. Bell's palsy is a neurological complication

19. Doxycycline is the treatment of choice in early cases

20. Vesicular lesions may develop as the disease progresses

Questions 21 through 24

   (A) *Salmonella* gastroenteritis

   (B) *Shigella*

21. The disease is usually self-limited

22. Antimicrobial treatment is unnecessary in uncomplicated cases

23. Associated with sexual transmission

24. Antibiotics do not shorten the course of the illness

Questions 25 through 26

   (A) hepatitis B

   (B) hepatitis C

25. Blood transfusions have been implicated as a cause

26. Associated with chronic active disease

Questions 27 and 28

   (A) gonococcal urethritis

   (B) nongonococcal urethritis

27. Diagnosis can be assisted by use of Gram stain

28. Onset of symptoms occur within one week of sexual contact

DIRECTIONS (Questions 29 through 43): For each of the items in this section, ONE or MORE of the numbered options is correct. Choose answer

   (A) if only (1), (2), and (3) are correct,

   (B) if only (1) and (3) are correct,

   (C) if only (2) and (4) are correct,

   (D) if only (4) is correct,

   (E) if all are correct.

Questions 29 through 43

29. Which of the following diseases are associated with desquamation of the skin?

   (1) scarlet fever

   (2) toxic shock syndrome

   (3) scalded skin syndrome

   (4) Kawasaki's disease

30. A patient you have seen for the first time presents with a petechial rash. She gives you a history of a possible tick bite 2 weeks earlier. You suspect Rocky Mountain spotted fever (RMSF). What other important findings may aid you in your diagnosis of RMSF?

   (1) She lives in North Carolina.

   (2) The patient responds favorably to a 10-day course of erythromycin.

   (3) Her lab values may show thrombocytopenia.

   (4) The disease is transmitted by the vector *Rickettsia rickettsii.*

31. Herpes simplex virus, type 2 (HSV-2), or genital herpes, is the most common cause for genital ulcers. What else is true regarding this disease?

    (1) Its occurrence as an STD now equals that of the human papillomavirus.
    (2) The incubation period is four to seven days.
    (3) Its recurrence rate is equal to that of herpes labialis (HSV-1).
    (4) An initial episode is less severe if there has been a prior HSV-1 infection.

32. Looking under the laboratory microscope you notice a "face and two large eyes" staring back at you. Realizing this is actually a *Giardia lamblia* trophozoite, you also know that this protozoa

    (1) primarily affects the large intestine
    (2) can be associated with sexual transmission in homosexuals
    (3) causes bloody stools
    (4) can cause malabsorption

33. Infant botulism differs from food-borne botulism in that

    (1) there is toxin production in vivo
    (2) constipation is common
    (3) the ingestion of honey has been implicated as a cause
    (4) it primarily affects those 6 to 12 months of age

34. One problem clinicians encounter when treating tuberculosis is resistance of the organism to standard treatment regimens. Which of the following statements are true regarding drug-resistant tuberculosis?

    (1) Rifampin is one of the drugs to which TB is most resistant.
    (2) Resistance is greater in the inner city.
    (3) Regarding age groups, resistance is greater among the elderly.
    (4) Regarding population groups, resistance is greater in immigrants from Southeast Asia or Latin America.

35. Malaria is relatively uncommon in the United States but individuals traveling abroad may return with the disease. You suspect a patient has malaria based on

    (1) the patient's complaint about cyclic episodes of chills, fever, and sweating
    (2) his/her recent trip to Somalia without prior chemoprophylaxis
    (3) splenomegaly during your physical examination
    (4) a normochromic, normocytic anemia

36. Hepatitis A (HAV) differs in many aspects from the other viral hepatic infections. Which of the following statements are true regarding HAV?

    (1) There is no known chronic carrier state.
    (2) Dark urine and clay-colored stools are first noticed after jaundice occurs.
    (3) The patient can show antibodies to HAV without ever having clinically apparent disease.
    (4) The IgM antibody indicates past infection and persisting immunity.

37. Fever of unknown origin is a diagnostic dilemma. Other than viral and bacterial causes, what other diseases can be uncovered during the work-up?

    (1) juvenile rheumatoid arthritis
    (2) factitious fever
    (3) leukemia
    (4) thyrotoxicosis

38. The tuberculin skin test is a useful diagnostic aid for the detection of tuberculosis. Which of the following statements are true regarding this test?

    (1) The preferred method is a subdermal injection of 0.1 ml of 25 tuberculin units (TU) of PPD
    (2) A palpable erythematous area of 10 mm or more, read at 48–72 hours posttest, is considered a positive test.
    (3) The tine test is preferred over the Mantoux test.
    (4) A 5- to 9-mm reaction is doubtful for diagnosis and may be due to other mycobacterium species.

39. The following have been associated as causes of nongonococcal urethritis

    (1) *Chlamydia trachomatis*
    (2) *Trichomonas vaginalis*
    (3) *Ureaplasma urealyticum*
    (4) herpes simplex virus

40. Recommendations for treating cases of tuberculosis prophylactically include

    (1) isoniazid as the drug of choice
    (2) therapy should be given for 6 to 12 months
    (3) multiple drug therapy may be needed in the SE Asian population
    (4) treatment should be given to close contacts of infected individuals, such as small children

41. On examination of a toddler, you notice small, irregular, grayish-white lesions on the upper buccal mucosa. You suspect these are Koplick spots and are concerned the child has rubeola. Of the following statements, which are true regarding rubeola?

    (1) The child was probably exposed to rubeola 9 to 12 days prior.
    (2) Koplick spots are pathognomonic.
    (3) Prodromal symptoms include conjunctivitis, coryza, nasal discharge, and a hacking cough.
    (4) There is a maculopapular brick-red rash, occurring simultaneously to the head, neck, trunk, and upper extremities.

42. Current treatment recommendations for initial uncomplicated pulmonary and extrapulmonary tuberculosis are

    (1) isoniazid daily for 12 months
    (2) rifampin and isoniazid without pyrazinamide daily for 9 to 12 months
    (3) ethambutol and streptomycin daily for 6 months in isoniazid-resistant cases
    (4) isoniazid and rifampin daily for 6 months, with pyrazinamide added during the first 2 months

43. Which of the following statements are true regarding infectious mononucleosis?

    (1) It is caused by a member of the herpes group of viruses.
    (2) Rupture of the spleen, either spontaneously or following trauma, may occur.
    (3) There is elevated liver function in almost all cases.
    (4) There is petechial rash associated with concurrent ampicillin therapy.

Answers and Explanations

1 **(B)** Frequently, the individual with mononucleosis presents with fever, sore throat, lymphadenitis, and malaise. The spleen is enlarged in more than half of the cases. Hepatomegaly may be found in 10% to 20% of cases; however, more frequently on examination, there may be percussion tenderness over the liver but no associated hepatomegaly. Laboratory values reveal elevated liver function tests in almost all cases. There is an increase in atypical lymphocytes noted on the differential, usually greater than 10%. *(Behrman, pp. 805–806; Berkow, pp. 2283–2285; Mandell et al, p. 1176; Rakel, pp. 109–110; Wilson et al, pp. 690–691; Wyngaarden et al, pp. 1838–1839)*

2. **(B)** Lyme disease is the leading cause of tick-borne disease in the United States. After the bite of the infected tick, a characteristic expanding annular rash develops, called erythema chronicum migrans. The rash may resolve spontaneously and advance to a second stage that includes neurologic and cardiac sequelae. A third stage may develop involving arthritis, which primarily affects the large joints, mostly the knees. The treatment of choice in early cases is, in order of preference, doxycycline, amoxicillin, and erythromycin. *(Abramowicz, pp. 95–97; Berkow, pp. 154–156; Mandell et al, pp. 1819–1825; Rankel, pp. 124–125; Tierney et al, pp. 72–76; Wilson et al, pp. 667–669; Wyngaarden et al, pp. 1772–1776)*

3. **(D)** Traveler's diarrhea is most often caused by an enterotoxigenic strain of *Escherichia coli*. Bottled, carbonated beverages are considered safe to drink, as well as fruit that can be peeled. Bismuth subsalicylate (Pepto-Bismol) provides symptomatic relief. Diphenoxylate (Lomotil) and loperamide (Imodium) provide symptomatic relief but should be discontinued if symptoms persist for more than 24 hours. The symptoms resolve in 1 to 5 days and rarely last 2 to 3 weeks. Prophylactic therapy may begin the day of the trip with either doxycyline 100 mg, double strength trimethoprim-sulfamethoxazole, norfloxacin 400 mg, or ciprofloxicin 500 mg, once daily for 3 days. However, many feel treatment should begin when symptoms develop.

The same treatment may be used for symptomatic patients but in twice daily doses for three days. *(Abramowicz, pp. 41–42; Berkow, pp. 819–820; Mandell et al, pp. 856–858; Rakel, pp. 13–14; Tierney et al, p. 1001; Wilson et al, pp. 523–524; Wyngaarden et al, pp. 705–706)*

4. **(A)** Human papillomavirus (HPV) has at least 60 subtypes that are recognized. Approximately 10 of these subtypes are responsible for the transmission of genital warts. There are also oncogenic strains that have been associated with cancer of the glans penis. In the past ten years STDs due to HPV infection has doubled that of those STDs secondary to genital herpes. After contact there is an incubation period of 1 to 6 months. The lesions are soft, minute, pink lesions that grow rapidly. In the male the most common site is the frenulum and the coronal sulcus. Diagnosis can be made by acetowashing the affected area for 3 to 5 minutes with 5% acetic acid. The lesions can be confused with molluscum contagiosum and condyloma lata of secondary syphilis. The treatment of choice is cryotherapy. The most common form of treatment is topical podophyllum. Other forms of treatment are electrodessication, surgical excision, laser therapy, or topical fluorouracil. No single treatment has been found to be effective in eradicating the virus. Recurrence is frequent. *(Abramowicz, pp. 119–124; Berkow, pp. 271–272; Mandell et al, pp. 1191–1197; Rakel, pp. 782,788; Tierney et al, pp. 102, 502,569; Wilson et al, pp. 742–743)*

5. **(D)** The stools of one infected with *Giardia lamblia* are generally foul-smelling, greasy in appearance, and float in the water. Blood or mucous is not typically present. In chronic cases, the stools tend to be mushy. *(Berkow, p. 228; Mandell et al, p. 2113; Tierney et al, pp. 1120–1121; Wilson et al, pp. 802–803; Wyngaarden et al, p. 1993)*

6. **(B)** Botulism is food poisoning caused by the ingestion of the toxin *Clostridium botulinum*. It primarily affects the neuromuscular system. The three types are food-borne, wound, and infant botulism. Home-canned foods, particularly vegetables, fruits, and condiments, are the most common sources of contamination. In adults, the first neurological manifestation is diplopia, dysarthria, and/ or dysphagia. The person is afebrile, and remains alert and oriented throughout the course of the illness. As the illness progresses, neuromuscular block may result in respiratory failure. *(Behrman, pp. 752–753; Berkow, pp. 817–818; Mandell et al, pp. 1847–1849; Tierney et al, pp. 782–783; Wilson et al, p. 579; Wyngaarden et al, pp. 1682–1683)*

7. **(D)** Hepatitis D, also known as the delta agent, is an incomplete RNA virus that replicates only in the presence of the hepatitis B virus (HBV). It cannot exist as an isolated infecting organism. It can be associated with a superinfection, which is more severe than infection with HBV alone. This can result in severe chronic hepatitis and cirrhosis. High-risk groups include IV-drug users, dialysis patients, and those receiving multiple transfusions. Male homosexuals have shown evidence of delta hepatitis, but the virus has not permeated the homosexual community and the incidence is low. *(Berkow, pp. 900,905; Mandell et al, pp. 1007–1008,1213; Tierney et al, pp. 506–510; Wilson et al, pp. 1327–1331; Wyngaarden et al, pp. 763–770)*

8. **(D)** When exposed to rubeola and having no previous history of vaccination or adequate antibodies for protection, gamma globulin given at 0.25 ml/kg within 6 days, will be preventative. It is not effective once symptoms have developed. If indicated, a live, attenuated virus vaccine should be given at least 3 months later. Routine immunization should be done using the same type of vaccine. The first dose is given at 15 months of age, usually with the mumps and rubella vaccines. A booster vaccine is also recommended at 4 to 6 years of age (CDCP guideline) or 12 years of age (American Academy of Pediatrics guideline). An individual does not need to be revaccinated if he or she was born prior to 1957, had measles previously, or has already received 2 doses of vaccine. In cases of outbreaks, a monovalent vaccine can be given initially at age 6 months or older. Routine immunization is carried out thereafter. *(Behrman, pp. 791–793; Berkow, pp. 2166–2170; Mandell et al, pp. 1279–1284; Rakel, pp. 133–135; Tierney et al, pp. 1036–1037; Wilson et al, pp. 705–707; Wyngaarden et al, pp. 1825–1827)*

9. **(C)** The treatment of choice for the initial episode of herpes simplex virus, type 2 (HSV-2) is acyclovir 200 mg five times per day for 7 to 10 days. Also effective is acyclovir 400 mg tid for 7 to 10 days. For recurring infections, acyclovir 200 mg five times per day for 5 days is used. This regimen for recurrence is not recommended for routine use of all recurring episodes. Preventive therapy should be considered. Treatment for prevention of HSV-2 is acyclovir 400 mg bid or 200 mg 2 to 5 times daily. Long-term use is considered safe, but treatment should be discontinued for 1 to 2 months to determine disease recurrence. Topical acyclovir offers little or no benefit in the treatment of HSV-2. *(Abramowicz, pp. 119–124; Berkow, p. 271; Mandell et al, pp. 1150–1151; Rakel, pp. 785–786; Tierney et al, p. 84; Wilson et al, p. 685; Wyngaarden et al, pp. 1833–1834)*

10. **(B)** Hepatitis B vaccine gives hepatitis B surface antibody response to approximately 90% of those vaccinated. The vaccine can be given before or after exposure. Pre-exposure vaccination should be given to those at risk of coming into contact with hepatitis B, such as health care workers who may come into contact with infectious blood (or blood products) and promiscuous heterosexuals, as well as homosexuals. Postexposure vaccination should be given to those who have been accidentally stuck with a needle contaminated with hepatitis B surface antigen (HBsAg) positive blood, or to infants born to HBsAg positive mothers. The vaccine is ineffective for those with currently active disease. *(Berkow, p. 903; Mandell et al, p. 1222; Rakel, p. 494; Tierney et al, p. 508; Wilson et al, p. 1333; Wyngaarden et al, p. 770)*

11. **(E)** Drug-resistant tuberculosis (DRTB) is occurring with greater frequency in the U.S. This is in part due to the increase in immigrants coming to the U.S. from areas where resistance is more common, such as Southeast Asia, Haiti, Latin America, and Africa. Treatment should begin in suspected cases with two drugs that the patient has not taken previously, provided that one of these two new drugs is either isoniazid or rifampin. The treatment of choice for DRTB is isoniazid, rifampin, pyrazinamide, and ethambutol initially, with modifications made after susceptibility testing is available. The regimen of isoniazid, rifampin, and streptomycin is inadequate because resistance to isoniazid and streptomycin is most common. Resistance to rifampin and ethambutol is less common. *(Abramowicz, pp. 10–11; Rakel, p. 221; Tierney et al, p. 216; Wilson et al, p. 644; Wyngaarden et al, p. 1738)*

12. **(D)** In recent years, gonococcal urethritis (GU) has been on the decline whereas nongonococcal urethritis (NGU) has been on the rise. Cases of NGU are three times more common than GU; however, among college students this ratio is 10:1. The most common cause of NGU is *Chlamydia trachomatis* which comprises 40% to 50% of cases. Diagnosis of NGU is often made by exclusion. On Gram stain, in the absence of gram-negative intracellular diplococci, a diagnosis of NGU can be made by seeing at least 5 PMNs/hpf. Treatment of GU should be aimed at eradication of both GU and NGU since 40% to 50% of those affected with GU

also have NGU. The treatment of choice for GU is ceftriaxone 250 mg IM once, ciprofloxacin 500 mg once, floxicin 400 mg once, or spectinomycin 2 g IM once. To any of the above regimens doxycycline 100 mg bid for seven days should be added to treat NGU since there is no one single treatment to simultaneously eradicate both GU as well as NGU. *(Abramowicz, pp. 119–124; Berkow, pp. 254–255,257–258, Mandell et al, pp. 942–948; Rakel, pp. 710–713; Tierney et al, pp. 1079–1080,1089; Wilson et al, pp. 524–525; Wyngaarden et al, pp. 1751–1752)*

13. **(B)** Hepatitis B surface antigen (HBsAg) is the first serologic marker of hepatitis B (HBV) infection. It usually occurs during the incubation period and disappears during the recovery phase. The HBV surface antibody (anti-HBs) develops after clinical recovery. It represents past HBV infection or past immunization. The HBV core antigen (HBcAg) represents the viral inner core. It is not detectable in serum by conventional lab methods, but only by specialized techniques. The HBV core antibody (anti-HBc) is a marker of acute, persistent, or past infection. The anti-HBc(IgM) will be positive for 6 to 18 months after infection, and the anti-HBc(IgG) will remain as the indicator of past infection. There is a "window" period in HBV. This occurs during the transition from the disappearance of HBsAg and the appearance of anti-HBs. Anti-HBc(IgM) will be the only indicator of infection during this time. The HBVe antigen (HBeAg) is only found in HBsAg positive serum. Its presence in the serum, along with HBsAg, for more than 10 weeks correlates with ongoing viral replication and may be a predictor of chronic disease. *(Berkow, pp. 899–900; Mandell et al, pp. 1219–1221; Tierney et al, p. 506; Wilson et al, pp. 1328–1330; Wyngaarden et al, pp. 763–770)*

14. **(B)** Childhood tuberculosis (TB) differs in several ways from TB in the adult. The child's symptoms may be mild or nonspecific. Some symptoms, such as a persistent, nonproductive cough, are associated with bronchial compression, due to enlarged hilar lymph nodes. When seen on a chest x-ray, enlarged hilar lymph nodes are considered the hallmark of childhood TB. The child that is less than 3 years old and elderly persons are particularly sensitive to becoming infected with TB. Rarely, a child will develop progressive primary TB, which may result in caseation and cavity formation. *(Behrman, p. 765; Berkow, p. 139; Mandell et al, pp. 1884–1886; Wyngaarden et al, pp. 1733–1736)*

15–17. 15. **(C)**; 16. **(B)**; 17. **(A)** Kawasaki's disease is a disease of unknown etiology. It consists of an exanthem, fever, lymphadenopathy, and polyarteritis. The coronary arteries may become involved, including the formation of aneurysms. The disease is also associated with mucous membrane changes, which include pharyngeal injection, fissured lips, and injected, nonpurulent conjunctiva. *(Behrman, pp. 629–630; Berkow, pp. 2201–2202; Mandell et al, pp. 2171–2172; Tierney et al, p. 1049; Wyngaarden et al, p. 2301)*

Toxic shock syndrome is believed to be caused by a strain of *S. aureus* that produces a toxin, thus causing the symptoms. Initial presenting symptoms include the sudden onset of fever, rash, pharyngitis, and nonpurulent conjunctivitis. There may also be headache, lethargy, and hypotension. There is no known coronary artery involvement. *(Behrman, pp. 629–630; Berkow, pp. 88–89; Mandell et al, pp. 2171–2172; Tierney et al, p. 1049; Wilson et al, p. 1462; Wyngaarden et al, p. 2301)*

18–20. 18. **(A)**; 19. **(C)**; 20. **(D)** Lyme disease begins with the tick bite from *Ixodes dammini* or *I. pacificans*, which transmits the spirochete *Borrelia burgdorferi*. The classic rash, erythema chronicum migrans, begins as a macular or maculopapular lesion that expands, leaving centralized clearing. This occurs within 1 month of the tick bite in most patients and can resolve spontaneously. Within a week to months, a second stage of the disease can occur, which includes cardiac and neurologic complications. Bilateral Bell's palsy may occur, as well as severe fatigue, peripheral neuropathy, and meningitis. Early manifestations of the disease are treated with doxycycline 100 mg bid for 10 to 21 days, or amoxicillin 250 mg or 500 mg for 10 to 21 days. *(Abramowicz, pp. 95–97; Berkow, pp. 154–156; Mandell et al, pp. 1819–1825; Rakel, pp. 124–125; Tierney et al, pp. 1104–1106; Wilson et al, pp. 666–667; Wyngaarden et al, pp. 1772–1776)*

Rocky Mountain spotted fever (RMSF) is transmitted by the bite of any one of the three vectors of the genus *Dermacentor*. The lone star tick, *Amblyomma americanum*, also is responsible in transmitting the disease. The disease-causing organism is *Rickettsia rickettsii*. The rash of RMSF typically begins as a macular or maculopapular lesion but progresses to form petechial lesions. The lesions may coalesce to form large hemorrhagic areas. In RMSF, the treatment of choice is either chloramphenicol 50 mg/kg/day, in children over 8 years old and pregnant females, or doxycycline 100 mg q12h. *(Berkow, pp. 174,181; Mandell et al, pp. 1465–1470; Rakel, pp. 128–130; Tierney et al, pp. 1054–1055; Wilson et al, pp. 756–758; Wyngaarden et al, p. 1790)*

21–24. 21. **(C)**; 22. **(C)**; 23. **(B)**; 24. **(A)** *Salmonella* gastroenteritis is usually transmitted by infected meat, poultry, eggs, egg products, and raw milk. Infections affecting the intestinal tract are manifested by watery stools, with occasional blood and mucus. The disease is usually self-limited in uncomplicated cases and does not necessarily warrant antibiotic use. Treatment with antibiotics may actually prolong the time in which *Salmonella* resides in the intestinal tract. *(Behrman, pp. 731–733; Berkow, pp. 105–106; Mandell et al, pp. 1700–1712; Rakel, p. 144; Tierney et al, p. 1075; Wilson et al, pp. 612–613; Wyngaarden et al, pp. 1691–1694)*

Shigella is usually transmitted by the stools of infected individuals, particularly the fecal-oral route. There is increasing incidence in the daycare centers. Homosexuals practicing anilingus, are considered a high-risk group. It can also be obtained from contaminated water and sanitation facilities. Shigellosis begins with infrequent, voluminous, watery stools. This later progresses to frequent stools with decreased volume, often containing mucus, pus, and blood. Treatment is variable. If left untreated, the disease is usually self-limited. In severe cases, antimicrobial treatment is recommended, because the disease can lead to dehydration. Infants are at greater risk for developing further complications. *(Behrman, pp. 734–736; Berkow, pp. 106–108; Mandell et al, pp. 1718–1719; Tierney et al, pp. 1075–1076; Wilson et al, pp. 613–615; Wyngaarden et al, pp. 1694–1696)*

25. (C) Hepatitis B infection use to make up the majority of cases associated with posttransfusion hepatitis. With the advent of blood screening by blood banks, now less than 5% of posttransfusion hepatitis cases are hepatitis B. The remainder of posttransfusion hepatitis cases are mostly hepatitis C, constituting approximately 90% of all cases. *(Berkow, pp. 900–901; Mandell et al, pp. 1214,1220; Tierney et al, pp. 505–506; Wilson et al, pp. 1326–1327; Wyngaarden et al, pp. 763–770)*

26. (C) Approximately 10% of hepatitis B-infected individuals will still have detectable HBsAg in their blood after 6 months. A small percentage (about 3%) of these will remain HBsAg positive for years. They may be asymptomatic carriers or develop chronic active disease. This is also confirmed by liver biopsy and failure of liver function tests to return to normal. Approximately 40% to 50% of those with posttransfusion hepatitis C will develop chronic active disease. This too, like hepatitis B, is confirmed by failure of the liver function tests to return to normal, and liver biopsy. Unlike hepatitis B, the HBsAg will not be detectable in the serum. *(Berkow, p. 905; Mandell et al, pp. 1408–1410; Tierney et al, p. 905; Wilson et al, p. 1331; Wyngaarden et al, pp. 763–770)*

27–28. 27. (C); 28. (A) In gonococcal urethritis (GU), the Gram stain reveals gram-negative intracellular diplococci in over 90% of the cases. This is a reliable finding in the diagnosis of GU. In nongonococcal urethritis (NGU) there are no intracellular diplococci found, but in the absence of this finding, a diagnosis of NGU can be made by exclusion, by finding at least 5 PMNs/hpf on the Gram stain.

From exposure to the onset of symptoms, GU has an incubation period of 2 to 8 days; for NGU it is 1 to 3 weeks. The discharge of GU is generally of greater quantity and purulence than NGU. There is more dysuria with GU as well. *(Berkow, pp. 254–255,257–258; Mandell et al, pp. 942–948; Rakel, pp. 710–713; Tierney et al, pp. 1079–1080,1089; Wilson et al, pp. 524–525; Wyngaarden et al, pp. 1751–1752)*

29. (E) Scarlet fever is associated with group A *Streptococcus*. Along with other symptoms, there is also a rash and fever. When the fever subsides, the upper layer of the epidermis desquamates where the rash was present.

Toxic shock syndrome is believed to be caused by a toxin-producing strain of *S. aureus*. There is a fever, rash, and often hypotension associated with this disease. Desquamation of the epidermis, particularly of the palms and soles, occurs 1 to 2 weeks from the onset of symptoms.

Scalded skin syndrome is associated with a coagulase-positive strain of staphylococci, which produces an epidermal toxin, causing the skin to slough. This condition is seen most often in infants and young children.

Kawasaki's disease is of unknown etiology, and consists of an exanthem, fever, lymphadenopathy, and polyarteritis. One to two weeks after the onset of symptoms, desquamation occurs to the palms, soles, and periungual areas. *(Berkow, pp. 88–89, 2201–2202; Mandell et al, pp. 2171–2172; Tierney et al, p. 1049; Wilson et al, p. 1462; Wyngaarden et al, p. 2301)*

30. (B) Rocky Mountain spotted fever (RMSF) has a high incidence of occurrence in the South Atlantic states, with a high percentage of the cases occurring in North Carolina, Virginia, Georgia, Maryland, Tennessee, and Oklahoma. The disease is transmitted by any one of three ticks from the genus *Dermacentor,* as well as from the Lone Star tick, *Amblyomma americanum.* These ticks act as vectors of the disease-causing organism, *Rickettsia ricketsii.* Clinically, the patient presents with a macular or maculopapular rash that develops into petechial lesions. Lab values often reveal a normal white blood cell count, but an increased quantity of immature myeloid cells. Thrombocytopenia is present in about one-third of the patients. The treatment of choice is either chloramphenicol, especially for pregnant women and children less than eight years old, or tetracycline. *(Berkow, pp. 174,181; Mandell et al, pp. 1465–1470; Rakel, pp. 129–130; Tierney et al, pp. 1054–1055; Wilson et al, pp. 756–758; Wyngaarden et al, pp. 1788–1790)*

31. (C) Herpes simplex virus, type 2 (HSV-2) is the most common source of genital ulcers. It is a frequently occurring STD; however, in the past 10 years the human papillomavirus, or genital warts, occurs at twice the rate of HSV-2. Initial episodes are usually accompanied by fever, headache, malaise and myalgia. These symptoms are usually less severe if the patient has had a prior HSV-1 infection. Lesions are preceded by itching and pain. Unlike herpes zoster virus there is bilateral distribution. The treatment of choice is oral acyclovir. HSV-2 frequently recurs, usually at the site of the initial infection. HSV-2 has a recurrence rate of 80% to 90% within 12 months, compared to a recurrence rate of 50% for HSV-1 for the same time period. *(Berkow, pp. 270–271; Mandell et al, pp. 1144–1148,1150–1151; Rakel, pp. 785–786; Tierney et al, p. 84; Wilson et al, pp. 683,685; Wyngaarden et al, pp. 1832–1834)*

32. (C) *Giardia lamblia* is spread from host-to-host by fecal–oral transmission. It has been associated with sexual transmission, particularly homosexuals practicing anilingus. It primarily affects the duodenum and jejunum. Malabsorption may occur, possibly from mechanical blockage of the intestinal mucosa. Regardless of frequency, the stools are free from pus or blood, but may contain mucus. *(Berkow, p. 228; Mandell et al, pp. 2110–2113; Tierney et al, pp. 1120–1121; Wilson et al, pp. 802–803; Wyngaarden et al, p. 1993)*

33. (A) Botulism is food poisoning caused by the ingestion of the toxin *Clostridium botulinum*. It primarily affects the nervous system. In infant botulism, the ingestion of *C. botulinum* spores alone can result in the disease because of toxin production in vivo. Most cases of infant botulism occur between 1 and 6 months of age, but most frequently between ages 2 and 3 months. Honey has been found to have *C. botulinum* spores; therefore, it is not recommended for infants less than 12 months old. Constipation may be one of the first presenting complaints in infants. *(Behrman, pp. 752–753; Berkow, pp. 817–818; Mandell et al, pp. 1847–1849; Tierney et al, p. 783; Wilson et al, pp. 579–580; Wyngaarden et al, pp. 1682–1683)*

34. (C) Drug-resistant tuberculosis (DRTB) occurs in two-thirds of those who were previously treated for TB. This is due to inadequate duration of therapy and sporadic dosing by the patient. There is greater risk for DRTB if one lives in the inner city. Immigrants from Haiti, Latin America, Africa, and Southeast Asia are also at greater risk. DRTB is more common in children less than three years old but is uncommon in the elderly. TB shows the most resistance to isoniazid first, then streptomycin second. *(Abramowicz, pp. 10–11; Rakel, p. 221; Tierney et al, p. 216; Wilson et al, p. 644; Wyngaarden et al, p. 1738)*

35. (E) Malaria is endemic to many areas of Africa, South America, and Oceania. It is a protozoan parasitic disease caused by one of the four species from the genus *Plasmodium*. It is transmitted most commonly by the bite of an infected *Anopheles* mosquito. After returning from an endemic area, most infected individuals will have recurring episodes of chills, fever, and sweating at regular intervals, but this depends upon the infecting parasite. A normochromic, normocytic anemia is usual. Lab findings may show a normal to low leukocyte count, decreased platelets, and an increased sedimentation rate. Demonstration of a parasite on stained blood smears is diagnostic. *(Berkow, pp. 229–231; Mandell et al, pp. 2058–2062; Tierney et al, pp. 1125–1126; Wilson et al, pp. 782–788; Wyngaarden et al, pp. 1972–1975)*

36. (B) Hepatitis A virus (HAV) is transmitted by the fecal–oral route. Compared to hepatitis B, it has a much shorter incubation period. The prodromal symptoms are varied, but include dark-colored urine and clay-colored stools prior to the onset of jaundice, which is the start of the clinical phase. The posticteric phase follows this, lasting 2 to 12 weeks. Lab indicators show a positive HAV antibody of the IgM class [anti-HA(IgM)] during an acute infection. During the disappearance of anti-HA(IgM), the anti-HA(IgG) remains as the only serologic marker of past infection and persisting immunity. Passive immunization is possible through immune globulin injections. Exposure to the virus without clinically apparent symptoms can produce antibodies as well. Unlike hepatitis B, there is no known chronic carrier state. *(Berkow, pp. 899,902; Mandell et al, pp. 1387–1390; Tierney et al, pp. 505,507; Wilson et al, pp. 1326–1330; Wyngaarden et al, pp. 763–770)*

37. (E) The definition of fever of unknown origin varies in regard to the degree of fever and the length of time the fever is present. A definition derived from various sources is a rectal temperature greater than 101°F for 2 to 3 weeks without an identifiable cause, after 1 week of intensive investigation.

Bacterial and viral infections are the usual causes of FUO in about 50% of cases. Of these, viral infections are the presumed etiology in most cases. The remaining causes are categorized into collagen vascular diseases, such as juvenile rheumatoid arthritis or SLE; neoplasms, such as leukemia or lymphoma; and miscellaneous causes, which include factitious fever, thyrotoxicosis, and pulmonary emboli, to name a few. *(Behrman, pp. 652–653; Berkow, p. 9; Mandell et al, pp. 468,472–477; Tierney et al, pp. 17–18; Wilson et al, pp. 128–133; Wyngaarden et al, pp. 1568–1569)*

38. (D) The tuberculin skin test may be used as a generalized screen for tuberculosis or for individuals who are suspected of harboring the disease. The preferred method of administration is 0.1 mL of 5 tuberculin units (TU) of PPD subdermally, most commonly on the volar aspect of the forearm. This is known as the Mantoux test. The multipuncture, or tine test, is used for large-scale screenings, as in schools. A positive reaction is an area of palpable induration, not erythema, of 10 mm or more at the test site 48 to 72 hours later. Induration of 5 mm to 9 mm is considered nondiagnostic and can be caused by other species of nontuberculous *Mycobacterium*. *(Behrman, p. 764; Berkow, p. 134; Mandell et al, pp. 1882–1883; Tierney et al, p. 215; Wilson et al, p. 642; Wyngaarden et al, pp. 1734–1735)*

39. **(E)** Several organisms have been implicated in causes of nongonococcal urethritis (NGU). *Chlamydia trachomatis* can be found in 40% to 50% of cases of NGU. *Ureaplasma urealyticum* and *Trichomonas vaginalis* make up an additional 30% of cases. HSV-2, as well as *Corynebacterium genitalium*, can also cause NGU. *(Berkow, pp. 257–258; Mandell et al, p. 944; Rakel, pp. 712–713; Tierney et al, p. 1089; Wilson et al, pp. 524–525; Wyngaarden et al, pp. 1751–52)*

40. **(E)** Isoniazid is the drug of choice for prophylactic treatment of tuberculosis. It is given in a daily dose of 300 mg for 6 to 12 months. Because of isoniazid-resistant strains of *Mycobacterium,* the Southeast Asian population may need multiple drug therapy for prophylactic treatment. The risk of developing tuberculosis is particularly high in close contacts of newly infected individuals, and also within 2 years after the development of a positive tuberculin skin test. The risk of developing serious tuberculosis infections, including meningitis, is particularly high among infants and adolescents. *(Abramowicz, pp. 10–11; Berkow, pp. 140–141; Rakel, p. 222; Tierney et al, p. 218; Wilson et al, pp. 641–642; Wyngaarden et al, pp. 1736–1737)*

41. **(A)** Rubeola is a highly infectious disease. There is an incubation period that ranges from 9 to 12 days. This is followed by a prodromal period where ocular symptoms are frequent. This includes mild conjunctivitis, edema of the eyelids, excessive lacrimation, as well as photophobia. There is usually rhinorrhea and a hacking cough present. Lastly, there is a sudden rise in temperature to the 104° to 105°F range, which is accompanied by a maculopapular rash. The rash is brick-red. It is irregularly confluent and in severe cases can be petechial. It starts about two weeks after exposure. It occurs first to the facial area, especially to the forehead and around the ears, spreading downward as the disease progresses, eventually affecting the neck, shoulders, trunk, and upper extremities. The rash resolves in about 6 days, but persists for about 3 days in each area, disappearing in the same order of appearance. Isolation is required 7 days after exposure until 5 days after the rash has appeared. *(Behrman, pp. 791–793; Berkow, pp. 2166–2170; Mandell et al, pp. 1279–1284; Rakel, pp. 133–135; Tierney et al, pp. 1036–1037; Wilson et al, pp. 705–707; Wyngaarden et al, pp. 1825–1827)*

42. **(C)** Isoniazid alone for 12 months can be given prophylactically for the treatment of tuberculosis (TB), but not to treat initial uncomplicated TB. The current treatment preferred is isoniazid and rifampin daily for 6 months, with pyrazinamide added during the first 2 months. Alternatively, isoniazid and rifampin without pyrazinamide may be given daily for 9 to 12 months. In isoniazid-resistant cases, isoniazid, rifampin, pyrazinamide and ethambutol are given for 12 months. Adjustments in this regimen can be made after drug sensitivity testing is available. *(Abramowicz, pp. 10–11; Berkow, p. 144; Tierney et al, p. 216; Wilson et al, pp. 641–642; Wyngaarden et al, pp. 1736–1737)*

43. **(A)** Infectious mononucleosis is caused by the Epstein–Barr virus, a herpes group virus. Clinically, there is pharyngitis, lymphadenitis, and splenomegaly. Rupture of the spleen may occur, either spontaneously or following trauma, but is rare. Elevated liver function tests are the norm. With concurrent ampicillin use, there is an associated erythematous macular or maculopapular rash in 80% to 100% of cases. *(Behrman, pp. 805–806; Berkow, pp. 2281–2285; Mandell et al, pp. 1172–1176; Rakel, pp. 109–110; Tierney et al, pp. 1033–1034; Wilson et al, pp. 690–691; Wyngaarden et al, pp. 1838–1839)*

REFERENCES

Abramowicz M (ed). Drugs for sexually transmitted diseases. *Med Letter.* 1991;33:119–124.

Abramowicz M (ed). Treatment of Lyme disease. *Med Letter.* 1992;34:95–97.

Abramowicz M (ed). Advice for travelers. *Med Letter.* 1992;34:41–42.

Abramowicz M (ed). Drugs for tuberculosis. *Med Letter.* 1992;34:10–11.

Behrman RE (ed). *Nelson Textbook of Pediatrics,* 14th ed. Philadelphia, PA: WB Saunders; 1992.

Berkow R (ed). *The Merck Manual of Diagnosis and Therapy,* 16th ed. Rahway, NJ: Merck; 1992.

Mandell GL, Douglass RG Jr, Bennett JE (eds). *Principles and Practice of Infectious Disease,* 3rd ed. New York, NY: Churchill Livingstone; 1990.

Rakel RE (ed). *Conn's Current Therapy,* Philadelphia, PA: WB Saunders; 1993.

Tierney LM Jr, McPhee SJ, Papadakis MA, Schroeder SA (eds). *Current Medical Diagnosis and Treatment.* Norwalk, CT: Appleton & Lange; 1993.

Wilson JD, Braunwald E, Isselbacher KJ, Petersdorf RG, Martin FB, Fauci AS, Root RK (eds). *Harrison's Principles of Internal Medicine,* 12th ed. New York, NY: McGraw Hill; 1991.

Wyngaarden JB, Smith LH, Bennet JC (eds). *Cecil Textbook of Medicine.* 19th ed. Philadelphia, PA: WB Saunders; 1992.

Subspecialty List: Infectious Diseases

QUESTION NUMBER AND SUBSPECIALTY

1. Infectious mononucleosis
2. Lyme disease
3. Traveler's diarrhea
4. Human papillomavirus
5. *Giardia lamblia*
6. Botulism
7. Hepatitis D
8. Rubeola
9. Genital herpes treatment
10. Hepatitis B vaccine
11. Tuberculosis
12. Urethritis
13. Hepatitis B
14. Tuberculosis
15. Kawasaki's disease/toxic shock syndrome
16. Kawasaki's disease/toxic shock syndrome
17. Kawasaki's disease/toxic shock syndrome
18. Lyme disease/Rocky Mountain spotted fever
19. Lyme disease/Rocky Mountain spotted fever
20. Lyme disease/Rocky Mountain spotted fever
21. *Salmonella/Shigella*
22. *Salmonella/Shigella*
23. *Salmonella/Shigella*
24. *Salmonella/Shigella*
25. Hepatitis B/hepatitis C
26. Hepatitis B/hepatitis C
27. Urethritis
28. Urethritis
29. Desquamating rashes
30. Rocky Mountain spotted fever
31. Genital herpes
32. *Giardia lamblia*
33. Infant botulism
34. Tuberculosis
35. Malaria
36. Hepatitis A
37. Fever of unknown origin
38. Tuberculin skin testing
39. Urethritis
40. Tuberculosis treatment
41. Rubeola
42. Tuberculosis treatment
43. Infectious mononucleosis

Internal Medicine: Cardiology
Questions

DIRECTIONS (Questions 1 through 32): For each of the items in this section, ONE or MORE of the numbered options is correct. Choose answer

    (A) if only (1), (2), and (3) are correct,
    (B) if only (1) and (3) are correct,
    (C) if only (2) and (4) are correct,
    (D) if only (4) is correct,
    (E) if all are correct.

Questions 1 through 32

1. Prolongation of the Q-T interval can be due to
   (1) hyperkalemia
   (2) disopyramide
   (3) digitalis
   (4) quinidine toxicity

2. Factors that can raise high-density lipoprotein are
   (1) exercise
   (2) cessation of cigarette smoking
   (3) therapy with gemfibrozil
   (4) estrogen

3. Sick sinus syndrome includes the following rhythm disturbances:
   (1) alternating slow atrial and ventricular rates with rapid atrial tachyarrhythmias
   (2) persistent sinus bradycardia
   (3) sinus arrest or exit block
   (4) a combination of SA or AV conduction abnormalities

4. Thromboembolism is a complication of
   (1) mitral regurgitation
   (2) pulmonic stenosis
   (3) mitral stenosis
   (4) aortic stenosis

5. Torsade de pointes, a pleomorphic ventricular tachycardia, can be seen with
   (1) severe bradycardia
   (2) quinidine
   (3) disopyramide
   (4) hypokalemia

6. Which of the following are necessary in a cholesterol-reducing diet?
   (1) weight reduction in an obese individual
   (2) saturated fat of less than 10% of calories
   (3) cholesterol of less than 300 mg/day
   (4) total fat intake of less than 30% of total calories

7. Which of the following are true regarding variant angina (Prinzmetal's angina)?
   (1) occurs at rest
   (2) transient ST-segment elevations on electrocardiogram
   (3) caused by coronary artery vasospasm
   (4) beta-adrenergic therapy is the treatment of choice

8. Which of the following foods have high cholesterol content?
   (1) soybeans
   (2) coconuts
   (3) salmon
   (4) liver

9. Which of the following therapeutic steps are used in the treatment of chronic congestive heart failure?
   (1) digoxin
   (2) low sodium diet
   (3) vasodilators
   (4) diuretics

10. The following drugs affect serum potassium levels:

    (1) captopril
    (2) diltiazem
    (3) hydrochlorothiazide
    (4) atenolol

11. In Mobitz type II second-degree AV block

    (1) every atrial impulse is conducted to a ventricle
    (2) a nonconducted P wave is preceded by sinus beats with constant P-R intervals
    (3) a progressive P-R prolongation ending in a nonconducted P wave
    (4) a permanent pacemaker may be necessary

12. The following are associated with Wolff–Parkinson–White syndrome?

    (1) delta wave
    (2) prolonged QRS
    (3) short PR intervals
    (4) paroxysmal atrial tachycardia

13. Electrocardiographic finding(s) in atrial fibrillation include

    (1) grossly irregular P waves
    (2) atrial rate 250–350 beats/min
    (3) ventricular rate 100–160
    (4) sawtooth contour to P waves

14. Precipitating causes of angina pectoris are

    (1) exercise
    (2) cold environment
    (3) walking after large meal
    (4) stress

15. In addition to medical therapy, which of the following nondrug therapies should be recommended for treating hypertension?

    (1) weight-reduction diet
    (2) reducing alcohol consumption to less than 2 oz daily
    (3) dietary sodium restriction
    (4) low cholesterol, low-fat diet

16. Inverted T waves can be seen with

    (1) myocardial ischemia
    (2) left ventricular hypertrophy
    (3) subendocardial infarction
    (4) hyperkalemia

17. In congestive heart failure, the following features may be seen on a chest roentgenogram:

    (1) increased size and shape of cardiac silhouette
    (2) pulmonary vascular redistribution
    (3) pleural effusions
    (4) Kerley's lines

18. High-output heart failure can be caused by

    (1) anemia
    (2) thyrotoxicosis
    (3) pregnancy
    (4) hypertension

19. Which of the following is/are true of one-man cardiopulmonary resuscitation for adults?

    (1) ratio of compressions to breaths is 15:2
    (2) ratio of compression to breaths is 5:1
    (3) rate of compressions is 80–100 times per minute
    (4) rate of compression is at least 100 times per minute

20. Which of the following statements is/are true regarding HDL cholesterol?

    (1) removes cholesterol from peripheral tissues
    (2) transports cholesterol to peripheral cells
    (3) low HDL cholesterol (35 mg/daily) is a risk factor for coronary heart disease
    (4) cigarette smoking raises HDL

21. When performing cardiopulmonary resuscitation for small children

    (1) the ratio is 5 compressions to 1 breath
    (2) the rate of compressions is 80–100 times per minute
    (3) depress the sternum 1 to 1½ inches
    (4) use the heel of one hand

22. The following adverse effects are associated with beta-adrenergic blocking agents

    (1) sexual dysfunction
    (2) masking of hypoglycemic symptoms
    (3) severe bradycardia
    (4) bronchospasm

23. Complications of hypertension are

    (1) dissecting aortic aneurysm
    (2) myocardial infarction
    (3) cerebral hemorrhage
    (4) aortic stenosis

24. Which of the following is/are true regarding abdominal aortic aneurysms?

    (1) pain located in hypogastrium and lower back
    (2) rupture of an aneurysm results in hypotension and shock
    (3) majority of abdominal aortic aneurysms are asymptomatic
    (4) surgery recommended for aneurysms 3 cm in width or wider

25. Clinical manifestations of thoracic aortic aneurysms is/are

    (1) dysphagia
    (2) chest pain
    (3) tracheal deviation
    (4) cough

26. Causes of sudden cardiac death include

    (1) hypertrophic obstructive cardiomyopathy
    (2) aortic stenosis
    (3) coronary heart disease
    (4) acute heart failure

27. A new, loud, systolic murmur in a patient with an acute myocardial infarction can be the result of

    (1) left ventricular aneurysm
    (2) ventriculoseptal defect
    (3) pericarditis
    (4) rupture of papillary muscle

28. A mechanical prosthetic heart valve

    (1) has an excellent record of durability
    (2) is associated with increased incidence of thromboembolism
    (3) requires patients to receive anticoagulation therapy
    (4) has limited durability

29. Which of the following is/are true regarding an atrial septal defect?

    (1) results in a left-to-right shunt
    (2) most common ASD is ostium secundum type
    (3) usually asymptomatic in early life
    (4) often diagnosed in early infancy

30. Indications for cardiac pacing include

    (1) first-degree AV block
    (2) asymptomatic bundle branch block
    (3) asymptomatic sick sinus syndrome
    (4) symptomatic bradycardia

31. Causes of atrial fibrillation include

    (1) rheumatic heart disease
    (2) thyrotoxicosis
    (3) coronary heart disease
    (4) pulmonary emboli

32. Adverse reactions associated with nitroglycerin administration are

    (1) headache
    (2) hypotension
    (3) flushing
    (4) nausea and vomiting

DIRECTIONS (Questions 33 through 53): Each of the numbered items or incomplete statements in this section is followed by answers or by completions of the statement. Select the ONE lettered answer or completion that is BEST in each case.

Questions 33 through 53

33. Mitral regurgitation may result from abnormalities of all of the following structures EXCEPT

    (A) mitral annulus
    (B) left atrium
    (C) papillary muscles
    (D) chordae tendinae
    (E) mitral leaflets

34. In severe aortic stenosis, all the following are indications for valve replacement EXCEPT

    (A) angina
    (B) dyspnea on exertion
    (C) palpitations
    (D) congestive heart failure
    (E) syncope

35. All the following physical findings are characteristic of an aortic regurgitation murmur EXCEPT

    (A) wide pulse pressure
    (B) diastolic murmur
    (C) waterhammer pulse
    (D) loud S1
    (E) bisferious pulse

36. The earliest symptom of left-sided heart failure is

    (A) orthopnea
    (B) pedal edema
    (C) paroxysmal nocturnal dyspnea
    (D) dyspnea on exertion
    (E) fatigue

37. All the following are causes of pericarditis EXCEPT

    (A) acute myocardial infarction
    (B) trauma
    (C) uremia
    (D) neoplasm
    (E) liver disease

38. All the following statements are true of hypertrophic cardiomyopathy EXCEPT

    (A) dyspnea is the most common
    (B) systolic ejection murmur is present
    (C) associated with sudden death
    (D) symptoms decrease with exertion
    (E) left ventricular hypertrophy is present on echocardiogram

39. All the following medications can aggravate hyperlipidemia EXCEPT

    (A) captopril
    (B) thiazide diuretic
    (C) oral contraceptives
    (D) anabolic steroids
    (E) progestins

40. Features of mitral valve prolapse include all the following EXCEPT

    (A) midsystolic clicks
    (B) nonspecific ST-T changes on ECG
    (C) mid-to-late crescendo systolic murmur
    (D) majority of patients are asymptomatic
    (E) S4 gallop

41. Elevated levels of the following lipoprotein increase the risk of coronary heart disease

    (A) chylomicrons
    (B) triglycerides
    (C) LDL
    (D) VLDL
    (E) HDL

42. All of the following are contraindications to stress testing EXCEPT

    (A) unstable angina
    (B) congestive heart failure
    (C) severe hypertension
    (D) severe aortic stenosis
    (E) premature ventricular contractions

43. The most common cause of mitral stenosis is

    (A) lupus
    (B) bacterial endocarditis
    (C) trauma
    (D) rheumatic fever
    (E) congenital

44. All the following are used in the management of unstable angina EXCEPT

    (A) bedrest
    (B) nitrates
    (C) beta-adrenergic blockers
    (D) calcium-channel blockers
    (E) digoxin

45. The most useful cardiac enzyme test for myocardial necrosis is

    (A) creatine kinase–MM
    (B) creatine kinase–MB
    (C) glutamic oxaloacetic transferase
    (D) lactic dehydrogenase
    (E) alkaline phosphatase

46. The major cause of cardiogenic shock is

    (A) perforation of the interventricular septum
    (B) acute myocardial infarction
    (C) atrioventricular block
    (D) pulmonary embolism
    (E) severe bradycardia

47. The standard endocarditis prophylaxis recommendation for dental procedures or surgery of the upper respiratory tract is

    (A) penicillin V 1.0 g orally on the day before procedure and 1.0 g 1 hour after procedure
    (B) penicillin V 2.0 g orally 6 hours before procedure and 1.0 g 6 hours later
    (C) penicillin V 2.0 g orally 1 hour before procedure and 1.0 g 1 hour later
    (D) penicillin V 2.0 g orally 1 hour before procedure and 1.0 g 6 hours later
    (E) penicillin V 1.0 g orally 1 hour before procedure and 1.0 g 6 hours later

48. Absolute contraindications to thrombolytic therapy include all of the following except

    (A) history of cerebrovascular disease
    (B) history of significant gastrointestinal bleeding
    (C) severe uncontrolled hypertension
    (D) diabetes
    (E) recent history of severe trauma

49. Following percutaneous transluminal coronary angioplasty (PTCA), 20% of patients will develop signs of restenosis after

    (A) 6 months
    (B) 8 months
    (C) 10 months
    (D) 12 months
    (E) 24 months

50. The most common cause of syncope is

    (A) seizure
    (B) arrhythmia
    (C) vasovagal hypotension
    (D) transient ischemic attack
    (E) hypoglycemia

51. The major side effect of bile acid sequestrants such as cholestyramine is

    (A) gastrointestinal
    (B) myositis
    (C) flushing
    (D) rash
    (E) reversible liver damage

52. Renovascular hypertension should be suspected with all the following clinical features EXCEPT

    (A) severe, rapidly accelerating hypertension
    (B) presence of an abdominal bruit
    (C) onset of hypertension before age 30, particularly in slender white women
    (D) headaches, sweating, and palpitations
    (E) onset of hypertension after renal trauma

53. Precipitating causes of heart failure include

    (A) systemic infection
    (B) arrhythmias
    (C) inappropriate reduction of therapy
    (D) dietary sodium excesses
    (E) all of the above

DIRECTIONS (Questions 54 through 58): Each group of items in this section consists of an electrocardiographic tracing followed by a set of letter headings. Select the ONE letter that is most closely associated with it.

Questions 54 through 58

54. Figure 4–1

    (A) atrial flutter
    (B) premature atrial contraction
    (C) atrial fibrillation
    (D) sinus rhythm

55. Figure 4–2

    (A) complete heart block
    (B) atrial fibrillation
    (C) Mobitz type I
    (D) atrial flutter

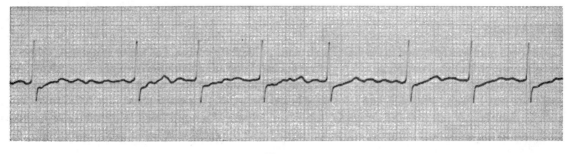

Fig. 4–1

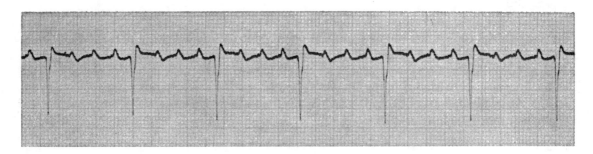

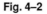

Fig. 4–2

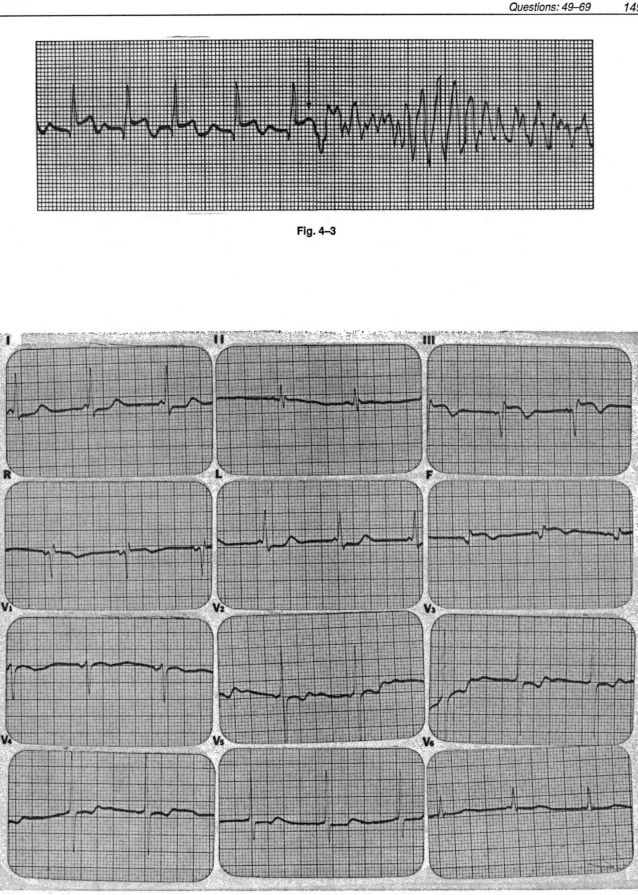

Fig. 4–3

Fig. 4–4

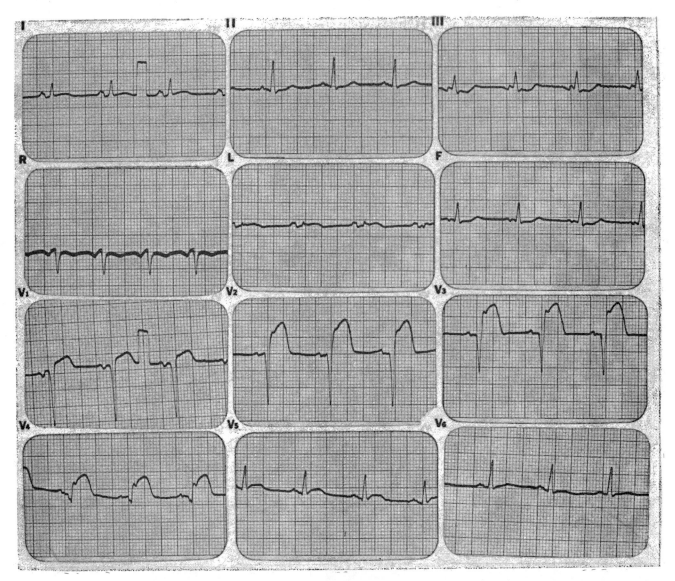

FIG. 4–5

56. Figure 4–3

    (A) ventricular tachycardia
    (B) Torsades de pointes
    (C) ventricular fibrillation
    (D) artifact

57. Figure 4–4

    (A) anterior myocardial infarction
    (B) anterior ischemia

(C) inferior myocardial infarction
(D) pericarditis

58. Figure 4–5

    (A) old anterior myocardial infarction
    (B) acute anteroseptal myocardial infarction
    (C) left ventricular hypertrophy with strain
    (D) apical aneurysm

DIRECTIONS (Questions 59 through 80): Each set of items in this section consists of a list of lettered options followed by several numbered words or phrases. For each numbered word or phrase, select the ONE lettered option that is most closely associated with it. Each lettered option may be selected once, more than once, or not at all.

Questions 59 through 62

    (A) aortic stenosis
    (B) mitral regurgitation
    (C) both
    (D) neither

59. Pansystolic murmur

60. Radiates to axilla

61. Bicuspid valve

62. Murmur reduced during Valsalva's maneuver

Questions 63 through 65

    (A) increases myocardial oxygen supply
    (B) decreases myocardial oxygen demand
    (C) both
    (D) neither

63. Propranolol

64. Diltiazem

65. Nitroglycerin

Questions 66 through 69

    (A) affects serum lipids
    (B) affects serum potassium levels
    (C) both
    (D) neither

66. Captopril

67. Hydrocholorothiazide

68. Diltiazem

69. Clonidine

Questions 70 through 73

For each of the antihypertensive drugs listed below, select the mechanism of action with which it is associated.

    (A) calcium channel blockers
    (B) beta-adrenergic blockers
    (C) angiotensin-converting enzyme inhibitor
    (D) alpha-adrenergic receptor blocker
    (E) vasodilator

70. Enalapril

71. Verapamil

72. Metoprolol

73. Prazosin

Questions 74 through 77

For each of the heart sounds listed below, select the appropriate origin of the sound.

    (A) S1
    (B) S2
    (C) S3
    (D) S4
    (E) opening snap

74. Caused by closure of aortic and pulmonic valves

75. Associated with atrial contraction in a hypertrophied heart

76. Caused by closure of mitral and tricuspid valve

77. Heart with left ventricular failure

Questions 78 through 80

Match the congenital heart defect with the appropriate description.

    (A) atrial septal defect
    (B) ventricular septal defect
    (C) coarctation of the aorta
    (D) patent foramen ovale
    (E) patent ductus arteriosus

78. Most common congenital malformation in infants and children

79. Cause of surgically correctable hypertension

80. Patient may remain asymptomatic until past the age of forty

Answers and Explanations

1. **(C)** Prolongation of the Q-T interval may occur with type Ia antiarrhythmic drugs, such as quinidine, procainamide, and disopyramide. It is also seen with hereditary syndromes. Hyperkalemia and digitalis will cause shortening of the Q-T interval. *(Braunwald, pp. 699,749)*

2. **(E)** High-density lipoproteins are produced by the liver and the gut and facilitate cholesterol removal from the tissues. There is an inverse relationship between high-density lipoproteins and coronary artery disease. Medical therapy with gemfibrozil has been shown to reduce triglyceride levels by 50% and increase HDLs by 20%. Estrogen, exercise, and ETOH (the three Es), and smoking cessation also increase serum HDL levels. *(Braunwald, pp. 1161–1162,1170–1172)*

3. **(E)** Sick sinus syndrome is the result of sinus node dysfunction. The rhythm disturbances include bradycardia–tachycardia syndrome, persistent sinus bradycardia, sinus arrest or exit block, or a combination of SA or AV conduction abnormalities. A patient can have more than one of these conductive disturbances. Patients with symptomatic sick sinus syndrome (such as syncope, dizziness) generally require a permanent pacemaker. *(Braunwald, p. 667)*

4. **(B)** Thromboembolism is a complication of mitral valve disease due to dilation of the left atrium and increased left atrial pressures. With left atrial enlargement, there is a predisposition to atrial fibrillation. *(Braunwald, pp. 1026,1027)*

5. **(E)** Torsade de pointes is a rapid pleomorphic ventricular tachycardia with rates of 200–250, in which the amplitude and polarity of QRS complexes continuously change and appear to be rotating around an isoelectric baseline. Torsade de pointes occurs in the setting of prolonged ventricular repolarization. The most common causes are potassium depletion, severe bradycardia, and type Ia antiarrhythmics, such as quinidine and disopyramide. *(Braunwald, pp. 698–699)*

6. **(E)** The National Cholesterol Education Program has recommended that the first step in lowering cholesterol is dietary treatment. Cholesterol can be reduced by following a diet with a cholesterol intake of less than 300 mg/day, a total fat intake of less than 30% of the total calories; 10% of the fat calories come from saturated fat. Weight reduction is recommended in the obese individual to help lower cholesterol. *(National Cholesterol Education Program, pp. 1–7)*

7. **(A)** Prinzmetal's angina, or variant angina, occurs more commonly during times of rest. It is caused by spasm of the major coronary artery. The spasm is usually superimposed upon a fixed atherosclerotic coronary stenosis, but it can also occur in individuals with coronary arteries that are free of significant narrowing. During episodes of vasospasm, there is transmural myocardial ischemia that leads to ST-segment elevation. Long-acting nitrates and calcium channel blockers are used to prevent vasospasm. *(Braunwald, pp. 1360–1361)*

8. **(D)** Cholesterol is found only in foods from animal origin (such as meats, whole milk, cheeses, butter, eggs, ice cream, lard). Soybeans have polyunsaturated fats, which are found in foods of plant origin and decrease cholesterol. Salmon contains omega-3 fatty acids, which are polyunsaturated fats and decrease cholesterol. Saturated fats will raise cholesterol. Saturated fats are generally derived from foods of animal origin. The exceptions are coconut oil and palm oil, which come from plant sources but are highly saturated. *(Braunwald, pp. 1167–1168)*

9. **(E)** When treating chronic heart failure, simple therapeutic means, such as diuretics and restricted sodium intake, are often the first line of therapy. If the symptoms or physical signs of heart failure continue, vasodilators and/or a digitalis glycoside may be used. Vasodilators are used to reduce the heart's workload. Digitalis helps to improve cardiac contractility. *(Braunwald, pp. 485–488)*

10. **(B)** Captopril is a potassium-sparing agent. It is an angiotensin-converting enzyme inhibitor and blocks the formation of angiotensin II, which stimulates aldosterone production. By decreasing aldosterone production, serum potassium levels may increase. Hydrochlorothiazide is a diuretic that can lower serum potassium levels. Hypokalemia can cause muscle weakness, polyuria, leg cramps, or increased ventricular ectopy. Diltiazem, a calcium channel blocker, and atenolol, a beta-adrenergic blocking agent, do not affect serum potassium levels. *(Braunwald, pp. 870,877)*

11. **(C)** In first-degree AV block, every atrial impulse is conducted to the ventricle. In second-degree AV block, every atrial impulse is not conducted to the ventricles. A nonconducted P wave is preceded by sinus beats with constant PR intervals in Mobitz type II second-degree AV block. Adams–Stokes syncope and complete AV block (atria and ventricle have independent pacemakers) are often preceded by Mobitz type II second-degree AV block, and a permanent pacemaker is necessary. *(Braunwald, pp. 702–706)*

12. **(E)** The classical electrocardiographic findings in Wolff–Parkinson–White syndrome are a short PR interval (less than 0.12 seconds), delta wave (initial slurring of the QRS complex), and wide QRS (greater than 0.12 seconds). These findings are caused by preexcitation of the ventricles. In Wolff–Parkinson–White syndrome, patients possess an accessory pathway that originates in one of the atria and terminates in one of the ventricles. The most common arrhythmia associated with Wolff–Parkinson–White syndrome is paroxysmal atrial tachycardia. The tachycardia is based upon a circus movement involving the myocardium, accessory pathway, and atrial myocardium. *(Braunwald, pp. 202–203,605–606)*

13. **(B)** In atrial fibrillation, the P waves are grossly irregular due to disorganized atrial depolarization. There is no effective atrial contraction. The atrial rate may be 350 to 600 beats per minute with a ventricular response of 100 to 160 beats per minute. In atrial flutter, the P waves are regular, with a sawtooth appearance. The atrial rate in atrial flutter is 250 to 350 beats per minute. *(Braunwald, pp. 660,672–673)*

14. **(E)** In angina, chest pain is related to an increase in myocardial oxygen demand that can occur with exercise, walking after a large meal, and exposure to cold weather. Stress causes a rise in heart rate and blood pressure, which also increases myocardial oxygen demand. Moreover, angina can occur during episodes of coronary vasoconstriction as a result of a transient decrease in myocardial oxygen supply. *(Braunwald, pp. 1316–1317)*

15. **(A)** Weight loss can be effective in lowering blood pressure and may delay or avoid the need for medical therapy. It has been shown that heavy alcohol consumption increases the risk of developing hypertension. It is recommended that alcohol be limited to less than 2 ounces per day. Dietary sodium restriction will help reduce blood pressure. Moderate sodium restriction can be accomplished by following simple guidelines such as not adding salt to food during cooking or at the table and avoiding obviously high-sodium foods (ie, processed foods). A low cholesterol, low-fat diet is beneficial in weight reduction, in addition to reducing the risk of developing cardiovascular heart disease. *(Braunwald, pp. 837,865–867)*

16. **(A)** Inverted T waves are caused by a number of conditions, including myocardial ischemia, subendocardial infarction, and left ventricular hypertrophy. A high serum potassium causes tall and peaked T waves. As the hyperkalemia worsens, the PR interval is prolonged and the QRS can widen. *(Clinical Synopsia–CIBA, pp. 27–30)*

17. **(E)** A chest roentgenogram in a patient with congestive heart failure may show an enlarged cardiac silhouette, pulmonary vascular redistribution, pleural effusions, and Kerley's lines. Pulmonary vascular redistribution is a result of interstitial and perivascular edema developing in the lung bases that leads to compression of the vessels in the lower lobes. With constriction of the lower lobe vessels, dilation of the vessels to the upper lobes occurs. With increased pulmonary and capillary pressures, pulmonary edema develops and may lead to pleural effusions or Kerley's lines. Kerley's lines are sharp, linear densities caused by edema. *(Braunwald, p. 483)*

18. **(A)** High-output heart failure can occur with anemia, thyrotoxicosis, and pregnancy. With these conditions, the cardiac output is markedly elevated, and the heart must pump an abnormally large volume. If the heart cannot adapt to the higher demands imposed by hypermetabolic or hyperkinetic states, then cardiac decompensation will occur. Hypertension can lead to a low cardiac output failure. *(Braunwald, pp. 778–790)*

19. **(B)** In cardiopulmonary resuscitation, one must open the airway and provide rescue breathing and artificial circulation. Artificial circulation is done by external chest compressions at a rate of 80 to 100 times per minute in an adult. Chest compressions are done at least 100 times per minute in an infant. The ratio of chest compressions to breaths

is 15:2 in one-man CPR. In two-man CPR, the ratio is 5 compressions to one breath. *(JAMA, p. 2905)*

20. **(B)** HDL removes cholesterol from peripheral tissues and carries it to the liver. In the liver, HDL/cholesterol complex is broken down into bile and acid salts and eliminated. Studies have indicated that a low HDL (35 mg/dL) is a risk factor for coronary artery disease. Cigarette smoking lowers HDL, and exercise can raise it. Low-density lipoproteins (LDLs) transport cholesterol to the peripheral cells. *(Braunwald, pp. 1161–1162; National Cholesterol Education Program, pp. 1–7)*

21. **(E)** When performing cardiopulmonary resuscitation in a small child, the heel of one hand should depress the sterum 1 to 1½ inches. The ratio of compressions to breaths is 5:1 at a rate of 80 to 100 compressions per minute. *(Effren, p. 33)*

22. **(E)** Beta-adrenergic blocking agents are used in the treatment of hypertension, coronary artery disease, and arrhythmias. Most of the side effects associated with beta-adrenergic blocking agents include myocardial effects (ie, severe bradycardia, sinus arrest, AV block). Fatigue, insomnia, and hallucinations are direct effects of the beta-blockers on the central nervous system. These side effects occur less often with lower lipid soluble agents (ie, atenolol) which may penetrate the brain in lower concentration. A beta-blocker can induce bronchospasm and is a contraindication in a patient with a history of asthma or bronchospasm. Other adverse effects include sexual dysfunction and gastrointestinal distress. Masking of hypoglycemic response (ie, tachycardia, palpitations, anxiety, tremor, diaphoresis) can occur with the use of beta-blockers and can lead to life-threatening hypoglycemia. Use of beta-blockers in diabetics should be avoided. *(Braunwald, pp. 1330–1332)*

23. **(A)** Aortic dissection, myocardial infarction, and cerebral hemorrhage are all complications of hypertension. Aortic dissections in hypertensives may result from a combination of atherosclerosis and high pulsative wave stress. The major cause of stroke is hypertension and is directly related to the blood pressure elevation. *(Kaplan, pp. 136–143)*

24. **(A)** The majority of abdominal aortic aneurysms are asymptomatic and may be found on routine physical exam. If pain is present, it may be steady and located in the hypogastrium and lower back. Rupture of an aneurysm is associated with severe abdominal and/or back pain, hypotension, and shock. A normal aorta is 2 cm in diameter. Surgery is recommended, if possible, when the aortic aneurysm is 6 cm in diameter or wider. Fifty percent of aneurysms greater than 6 cm in diameter may rupture in 1 year. *(Braunwald, pp. 1548–1550)*

25. **(E)** Signs and symptoms of thoracic aneurysms are related to their size and location. Cough and deviation of the trachea occur with aneurysms of the descending thoracic aorta as a result of compression of the tracheobronchial tree and lung. Dysphagia occurs when there is compression of the esophagus, and chest pain is related to compression of musculoskeletal structures. *(Braunwald, pp. 1551–1552)*

26. **(E)** Sudden cardiac death is defined as an unexpected natural death that is due to cardiac problems and associated with abrupt loss of consciousness. The most common cause of sudden cardiac death is coronary heart disease. Sudden cardiac disease in hypertrophic obstructive cardiomyopathy and aortic stenosis may be related to cardiac arrhythmias. Acute heart failure may cause sudden cardiac death as a result of circulatory failure or secondary arrhythmia. *(Braunwald, pp. 742–749)*

27. **(C)** Serious complications of an acute myocardial infarction are rupture of the interventricular septum and rupture of a papillary muscle. A loud systolic murmur may be associated with both these complications. A differentiation can be made with a two-dimensional echocardiogram with Doppler. *(Braunwald, pp. 1283–1287)*

28. **(A)** Two major types of artificial valves are mechanical prostheses and bioprostheses (tissue valves). Mechanical valves have an excellent record of durability but are also associated with an increased risk of thromboembolism. With the hazard of thromboembolism, patients require anticoagulation therapy. Tissue valves were developed to decrease the risk of thromboembolism but are not as durable as mechanical valves. *(Braunwald pp. 1078–1081)*

29. **(A)** An atrial septal defect causes left-to-right shunt. The most common ASD is the ostium secundum type that is located in the region of the foramen ovale. An atrial septal defect is rarely diagnosed or causes symptoms in early life. Symptoms often develop in adults and include dyspnea, fatigue, supraventricular arrhythmias, and respiratory illness. *(Braunwald, pp. 915–916,982)*

30. **(D)** One indication for cardiac pacing is symptomatic bradycardia. Medical therapy is usually not successful in speeding up the heart, so a pacemaker is indicated. Patients with asymptomatic bundle branch block and first-degree AV block do not require cardiac pacing. Cardiac pacing is not indicated in asymptomatic sick sinus syndrome. If

symptoms appear, however, a permanent pacemaker is indicated. *(Braunwald, pp. 667,717–718)*

31. **(E)** Atrial fibrillation can occur in normal hearts or be associated with heart disease. Atrial fibrillation is associated with rheumatic heart disease, pulmonary emboli, coronary heart disease, hypertensive cardiovascular disease, cardiomyopathy, atrial septal defect, and following cardiac surgery. Thyrotoxicosis can also be a precipitating cause of atrial fibrillation. *(Braunwald, p. 673)*

32. **(A)** Headache, flushing, and hypotension are adverse reactions that are associated with nitroglycerin administration. The action of nitrates is to relax vascular and smooth muscle, causing vasodilation of both peripheral and coronary arteries. The side effects are a result of the vasodilatory properties of nitrates. *(Braunwald, pp. 1327–1329)*

33. **(B)** Mitral regurgitation can be associated with abnormalities of the mitral annulus, papillary muscles, chordae tendinae, and mitral leaflets. Disorders of the mitral annulus (ie, rheumatic heart disease abscess) or dilation of the left ventricle from heart disease result in dilation of the mitral annulus. Papillary muscle dysfunction causes mitral regurgitation. This can be seen with an acute myocardial infarction or ischemia, because the papillary muscles are perfused by the coronary arteries. The chordae tendinae can rupture as a result of trauma, rheumatic fever, myxomatous degeneration, endocarditis, or a congenital abnormality. Abnormalities of the mitral leaflets are seen most frequently in rheumatic heart disease. *(Braunwald, pp. 1034–1037)*

34. **(C)** Angina, dyspnea on exertion, congestive heart failure, and syncope are indicators for valve replacement in aortic stenosis. Angina is due to the increased oxygen needs of the hypertrophied left ventricle and decreased oxygen delivery as a result of compression of the coronary arteries. Dyspnea on exertion and congestive heart failure are late symptoms and are caused by pulmonary venous hypertension. Syncope usually occurs during exertion as a result of a drop in cardiac output or a ventricular arrhythmia. *(Braunwald, pp. 1057–1059)*

35. **(D)** The murmur of aortic regurgitation is a high-pitched diastolic murmur. It begins immediately after A2 and is best heard along the left sternal border, 3rd and 4th intercostal spaces; a soft S1 is heard. The systolic arterial pressure is elevated and the diastolic pressure is low, resulting in a wide pulse pressure. The pulses are abrupt with a quick collapse and are often described as a waterhammer pulse. A bisferious pulse is present. It is a dicrotic pulse, two pulsations; the second

pulsation is during diastole and is felt following S2. This is best appreciated in the brachial or femoral pulse. A loud S1 is present with high-velocity closure of the mitral valve, as seen with mitral valve prolapse. *(Braunwald, pp. 1064–1605)*

36. **(D)** Dyspnea on exertion is usually the earliest symptom of left-sided heart failure. Patients with left ventricular disease develop high left ventricular filling pressures with exercise. This results in increased pulmonary capillary and pulmonary venous pressures causing shortness of breath with exertion. Orthopnea and paroxysmal nocturnal dyspnea usually develop at a later stage of left ventricular failure. Fatigue is often a complaint in patients with heart failure and low cardiac output. *(Cohn, pp. 129–131)*

37. **(E)** Liver disease is not a cause of acute pericarditis. Following an acute myocardial infarction, pericarditis can develop during the first week after infection—acute postinfarction pericarditis. Or it can develop weeks to months following an MI, as seen with Dressler's syndrome, which is characterized by acute illness with fever, pericarditis, and pleuritis. Chest trauma may result in the development of an acute pericarditis. Uremic pericarditis is a complication of chronic renal failure. The exact cause is unknown. Patients with malignant neoplasms may present with an acute pericarditis. Pericardial effusions can occur as a result of metastatic involvement of the pericardium. Primary tumors of the pericardium are rare. *(Braunwald, pp. 1488,1521–1522)*

38. **(D)** Hypertrophic cardiomyopathy is a disease characterized by hypertrophy of the cardiac muscle without any identifiable cause. On physical exam, a systolic ejection murmur is best heard at the lower left sternal border and apex. Dyspnea is the most common symptom. Angina and syncope are also common complaints. Syncopal episodes are often related to arrhythmias. Ventricular arrhythmias are probably responsible for the majority of sudden death cases. The symptoms are increased with exertion. Syncope and sudden death have been associated with extreme exertion. Left ventricular hypertrophy is seen on the echocardiogram. *(Braunwald, pp. 1422–1426)*

39. **(A)** Captopril is an angiotension-converting enzyme inhibitor. It does not affect serum lipid levels. A thiazide diuretic can cause an elevation of low-density lipoprotein cholesterol, which is an atherogenic class of lipoproteins. Oral contraceptives, progestins, and anabolic steroids can also raise serum levels of lipoproteins. *(Braunwald, pp. 515–516,1167)*

40. (E) Mitral valve prolapse syndrome is one of the most common valvular abnormalities. The majority of patients with MVP are asymptomatic. Symptomatic patients may complain of chest pain and palpitations. The chest pain is often atypical and is not related to exertion and can be prolonged. Palpitations can be associated with atrial and ventricular premature contractions, as well as supraventricular and ventricular tachyarrhythmias. The auscultatory findings associated with MVP syndrome are a midsystolic click and late systolic murmur. There is a great variability in physical findings. Patients may have both a click and a murmur or only one of the findings. The electrocardiogram can show nonspecific ST-T wave changes. An S4 gallop is not associated with MVP. It is associated with a noncompliant heart such as hypertrophic cardiomyopathy. *(Braunwald, pp. 1044–1049)*

41. (C) Patients with high LDL cholesterol (106 mg/dL) are at increased risk for developing coronary heart disease. LDL cholesterol transports cholesterol to peripheral cells. Very low-density lipoproteins (VLDLs) (ie, triglycerides) are produced by the liver and small intestine. High levels of triglycerides can cause pancreatitis. Chylomicrons are large lipoprotein particles that consist of cholesterol and triglycerides. HDL cholesterol is inversely related to the risk of coronary heart disease. HDL cholesterol removes cholesterol from peripheral tissues and carries it back to the liver, where it is eliminated. *(National Cholesterol Education Program, p. 17; Braunwald, pp. 1154–1162)*

42. (E) Contraindications to stress testing include unstable angina, congestive heart failure, severe hypertension, and severe aortic stenosis. Exercise can aggravate any of these clinical conditions. A patient with mild to moderate aortic stenosis may exercise safely, but there is a risk of syncope or sudden death with aortic stenosis during vigorous exercise. A patient with premature ventricular contractions can safely do an exercise stress test. *(Braunwald, p. 238)*

43. (D) Rheumatic fever is the major cause of mitral stenosis. Most patients do not develop symptoms of mitral stenosis for at least a decade after the onset of acute rheumatic fever. *(Braunwald, p. 1023)*

44. (E) Unstable angina is a serious condition and may be a warning of an impending myocardial infarction. The management of unstable angina includes bedrest, nitrates, beta-adrenergic blockers, and calcium channel blockers. Nitrates are the mainstay of therapy. They relieve pain and may improve global and left ventricular function. Digoxin increases myocardial contractions; this in-

creases myocardial oxygen demand. *(Braunwald, pp. 1353–1358)*

45. (B) Enzymes are released into the circulation by injured myocardial cells. Elevations of serum glutamic oxaloacetic transferase (SGOT), lactic dehydrogenase, and creatine kinase–MB (CK–MB) are used in the diagnosis of an acute myocardial infarction. There are three isoenzymes of creatine kinase—MM, BB, and MB. MM isoenzyme is present primarily in skeletal muscle. Brain and kidney contain BB isoenzyme, and cardiac muscle contains MM isoenzyme and MB isoenzyme. Elevated CK–MB is usually the result of an acute myocardial infarction and is the most sensitive enzyme test for myocardial necrosis. *(Braunwald, pp. 1239–1241)*

46. (B) The major cause of cardiogenic shock is acute myocardial infarction. Cardiogenic shock occurs primarily with an anterior and anteroseptal myocardial infarction. The onset and severity of cardiogenic shock is related to the amount of functional myocardium that is lost. *(Braunwald, p. 572)*

47. (D) The present recommended antibiotic regimen for dental procedures and surgery of the upper respiratory tract is penicillin V 2.0 g orally 1 hour before the procedure, then 1.0 g 6 hours later. Patients allergic to penicillin can take erythromycin 1.0 g orally 1 hour before and 50 mg 6 hours later. *(Shulman et al, pp. 1124A–1125B)*

48. (D) Thrombolytic agents (ie, streptokinase, tissue plasminogen activator (t-PA), have been used to lyse clots in an effort to limit myocardial damage during infarction. There is a possibility of bleeding complication with thrombolytic agents, so patients must be screened carefully. Absolute contraindications include a history of cerebrovascular disease, gastrointestinal bleeding, severe uncontrolled hypertension, bleeding diathesis, and recent severe trauma. *(Braunwald, pp. 1253–1257)*

49. (A) In PTCA, restenosis will occur within 6 months in approximately 20% of patients. Patients should be closely followed clinically and with exercise tests in the 6 months after PTCA. If restenosis develops, repeat catheterization with repeat PTCA is often successful. *(Braunwald, p. 1387)*

50. (C) Vasovagal hypotension, which is the common faint, is the most common type of syncope. This is often precipitated by the sight of blood, a stressful or painful experience (ie, venipuncture, trauma), crowding, and prolonged standing. The signs and symptoms associated with vasovagal syncope are pallor, weakness, nausea, and diaphoresis. The symptoms usually occur when the patient is in an upright position. It can usually be differentiated from other causes of syncope by the type of setting in which it happens, appearance of the patient, and knowledge of the onset. *(Braunwald, pp. 887–892)*

51. **(A)** Bile acid sequestrants are used in the treatment of lipid disorders. They are often difficult to take because of the frequent gastrointestinal side effects, such as constipation, abdominal distention, nausea, vomiting, or diarrhea. Myositis and reversible liver damage are side effects associated with lovastatin. Flushing is a side effect of nicotinic acid. *(Braunwald, p. 1169)*

52. **(D)** The two major types of renovascular hypertension are caused by atherosclerotic disease and fibroplastic disease. Atherosclerotic disease is seen mostly in older men, whereas fibroplastic disease is seen more frequently in younger women. Renovascular disease should be suspected if the following clinical features are present: (1) abdominal bruit, particularly if lateral to midline; (2) severe, rapidly accelerating hypertension; (3) onset of hypertension before age 30, particularly in white women, as it may be due to fibroplastic disease; (4) onset after renal trauma; (5) rapidly deteriorating renal function. Headache, flushing, and palpitations are associated with a pheochromocytoma. *(Braunwald, pp. 842–843,847)*

53. **(E)** A number of events may precipitate heart failure in a previously compensated individual. The most common events are reductions in therapy or dietary sodium excess. A patient may adjust his or her own medication as he/she begins to feel better or be more lenient with the sodium intake and precipitate heart failure. Tachyarrhythmias, bradycardia, atrial-ventricular dissociation, and abnormal intraventricular conduction can all intensify heart failure. Systemic infections can increase the hemodynamic burden of the heart and precipitate heart failure. *(Braunwald, pp. 474–475)*

54. **(C)** The ECG tracing shows atrial fibrillation. The ventricular rate is 80 and the rhythm is irregular. P waves are absent and there are fibrillatory waves (f waves) of different size and shape. Atrial fibrillation can be chronic, as a result of underlying heart disease, or intermittent, which may occur in normal hearts. Hypertension is the most common disease process that causes atrial fibrillation. *(Braunwald, pp. 672–674)*

55. **(D)** The ECG tracing is of atrial flutter. Note the regular sawtooth flutter wave and the regular ventricular response. This is a 4:1 block. Atrial flutter occurs less commonly than atrial fibrillation. Paroxysmal atrial flutter may occur in patients without organic heart disease, while chronic atrial flutter is associated with heart disease, such as

rheumatic or ischemic heart disease. *(Braunwald, pp. 671–672)*

56. **(C)** The ECG shows ventricular fibrillation. Note the R on T phenomenon. This represents severe derangement of the heartbeat and usually terminates fatally within 3 to 5 minutes. *(Braunwald, pp. 701–702)*

57. **(C)** This ECG shows an inferior myocardial infarction. The inferior leads on an ECG are II, III, and aVF. On this tracing there is ST segment elevation, indicative of infarction, in leads III and aVF. There are also reciprocal changes, ST depression, in the anterior leads. *(Braunwald, pp. 1241–1242)*

58. **(B)** This ECG tracing indicates an acute anteroseptal myocardial infarction. There is marked ST segment elevation, as well as Q waves in leads V2, V3, and V4. *(Braunwald, pp. 1241–1242)*

59. **(B)** Mitral regurgitation is a pansystolic murmur. It usually begins immediately after S1 and continues throughout systole. It is blowing, high-pitched, and of constant intensity. Aortic stenosis is a crescendo decrescendo ejection murmur. It usually begins after the onset of S1 and ends before A2. *(Braunwald, pp. 70,1055–1057)*

60. **(B)** The murmur of mitral regurgitation is best heard at the apex but can radiate to the axilla and occasionally the base of the heart. The murmur of aortic stenosis is best heard at the base of the heart but can radiate to the neck and apex. *(Braunwald, pp. 1040–1042,1055–1057)*

61. **(A)** The normal aortic valve is tricuspid. Aortic stenosis can occur as a result of a congenital bicuspid valve. The bicuspid valve causes turbulent flow, resulting in fibrosis and narrowing of the aortic valve. *(Braunwald, pp. 1052–1054)*

62. **(C)** With Valsalva's maneuver, there is a decline in systemic venous return, resulting in decreased filling of the right and left side of the heart. This results in a fall in stroke volume and arterial pressure that diminishes the murmurs of aortic stenosis and mitral regurgitation. *(Braunwald, pp. 1040–1042,1055–1057)*

63. **(B)** Propranolol is a beta-adrenergic blocking agent which acts by decreasing heart rate, blood pressure, and contractility, thereby decreasing myocardial oxygen demand. *(Braunwald, pp. 1330–1332)*

64. **(C)** Diltiazem, a calcium channel blocker, relaxes vascular smooth muscle which causes coronary vasodilation that will increase myocardial

oxygen supply. Diltiazem will also lower blood pressure, which will decrease myocardial oxygen demand. *(Braunwald, pp. 1332–1335)*

65. **(C)** Nitroglycerin is a coronary vasodilator that increases myocardial oxygen supply. It is also a venodilator that reduces preload and can lower blood pressure, which decreases myocardial oxygen demand. *(Braunwald, pp. 1328–1330)*

66. **(B)** Captopril is an angiotensin-converting enzyme inhibitor. It blocks the formation of angiotensin II, which stimulates aldosterone production. By decreasing aldosterone production, serum potassium levels may increase. Angiotensin-converting enzyme inhibitors should be used cautiously with potassium-sparing diuretics because of the potential for hyperkalemia. *(Braunwald, pp. 52,877–878)*

67. **(C)** Hydrochlorothiazide is a diuretic and can cause an elevation of low-density lipoprotein cholesterol and a fall in serum potassium. Patients with hypokalemia may experience muscle weakness, polyuria, leg cramps, or increased ventricular ectopy. *(Braunwald, p. 516)*

68. **(D)** Diltiazem is a calcium channel blocker. It is used in the treatment of angina and hypertension. Calcium channel agents cause relaxation of the vascular smooth muscles in the coronary arteries and systemic arterial beds. Side effects include headache, dizziness, flushing, hypotension, leg edema, and gastrointestinal complaints. *(Braunwald, pp. 1332–1333,1667)*

69. **(D)** Clonidine is an alpha-receptor agonist used in the treatment of hypertension. It does not affect serum potassium or serum lipid levels. Some of the side effects include dry mouth and drowsiness. *(Braunwald, pp. 873,1167)*

70. **(C)** Enalapril is an angiotensin-converting enzyme inhibitor. It lowers blood pressure by blocking the action of angiotensin-converting enzyme, which is involved in converting angiotensin I to angiotensin II. Angiotensin II is a vasoconstrictor and stimulates aldosterone production. *(Braunwald, pp. 877–878)*

71. **(A)** Verapamil is a calcium channel blocker. It lowers blood pressure by decreasing systemic vascular resistance. *(Braunwald, pp. 394,1332–1333)*

72. **(B)** Metoprolol is a beta-adrenergic blocking agent. It lowers blood pressure by decreasing cardiac output, reducing renin activity, and decreasing sympathetic discharge. *(Braunwald, pp. 872,874)*

73. **(D)** Prazosin is an alpha-adrenergic receptor blocker with its primary action as a postsynaptic alpha-blocker. The antihypertensive effect of the drug is a result of blocking alpha-mediated vasoconstriction. *(Braunwald, pp. 873,874,877)*

74. **(B)** S2 is also high-pitched and is the result of the closure of the pulmonic and aortic valves. *(Braunwald, pp. 29–30,46–48)*

75. **(D)** S3 is a low-pitched heart sound and occurs as passive ventricular filling begins. An S3 is heard with ventricular dysfunction or with marked left ventricular volume overload. *(Braunwald, pp. 31–32,50–51)*

76. **(A)** S1 is a high-pitched sound caused by the closure of the mitral and tricuspid valves. *(Braunwald, pp. 29–30,43–46)*

77. **(C)** An S2 is a low-pitched heart sound that occurs with atrial contraction. S4 is heard when there is increased left ventricular hypertrophy and restricted diastolic filling. *(Braunwald, pp. 31–32,50–51)*

78. **(B)** Ventricular septal defect is the most common congenital malformation seen in children and infants. A ventricular septal defect can present anywhere in the interventricular septum and may vary in size. Symptoms are related to the size of the shunt and pulmonary vascular resistance. *(Braunwald, pp. 920–923,985–988)*

79. **(C)** Coarctation of the aorta is narrowing of the thoracic aorta just distal to the insertion of the ligamentum arteriosum or just beyond the origin of the left subclavian artery. Features of coarctation include hypertension in the arms and weak or absent femoral pulses. Coarctation is a cause of hypertension and is surgically correctable. *(Braunwald, pp. 994–996)*

80. **(A)** A patient with an atrial septal defect may remain asymptomatic until the fourth or fifth decade. Symptoms of an atrial septal defect are dyspnea on exertion, fatigue, and palpitations secondary to supraventricular tachyarrhythmias. *(Braunwald, pp. 848,982,985)*

REFERENCES

Braunwald E (ed). *Heart Disease: A Textbook of Cardiovascular Medicine*, 3rd ed. Philadelphia, PA: WB Saunders; 1988.

Cohn JN. *Drug Treatment of Heart Failure*, 2nd ed. Secaucus, NJ: Advanced Therapeutics Communications International; 1988.

Effren D. *Cardiopulmonary Resuscitation,* 3rd ed. Tulsa, OK: CPR Publishing; 1989.

Kaplan NM. *Clinical Hypertension,* 4th ed. Baltimore, MD: Williams & Wilkins; 1986.

National Cholesterol Education Program. Highlights of the report of the expert panel on detection, evaluation, and treatment of high blood cholesterol in adults. NIH Publication No. 88-2926. Washington, DC: Public Health Service; 1987.

Rautaharju PM, Prince RJ, Eifler J, et al. Prognostic value of exercise ECG in men at high risk of future coronary heart disease: Multiple risk factor intervention trial experience. *J Am Coll Cardiol.* 1986;8:1–10.

Scheidt S. Basic electrocardiography. Abnormalities in electrocardiographic patterns. *CIBA Clin Symp.* 1984; 36:1–32.

Shulman ST, Amren DP, Bisro AL, et al. Prevention of bacterial endocarditis. A statement for health professionals by the Committee on Rheumatic Fever and Infective Endocarditis of the Council on Cardiovascular Disease in the Young. *Circulation.* 1984;70:1123–1127A.

Subspecialty List: Cardiology

QUESTION NUMBER AND SUBSPECIALTY

1. ECG findings
2. Cholesterol physiology
3. Cardiac arrhythmias
4. Mitral valve disease—complications
5. Cardiac arrhythmias
6. Cholesterol
7. Cardiac arrhythmias
8. Cholesterol
9. Congestive heart failure—treatment
10. Medication
11. Cardiac arrhythmias
12. Wolff–Parkinson–White syndrome—features
13. ECG findings
14. Angina—exacerbation
15. Hypertension—nonmedical treatment
16. ECG findings
17. Congestive heart failure—x-ray findings
18. Cardiac failure—causes of
19. Cardiopulmonary resuscitation
20. Cholesterol physiology
21. Cardiopulmonary resuscitation
22. Medications
23. Hypertension—complications
24. Aortic aneurysms—characteristics
25. Thoracic aneurysms—clinical findings
26. Sudden cardiac death—causes
27. Murmurs
28. Prosthetic heart valves
29. Atrial septal defects
30. Cardiac pacemakers—indications
31. Atrial fibrillation—causes
32. Medications
33. Murmurs—causes
34. Murmurs—indications for treatment
35. Murmurs—physical findings
36. Heart failure—symptoms
37. Pericarditis—causes
38. Cardiomyopathy—characteristics
39. Medications
40. Mitral valve prolapse—characteristics
41. Coronary heart disease—risk factors
42. Stress testing—contraindications
43. Mitral stenosis—causes
44. Angina—treatment
45. Myocardial necrosis—laboratory evaluation
46. Cardiogenic shock—causes
47. Endocarditis—prophylaxis
48. Thrombolytic therapy—contraindications
49. Coronary angioplasty—results
50. Syncope—causes
51. Medications
52. Renovascular hypertension—clinical findings
53. Heart failure—exacerbation
54. ECG interpretation
55. ECG interpretation
56. ECG interpretation
57. ECG interpretation
58. ECG interpretation
59. Murmurs
60. Murmurs
61. Murmurs
62. Murmurs
63. Medications
64. Medications
65. Medications
66. Medications
67. Medications
68. Medications
69. Medications
70. Medications
71. Medications
72. Medications
73. Medications
74. Heart sounds
75. Heart sounds
76. Heart sounds
77. Heart sounds
78. Congenital heart defects
79. Congenital heart defects
80. Congenital heart defects

Internal Medicine: Endocrinology
Questions

DIRECTIONS (Questions 1 through 11): Each set of items in this section consists of a list of lettered options followed by several numbered words or phrases. For each numbered word or phrase, select the ONE lettered option that is most closely associated with it. Each lettered option may be selected once, more than once, or not at all.

Questions 1 through 4

Match the following hormones with the site where they are produced.

    (A) posterior pituitary
    (B) anterior pituitary
    (C) both
    (D) neither

1. Luteinizing hormone and follicle-stimulating hormone

2. Thyroid-stimulating hormone and adrenocorticotropic hormone

3. Antidiuretic hormone and thyroid-stimulating hormone

4. Corticotropin-releasing factor and melanocyte-stimulating hormone

Questions 5 through 7

Match the substance secreted by this section of the adrenal gland.

    (A) aldosterone
    (B) cortisol
    (C) both
    (D) neither

5. Zona glomerulosa

6. Zona reticularis

7. Zona fasciculata

Questions 8 through 11

Match the following with its cause or symptom.

    (A) nephrogenic diabetes insipidus
    (B) neurogenic diabetes insipidus
    (C) both
    (D) neither

8. Polyuria

9. Psychogenic polydipsia

10. Lithium

11. Urinary tract obstruction

DIRECTIONS (Questions 12 through 38): For each of the items in this section, ONE or MORE of the numbered options is correct. Choose answer

    (A) if only (1), (2), and (3) are correct,
    (B) if only (1) and (3) are correct,
    (C) if only (2) and (4) are correct,
    (D) if only (4) is correct,
    (E) if all are correct.

Questions 12 through 38

12. Myxedema may present with which of the following symptoms?
    (1) arthralgias
    (2) anovulation
    (3) hoarseness
    (4) diarrhea

13. NIDDM (noninsulin-dependent diabetes mellitus) is characterized by a variety of metabolic defects, including
    (1) deficient beta cell function
    (2) a reduction of insulin receptors
    (3) impaired transport of glucose into cells
    (4) postreceptor intracellular defects

14. Prolactin secretion is enhanced by a variety of factors, including

   (1) opiate narcotics
   (2) bromocryptine therapy
   (3) pregnancy
   (4) L-dopa therapy

15. Treatment of DKA (diabetic ketoacidosis) may result in

   (1) hypoglycemia
   (2) hypokalemia
   (3) hypophosphatemia
   (4) hypocalcemia

16. Causes of hyperthyroidism can include

   (1) subacute thyroiditis
   (2) painless thyroiditis
   (3) toxic multinodular goiter
   (4) struma ovarii

17. Hypothroidism may be caused by

   (1) Hashimoto's thyroiditis
   (2) iodine excess (large dose)
   (3) iodine deficiency
   (4) chronic steroid therapy

18. Triiodothyronine (T_3) in the serum is derived from

   (1) secretion from the thyroid gland
   (2) iodination of tyrosine in the periphery
   (3) deiodination of T_4 in the periphery
   (4) oxidation of T_4 in the thyroid

19. T_4 is highly bound (more than 99%) in the plasma to

   (1) albumin
   (2) thyroid-binding globulin
   (3) thyroid-binding prealbumin
   (4) calmodulin-binding globulin

20. Fasting hypoglycemia may occur with

   (1) uremia
   (2) Addison's disease
   (3) insulin-producing islet cell tumors
   (4) acute hepatic necrosis

21. Clinical symptoms of acute adrenal insufficiency include

   (1) abdominal pain
   (2) hyponatremia
   (3) hypotension
   (4) hyperthermia

22. Endocrine causes for systolic and diastolic hypertension could include

   (1) primary aldosteronism
   (2) hyperthyroidism
   (3) hypercalcemia
   (4) Cushing's syndrome

23. Hypercalciuria (excretion rate greater than 300 mg in males and greater than 250 mg in females in 24 hours) may be due to

   (1) primary hyperparathyroidism
   (2) sarcoidosis
   (3) vitamin D intoxication
   (4) thyrotoxicosis

24. Risk factors for nephrolithiasis include

   (1) hypercalciuria
   (2) hyperuricosuria
   (3) urine volume less than 1 L per day
   (4) high protein intake

25. Multiple endocrine neoplasia type I may include the following types of tumors:

   (1) pituitary
   (2) parathyroid
   (3) pancreatic
   (4) medullary carcinoma of the thyroid

26. ACTH is stimulated by

   (1) TSH (thyroid-stimulating hormone)
   (2) CRF (corticotropin-releasing factor)
   (3) low cortisol
   (4) AVP (arginine vasopressin)

27. Aldosterone causes the kidney to

   (1) secrete potassium
   (2) absorb potassium
   (3) absorb sodium
   (4) secrete sodium

28. Short stature is a common endocrine problem seen in pediatric clinics. Differential diagnosis could include

   (1) familial
   (2) CNS tumors
   (3) hypothyroidism
   (4) growth hormone deficiency

29. Background diabetic retinopathy consists of

   (1) exudate
   (2) hemorrhages

(3) microaneurysms

(4) neovascularization

30. The Somogyi phenomenon is early morning hyperglycemia and ketonuria secondary to

(1) excessive insulin administration

(2) elevated epinephrine level

(3) elevated growth hormone level

(4) elevated cortisol level

31. First generation oral hypoglycemic agents include

(1) tolbutamide

(2) glipizide

(3) acetohexamide

(4) glyburide

32. SIADH (syndrome of inappropriate antidiuretic hormone release) can be caused by

(1) narcotics

(2) low serum osmolarity

(3) adenocarcinoma of the lung

(4) excessive H_2O drinking

33. Renal osteodystrophy refers to metabolic bone disease seen in end-stage renal disease. Possible bone lesions secondary to renal disease could include

(1) osteomalacia

(2) osteopetrosis

(3) hyperparathyroid bone disease

(4) fibrous dysplasia

34. Pheochromocytomas may be present in the

(1) adrenals

(2) organ of Zucherkandle

(3) paravertebral sympathetic ganglion

(4) kidney

35. Treatment for Cushing's disease can include

(1) pituitary surgery

(2) ketoconazole

(3) op DDD

(4) dexamethasone

36. Osteomalacia is defined as excess unmineralized bone due to impaired bone mineralization. The possible etiologies include

(1) vitamin D deficiency

(2) hyperparathyroidism

(3) hypophosphatemia

(4) hyperthyroidism

37. A 21-hydroxylase deficiency in the newborn needs to be considered when there is

(1) rapid weight gain

(2) ambiguous genitalia

(3) a breech delivery

(4) the occurrence of shock or death

38. Complications of diabetes include

(1) microangiopathy

(2) gastroparesis

(3) nocturnal diarrhea

(4) segmental demyelinization

DIRECTIONS (Questions 39 through 63): Each of the numbered items or incomplete statements in this section is followed by answers or by completions of the statement. Select the ONE lettered answer or completion that is BEST in each case.

Questions 39 through 63

39. A patient has a nodule on palpation over the thyroid gland. Factors indicating possible carcinoma include

(A) a scan with a hot nodule

(B) a scan with a cold nodule

(C) an echo with a clean cystic mass

(D) biopsy with chronic lymphocytic infiltration

(E) biopsy with a granulomatous lesion

40. ACTH (corticotropin) is a potent stimulatory for

(A) estrogen release

(B) testosterone release

(C) cortisol production

(D) ammonia generation

(E) aldactone release

41. ACTH is inhibited by

(A) high CRF

(B) high cortisol

(C) low cortisol

(D) high estrogen

(E) adrenalectomy

42. Adequacy of levothyroxine replacement dose in primary hypothyroidism can be best determined by which of the following laboratory values?

(A) T_3 RIA

(B) reverse T_3

(C) TBG

(D) T_3 stimulation test

(E) TSH

43. Klinefelter's syndrome is characterized by

    (A) a tall male
    (B) a short female
    (C) an abnormal XY chromosome
    (D) an XXY male
    (E) an XXY female

44. Infiltrative ophthalmopathy secondary to thyroid dysfunction is seen with

    (A) Graves' disease
    (B) Hashimoto's thyroiditis
    (C) toxic multinodular goiter
    (D) hypothyroidism
    (E) medullary carcinoma of the thyroid

45. The major clinical features of Turner's syndrome are

    (A) baldness with short stature
    (B) gigantism alone
    (C) webbed neck, low hairline, and short stature
    (D) gigantism with low hairline
    (E) short stature alone

46. Vitamin D is essential for normal calcium homeostasis and absorption. Of the following vitamin D sterols, which is the most important for calcium absorption?

    (A) $1,25\text{-}(OH)2D_3$
    (B) vitamin D_2
    (C) vitamin D_3
    (D) $24,25(OH)2D_3$
    (E) $25\text{-}OHD_{32}$

47. Magnesium ammonium phosphate stones (struvite stones) are usually caused by

    (A) hyperparathyroidism
    (B) hyperthyroidism
    (C) renal tubular acidosis
    (D) infection
    (E) trauma

48. Parathyroid hormone can increase serum calcium

    (A) by directly stimulating the GI tract
    (B) by stimulating nephrogenic cyclic AMP
    (C) by decreasing bone turnover
    (D) by increasing serum $1,25\text{-}(OH)2D_3$
    (E) by stimulating $25\text{-}OHD_3$

49. Single-drug therapy for pheochromocytoma should NOT include

    (A) propranolol
    (B) prazosine

    (C) phenoxybenzamine
    (D) phentolamine
    (E) nitroprusside

50. The pituitary gland is located in the

    (A) glenoid fossa
    (B) sphenoid fossa
    (C) sella turcica
    (D) anterior skull
    (E) median eminence

51. Release of antidiuretic hormone (ADH) from the posterior pituitary is determined by the

    (A) serum osmolarity
    (B) serum viscosity
    (C) plasma ADH level
    (D) urine osmolarity
    (E) serum potassium level

52. Elevated VLDL with normal LDL is found to fit into which of the following Fredrickson classifications?

    (A) Type IIa
    (B) Type IIb
    (C) Type III
    (D) Type IV
    (E) Type V

53. The dawn phenomenon is

    (A) hypoglycemia in the early AM
    (B) hypoglycemia in the late AM
    (C) hyperglycemia in early AM
    (D) ketoacidosis in the early AM
    (E) when NPH insulin peaks in patients

54. Oral hypoglycemic agents improve glucose control in diabetic patients by

    (A) improving insulin distribution
    (B) enhancing beta cell function
    (C) preventing gastric glucose absorption
    (D) enhancing glycogenolysis
    (E) preventing gluconeogenesis

55. The laboratory diagnosis of diabetes mellitus includes

    (A) a fasting glucose of <140
    (B) a fasting glucose of <100
    (C) a fasting glucose of >140
    (D) a fasting glucose of >100
    (E) 2-hour postprandial glucose of >100

56. The highly characteristic renal lesion of diabetes mellitus is called

   (A) membranous nephropathy
   (B) minimal change
   (C) Kimmelstiel–Wilson lesion
   (D) Pendred lesion
   (E) focal glomerular sclerosis

57. As a patient with diabetic ketoacidosis is being treated, the BP, pH, anion gap, and blood sugar improve except for the serum acetone level. With treatment, the acetone level increases. The most likely etiology for this phenomenon is

   (A) laboratory error
   (B) lactate is being converted to acetone
   (C) glucose is being converted to acetone
   (D) B-hydroxybutyrate is being converted to acetone
   (E) glycogen is being converted to acetone

58. Appropriate laboratory work-up for adrenal insufficiency includes

   (A) a TSH level
   (B) an ACTH stimulation test
   (C) a TRH stimulation test
   (D) a CRF level
   (E) a urine for ACTH level

59. TSH (thyrotropin) is stimulated by

   (A) glucagon
   (B) TRH (thyrotropin-releasing hormone)
   (C) prolactin
   (D) ADH (antidiuretic hormone)
   (E) ACTH (adrenocorticotrophic hormone)

60. Hyponatremia may be a presenting sign of

   (A) ADH deficiency
   (B) Graves' disease
   (C) Cushing's syndrome
   (D) hypothyroidism
   (E) lithium therapy

61. Appropriate laboratory evaluation of Cushing's syndrome would include

   (A) random ACTH level
   (B) random cortisol level
   (C) cortisol level at 4 PM
   (D) 24-hour urine for cortisol
   (E) cortisol level at 9 AM

62. Which of the following laboratory data would be most useful in the evaluation of nephrolithiasis?

   (A) urine culture
   (B) urine phosphate level
   (C) plasma to urine calcium ratio
   (D) urine citric acid level
   (E) 24-hour urine for osmolarity

63. A 25-year-old female on birth control pills is found to have an elevated T_4 of 17.2 mcg/dL (normal range 4.5 to 12.0 mcg/dL) on routine laboratory testing. The most likely etiology for the elevated T_4 is

   (A) decreased T_4 clearance
   (B) an elevated TBG level
   (C) daily levothyroxine intake of 0.025 mcg
   (D) an elevated TSH level
   (E) decreased T_4 metabolism

Answers and Explanations

1. (B) LH (luteinizing hormone) and FSH (follicle-stimulating hormone) are secreted from the anterior pituitary. *(Felig et al, pp. 249–259)*

2. (B) TSH (thyroid-stimulating hormone) and ACTH (adrenocorticotropic hormone) are secreted from the anterior pituitary. *(Felig et al, pp. 249–259)*

3. (C) ADH (antidiuretic hormone) is secreted from the posterior pituitary and TSH (thyroid-stimulating hormone) is secreted from the anterior pituitary. *(Felig et al, pp. 249–259)*

4. (D) CRF (corticotropin-releasing factor) is released by the hypothalamus and MSH (melanocyte-stimulating hormone) is part of the ACTH molecule. *(Felig et al, pp. 249–259)*

5. (A) Layers of the adrenal gland are glomerulosa (outermost layer), fasciculata, and reticularis. The glomerulosa secretes only aldosterone. *(Felig et al, p. 514)*

6. (B) The reticularis secretes androgens, estrogens, and cortisol. *(Felig et al, p. 514)*

7. (B) The fasciculata makes up approximately 75% of the adrenal gland and secretes cortisol, androgens, and estrogen. *(Felig et al, p. 514)*

8. (C) Nephrogenic diabetes insipidis and neurogenic diabetes insipidis by definition imply a polyuric state. *(Felig et al, pp. 361–364)*

9. (D) Psychogenic polydipsia is seen with mental disorders, and these patients drink an inordinate amount of fluid. *(Felig et al, pp. 361–364)*

10. (A) Lithium will cause distal tubular injury, thus making these cells insensitive to ADH. *(Felig et al, pp. 361–364)*

11. (A) Urinary tract obstruction will cause distal tubular injury, thus making those cells poorly responsive to ADH. *(Felig et al, pp. 361–364)*

12. (A) Symptoms of hypothyroidism can at times be difficult to detect, particularly if there is gradual progression of the disease or if another disease (ie, CHF, sepsis) dominates. The severe form of hypothyroidism, called *myxedema*, may present with hoarseness, constipation, edema, arthralgias, anovulation, fatigue, and headaches. Diarrhea is not a symptom of myxedema; it can be seen with hyperthyroidism. *(Federman, p. 16)*

13. (E) Noninsulin-dependent diabetes mellitus has a variety of etiologies. Beta cell function tends to decline over time in association with increased peripheral resistance to insulin. This resistance is composed of a reduction in insulin receptors, impaired cellular glucose uptake, and postreceptor defects. *(DeFronzo et al, pp. 52–81; Berger et al, p. 82)*

14. (B) Release of prolactin is accomplished by interrupting the normal inhibitory control mechanism that at present is felt to be dopamine. Bromocriptine (a dopaminergic agonist) and L-dopa will, therefore, inhibit prolactin release. Pregnancy with elevated estrogens directly stimulates prolactin. Opiates inhibit central dopamine release, thus increasing prolactin. *(Felig et al, pp. 272–273)*

15. (A) Treatment of DKA may cause hypoglycemia if vigorous insulin therapy is used. The incidence of hypoglycemia has been reduced with low-dose insulin regimens. Hypokalemia presents secondary to renal potassium wasting due to renal glycosuria with associated polyuria, poor intake, and cellular shifts (insulin therapy and correction of acidosis cause potassium to shift into the cell). Hypophosphatemia can be severe in DKA (rarely fatal), but is usually clinically silent. Hypocalcemia is not generally a condition associated with DKA. *(Kreisberg, pp. 681–695; Barrett et al, pp. 899–1104)*

16. (E) All options given can cause hyperthyroidism. Transient hyperthyroidism in subacute thyroiditis occurs in more than 50% of patients secondary to tissue injury to the gland and release of endogenous T_4 stores. Painless thyroiditis may be the second most common cause of hyperthyroidism due to lymphocytic infiltration of the gland. Autonomous hot nodules in the thyroid gland (toxic multinodular goiter) can cause marked hyperthyroidism. Struma ovarii (ovarian tumor) can cause ectopic thyroid production. *(Felig et al, p. 421)*

17. **(A)** Hashimoto's thyroiditis is an autoimmune thyroid disease that is the most common cause of hypothyroidism. Iodine excess will inhibit organification in large doses (Wolff–Chaikoff effect). Chronic iodine deficiency may result in goiter and hypothyroidism. Chronic steroid therapy does not cause hypothyroidism. *(Felig et al, p. 445)*

18. **(B)** T_3 is directly secreted by the thyroid gland and by peripheral conversion of T_4 to T_3 (liver, muscles). Iodination of thyrosine in the periphery does not occur. Oxidation of T_4 does not occur. *(Felig et al, p. 392)*

19. **(A)** T_4 is approximately 80% bound to thyroid-binding globulin (TBG), 15% to thyroid-binding prealbumin (TBPA), and 5% to albumin. Calmodulin-binding globulin does not exist. *(Felig et al, p. 396)*

20. **(E)** Insulin is broken down by the kidney; thus, more insulin can remain in circulation in patients with uremia. To maintain adequate glucose homeostasis, cortisol (a counterregulatory hormone) is one of the primary hormones necessary to prevent hypoglycemia. Islet cell tumors of the pancreas are classic for causing fasting hypoglycemia. With total liver necrosis, gluconeogenesis will be absent, thus causing hypoglycemia. *(Felig et al, p. 1184)*

21. **(E)** Abdominal pain, even presenting as an acute abdomen, can be due to acute adrenal insufficiency. Hyponatremia with secondary increased ADH (antidiuretic hormone) and impaired free water clearance is common with Addison's disease. Both cortisol and mineralocorticoid are needed to maintain blood pressure. Fever can accompany adrenal crisis. *(Felig et al, p. 590)*

22. **(E)** Primary aldosteronism and Cushing's syndrome can increase blood pressure as the secretion of mineralocorticoid and the mineralocorticoid effect of cortisol cause sodium retention. Hypercalcemia by itself can increase blood pressure because it mediates the contractile elements of the vascular system. Hyperthyroidism increases metabolic rate and cardiac output, thus increasing blood pressure. *(Felig et al, pp. 695,713–714,751–795)*

23. **(E)** Primary hyperparathyroidism can cause increased bone and gastrointestinal tract calcium absorption. Sarcoidosis and vitamin D intoxication enhances GI calcium absorption. Thyrotoxico-

sis causes increased bone turnover with release of calcium. Hence, all can cause hypercalcuria. *(Felig et al, pp. 1531–1536)*

24. **(E)** Risk factors for kidney stone formation have been established (similar to the principle of coronary risk factors). Low-urine volume, high concentration of solute (calcium, urate, phosphate), pH (low for uric acid, high for infection or calcium phosphate) are all separate risk factors. High protein intake increases urate load and decreases pH. *(Felig et al, pp. 1500–1578)*

25. **(A)** Multiple endocrine neoplasia type I is usually made up of the 3 Ps—pituitary, pancreatic, and parathyroid neoplasia. MEN type IIa includes medullary cancer of the thyroid. (Components of MEN type IIa are medullary carcinoma, pheochromocytoma, and hyperparathyroid.) MEN type IIb consists of pheochromocytoma, medullary carcinoma, and marfanoid habitus. *(Felig et al, p. 1663)*

26. **(C)** Corticotropin-releasing factor (CRF) and arginine vasopressin (AVP) both can stimulate ACTH (corticotropin or adrenocorticotropin). CRF and AVP are both produced in the hypothalamus, passed into the portal vessels of the anterior pituitary, and stimulate ACTH release. TSH stimulates the thyroid. Low cortisol by itself does not stimulate ACTH. It is through CRF or AVP; remember with the circadian rhythm, the afternoon cortisol level may be zero without causing release of ACTH. *(Felig et al, p. 523)*

27. **(B)** The effect of aldosterone at the renal tubule is potassium secretion and sodium retention. Retention of sodium, in turn, causes the kidney to retain fluid. *(Felig et al, p. 531)*

28. **(E)** Causes for short stature are quite extensive and are a common reason for childhood visits to a pediatrician, especially in the early adolescent years. Etiology for short stature has been separated into congenital growth hormone deficiency (ie, embryologic defects, inactive growth hormone) or acquired growth hormone deficiency (trauma, inflammatory disease, autoimmune) and CNS tumors that cause destruction of the pituitary. Hypothyroidism can also cause short stature. *(Felig et al, p. 1605)*

29. **(A)** Retinopathy is usually divided into background or proliferative. Background retinopathy has evidence of retinal injury from diabetic vessel damage. Findings include hemorrhages, exudates, and microaneurysms. Laser therapy can be of great value. Neovascularization with vessels growing into the vitreous is called proliferative retinopathy. *(Felig et al, p. 1116)*

30. **(E)** The underlying problem with Somogyi phenomenon is the excessive insulin doses resulting in hyperglycemia after counterregulatory hormones (epinephrine, growth hormone, and cortisol) are released. The overdosed patient will become hypoglycemic and the resultant events cause a relative hyperglycemia. This frequently occurs in the early AM with elevated fasting blood sugars that may in fact be treated with a larger dose of insulin when the opposite is needed. *(Felig et al, p. 1137)*

31. **(B)** First-generation sulfonylureas are tolbutamide, chlorpropamide, acetohexamide, and tolazamide. Second-generation agents are glipizide and glyburide. *(Cahill et al, p. 14)*

32. **(B)** Inappropriate release of ADH has numerous etiologies including CNS lesion, adenocarcinoma of the lung, drugs (narcotics, phenothiazines), and pain. Low serum osmolarity or excessive H_2O drinking do not cause SIADH. *(Felig et al, pp. 368–374)*

33. **(B)** Renal osteodystrophy is a complicated disease process that may involve numerous etiologies and cause a variety of bone lesions. The most common lesions found are osteomalacia (from vitamin D deficiency or aluminum induction) and hyperparathyroid bone disease from secondary hyperparathyroidism. Less frequently, osteoporosis is seen. Osteopetrosis and fibrous dysplasia are not associated with renal failure. *(Felig et al, p. 1480)*

34. **(A)** Chromaffin cells are usually found in the adrenal glands and they can grow into pheochromocytomas. These cells are also found in the sympathetic nerve chain and on the organ of Zuckerkandle near the aortic bifurcation. They are not found in the kidney. *(Felig et al, p. 667)*

35. **(A)** Therapy of Cushing's disease can be quite difficult. If an ACTH-producing tumor is present in the pituitary, it can be surgically resected. Ketoconazole and op DDD (mitotane) both can prevent adrenal cortisol production. Dexamethasone, a steroid, is used only in diagnosis, not as a treatment. *(Felig et al, pp. 615–617)*

36. **(B)** Both vitamin D deficiency and hypophosphatemia are the broad categories that head a long list of causes for osteomalacia. Hyperparathyroidism and hyperthyroidism do not cause osteomalacia. *(Felig et al, p. 1462)*

37. **(C)** A 21-hydroxylase block in the pathway of cortisol formation will result in low serum cortisol and aldosterone levels. The pathway is then shifted to the androgen excess. Clinical features include ambiguous genitalia in the male, severe salt washing, hypotension, shock, or death. It is important to determine this in a newborn, as death can occur rapidly if undetected. Weight gain and type of delivery are not associated with a 21-hydroxylase block. *(Felig et al, p. 626)*

38. **(E)** Complications of diabetes are numerous, including accelerated atherosclerosis and diabetic neuropathy that may present with carpal tunnel syndrome, gastroparesis, GI motility disorders, decreased sensation, and nocturnal diarrhea. Segmental demyelination of the peripheral nerves and sorbitol deposition are the main causes of the neuropathy. *(Cahill et al, p. 17)*

39. **(B)** Thyroid tumors are classified into papillary, follicular, medullary, or undifferentiated. On scan they appear cold (they are usually nonfunctional). On echo they tend to be solid or have evidence of blood or fragments of tissue within the cyst. Chronic lymphocytic infiltration is seen with Hashimoto's thyroiditis. Granulomatous lesions are not seen with thyroid cancer. *(Felig et al, pp. 494–504)*

40. **(C)** ACTH is mainly responsible for stimulating cortisol. ACTH does help with the stimulation of cholesterol to pregnenolone, which is the steroid needed for all subsequent steroid generation, including estrogen and testosterone. It is not a stimulator of estrogen or testosterone release. Ammonia generation as well as aldosterone release are not under ACTH control. Aldactone is a drug that blocks aldosterone. *(Felig et al, pp. 513–518)*

41. **(B)** A high serum cortisol level will inhibit ACTH release. Also, high CRF or an adrenalectomy will stimulate ACTH. High estrogen or low cortisol do not inhibit ACTH release. *(Felig et al, p. 530)*

42. **(E)** In primary hypothyroidism, when the TSH is elevated prior to replacement therapy following the decrease in TSH, is the most sensitive laboratory assay. The goal is to achieve a normal TSH level (unless clinically contraindicated). T_3 RIA should normalize with T_4 therapy; however, it is not sensitive enough because of the binding protein TBG. Reverse T_3 is presently a research tool. It may be of great value in diagnosis of sick euthyroid syndrome. The T_3 stimulation test does not exist. *(Felig et al, p. 458)*

43. **(D)** Klinefelter's is usually caused by an extra chromosome, thus forming an XXY male with hypogonadism, usually associated with short stature and subnormal intelligence. This diagnosis needs to be entertained in a male with small firm testes, gynecomastia, and abnormal arm-to-body length. *(Felig et al, p. 1000)*

44. (A) Graves' ophthalmopathy can be seen with hyperthyroid or euthyroid Graves' disease. The etiology is unclear, but pathologically a lymphocytic and plasma cell infiltration occurs in the retroorbital space. Because the eye lies in the socket compartment, any additional mass added to the retroorbital space results in anterior displacement of the eye with resultant proptosis. *(Felig et al, p. 440)*

45. (C) Classic Turner's syndrome is a result of gonadal dysgenesis with streak gonads and they present with low hairline, low-set ears, webbed neck, broad chest, short stature, shortening of the fourth metacarpal, and commonly with renal abnormalities. They usually have a 45,X karyotype. *(Felig et al, p. 1006)*

46. (A) $1,25-(OH)2D_3$ acts on the GI tract to cause calcium absorption and in concert with parathyroid hormone help maintain normal bone homeostasis. Vitamin D_2 and D_3 are metabolized to 25-OH D_3 in the liver and then hydroxylated to $1,25-(OH)2D_3$ or $24,25(OH)2D_3$ in the kidney. The true function of $24,25-(OH)2D_3$ is not clear at present, but it may be quite important in new bone formation. *(Felig et al, p. 1346)*

47. (D) Struvite (infection, triple phosphate) stones occur when the urine is supersaturated with magnesium, ammonium, and phosphate in the presence of urea-splitting bacteria. Proteus is the most common bacterium, although *Klebsiella, Pseudomonas, Bacteroides,* and *Staphylococcus aureus* also have been implicated. *(Felig et al, pp. 1521–1524)*

48. (D) Hypercalcemia of hyperparathyroidism is due to increased GI absorption of calcium mediated by $1,25-(OH)2D_3$. Parathormone (PTH) stimulates increased $1,25-(OH)2D_3$ formation. Remember, this is in contrast to the hypercalcemia of malignancy (either through bone metastasis or humoral causes) in which the hypercalcemia is due to bone calcium release, not increased GI absorption. PTH does not stimulate the GI tract directly, nor stimulate $25-OHD_3$. Nephrogenic cyclic AMP is a marker of PTH action at the kidney, but cyclic AMP does not cause hypercalcemia. *(Felig et al, pp. 1377–1384).*

49. (A) Prazosine, phenoxybenzamine, phentolamine, or nitroprusside can be first-line drugs in the treatment of pheochromocytoma as they are all alpha-adrenergic antagonists. Propranolol, a beta-adrenergic antagonist, should never be used alone. By only blocking the vasodilator beta receptors with propranolol, there will then be unopposed alpha stimulation resulting in vasoconstriction and a rapid rise in blood pressure. *(Felig et al, p. 671)*

50. (C) The pituitary gland is located at the base of the skull in a saddle-shaped cavity termed the *sella turcica.* It is divided into anterior and posterior components. Along with the hypothalamus it provides the major components to a number of autoregulatory functions of the endocrine system. *(Felig et al, p. 247)*

51. (A) Serum osmolarity is the most potent stimulus for ADH release. Serum osmolarity that is greater than 285 will cause a strong stimulus for ADH release. None of the other choices linked have any influence on the ADH reflex. *(Felig et al, p. 341)*

52. (E) Fredrickson's classification is based on the following table:

Type	Lipoprotein Abnormality
I	Chylomicrons markedly increased; VLDL and LDL are normal
IIa	LDL increased, VLDL normal
IIb	Both LDL and VLDL are increased
III	Abnormal cholesterol, normal VLDL, and increased beta-VLDL
IV	VLDL increased and LDL normal
V	Chylomicrons markedly increased, VLDL increased, LDL normal

Type IV is also commonly seen in poorly controlled diabetics. *(Grundy, p. 2045)*

53. (C) Hyperglycemia in the early morning in those patients on insulin may be due to the dawn phenomenon. It is felt to be secondary to early morning rise in growth hormone secretion, which is a counterregulatory hormone and thus raises serum glucose. This is in contrast to the Somogyi effect, causing early morning hyperglycemia due to insulin overdose and release of all counterregulatory hormones. In patients with dawn phenomenon, the insulin dose is not excessive. *(Felig et al, p. 13)*

54. (B) Oral agents enhance beta cell function and thus increase insulin release. They also improve peripheral sensitivity to insulin. Both of these actions tend to normalize blood sugar levels in the noninsulin-dependent diabetic. *(Cahill et al, p. 13)*

55. (C) A fasting blood sugar of >140 mg/dL on two occasions is diagnostic of diabetes mellitus. A ½ hour, 1 hour, or 1½ hour blood sugar of >200 mg can be diagnostic of diabetes during a glucose tolerance test. A 2-hour postprandial of >200 is also diagnostic of diabetes. *(Cahill et al, p. 7)*

56. (C) Kimmelstiel–Wilson lesions include spherical nodular hyaline masses and sclerosis of the renal glomerulus. This is characteristic of diabetes mellitus. No other disease process is known to cause this lesion. *(Felig et al, pp. 1115–1116)*

57. (D) As diabetic ketoacidosis worsens, especially if there is concomitant lactic acidosis, B-hydroxybucerate is more likely to be formed. B-hydroxybucerate is not measured in the acetone assay. As DKA is treated, the B-hydroxybucerate will be converted to acetone, thus giving the paradoxical rise in serum acetone as the patient improves. *(Felig et al, p. 1150)*

58. (B) Appropriate tests would be a serum ACTH level and an ACTH stimulation test to measure adrenal reserve. The TSH level is to evaluate the thyroid, not the adrenal gland. CRF is a research tool and is not needed, as ACTH level can be measured directly. Urine for ACTH cannot be done. *(Felig et al, p. 592)*

59. (B) TRH (thyrotropin-releasing hormone) stimulates TSH (thyrotropin). Glucagon, prolactin, ADH, and ACTH do not stimulate TSH. When T_4 and T_3 levels rise slightly above normal, they suppress TSH. *(Felig et al, p. 400)*

60. (D) Hypothyroidism will cause an inability to secrete a water load secondary to elevated ADH level. Poor myocardial function with impaired cardiac output, often associated with hypothyroidism, will also prevent adequate free water excretion through the renal tubules. ADH deficiency and lithium therapy cause hypernatremia. Graves' disease and Cushing's disease are usually not associated with the inability to excrete a water load. *(Felig et al, pp. 453–454)*

61. (D) Glucocorticoid excess secondary to pituitary ACTH hypersecretion is labeled *Cushing's disease.* Cushing's syndrome has numerous etiologies (iatrogenic, tumor, etc). Laboratory work-up would include a 24-hour urine for cortisol (normal <100 mg/24-hour). Random ACTH, random cortisol, and a 4 PM cortisol are of no diagnostic aid because they do not establish a cortisol excess state. ACTH has a wide daily fluctuation; cortisol is usually high in the early morning and low in the late afternoon (usual circadian rhythm). *(Felig et al, pp. 609–611)*

62. (A) The appropriate laboratory work-up for kidney stones should include a urine culture to rule out infection as the etiology for the stone disease. Staghorn calculi in the renal pelvis are composed of struvite and are caused by infection. Urine phosphate and citric acid levels are nonexistent tests. A plasma-to-urine calcium ratio has no clinical relevance. The urine osmolarity only tells you if ADH is being secreted. *(Felig et al, pp. 1521–1524)*

63. (B) Isolated elevations of T_4 do not imply that the patient is hyperthyroid. The serum T_4 assay will measure both bound and free T_4. More than 99.95% of T_4 is bound; thus, if TBG is elevated, so too will the measurable T_4 in the serum. Increases in TBG can be seen with any elevated estrogen state (ie, pregnancy, birth control pills, etc), heredity and acute hepatitis. Elevated TSH levels causing high T_4 is exceedingly rare. Decreased T_4 metabolism or clearance will not increase T_4. A levothyroxine dose of 0.025 mg is miniscule (usual replacement dose is 100 to 150 mg/day). *(Felig et al, pp. 395,411,458)*

REFERENCES

Barrett E, DeFronzo R. Diabetic ketoacidosis: Diagnosis and treatment. *Hosp Pract.* 1984;19:89–104.

Berger M, Birchtold P. Insulin transport and action at target cells. *Joslin's Diabetes Mellitus,* 12th ed. Philadelphia, PA: Lea and Febiger; 1985.

Cahill F, Arky A, et al. VI diabetes mellitus. *Sci Am.* January 1987.

DeFronzo RA, Ferrannin E, et al. New concepts in the pathogenesis and treatment of noninsulin-dependent diabetes mellitus. *Am J Med.* 1983;74(1a):52–81.

Federman D. Thyroid. *S AM M.* 1 May 1989.

Felig P, Baster D, et al (eds). *Endocrinology and Metabolism.* New York: McGraw-Hill; 1987.

Grundy M. Disorders of lipids and lipoproteins. In Stein Jay H, et al (eds). *Internal Medicine,* 2nd ed. Boston, MA: Little, Brown; 1987.

Kreisberg A. Diabetic ketoacidosis: New concepts and trends in pathogenesis and treatment. *Ann Intern Med.* 1978;88:681–695.

Wilson JD, Foster WD (eds). *Williams Textbook of Endocrinology,* 8th ed, Philadelphia, PA: WB Saunders; 1992.

Subspecialty List: Endocrinology

QUESTION NUMBER AND SUBSPECIALTY

1. Pituitary
2. Pituitary
3. Pituitary
4. Pituitary
5. Adrenal
6. Adrenal
7. Adrenal
8. Pituitary/ADH
9. Pituitary/ADH
10. Pituitary/ADH
11. Pituitary/ADH
12. Thyroid
13. Diabetes
14. Pituitary function
15. Diabetic ketoacidosis
16. Thyroid
17. Thyroid
18. Thyroid
19. Thyroid
20. Hypoglycemia
21. Adrenal
22. Hypertension
23. Adrenal
24. Nephrolithiasis
25. Endocrine tumors
26. Pituitary
27. Aldosterone
28. Growth hormone
29. Diabetes mellitus
30. Diabetes mellitus
31. Diabetes mellitus
32. Adrenal
33. Metabolic bone disorders
34. Adrenal
35. Adrenal
36. Metabolic bone disorders
37. Adrenal
38. Diabetes mellitus
39. Thyroid
40. Adrenal
41. Adrenal
42. Thyroid
43. Developmental genetics
44. Thyroid
45. Developmental genetics
46. Calcium regulation
47. Nephrolithiasis
48. Parathyroid
49. Pheochromocytoma
50. Pituitary anatomy
51. Pituitary
52. Lipoproteins
53. Diabetes mellitus
54. Diabetes mellitus
55. Diabetes mellitus
56. Diabetes mellitus
57. Diabetes mellitus
58. Adrenal insufficiency
59. Thyroid regulation
60. Hyponatremia
61. Adrenal
62. Nephrolithiasis
63. Thyroid

Internal Medicine: Gastroenterology
Questions

DIRECTIONS (Questions 1 through 24): For each of the items in this section, ONE or MORE of the numbered options is correct. Choose answer

    (A) if only (1), (2), and (3) are correct,
    (B) if only (1) and (3) are correct,
    (C) if only (2) and (4) are correct,
    (D) if only (4) is correct,
    (E) if all are correct.

Questions 1 through 24

1. Acute esophageal obstruction is generally seen secondary to food impaction. Treatment consists of which of the following?

   (1) IV glucagon (1 mg)
   (2) nitroglycerin sublingually (0.6 mg)
   (3) endoscopy
   (4) barium swallow

2. Treatment of gastroesophageal reflux disease (GERD) consists of

   (1) H-2 blockers (ranitidine, famotidine, cimetidine)
   (2) dietary adjustment
   (3) prokinetic agents (metaclopramide, bethanecol, domperidone)
   (4) Nissen fundoplication

3. In the U.S., esophageal cancer accounts for about four percent of all cancers. It is also three to four times more common in blacks than in whites. Which of the following conditions are associated with increased risk of the development of esophageal cancer?

   (1) consuming more than 8 oz ETOH/day
   (2) tobacco abuse
   (3) achalasia
   (4) Barrett's esophagus

4. Which of the following are associated with gastric ulcer?

   (1) aspirin use
   (2) nonsteroidal agents
   (3) smoking
   (4) *Helicobacter pylori*

5. Pseudomembranous colitis, an antibiotic-related disorder caused by an overgrowth of *Clostridium difficile,* usually manifesting as severe diarrhea, can be treated with which of the following?

   (1) oral vancomycin 125–500 mg PO tid–qid
   (2) Lomotil prn loose stools
   (3) Flagyl 250–500 mg PO qid
   (4) colectomy or diverting colostomy

6. Which of the following are true regarding Zollinger–Ellison syndrome?

   (1) dramatic symptomatic response to Omeprazole
   (2) rarely associated with development of peptic disease
   (3) due to a non-beta islet cell tumor of the pancreas that secretes gastrin
   (4) initial manifestations most common in the teenage years

7. Malabsorption syndromes are characterized by weight loss, diarrhea, nutritional deficiency and, often, abdominal distention. Which of the following disorders is/are associated with an immunological reaction to gluten?

   (1) afferent loop syndrome
   (2) radiation enteritis
   (3) tropical sprue
   (4) celiac sprue

8. Well-known complications of ulcerative colitis include

   (1) toxic megacolon
   (2) iron deficiency anemia

(3) carcinoma

(4) arthritis

9. What is/are the most common complication(s) of a Meckel's diverticulum?

    (1) diverticulitis

    (2) intestinal obstruction

    (3) intussusception

    (4) hemorrhage

10. The ileum is primarily responsible for which of the following digestive functions?

    (1) water absorption

    (2) bile salt absorption

    (3) nutrient and electrolyte absorption

    (4) B_{12} absorption

11. Colon cancer is the most common GI malignancy. Which of the following is/are true regarding colon cancers?

    (1) Most cancers are felt to develop in hyperplastic polyps.

    (2) A family history of colon cancer triples the risk.

    (3) Most colon cancers develop in the cecum.

    (4) 90% of symptomatic patients have at least a Duke's B lesion.

12. A 45-year-old white female presents to your office with a two-day history of generalized lower abdominal pain, subjective fever, and intermittent minor rectal bleeding. A CBC drawn in your office reveals a WBC of 16,000 and oral temperature is 100.8°F. Your differential diagnosis includes which of the following?

    (1) inflammatory bowel disease

    (2) ischemic colitis

    (3) diverticulitis

    (4) irritable bowel syndrome

13. Which of the following is/are associated with the development of acute pancreatitis?

    (1) alcohol use

    (2) choledocholithiasis

    (3) hyperlipidemia

    (4) drug sensitivity

14. Pancreatitis is suggested by which of the following findings?

    (1) elevated serum lipase

    (2) left pleural effusion

    (3) sentinel loop on plain abdominal film

    (4) midepigastric pain radiating to the back

15. Management of acute pancreatitis consists of which of the following measures?

    (1) NPO status

    (2) NG suction

    (3) fluid and electrolyte replacement

    (4) antibiotics

16. Severe folate deficiency is found in which of the following cases?

    (1) alcoholism

    (2) Crohn's disease

    (3) celiac sprue

    (4) partial gastrectomy state

17. Which of the following is/are true regarding biliary colic?

    (1) Pain is generally postprandial.

    (2) Pain is produced by stone impaction in the common duct.

    (3) CCK (cholecystokinin) release from the small bowel stimulates contraction of the gallbladder.

    (4) Fever and chills are characteristic.

18. Factors and/or disease states felt to contribute to the development of gastric carcinoma include

    (1) atrophic gastritis

    (2) hypertrophied gastric ruggal folds

    (3) prior gastric surgery

    (4) dietary factors

19. Which of the following is/are true regarding acute cholecystitis?

    (1) It is usually associated with fever and localized tenderness.

    (2) OCG generally demonstrates opacification of the gallbladder.

    (3) Immunocompromised or elderly patients may be asymptomatic.

    (4) It results from obstruction of the common bile duct.

20. Ascites is caused by which of the following conditions?

    (1) tuberculosis

    (2) cirrhosis

    (3) congestive heart failure

    (4) neoplasm

21. Which of the following disorders have been associated with chest pain of uncertain etiology (or central chest pain syndrome)?

    (1) neoplasm

    (2) gastroesophageal reflux disease

    (3) esophageal inflammation

    (4) scleroderma

22. Jaundice due to extrahepatic obstruction would be suggested by which of the following?

    (1) palpable gallbladder or abdominal mass

    (2) elevated serum amylase

    (3) occult blood in the stool

    (4) disproportionate elevation of the bilirubin and alkaline phosphatase

23. Which of the following are true regarding carcinoid tumors?

    (1) Elevated 5-HIAA levels are characteristic.

    (2) Diarrhea, flushing, and cramping are common due to oversecretion of serotonin by the tumor cells.

    (3) The appendix is the most common site, followed by the terminal ileum.

    (4) They are fast growing tumors.

24. Clinical features of achalasia include which of the following?

    (1) dysphagia

    (2) regurgitation

    (3) chest pain

    (4) gastroesophageal reflux

DIRECTIONS (Questions 25 through 37): Each question in this section consists of two lettered choices followed by several numbered words or phrases. For each word or phrase, choose the ONE lettered heading that is most closely associated with it. Each lettered heading may be selected once, more than once, or not at all.

Questions 25 through 28

Match the following cause of upper GI bleeding with the most common presentation.

    (A) painful

    (B) painless

25. Esophageal varices

26. Mallory–Weiss tear

27. Angiodysplasia

28. Peptic ulcer disease

Questions 29 through 33

Match the following clinical features, presentations, or complications with the most commonly associated form of inflammatory bowel disease.

    (A) ulcerative colitis

    (B) Crohn's disease

29. Intestinal obstruction

30. Bloody diarrhea

31. Fistulization

32. Toxic megacolon

33. Colon cancer

Questions 34 through 37

Select the type of hepatitis described best by the following statements.

    (A) hepatitis A

    (B) hepatitis B

34. Intravenous drug use or homosexuality are risk factors

35. Transmitted via the fecal–oral route

36. Gammaglobulin prophylaxis is felt to be beneficial

37. 3% to 10% develop chronic active hepatitis or cirrhosis

DIRECTIONS (Questions 38 through 44): Each of the numbered items or incomplete statements in this section is followed by answers or by completions of the statement. Select the ONE lettered answer or completion that is BEST in each case.

Questions 38 through 44

38. A 75-year-old male with a history of CAD and COPD presents to you complaining of weight loss and crampy, dull, periumbilical pain occurring 15 to 20 minutes postprandially and lasting for hours. Stool is negative for occult blood, CBC is normal, and abdominal exam reveals only the presence of a soft abdominal bruit. The most likely diagnosis is

    (A) gallstones

    (B) mesenteric ischemia

    (C) pancreatitis

    (D) abdominal aneurysm

    (E) peptic ulcer disease

39. The most common type of small bowel tumor is

(A) carcinoid

(B) lymphoma

(C) adenocarcinoma

(D) sarcoma

(E) neurofibroma

40. A 30-year-old female presents to you with a 2-week history of nausea, epigastric distress, crampy abdominal discomfort, flatulence, and diarrhea. No blood has been noted in her stool, but she has lost 6 pounds. CBC drawn in your office is normal. She offers one additional bit of history—she recently returned from a camping trip. What is the most likely diagnosis?

(A) enterotoxigenic *E. coli*

(B) giardiasis

(C) *Campylobacter*

(D) *Salmonella*

(E) irritable bowel syndrome

41. A 55-year-old white female smoker presents to you complaining of a 10-pound weight loss, weakness, and dull upper abdominal pain radiating into her back. Physical exam is unremarkable. Lab values show a Hgb of 10, serum amylase of 90, and alkaline phosphatase of 240 (elevated). ERCP shows a single, focal, irregular stricture of the pancreatic duct. The most likely diagnosis is

(A) acute pancreatitis

(B) pancreatic carcinoma

(C) chronic pancreatitis

(D) ampullary carcinoma

(E) choledocholithiasis

42. Gastroparesis, or delayed gastric emptying, can be due to obstructive or nonobstructive causes. From the following list, which is the most common cause of nonobstructive delay?

(A) medications such as narcotics and antidepressants

(B) diabetes

(C) connective tissue diseases

(D) gastric surgery

(E) primary chronic intestinal pseudo-obstruction

43. A 65-year-old white male is hospitalized in an intensive care setting for a serious pneumonia. He is diabetic and hypertensive. He develops recurrent spiking fever and poorly localized abdominal discomfort after initial treatment for his pneumonia. Leukocytosis is present, with a WBC of 12,000. HIDA scan is negative, and ultrasound shows a gallbladder wall measuring 7 mm with no stones seen. Your diagnosis is

(A) acute cholecystitis

(B) emphysematous cholecystitis

(C) acute cholangitis

(D) acute acalculous cholecystitis

(E) ileus

44. A 23-year-old female with a history of previously diagnosed irritable bowel syndrome presents with small amounts of painful rectal bleeding on defecation. The most likely etiology for this is

(A) inflammatory bowel disease

(B) hemorrhoids

(C) anal fissure

(D) anorectal abscess

(E) rectovaginal fistula

45. Charcot's triad consists of fever, abdominal pain, and jaundice and is the clinical hallmark of

(A) chronic cholecystitis

(B) acute cholecystitis

(C) acute cholangitis

(D) acalculous cholecystitis

(E) carcinoma of the gallbladder

Answers and Explanations

1. **(A)** Pharmacologic agents, such as glucagon and nitroglycerin, help relax the lower esophageal sphincter and may allow passage of a bolus of food. Endoscopy is used for diagnostic and therapeutic purposes by allowing extraction of an impacted foreign body. Endoscopy will also allow diagnosis of occult esophageal carcinoma or strictures as the causative agent of the obstruction. Barium swallow will increase the risk of aspiration and, therefore, should be avoided. *(Sachar et al, p. 16)*

2. **(E)** GERD is exceedingly common. Dietary management is usually the first order of treatment. Avoidance of foods which reduce the lower esophageal sphincter pressure (eg, coffee, chocolate, mints, alcohol, tomatoes) is important. Mechanical measures, such as weight reduction, elevation of the head of the bed, and loose-fitting garments, are also beneficial. The next step generally includes addition of antacids, H-2 blockers, or Prilosec. If these are not helpful, the addition of a prokinetic agent may be useful. Reglan, a dopamine antagonist, and bethanechol, a cholinergic agent, are two common examples of medication often used. Cisapride and domperidone are the newest agents, both of which are said to have a more favorable side effect profile but are not yet widely available. If symptoms are truly intractable and/or are complicated by aspiration, severe esophagitis, or other difficulties, then antireflux surgery (ie, Nissen fundoplication) should be considered. *(Sachar et al, p. 11)*

3. **(E)** In the U.S., the risk of esophageal cancer is increased by a factor of 18 in alcoholics who drink more than 80 g (8 oz) of alcohol per day, and by a factor of 44 in those who also have a tobacco consumption of 2 packs per day. Barrett's esophagus, a complication of chronic gastroesophageal reflux, results from replacement of the original squamous epithelium with a metaplastic columnar epithelium, and is thought to be associated with a 10% risk of developing esophageal cancer. The prevalence of esophageal cancer in patients with achalasia is low at 2% to 7%. *(Sleisenger and Fordtran, pp. 580,599,619–620)*

4. **(E)** The incidence of gastric ulcer in the U.S. is estimated at 0.5 per 1000 and is one-fourth as common as duodenal ulcers. The primary event is disruption of the gastric mucosal barrier, with consequent damage by acid, pepsin, or other destructive agents. Aspirin alters ion transport and the potential difference across the gastric mucosa and inhibits prostaglandin synthesis. Nonsteroidals also inhibit prostaglandin synthesis. The relationship between smoking and gastric ulceration is controversial. There is a positive correlation between smokers and ulcers, and also the quantity of smoking and prevalence of gastric ulcer disease. The mechanism is not clear but is possibly due to inhibition of pancreatic secretion of bicarbonate, thus diminishing the buffering capacity of the duodenal gastric reflux and subsequent ulceration. *Helicobacter pylori* has recently been implicated in the pathogenesis of gastritis and the formation of gastric ulcers. *(Sleisenger and Fordtran, pp. 885–887; Chobanian and Van Ness, pp. 43–44)*

5. **(B)** The therapy for pseudomembranous colitis consists mainly of discontinuation of any implicated agents and IV fluids to correct fluid losses. Antibiotic treatment has been shown to be successful with oral vancomycin, oral metronidazole, and more recently, oral bacitracin. These are all poorly absorbed in oral forms and deliver high concentrations to the colon without the risk of systemic toxicity. A newer therapy that may prove effective is the use of anion exchange resins (ie, cholestyramine), which have been shown to bind the toxins produced by *Clostridium difficile*. Lomotil and other antispasmodics should routinely be avoided because they have been shown to actually increase the incidence of antibiotic-related diarrhea and to worsen the symptoms. Colectomy and diverting ileostomy should be reserved for the very few patients who develop fulminant or intractable symptoms (usually in patients with profound ileus and toxic megacolon). *(Sleisenger and Fordtran, pp. 1310–1316)*

6. **(B)** Zollinger–Ellison syndrome bears the name of two patients with the clinical triad characteris-

tic of this disease, that is, gastric acid hypersecretion, severe ulcer disease, and non-beta islet cell tumors of the pancreas. Ninety to ninety five percent of patients with ZE will develop ulceration of the UGI tract that usually manifests between the ages of 30 and 50. Patients often become resistant to treatment with H-2 blockers. Prilosec (Omeprazole), however, has proven very effective in inducing striking symptom relief and ulcer healing. (Prilosec is an inhibitor of hydrogen potassium ATPase, which is the proton pump considered the terminal step in parietal cell secretion of hydrogen ions.) *(Sleisenger and Fordtran, pp. 909,912,918)*

7. **(D)** Celiac sprue is primarily a disorder of the jejunum. It appears to be associated with an immunological reaction to gluten, the protein contained in wheat, barley, rye, and oats. Most patients have onset of symptoms in the third or fourth decade, and presentation is either with features of steatorrhea or a more subtle finding of iron or folate deficiency. Celiac sprue is suggested by a low D-xylose test, small bowel dilatation on plain films, and biopsy of the small bowel showing subtotal villous atrophy. Primary treatment is adherence to a gluten-free diet. *(Sachar et al, pp. 184, 189–192)*

8. **(E)** There are many complications of ulcerative colitis that can be divided into two categories: local and systemic. Local complications include massive colonic hemorrhage, colonic stricture (usually seen in long-standing and extensive colitis and seen most commonly in the rectum and transverse colon), toxic megacolon (the most severe life-threatening complication of ulcerative colitis that is caused by diffuse inflammation and destruction of colonic musculature), colonic perforation, and colon cancer. Systemic complications are multiple and include liver disease (pericholangitis, sclerosing cholangitis, bile duct carcinoma, fatty infiltration, chronic active hepatitis, and postnecrotic cirrhosis), iron deficiency anemia (the most common hematologic defect in this disease), thromboembolic diseases (including pulmonary emboli and DVT), arthritis (peripheral or seronegative arthritis and ankylosing spondylitis), dermatologic diseases (classically pyoderma gangrenosum), uveitis and iritis and, finally, renal abnormalities of pyelonephritis and nephrolithiasis. *(Sleisenger and Fordtran, pp. 1460–1470)*

9. **(D)** Meckel's diverticulum is the most common congenital anomaly of the intestinal tract, with an incidence of 0.3% to 3.0%. It is often asymptomatic throughout life. It is an ileal diverticulum and contains all layers of the intestinal tract. Gastric mucosa is present in about 40% of Meckel's. Bleeding is the most common complication, resulting from ulceration of ileal mucosa adjacent to ectopic gas-

tric mucosa. It is often painless and usually encountered in children. If a Meckel's diverticulum is suspected, a technetium-99 scan may be helpful in cases of bleeding. *(Sleisenger and Fordtran, pp. 1014–1015)*

10. **(C)** The proximal small bowel is primarily responsible for water, electrolyte, and nutrient absorption. The ileum is responsible for bile salt and B_{12} absorption. Resection or disease of the distal small bowel may cause serious diarrhea and steatorrhea. Conjugated bile salts, essential for normal fat absorption, are absorbed most effectively by an active transport mechanism present only in the ileum. *(Sleisenger and Fordtran, pp. 1049,1107)*

11. **(C)** Colon cancer is felt to be a disease of Western civilization in association with high-fat, low-fiber diets. Two-thirds of cancers occur in the left colon, about 15% in the cecum. The risk of developing colon cancer is increased threefold in patients with a family history (first-degree relative). Familial polyposis, inflammatory bowel disease, and a history of female genital cancer are all associated with an increased risk. Most cancers are thought to develop in adenomatous polyps. (Hyperplastic polyps are small polyps containing long dilated glands and do not have malignant potential.) Most patients do not develop bowel symptoms until the tumor is large and advanced and, therefore, 90% of symptomatic patients will have a Duke's B lesion or worse (tumor extending into the submucosa but not involving local lymph nodes). *(Sachar et al, pp. 272–275)*

12. **(A)** Inflammatory bowel disease, ischemic colitis, and diverticulitis all have pain, fever, and leukocytosis as prominent clinical features during a patient's presentation. Rectal bleeding may or may not be a part of each of these three disease states but is always a possibility. Irritable bowel syndrome, on the other hand, is a motor disorder characterized by altered bowel habits and is the most common GI disorder encountered by practitioners. Although abdominal pain is one of the major complaints, the presence of fever, elevated WBC, and rectal bleeding all argue strongly against this diagnosis. *(Sleisenger and Fordtran, pp. 1402–1410,1430–1431)*

13. **(E)** Acute pancreatitis ensues when there is damage to the pancreatic acinar cell. The most common cause is alcohol—generally due to prolonged rather than binge drinking. Biliary tract disease is the second most common cause. Acute cholecystitis, choledocholithiasis or obstructive lesions in the region of the ampulla of Vater may cause acute pancreatitis. Drug hypersensitivity has been implicated, especially to estrogens, thiazide diuretics, furosemide, sulfonamides, and

steroids. Pancreatitis can also result from abdominal trauma, viral infection, hyperparathyroidism, hyperlipidemia and following ERCP. Although all of the above are known causes, about one-third of all cases are idiopathic. *(Sachar et al, pp. 76–77)*

14. **(E)** The primary symptom of acute pancreatitis is midepigastric abdominal pain which radiates into the back. Nausea and vomiting are common. Fever, tachycardia, hypotension, and shock may result. The classic Grey–Turner's sign (flank ecchymosis) and Cullen's sign (ecchymosis of the periumbilical region) are quite rare. Pulmonary findings are present in up to one-third of cases, and an isolated left pleural effusion is highly suggestive of acute pancreatitis. Elevated serum amylase is the hallmark, but an elevated serum lipase is actually more helpful as it is more specific to the pancreas. Abdominal films may show signs of a gas-filled abscess, ascites, or a localized ileus called the "sentinel loop." *(Sachar et al, pp. 78–79)*

15. **(B)** The primary goal of medical management of acute pancreatitis is to stop autodigestion of the pancreas by reducing pancreatic enzyme synthesis and secretion (ie, putting the pancreas to rest by not eating). There is no evidence that any treatment method thus far has any clinical benefit (ie, antibiotics, H-2 blockers, somatostatin, NG suction). Supportive care is the primary treatment with careful attention to intravascular volume repletion and electrolyte balance. These patients are at risk for severe diseases, such as ARDS and DIC, as well as localized complications, such as abscesses or pseudocyst formation. NG suction is only helpful if vomiting or ileus develops. *(Sleisenger and Fordtran, pp. 1832–1833)*

16. **(B)** Folate absorption is largely confined to the upper small intestine and, therefore, malabsorption will be expected in disorders that affect the upper gut. Alcoholism and celiac sprue are two examples of such disorders that result in severe folate deficiency secondary to the significant inability to adequately absorb folate. Partial gastrectomy states usually result in rapid transit through the upper part of the GI tract and will, therefore, result in only mild folate deficiency. Crohn's disease also has only mild affects on folate absorption. *(Sleisenger and Fordtran, p. 1047)*

17. **(A)** Biliary colic results from a struggle between the flow of bile through the cystic duct and a stone in the cystic duct. The clinical feature of biliary colic is acute pain, usually in the right upper quadrant or epigastrium, sometimes with radiation to the right scapula. Pain often occurs at night, usually within a few hours of a heavy meal. Proteins and fats activate CCK release from the small bowel and thereby produce contraction of the gallbladder. If a stone moves or lodges in the neck of the gallbladder, pain is the result. Fever and, occasionally, chills occur when acute cholecystitis develops. *(Sachar et al, pp. 109–110)*

18. **(E)** All of the conditions listed are felt to contribute to the development of gastric carcinoma. Chronic atrophic gastritis, often a complication of pernicious anemia, results in decreased or absent normal gastric glands leading to a variable degree of inflammation and intestinal metaplasia. Although this can be seen in older but normal individuals without gastric cancer, many observations have been made that these two entities occur at a rather high rate in patients with gastric carcinoma—especially in autopsy specimens from the Japanese where there is an increased rate of gastric cancer. Ménétrier's disease, which is characterized by hypertrophic gastropathy, has been associated with a striking frequency of malignant transformation. This is a rather rare condition. Patients who have undergone prior gastric surgeries have been found to have gastric cancer at a rate of 5 to 16 times normal individuals. One theory for this is that intestinal metaplasia is more common in the gastric remnant after surgery and that the increased pH could allow for overgrowth of nitrate-producing bacteria. Lastly, dietary factors implicate long-term ingestion of a high concentration of nitrates in dried, smoked, and salted foods. These nitrates are thought to be converted to carcinogenic nitrites by bacteria. *(Sleisenger and Fordtran, pp. 745–760)*

19. **(B)** Acute cholecystitis consists of acute inflammation of the gallbladder wall and is accompanied usually by abdominal pain and fever. Elderly, debilitated, or immunocompromised patients may be completely asymptomatic and may present as fever of unknown etiology. Acute cholecystitis results from stasis, bacterial infection, or ischemia of the gallbladder. Most cases result from cystic duct obstruction by a stone. Ultrasound is usually helpful to identify stones and demonstrate wall thickening (>3 mm). OCG can be useful as opacification of the gallbladder largely rules out acute cholecystitis. *(Sleisenger and Fordtran, pp. 1701–1704)*

20. **(E)** Ascites is an accumulation of fluid within the peritoneal cavity. It is a common clinical finding with a wide variety of causes. Large amounts of ascites causes abdominal distention and a "fluid wave" on exam. However, it is difficult to detect less than two liters on physical exam. Abdominal ultrasound, CT scan, and paracentesis are helpful. Over 90% of cases are due to either cirrhosis, neoplasms, congestive heart failure, or tuberculosis. *(Sleisenger and Fordtran, pp. 428,433)*

21. (E) Chest pain can be caused by a variety of clinical states. Mucosal lesions such as neoplasms, esophageal inflammation secondary to bacterial/viral/fungal infections, or caustic damage have clearly been implicated in the development of chest pain, as has GERD. Scleroderma, as well as all distal esophageal motility disorders, have pain as a predominant feature. It must be remembered, however, that cardiac angina and pain of the esophageal disease are of sufficient similarity that differentiation on historical basis alone is not often possible. *(Sleisenger and Fordtran, pp. 560–561)*

22. (E) The causes of jaundice can generally be diagnosed by clinical history, physical exam, and routine lab studies. Itching usually suggests cholestasis. Extrahepatic obstruction with secondary cholestasis is suggested by a palpable gallbladder or abdominal mass (possibly pancreatic in origin). Occult blood in the stool may be due to periampullary neoplasm or hemobilia from a pancreatic cancer. Disproportionate elevations of bilirubin and alkaline phosphatase, as compared to other hepatic parameters, suggest extrahepatic obstruction as does an elevated amylase when associated with jaundice. *(Sleisenger and Fordtran, pp. 457–460)*

23. (A) Carcinoid tumors originate from neuroendocrine cells. At least 90% are located in the GI tract. The appendix is the most common site, followed by the terminal ileum and rectum. They are slow growing, often allowing more than 10-year survival even in patients with liver metastases. Appendiceal tumors, however, rarely metastasize. Carcinoid syndrome refers to the systemic effects of agents released by the tumor, namely serotonin and histamine. Signs and symptoms include diarrhea, abdominal pain, flushing, bronchospasm, and telangiectasias. Diagnosis is aided by the finding of elevated 5-HIAA levels in a 24-hour urine collection. Therapy currently is aimed at symptom control with use of somatostatin, which inhibits hormone secretion. *(Sachar et al, pp. 271–274)*

24. (A) Dysphagia, chest pain, and regurgitation are the main symptoms of achalasia. Dysphagia occurs early with both solids and liquids and is worsened by emotional factors, stress, or hurried eating. This may lead to chest pain, which appears to be more pronounced in vigorous achalasia than in classic achalasia. Regurgitation and pulmonary aspiration occur secondary to large amounts of retained foods and saliva in the esophagus. The presence of gastroesophageal reflux argues against achalasia secondary to the presence of high resting pressures of the lower esophageal sphincter and its inherent inability to relax normally. *(Wilson et al, p. 1225)*

25–28. 25. (B); 26. (B); 27. (B); 28. (A) Esophageal variceal hemorrhage is usually massive, life-threatening, and painless. Mallory–Weiss tears are mucosal tears at the GE junction and are generally due to vigorous retching and vomiting. These also present with painless hematemesis. Bleeding due to angiodysplasia is painless and often associated with renal disease and hereditary telangiectasia. Peptic ulcer disease is often accompanied by abdominal pain, but bleeding may be the presenting symptom in 15% of cases. *(Sachar et al, pp. 18,32–42)*

29–33. 29. (B); 30. (A); 31. (B); 32. (A); 33. (A) The hallmark of ulcerative colitis is bloody diarrhea. Complications of UC include toxic fulminant colitis due to deep transmural dissection of the ulcerative inflammatory process resulting in peritoneal signs, systemic toxicity, paralysis of bowel motility, and so-called "toxic megacolon." After 10 years of ulcerative colitis, there is a 20-fold increase in the risk of colon cancer, and the risk increases with the extent of the disease. Crohn's disease most frequently presents with diarrhea, abdominal pain, fever, RLQ fullness, or mass. Crohn's often results in small bowel obstruction from edema, fibrotic stricturing, or abscess formation. Fistulization results from deep sinus tracts and transmural inflammation penetrating the bowel wall and burrowing into adjacent structures. Complications of Crohn's include kidney stone formation due to increased colonic oxalate absorption and/or increased metabolism of uric acid. Gallstone disease is increased due to impaired bile salt reabsorption from the terminal ileum. Sclerosing cholangitis is also thought to be associated with Crohn's disease. *(Sachar et al, pp. 204–210)*

34–37. 34. (B); 35. (A); 36. (A); 37. (B) The typical symptoms of acute viral hepatitis are acute or subacute onset of fatigue, anorexia, RUQ discomfort, and possibly jaundice. Hepatitis A is caused by a picornavirus with incubation of 15 to 50 days and is usually asymptomatic in children. It is transmitted via the fecal–oral route. Its course is generally benign with symptoms lasting 3 to 6 weeks. Household contacts as well as sexual contacts are advised to receive prophylaxis with gamma globulin IM (0.02 ml/kg). Hepatitis B is usually spread parenterally or sexually via whole blood, semen, or saliva. The usual clinical attack is similar to that of hepatitis A, though it is more often severe. Patients may develop a serum sickness pneumonia characterized by fever, urticaria, and arthralgias due to immune complex involvement. The incubation period is 1 to 6 months. About 10% of people contracting hepatitis B will become carriers. These patients may show hepatic damage ranging from persistent hepatitis to chronic hepatitis with cirrhosis. Hepatitis B vaccine is currently available for health care workers, sexual contacts, and other high-risk persons. Interferon is now being used for the treatment of hepatitis B as well. (*Chobanian and Van Ness, pp. 142–144; Sachar et al, pp. 123–127*)

38. **(B)** Mesenteric ischemia, otherwise known as abdominal angina, reflects an imbalance of blood supply and demand. Patients with significant atherosclerotic narrowing of the splanchnic arteries cannot increase blood flow to match demand during ingestion of food and thus develop abdominal pain. Clinically, patients complain of dull or crampy abdominal pain periumbilically occurring within minutes of eating and often lasting for hours. Fear of eating is common, due to the pain and, therefore, weight loss is associated. The abdominal exam is usually normal, although soft bruits may be heard. The lab studies are also within normal ranges. Angiography is the diagnostic test of choice. (*Sachar et al, pp. 224–225*)

39. **(C)** Tumors of the small bowel are rare, accounting for only 5% of benign and malignant GI tract neoplasms. Only 1% of malignant GI carcinomas are found in the small bowel. Although all of the choices listed are clearly found in the small bowel, adenocarcinomas account for nearly 50% of all small bowel tumors. Most commonly seen in the duodenum, two-thirds of the adenocarcinomas diagnosed are noted in the region of the ampulla of Vater. The exact etiology of small bowel cancer is unknown, however there appears to be an increased incidence in patients with familial polyposis, Gardner's syndrome, and Crohn's disease. Other less common tumors of the small bowel include neurofibromatosis and Peutz–Jehgers syndrome. (*Sleisenger and Fordtran, pp. 1547–1548*)

40. **(B)** Giardiasis is the most common cause of water-borne diarrhea in the U.S. Although travel history is common, as many as half of affected patients have no obvious risk factors. Incubation period is 12 to 15 days. Giardiasis is associated with nausea, flatulence, and non-bloody diarrhea. Conversely, *Salmonella* and *Campylobacter* generally invade the colonic mucosa and therefore cause bloody, mucoid diarrhea. *Campylobacter* generally causes fever and headache as well. Toxigenic *E. coli* usually has a short incubation period of 1 to 3 days and runs its course quickly. Giardiasis may be difficult to culture, but endoscopic aspiration for organisms is sometimes helpful. Treatment consists of Metronidazole 250 mg tid for 5 to 7 days or Quinacrine 100 mg tid for 7 days. (*Clearfield and Borowsky, pp. 206–207*)

41. **(B)** Carcinoma of the pancreas is an insidiously developing and nearly universally fatal malignancy. For most patients there are few characteristic signs or symptoms early in the course of the disease. Insidious onset of weight loss, anorexia, and abdominal pain are often seen. Pain radiating into the back suggests invasion of retroperitoneal organs or nerves. Most patients have a mild anemia from blood loss into the bowel and/or nutritional deficiency. Elevated amylase is rare; alkaline phosphatase elevation is common from either hepatic metastasis or bile duct obstruction. ERCP characteristically shows a single irregular, abrupt focal stricture of the pancreatic duct with a smooth remaining system. Biopsy will confirm endoscopic findings. (*Sleisenger and Fordtran, p. 1872*)

42. **(B)** Although all of the listed choices are clearly implicated as causes of nonobstructive gastroparesis, the most common cause is diabetes. It is thought that abnormal neural control of gastric muscular action may be a significant component in the pathogenesis of this disease. It is also felt that the resulting complication of gastroparesis may in turn be partly responsible for poor diabetic control that is frequently seen in these patients. Other causes of gastroparesis—both obstructive and nonobstructive—are post-gastric surgical states (especially truncal vagotomy); pernicious anemia; psychiatric disorders, such as anorexia nervosa and bulimia; peptic ulcer disease; pyloric hypertrophy; gastric antral carcinoma; and pancreatic cancer. Treatment consists of the administration of prokinetic agents such as metoclopramide, bethanechol, and two not yet widely available agents—domperidone and cisapride. (*Sleisenger and Fordtran, pp. 244–247*)

43. **(D)** Acalculous cholecystitis is an important entity because it often progresses to gangrene and perforation. It most often occurs as a complication of another serious illness, surgery, or other trauma. Sepsis from another condition and diabetes mellitus are common associated findings. RUQ pain and fever are helpful, but as many as 25% of cases will have fever only. Leukocytosis is also helpful but again not always present. Ultrasound findings of gallbladder wall thickening (>3 mm), and/or gallbladder enlargement, and/or pericholecystic fluid are diagnostic (without the presence of stones, of course). As many as 20% of all cases of acalculous cholecystitis will have a false negative HIDA scan. (*Sleisenger and Fordtran, p. 1706*)

44. **(C)** Anal fissures are longitudinal defects in the anoderm, common in young and middle-aged adults, and usually caused by the trauma of passing a large, firm stool. Irritable bowel syndrome with its characteristic cycle of diarrhea and constipation can predispose a patient to the development of an anal fissure. Treatment is usually symptomatic with stool softeners, careful attention to diet, and topical creams. In more severe or non-

healing cases, surgical evaluation may be helpful. Hemorrhoids have bleeding as their cardinal symptom, but this is always painless unless the hemorrhoid is thrombosed. Inflammatory bowel diseases and anorectal abscesses usually do not have painful rectal bleeding as a presenting symptom. *(Sleisenger and Fordtran, pp. 1576–1580)*

45. **(C)** The classic presentation of acute cholangitis is fever, pain, and obstructive jaundice. The patient generally is ill appearing, often with rigors and upper abdominal tenderness. Cholangitis is caused by bacterial infection of the bile in the bile ducts. The most common causes are choledocholithiasis, neoplasm, or stricture. Antibiotics are the initial treatment, followed by diagnostic tests to determine the cause of obstruction, then possibly decompression via endoscopic sphincterotomy, biliary stent placement, or surgery, depending on the nature of the obstruction. *(Sleisenger and Fordtran, pp. 1717–1718)*

REFERENCES

Chobanian SJ, Van Ness MM. *Manual of Clinical Problems in Gastroenterology.* Boston, MA: Little, Brown; 1988.

Clearfield HR, Borowsky LM. *Case Studies in Gastroenterology.* Baltimore, MD: Williams & Wilkins; 1989.

Sachar DB, Waye JD, Lewis BS. *Pocket Guide to Gastroenterology.* Baltimore, MD: Williams & Wilkins; 1991.

Sleisenger MH, Fordtran JS. *Gastrointestinal Disease: Pathophysiology and Management,* 4th ed. Philadelphia, PA: WB Saunders; 1989.

Wilson JD, Braunwald E, Isselbacher KJ, et al (eds). *Harrison's Principles of Internal Medicine,* 12th ed. New York: McGraw-Hill; 1991.

Subspecialty List: Gastroenterology

QUESTION NUMBER AND SUBSPECIALTY

1. Esophageal obstruction
2. Gastroesophageal reflux
3. Esophageal cancer
4. Pseudomembranous colitis
5. Zollinger–Ellison syndrome
6. Malabsorption
7. Ulcerative colitis
8. Meckel's diverticulum
9. Ileal function
10. Colon cancer
11. Inflammatory bowel disease
12. Acute pancreatitis
13. Acute pancreatitis
14. Acute pancreatitis
15. Etiology of folate deficiency
16. Biliary colic
17. Gastric carcinoma
18. Acute cholecystitis
19. Ascites
20. Differential diagnosis of chest pain
21. Jaundice
22. Carcinoid
23. Achalasia
24. UGI bleeding
25. UGI bleeding
26. UGI bleeding
27. UGI bleeding
28. Ulcerative colitis and Crohn's disease
29. Ulcerative colitis and Crohn's disease
30. Ulcerative colitis and Crohn's disease
31. Ulcerative colitis and Crohn's disease
32. Ulcerative colitis and Crohn's disease
33. Hepatitis
34. Hepatitis
35. Hepatitis
36. Hepatitis
37. Mesenteric ischemia
38. Small bowel tumors
39. Diarrhea
40. Pancreatic carcinoma
41. Gastroparesis
42. Acalculous cholecystitis
43. Rectal bleeding
44. Cholangitis

Internal Medicine: Neurology
Questions

Questions 1 through 16

1. A 25-year-old patient presenting with acute low back pain, lateral thigh and leg pain after lifting a heavy object may require

    (A) lumbar brace for compression fracture
    (B) work-up for peripheral neuropathy
    (C) lumbar puncture
    (D) removal of herniated disc
    (E) rehabilitation for spinal cord injury

2. A patient who presents with ipsilateral ocular miosis, mild ptosis, and anhidrosis has findings indicative of

    (A) Horner's syndrome with parasympathetic paresis
    (B) Horner's syndrome with a sympathetic paresis
    (C) Argyll–Robertson syndrome with a parasympathetic paresis
    (D) Argyll–Robertson syndrome with a sympathetic paresis
    (E) pupillary-sparing III nerve palsy

3. Which of the following is LEAST likely to be diagnostic for multiple sclerosis?

    (A) CT scan
    (B) somatosensory-evoked responses
    (C) history and physical examination
    (D) MRI
    (E) CSF studies

4. The differential diagnosis for Alzheimer's disease includes which of the following?

    (A) normal pressure hydrocephalus
    (B) depression
    (C) cerebral mass lesion
    (D) AIDS dementia
    (E) all of the above

5. A child who is noted to have brief lapses in consciousness (without falling) should be evaluated for

    (A) generalized seizure disorder
    (B) partial seizure disorder
    (C) attention deficit disorder
    (D) complex partial seizure disorder
    (E) simple motor seizure disorder

6. A 50-year-old male presents with new onset seizures. Etiologic considerations include all of the following EXCEPT

    (A) metastatic cancer
    (B) cerebral mass lesion
    (C) idiopathic
    (D) diabetes mellitus
    (E) hyponatremia

7. A patient presents with a chief complaint of a left visual field cut involving both eyes. The anatomic source of the lesion is

    (A) right optic nerve
    (B) left optic nerve
    (C) optic chiasm
    (D) left optic tract
    (E) right optic tract

8. The most common type of intracerebral neoplasm is

    (A) glioma
    (B) metastasis
    (C) meningioma
    (D) lymphoma
    (E) abscess

9. Minor head injury (brief loss of consciousness with an initial Glasgow coma scale of 13 or greater) may be followed by a post-concussive syndrome. Symptoms may include all of the following EXCEPT

    (A) dizziness
    (B) headache
    (C) memory problems
    (D) diplopia
    (E) all of the above

10. A patient arrives in the emergency department complaining of nausea and vomiting. History reveals that the patient has eaten some home-canned food. What neurologic manifestations may develop?

    (A) incontinence
    (B) no neurologic symptoms are likely to develop
    (C) paralysis of extraocular muscles
    (D) intracerebral hemorrhage
    (E) seizure

11. Which of the following would be associated with Alzheimer's disease?

    (A) focal neurologic finding
    (B) sudden, stepwise progression of symptoms
    (C) depressed state preceding memory disturbance
    (D) nutritional deficiency
    (E) none of the above

12. Allowing hypophosphatemia to develop when providing hyperalimentation to a patient may lead to

    (A) encephalopathy
    (B) peripheral neuropathy
    (C) cranial nerve palsy
    (D) ataxia
    (E) all of the above

13. The most common symptom in a patient with spinal cord metastasis is

    (A) paresthesia
    (B) pain
    (C) numbness
    (D) urinary retention
    (E) focal weakness

14 Gower's maneuver is most indicative of

    (A) cranial nerve dysfunction
    (B) distal extremity weakness
    (C) sensory impairment
    (D) truncal ataxia
    (E) proximal extremity weakness

15. Intracerebral hemorrhage may be caused by all of the following EXCEPT

    (A) arteriovenous malformation
    (B) atrial fibrillation
    (C) aplastic anemia
    (D) anticoagulant therapy
    (E) mycotic aneurysm

16. The most likely diagnosis in a patient whose CSF reveals a glucose of 20 and a protein of 400 with a WBC of 1200 with 90% polys is

    (A) acute bacterial meningitis
    (B) partially treated bacterial meningitis
    (C) neoplastic meningitis
    (D) aseptic meningitis
    (E) cryptococcal meningitis

DIRECTIONS (Questions 17 through 23): For each of the items in this section, ONE or MORE of the numbered options is correct. Choose answer

    (A) if only (1), (2), and (3) are correct,
    (B) if only (1) and (3) are correct,
    (C) if only (2) and (4) are correct,
    (D) if only (4) is correct,
    (E) if all are correct.

Questions 17 through 23

17. A patient who complains of episodic unilateral hearing loss associated with tinnitus, vertigo, nausea, and vomiting has symptoms consistent with

    (1) oscillopsia
    (2) vestibular neuritis
    (3) benign positional vertigo
    (4) Ménière's disease

18. Immediate diagnosis and treatment is required for which of the following headaches?

    (1) migraine
    (2) cluster
    (3) tension
    (4) temporal arteritis

19. Parkinsonism is characterized by

    (1) rigidity
    (2) bradykinesia
    (3) rhythmic tremor
    (4) postural abnormalities

20. Argyll–Robertson pupils

   (1) react equally to light

   (2) should suggest a serologic test for syphilis

   (3) suggest the possibility of diabetes mellitus

   (4) react to near vision

21. Risk factors for cerebrovascular accident include all of the following EXCEPT

   (1) atrial fibrillation

   (2) diabetes mellitus

   (3) hyperlipidemia

   (4) mitral valve prolapse

22. A patient with an unknown past history who has been involved in a recent motor vehicle accident is drowsy, hypertensive, bradycardic, and vomiting. The patient should be immediately evaluated for

   (1) alcohol abuse

   (2) hypovolemic shock

   (3) perforated viscus

   (4) increased intracranial pressure

23. Contributing factors for migraine include

   (1) chocolate

   (2) alcohol

   (3) stress

   (4) refractive errors

DIRECTIONS (Questions 24 through 37): Each set of items in this section consists of a list of lettered options followed by several numbered words or phrases. For each numbered word or phrase, select the ONE lettered option that is most closely associated with it. Each lettered option may be selected once, more than once, or not at all.

Questions 24 through 28

For each of the following sets of signs/symptoms choose the neurologic process MOST likely responsible.

   (A) myelopathy

   (B) radiculopathy

   (C) peripheral neuropathy

   (D) myopathy

   (E) none of the above

24. Pain, numbness, weakness confined to a nerve root distribution

25. Trunk and proximal limbs involved early in course

26. Sphincter involvement

27. Begins in the distal aspect of the extremities

28. Diplopia is a cardinal feature

Questions 29 through 33

Choose the seizure category MOST closely associated.

   (A) generalized seizure

   (B) Jacksonian epilepsy

   (C) temporal lobe seizure

   (D) partial seizure

   (E) not a seizure

29. Petit mal (absence)

30. Déjà vu

31. Numbness confined to one extremity

32. Tonic-clonic

33. Shaking which begins in one extremity and spreads proximally

Questions 34 through 37

Choose the following headache group MOST closely associated.

   (A) cluster headache

   (B) classic migraine

   (C) both

   (D) neither

34. Have a serotonin-enhanced vascular etiology

35. May be relieved at menopause

36. Associated with elevated sedimentation rate

37. Occurs same time daily for days to weeks

Answers and Explanations

1. **(D)** This patient has symptoms classic of nerve root compression from a herniated disc causing a lumbar radiculopathy (nerve root pain). On examination, the patient may have reflex abnormality, weakness, or decreased sensation within a dermatomal/myotomal distribution. The straight leg testing maneuver is frequently positive. Compression fracture is unlikely in a 25-year-old without a pathologic cause. Peripheral neuropathy is not related to trauma. There is no symptoms of spinal cord injury (eg, gait or incontinence) and lumbar puncture would add no useful diagnostic or therapeutic information. *(Youman's, pp. 2678–2679)*

2. **(B)** A Horner's syndrome is caused by a sympathetic paresis. The pupil dilates more slowly (or less completely) in the dark and is associated with miosis, mild ptosis, and anhidrosis. Common causes of a Horner's syndrome include obstetrical/perinatal trauma, malignancy, cervical spine injury, thyroid disease, or thoracic outlet syndrome. *(Youman's, pp. 554–555)*

3. **(A)** A thorough history and physical examination remain the cornerstone in the diagnosis of multiple sclerosis. The waxing and waning of neurologic symptoms suggest the diagnosis. Evoked responses can localize lesions, and CSF studies may reveal an elevated IgG disproportionate to the serum protein, or the presence of oligoclonal bands. An MRI is capable of demonstrating the white matter lesions, and this confirms the clinical diagnosis. CT scanning may not reveal the lesions and does not add useful diagnostic information. *(Adams and Victor, pp. 787–789; Greenberg et al, pp. 157–158,307–308)*

4. **(E)** The diagnosis of Alzheimer's is one of exclusion. Potentially reversible causes of dementia need to be ruled out. The differential diagnosis of Alzheimer's includes normal pressure hydrocephalus, alcohol abuse, depression, cerebral mass lesion, AIDS dementia, and stroke. *(Adams and Victor, pp. 959–966)*

5. **(A)** This child likely has petit mal or absence type seizures. These are classified as generalized seizure disorders as they affect the entire brain. The seizure is fleeting, sometimes only lasting a few seconds, so no loss of consciousness occurs and the patient may be unaware of any abnormality. Petit mal epilepsy commonly presents in childhood. *(Brain and Bannister, pp. 171–199)*

6. **(C)** Idiopathic seizures are rare in anyone over the age of 25. A thorough work-up must be performed to evaluate the cause. Any condition which serves to irritate the cerebral cortex may initiate a seizure. The greatest concern is that of a neoplastic process, most likely a metastatic tumor. *(Brain and Bannister, pp. 171–199)*

7. **(E)** Because fibers originating in the nasal half of the retina cross at the chiasm and temporal fibers do not cross, a lesion in the *right* optic tract will block *right* temporal and *left* nasal fibers. This produces a *left* homonymous hemianopsia. (Remember that visual stimuli are transmitted to the retina reversed.) *(Greenberg et al, pp. 121–129)*

8. **(B)** Although glioma is the most common *primary* intracerebral neoplasm, metastatic disease is overall the most common, accounting for 10% to 15% of intracerebral neoplasms. The most common sources are those from the lung or breast. Definitive diagnosis is made by either locating a primary source or biopsying the lesion. Survival is determined by primary tumor type. *(Adams and Victor, pp. 554–555)*

9. **(E)** Symptoms of the postconcussive syndrome include headache, dizziness, memory problems, weakness, nausea, numbness, diplopia, tinnitus, and hearing problems. Symptoms vary from case to case but usually decrease in severity over time. Occasionally, these complaints will last for greater than one year. *(Youman's, pp. 2236–2237)*

10. **(C)** The patient has ingested *Clostridium botulinum* from inadequately sterilized and canned food. The toxin impairs release of acetylcholine at

the peripheral nerve synapse. This initially leads to problems with convergence, followed by ptosis, extraocular muscle paralysis, dilated pupils, weakness of the muscles of the mandible, dysphagia, dysarthria, and eventually limb and truncal weakness. *(Adams and Victor, pp. 943–944)*

11. **(E)** Alzheimer's disease is characterized by progressive dementia, increased loss of memory and intellect, speech disturbances, and shuffling gait. A focal neurologic finding suggests a neurologic lesion. The stepwise progression of symptoms suggests multi-infarct dementia which may be treated with anticoagulants to halt progression. Depression can mask dementia, but patients with Alzheimer's are actually unaware of their condition and not likely to be depressed. Nutritional deficiencies, such as Vitamin B_{12} deficiency, may lead to symptoms of dementia but can be treated with supplementation. *(Adams and Victor, pp. 959–966)*

12. **(E)** When providing hyperalimentation to a patient, careful monitoring of the chemistry profile is essential. Numerous complications are inherent in nutritional replacement, such as hyperglycemia, electrolyte imbalance, sepsis, etc. Hypophosphatemia may lead to encephalopathy, peripheral neuropathy, ataxia, and cranial nerve palsy. *(Tierney et al, pp. 984–986)*

13. **(B)** Pain is the most common symptom of spinal cord metastasis. The pain is frequently well localized back pain but may be radicular. The pain may precede neurologic deficit by several weeks and the goal is to institute treatment prior to the onset of weakness. *(Adams and Victor, pp. 1104–1108)*

14. **(E)** Gower's maneuver is used to compensate for proximal muscle weakness. In the act of rising from the floor, patients use their hands to push off and lean on their lower extremities to facilitate getting up. *(Weiner and Goetz, p. 228)*

15. **(B)** All the choices can lead to a cerebrovascular accident. However, atrial fibrillation is associated with embolic cerebrovascular events and not with hemorrhage. This frequently occurs in patients who fluctuate from atrial fibrillation to sinus rhythm. *(Weiner and Goetz, pp. 54–55; Adams and Victor, pp. 669–672)*

16. **(A)** CSF glucose may be low in any of the meningitides listed. Protein as high as 400 is a good indication of acute bacterial meningitis, although it can be that high in cryptococcal or neoplastic meningitis. However, the WBC clearly identifies acute bacterial meningitis. Counts greater than 500 are rare in other diseases and 90% polys ex-

cludes the other diagnoses. *(Weiner and Goetz, p. 17; Adams and Victor, pp. 604–605)*

17. **(D)** The symptoms of episodic unilateral hearing loss, tinnitus, and vertigo with nausea and vomiting are classic for Ménière's disease (also known as endolymphatic hydrops). Vestibular neuritis is NOT associated with a hearing loss. Benign positional vertigo is characterized by short duration vertigo exacerbated by head movements. Oscillopsia is the complete absence of peripheral vestibular function. These patients have disequilibrium without vertigo. *(Youman's, pp. 4328–4329)*

18. **(D)** Migraine and cluster headaches are chronic, and most patients have a management regimen focused on pain relief. Tension headaches can be managed at home and involve avoidance of the triggers, when possible, and pain management techniques. Temporal arteritis is an inflammatory process, usually with an elevated sedimentation rate, and may indicate a systemic vascular disorder. It is very responsive to steroid therapy, which should be initiated immediately to avoid irreversible blindness, which can result. *(Weiner and Goetz, p. 1443; Greenberg et al, pp. 70–90; Johnston et al, p. 162)*

19. **(E)** These symptoms are the hallmark of Parkinson's disease. Other disorders affecting the basal ganglia may demonstrate some of these findings. Encephalitis, particularly herpetic encephalitis, often affects the basal ganglia, but history and viral titers easily make the distinction. On the other hand, parkinsonism is often associated with depression and later dementia. Careful examination of depressed and demented patients will rule out parkinsonism. Treatment is aimed at restoring dopamine to the brain. Supportive and therapeutic assistance is maintained in conjunction with pharmacologic therapy. *(Weiner and Goetz, pp. 109–114; Adams and Victor, pp. 976–979; Johnston et al, p. 67)*

20. **(C)** Argyll–Robertson pupils are bilaterally small but may be irregular. They do not react to light, but do react to accommodation. They are characteristically seen in neurosyphilis. *(Weiner and Goetz, pp. 319–320)*

21. **(E)** Atrial fibrillation and mitral valve prolapse (by embolic means), diabetes, obesity, hyperlipidemia, and hemolytic disorders are among risk factors for stroke. Congenital malformations, such as aneurysms and arteriovenous malformations, can lead to devastating, sudden cerebrovascular events. *(Weiner and Goetz, p. 54; Adams and Victor, p. 672)*

22. **(D)** The presence of decreased level of consciousness, hypertension associated with bradycardia

(the reverse of hypovolemic shock), and nausea and vomiting should immediately alert the examiner to the presence of increased intracranial pressure and the possibility of uncal herniation. *(Youman's, p. 1992)*

23. (E) Migraines can be avoided to some degree by avoiding precipitating factors such as stress, refractive errors, dietary changes (eg, fats, eggs, chocolate, raw fruit, beef, etc), alcohol, and oral contraceptives. *(Brain and Bannister, pp. 205–210).*

24–28. 24. (B); 25. (D); 26. (A); 27. (C); 28. (E) Myelopathy is a disorder of the spinal cord. Motor function is affected from the site of the lesion distally. There is a sensory level suggesting the location of the lesion or a "suspended" sensory level on the trunk (eg, shawl distribution). Reflexes are usually hyperactive, the Babinski sign is positive and the urethral and anal sphincters are affected.

Peripheral neuropathy is a lower motor neuron disease distal to the nerve roots. There is a flaccid weakness, reflexes are hypoactive, and sensory findings are confined to the distribution of the peripheral nerve(s). Distal extremities are affected first. Sphincters are rarely involved.

Myopathy (muscle disease) involves the trunk and proximal musculature initially. There is a flaccid weakness; no sensory abnormality; reflexes are initially unaffected, then become hypoactive; and there is no sphincter disturbance.

Radiculopathy is a disorder of the nerve root. Pain, numbness, weakness, and reflex change are confined to a specific dermatome/myotome. *(Youman's, pp. 3,2678–2679)*

29–33. 29. (A); 30. (C); 31. (D); 32. (A); 33. (B) Generalized seizures include petit mal (absence) and tonic-clonic seizures. The abnormal discharge impairs consciousness. Petit mal involves only brief lapses in consciousness, while a tonic-clonic (or variation) leads to "convulsions."

Partial seizures include simple motor, simple sensory, and complex partial temporal lobe epilepsy). Simple motor seizures are characterized by a Jacksonian March in which the distal portion of the contralateral (to the seizure focus) extremity begins to shake. This shaking progresses proximally and may develop into a tonic-clonic event. The initial seizure activity, however, is focal. The patient may be left with a transient weakness of the extremity(s) initially involved. This is known as a Todd's paralysis.

A simple sensory seizure is similar to a simple motor seizure, but the initial focus is of a sensory nature.

Complex partial seizures exhibit unusual findings of aberrant smells or taste; a sense of déjà vu; vivid recall of minor past events; extreme fear or depression; or automatic movements, such as chewing, smacking lips, or even performing routine daily tasks. *(Brain and Bannister, pp. 171–199)*

34–37. 34. (C); 35. (B); 36. (D); 37. (A) Both migraine headaches and cluster headaches are vascular in origin. Cluster headaches are unilateral and orbital but also demonstrate ipsilateral lacrimation. Cluster headaches cluster, that is, occur frequently but give way to longer periods which are headache-free. They are more common in males, particularly those with blue or hazel eyes who smoke and use alcohol. During periods of attack, alcohol use is a common trigger and should be avoided. Cluster headaches are very severe, occur at the same time over days to weeks, and generally last 30 minutes to 2 hours and are not associated with nausea. Migraine headaches also tend to be ipsilateral, but nausea is common, and they are more likely to occur in females. They may decrease significantly with menopause. Migraines are often preceded by an aura and can last for a few hours or days. Ergotamine is useful for migraines, but if used frequently produces a dependency that in turn causes a migraine-like headache. Elevation of the sedimentation rate suggests temporal arteritis. *(Weiner and Goetz, pp. 71–72,79,68–70; Brain and Bannister, pp. 205–210; Johnston et al, p. 162)*

REFERENCES

Adams RD, Victor M. *Principles of Neurology,* 5th ed. New York: McGraw-Hill; 1993.

Bannister R, Brain R. *Brain and Bannister's Clinical Neurology,* 7th ed, Oxford: Oxford Medical Publications; 1992.

Greenberg DA, Aminoff MJ, Simon RP. *Clinical Neurology,* Norwalk, CT: Appleton & Lange; 1993.

Johnston MV, MacDonald RL, Young AB (eds). *Principles of Drug Therapy in Neurology,* Boston, MA: FA Davis; 1992.

Tierney LM Jr, McPhee SJ, Papadakis MA, Schroeder SA. *Current Medical Diagnosis & Treatment.* Norwalk, CT: Appleton & Lange; 1993.

Weiner W Jr, Goetz CG (eds). *Neurology for the Non-Neurologist,* 2nd ed. Philadelphia, PA: JB Lippincott; 1989.

Youmans JR (ed). *Neurological Surgery,* 3rd ed, Philadelphia, PA: WB Saunders; 1990.

Subspecialty List: Neurology

QUESTION NUMBER AND SUBSPECIALTY

1. Back pain
2. Ocular physiology
3. Multiple sclerosis
4. Alzheimer's
5. Seizure disorders
6. Seizure disorders
7. Ocular physiology
8. Cerebral neoplasms
9. Head trauma
10. Neurologic signs of botulism
11. Alzheimer's
12. Wernicke–Korsakoff syndrome
13. Spinal cord metastases
14. Neurologic examination
15. Stroke
16. Meningitis
17. Vertigo
18. Headache
19. Parkinsonism
20. Argyll–Robertson pupils

21. Stroke
22. Head injury
23. Migraine headache
24. Myelopathy, peripheral neuropathy, myopathy, radiculopathy
25. Myelopathy, peripheral neuropathy, myopathy, radiculopathy
26. Myelopathy, peripheral neuropathy, myopathy, radiculopathy
27. Myelopathy, peripheral neuropathy, myopathy, radiculopathy
28. Myelopathy, peripheral neuropathy, myopathy, radiculopathy
29. Seizure disorders
30. Seizure disorders
31. Seizure disorders
32. Seizure disorders
33. Seizure disorders
34. Headaches
35. Headaches
36. Headaches
37. Headaches

Internal Medicine: Rheumatology
Questions

DIRECTIONS (Questions 1 through 11): For each of the items in this section, ONE or MORE of the numbered options is correct. Choose answer

    (A) if only (1), (2), and (3) are correct,
    (B) if only (1) and (3) are correct,
    (C) if only (2) and (4) are correct,
    (D) if only (4) is correct,
    (E) if all are correct.

Questions 1 through 11

1. Which of the following are frequently found in patients with osteoarthritis in the early stages?

    (1) pain on motion with stiffness
    (2) Heberden's nodes
    (3) night pain
    (4) swan neck deformities

2. Which of the following laboratory and radiology findings suggests the diagnosis of osteoarthritis?

    (1) normal to slightly elevated sedimentation rate
    (2) joint space narrowing, osteophytes, and subchondral sclerosis
    (3) clear synovial fluid on joint aspiration
    (4) elevated antinuclear antibody test (ANA)

3. Signs of bacterial septic arthritis include

    (1) fever and chills
    (2) slow insidious onset
    (3) involves primarily large weight-bearing joints and the wrist
    (4) usually is polyarticular

4. Some of the signs and symptoms associated with psoriatic arthritis are

    (1) pitting of the fingernails
    (2) pain and stiffness of the distal interphalangeal joints
    (3) scaling plaques of the elbows and knees
    (4) urethritis

5. Which of the following would you consider important objectives in the treatment of rheumatoid disease?

    (1) relief of pain
    (2) suppression of inflammation
    (3) preservation of function
    (4) patient education

6. The most common neurologic problem seen in rheumatoid arthritis results from

    (1) peripheral neuropathy
    (2) nerve root irritation
    (3) myelopathy secondary to vertebral involvement
    (4) cerebellar cortical degeneration

7. Which of the following lab findings are consistent with the 11 criteria for the diagnosis of rheumatoid arthritis?

    (1) positive rheumatoid factor
    (2) elevated sedimentation rate
    (3) a poor mucin precipitation for synovial fluid (with shreds and cloudy solution obtained by adding synovial fluid to dilute acetic acid)
    (4) anemia

8. Which of the following are potential side effects from the use of nonsteroidal, anti-inflammatory medications?

    (1) gastrointestinal upset
    (2) rash
    (3) edema
    (4) elevated liver function test

9. Possible complications from the use of adrenocorticosteroid in patients with rheumatoid arthritis include

   (1) decreased hypoglycemic effects when used with insulin or oral hypoglycemics

   (2) osteoporosis

   (3) increased risk of digitalis toxicity in patients on digoxin

   (4) reactivated infectious processes

10. Drug-related lupus-like syndrome can occur with which of the following drugs?

   (1) hydralazine

   (2) procainamide (Procan, Pronestyl)

   (3) phenytoin (Dilantin)

   (4) indomethacin (Indocin)

11. Which of the following are correct concerning rheumatoid arthritis?

   (1) occurs predominantly in the second or third decade of life

   (2) is a highly predictable disease

   (3) the extent of articular involvement correlates well with the patient's complaints

   (4) affects women more often than men

DIRECTIONS (Questions 12 through 21): Each of the numbered items or incomplete statements in this section is followed by answers or by completions of the statement. Select the ONE lettered answer or completion that is BEST in each case.

Questions 12 through 21

12. Which of the following criteria would suggest clinical remission of rheumatoid arthritis according to the ARA?

   (A) duration of morning stiffness not exceeding 15 min

   (B) mild fatigue

   (C) decreased joint pain

   (D) decreased joint tenderness with less pain on motion

   (E) sedimentation rate (westergren method) less than 40 mm

13. In "rheumatoid disease" the majority of clinical and pathologic findings are a result of chronic inflammation of

   (A) synovial membranes

   (B) epiphyseal disc

   (C) articular cartilage

   (D) periosteal membrane

   (E) subchondral bone

14. Which of the following tests is most useful in assessing the response in the treatment of rheumatoid arthritis?

   (A) Hgb and Hct (hemoglobin and hematocrit)

   (B) sedimentation rate

   (C) rheumatoid factor

   (D) synovial fluid exam

   (E) WBC count

15. The therapy for rheumatoid disease is based primarily on the use of modalities that perform what function?

   (A) stimulate phagocytosis

   (B) fight infection

   (C) reverse histamine reaction

   (D) inhibit prostaglandin production

   (E) suppress phagocytosis

16. All of the following are criteria for the classification of systemic lupus erythematosus EXCEPT

   (A) elevated blood sugar

   (B) discoid rash

   (C) elevated ANA (antinuclear antibody)

   (D) arthritis

   (E) psychosis

17. Patients with rheumatoid arthritis can present with many types of deformities of the hand. Hyperextension of the PIP joint, in conjunction with flexion at the DIP joint, constitutes what deformity?

   (A) Dupuytren's contracture

   (B) mallet finger

   (C) swan neck deformity

   (D) boutonniere deformity

   (E) trigger finger

18. Ossification of the annulus, fibrosis of the intervertebral disc, and longitudinal ligament (bamboo spine) appearing on x-ray are classically associated with which of the following diseases?

   (A) systemic lupus erythematosus

   (B) osteoarthritis

   (C) degenerative disc disease

   (D) ankylosing spondylitis

   (E) posttraumatic changes from a compression fracture

19. A 52-year-old man presents with severe right ankle pain for 2 days and no other complaints. During the exam, the joint is erythematous and warm, and an effusion is noted. The patient is afebrile; WBC: 9000, with normal differential; BUN and creatinine are within normal limits. Uric acid level is 9.6 mg/dL (normal is 2.5 to 8 mg/dL). The most likely diagnosis is

(A) rheumatoid arthritis

(B) osteoarthritis

(C) pseudogout

(D) gouty arthritis

(E) bacterial septic arthritis

20. A 40-year-old female presents with a history of acute onset of right knee pain, chills, and sweats. Her temperature is 103.0°F. The right knee is erythematous and swollen with an effusion, and x-rays reveal only soft tissue swelling. Arthrocentesis reveals 80,000/μL leukocytes with 90% polymorphonuclear cells. The patient's symptoms, physical and laboratory findings are most consistent with

(A) gouty arthritis

(B) osteoarthritis

(C) rheumatoid arthritis

(D) bacterial septic arthritis

(E) Lyme disease

21. A 10-year-old child presents with acute onset of right knee pain, inflamed conjuctiva, mild burning with urination, and a history of fever and diarrhea one week prior. The most likely diagnosis is

(A) JRA (juvenile rheumatoid arthritis)

(B) joint sepsis

(C) Reiter's syndrome

(D) ankylosing spondylitis

(E) SLE (systemic lupus erythematosis)

DIRECTIONS (Questions 22 through 26): Each set of items in this section consists of a list of lettered options followed by several numbered words or phrases. For each numbered word or phrase, select the ONE lettered option that is most closely associated with it. Each lettered option may be selected once, more than once, or not at all.

Questions 22 through 26

Match the following diseases with the most appropriate description and physical findings.

(A) A multisystem disease characterized by persistent inflammatory synovitis, usually symmetrical and polyarticular, with morning stiffness. PIP and MCP are joints frequently involved.

(B) A multisystem disorder characterized by fibrotic infiltration of the skin and various organ systems. Raynaud's phenomenon, fibrosis of the skin (scleroderma), and hypomotility of the esophagus is common.

(C) The earliest changes in this disease are frequently found in the sacroiliac joints of young men, and it is strongly associated with histocompatibility antigen HLA-B27.

(D) It may affect any joint, usually limited to one or few joints, and laboratory investigation is usually unremarkable.

(E) It may involve virtually any organ system; common features include fatigue, fever, weight loss, and skin rashes (particularly malar rashes over both cheeks).

22. Progressive systemic sclerosis (PSS)

23. Rheumatoid arthritis (RA)

24. Systemic lupus erythmatosus (SLE)

25. Ankylosing spondylitis (AS)

26. Osteoarthritis (OA)

Answers and Explanations

1. **(B)** Osteoarthritis is divided into different stages —early and late. Early stages are characterized by pain with motion and stiffness, and night pain with response to anti-inflammatories. Late stages are dominated by joint instability, pain at rest with increased pain on weight bearing, and failure to respond to anti-inflammatories. Heberden's nodes refer to the osteoarthritic disfigurements of distal interphalangel joints, usually soft early on but becoming enlarged and angular later on. Swan neck deformities are frequently found with rheumatoid arthritis. *(Howell, pp. 1554–1557)*

2. **(A)** The laboratory investigation in osteoarthritis (OA) is helpful in excluding other joint disease. There is no single diagnostic test for OA. Rheumatoid factors and antinuclear antibody (ANA) tests are negative; the erythrocyte sedimentation rate is usually normal to slightly elevated in patients with generalized or erosive OA. Synovial fluid exam reveals clear, straw-colored fluid with a low leukocyte count. The peripheral WBC count is usually normal. Roentgenographic exam usually shows narrowing of the interosseous joint space resulting from destruction of articular cartilage, osteophytes at the margins of affected joints, and subchondral sclerosis. *(Howell, pp. 1554–1557)*

3. **(B)** Septic arthritis is a medical emergency. Failure to rapidly diagnose this condition has the potential to cause permanent damage to the involved joint. Septic arthritis typically affects one joint or a few asymmetric joints. Patients with septic arthritis usually present with an acute onset of pain, fever, erythema, and swelling of the affected joint; systemic signs of infection are common. Weight-bearing joints (most commonly the knee) and the wrist are most commonly involved. *(Schwartz, pp. 1354–1355)*

4. **(A)** Psoriatic arthropathy is a common disease, occurring in about 20% of individuals with psoriasis, particularly in those patients with psoriatic nail disease. It is associated with a synovitis generally indistinguishable from RA. Arthritis of the distal interphalangeal joints of the hands and the metatarsophalangeal joints of the feet are usually involved. The hips, knees, ankles, and wrists may also be affected. In some individuals there can be erosive, inflammatory joint changes that are usually polyarticular and occasionally can be severe, even mutilating. Psoriasis classically presents with plaques over the elbows and knees, but can appear over the thorax as well. Pitting of fingernails with lifting and flaring can be associated with psoriasis, though urethritis is not. *(Conn et al, pp. 1053–1061)*

5. **(E)** The treatment of rheumatoid diseases can be complex, with a wide variety of medications, and surgical and nonsurgical procedures available. The health care provider must be familiar with all treatment modalities; however, important general objectives must be kept in mind. The principal objectives of management must include: (1) relief of pain, (2) reduction or suppression of inflammation, (3) minimizing undesirable effects of the disease and treatment, (4) preservation of muscle and joint function, and (5) return to desirable and productive life. *(Arnett, pp. 1512–1513)*

6. **(A)** Neurologic involvement in RA usually involves peripheral nerve function secondary to chronic inflammation, which causes compression of the nerves. Rheumatoid vasculitis may cause a mononeuritis multiplex with patchy sensory loss in the extremities. Myelopathy due to vertebral involvement frequently involves the C1 and C2 area and is a neurosurgical emergency. As the name implies, cerebellar cortical degeneration is a central nervous system disorder due to chronic nutritional depletion commonly seen in alcoholics. *(Arnett, pp. 1512–1513)*

7. **(B)** Although mild normocytic, normochromic, or hypochromic-type anemia and elevated sedimentation rate are findings associated with RA, the 11 criteria set down for the purpose of classification and uniformity of diagnosis by the ARA are:

1. morning stiffness
2. pain on motion or tenderness in at least one joint (observed by a physician)
3. swelling in at least one joint (observed by a physician)
4. swelling of at least one other joint (any interval free of joint symptoms between the two joint involvement may not be more than 3 months)
5. symmetric joint swelling (with simultaneous involvement of the same joint on both sides of the body)
6. subcutaneous nodules on bony prominences, extensor surfaces, or in juxta-articular regions
7. roentgenographic changes typical of rheumatiod arthritis
8. a positive agglutination test result to demonstrate the presence of rheumatoid factor
9. a poor mucin precipitate from synovial fluid (with shreds and cloudy solution obtained on adding synovial fluid to dilute acetic acid)
10. characteristic histologic changes in the synovium
11. characteristic histological changes in the nodules. *(Arnett, pp. 1508–1513)*

8. **(E)** All the answers are correct. The side effects of nonsteroidal anti-inflammatory medications must be known by all who treat inflammatory diseases. The side effects vary greatly with the individual drug types. Gastrointestinal problems occur in 1% to 10% of patients, rash occurs in 3% to 9% of patients, and edema occurs in 1% to 3% of patients and may aggravate congestive heart failure. Elevation of liver function test can occur and should be followed at regular intervals. *(McCarren, Chap. 8)*

9. **(E)** Regardless of the therapy, the frequency and severity of osteoporosis, a feature of RA, are increased by adrenocorticosteroid treatment. Compression fractures of the vertebral bodies are common. Decreased host resistance to acquired or reactivated infections is a well-documented feature of adrenocorticosteroid therapy. The use of these drugs aggravates latent or overt diabetes mellitus, and the dose of insulin or oral hypoglycemics may need to be increased during therapy. Serum digoxin levels can be increased during therapy and rise to toxic levels; therefore, serum digoxin levels should be followed during therapy with adrenocorticosteroid medication. Prolonged therapy may lead to suppression of pituitary-adrenal function. Too rapid a withdrawal can cause adrenal insufficiency (eg, fever, myalgia, arthralgia, and malaise). *(Hayes, p. 104)*

10. **(A)** Drug-related lupus-like syndromes have been documented since 1953, with the use of hydralazine. There has been a steady accumulation of reports of lupus-like syndrome induced by various drugs. The syndrome occurs most commonly today with the use of procainamide (Procan, Pronestyl) and antiseizure medication such as phenytoin (Dilantin). Other medications that cause lupus-like syndromes are penicillamine, tetracycline, isonazide, chlorpromazine, and methyldopa. *(Schur, p. 1121)*

11. **(D)** RA affects women two to three times more often than men. Although the disease can occur at any age, the peak incidence is in the fourth to the sixth decade of life. RA is not at all predictable. The disease can vary from intermittent and mild to unrelenting and eventually fatal. Because RA can involve periarticular structures, the extent of articular involvement does not correlate with the patient's complaints. *(Hellman, pp. 654–659)*

12. **(A)** Clinical remission according to the ARA would require 5 or more of the following criteria: (1) duration of morning stiffness not exceeding 15 min; (2) no fatigue; (3) no joint pain (by history); (4) no joint tenderness or pain on motion; (5) no soft tissue swelling in joints or tendon sheaths; and (6) erthrocyte sedimentation rate (westergren method) less than 30 mm per hr for females or 20 mm per hr for males. However, spontaneous remission is not likely beyond 2 years of the disease. *(Harris, p. 971)*

13. **(A)** The classic presentation of RA is the result of chronic inflammation of synovial membranes. It is the formation of chronic granulation tissue (pannus) resulting from chronic synovitis that produces hydrolytic enzymes. These enzymes are capable of eroding articular cartilage, subchondrial bone, ligaments, and tendons. *(Arnett, p. 1509)*

14. **(B)** The erythrocyte sedimentation rate (ESR) is diversely elevated in most patients and roughly parallels the disease activity. Therefore, it becomes a useful parameter for assessing response to therapy. WBC counts are most often normal; only 25% of patients are considered as having leukocytosis. Rheumatoid factor is not present in everyone with RA, but those that are seropositive usually have a poor prognosis. There is some correlation between the degree of anemia and the initial severity of the illness in RA, but it does not correlate with disease activity. *(Harris, pp. 967–974)*

15. **(D)** The basis of therapy for RA is to suppress inflammation, because it is this process that leads to the destruction of skeletal and extraskeletal tissues. Prostaglandins are thought to act as mediators to stimulated inflammation. Inhibiting prostaglandin production is the major pharmacologic effect of aspirin, nonsteroidal anti-inflammatory drugs, and corticosteroids. Gold-containing

compounds, penicillamine, and antimalarials have a more specific anti-inflammatory action and no inhibitory effects on the synthesis of prostaglandins. *(Rodman et al, pp. 16–19)*

16. **(A)** Although it is possible to have the criteria for SLE and still not have SLE, the criteria are helpful in making the diagnosis. Not all the criteria must be present.

   1. malar rash
   2. discoid rash
   3. photosensitivity
   4. oral ulcers
   5. arthritis (two or more joints)
   6. serositis (pleuritis, pericarditis)
   7. renal disorder (proteinuria, cellular cast)
   8. neurologic disorder (seizures, psychosis)
   9. hematologic disorder (hemolytic anemia, leukopenia, lymphopenia, or thrombocytopenia)
   10. immunologic disorder (positive LE cell prep, anti-DNA, anti-SM, false-positive serologic test for syphilis)
   11. antinuclear antibody. *(Steinburg, p. 1526)*

17. **(C)** A hyperextension of the PIP joint in conjunction with flexion of the DIP joint describes a swan neck deformity. This deformity usually occurs in the index and middle fingers due to contraction of the interosseous and flexor muscles and tendons. Dupuytren's contracture is caused by thickening and shortening of the palmar and sometimes the plantar fascia. A mallet finger deformity is usually the result of a traumatic injury in which the extensor tendon of the distal phalanx is ruptured. Boutonniere deformity is also common in RA, but is a flexion deformity of the PIP joint and extension of the DIP joint. A trigger finger refers to flexor tendon sheath inflammation in association with the development of a tendon nodule, giving rise to a "locking" of the digit in flexion. *(Turek, pp. 1034,1044,1052,1063)*

18. **(D)** "Bamboo spine," as described in the question is seen in patients with ankylosing spondylitis with the greatest frequency. SLE has no classical radiographic pattern; however, 15% of patients with SLE develop deforming arthritis, and 5% to 8% develop aseptic necrosis. Osteoarthritis radiographically reveals joint space narrowing, subchrondral sclerosis, and osteophyte formation. Degenerative disc disease also shows joint space narrowing and osteophyte formation and spondylolisthesis may be present. Posttraumatic changes from compression fractures usually involve anterior wedging of the vertebral body. *(Calin, pp. 1516–1518)*

19. **(D)** The patient presents with a monoarticular arthritis involving the ankle joint. The laboratory investigation reveals an elevated uric acid level, and synovial fluid exam shows urate crystals classically seen in gouty arthritis. Bacterial septic arthritis is easily ruled out, as the patient has no fever, and one would expect a synovial white cell count in the range of 50,000 to 200,000. In rheumatoid arthritis, a monoarticular presentation is unlikely. Normal x-ray and urate crystals make the diagnosis of osteoarthritis remote. Pseudogout presents similarly, but crystal exam of the synovial fluid yields the rod-shaped crystals of calcium pyrophosphate. Also, one may find cartilaginous calcification on x-ray in pseudogout. Acute, gouty arthritis tends to affect the lower extremities, particularly the metatarsal phalangeal (MTP) joint (75% of patients), but is also frequently seen in the tarsal joints and ankle. The joints of the upper extremities can be affected, particularly the elbow, wrist, and metacarpal phalangeal joints. Shoulder, hip, and sacroiliac joint involvement are rare in pseudogout. *(Wyngaarden, pp. 1108–1111)*

20. **(D)** This patient presents with an acute onset of right knee pain, fever, and a swollen right knee. There are no x-ray findings consistent with bony pathology of intra-articular foreign body. There is an elevated synovial white count. These findings are most consistent with the diagnosis of bacterial septic arthritis. There are no urate crystals in the synovial fluid to accompany a diagnosis of gouty arthritis. Lyme disease is usually recognized clinically by an early, expanding, erythematous skin lesion (erythema chronicum migrans). One would not expect to find fever and an elevated synovial white count with osteoarthritis. *(Malawista, p. 1520)*

21. **(C)** Reiter's syndrome has a classic triad of urethritis, conjuctivitis, and arthritis. It usually follows a venereal infection (both chlamydia and mycoplasma have been indicated) or dysentery (*Shigella* or *Yersinia* may be implicated), and in many cases associated with HLA-B27. There can be involvement of ligaments and tendons, along with joint involvement. It can manifest itself in skin lesions (keratoderma blennorrhagicum), which can be misdiagnosed. No cure exists for Reiter's syndrome, and symptomatic management includes the use of NSAIDs, and steroid eye drops for recurrent uveitis. For patients with progressive disease, asathioprine or methotrexate may be effective. *(Calin, pp. 1038–1051)*

22. **(B)** Progressive systemic sclerosis (PSS) is a multisystem disorder characterized by inflammation, fibrosis, and degeneration of the integument. These problems are associated with similar changes and prominent vascular lesions in the gastrointestinal tract, synovium, heart, lung, and

kidneys. Raynaud's phenomenon, fibrosis of the skin (scleroderma), and hypomotility of the esophagus are common. *(LeRoy, pp. 1530–1531)*

23. **(A)** RA is a multisystem disease characterized by persistent inflammatory synovitis that is usually symmetrical, polyarticular, and associated with morning stiffness. RA is often associated with extra-articular involvement of other organ systems. Organs frequently affected include the skin, eye, cardiovascular system, respiratory system, spleen, and nervous system. *(Arnett, pp. 1512–1513)*

24. **(E)** SLE is an acute and chronic inflammatory process of unknown etiology that may involve virtually every organ system. The clinical presentation of SLE is highly variable, and common features include fatigue, fever, weight loss, and the classic butterfly rash. Polyarthralgias and polyarthritis are the most common manifestations of SLE, occurring in 95% of patients. *(Steinburg, p. 1522)*

25. **(C)** Anklylosing spondylitis (AS) usually presents during young adulthood in a male-to-female ratio of 3:1. The earliest changes in this disease are frequently found in the sacroiliac joints. There is an association with histocompatibility antigen HLA-B27. Inflammatory ocular disease, particularly acute anterior uveitis, occurs in approximately one quarter of those patients with AS. *(Calin, pp. 1516–1518)*

26. **(D)** Osteoarthritis is the most frequently encountered disorder of connective tissue affecting the joints in humans. It is a disease of both the articular cartilage and the subchondral bone. Osteoarthritis may affect any joint but is usually limited to one or a few. There are no specific laboratory features of osteoarthritis. *(Howell, pp. 1554–1557)*

REFERENCES

Arnett FC. Rheumatiod arthritis. In Wyngaarden JB, Smith LH, Bennett JC (eds). *Cecil Textbook of Medicine,* 19th ed. Philadelphia, PA: WB Saunders; 1992.

Calin A. The spondyloarthropathies. In Wyngaarden JB, Smith LH, Bennett JC (eds). *Cecil Textbook of Medicine,* 19th ed. Philadelphia, PA: WB Saunders; 1992.

Conn DL, Michet CJ. Psoriatic arthritis. In Kelly WN, Harris ED Jr, Ruddy S, Sledge CB (eds). *Textbook of Rheumatology.* Philadelphia, PA: WB Saunders; 1989.

Harrelson JM, Callaghan JJ. Infections and neoplasms of the bone. In Sabiston DC Jr (ed). *Textbook of Surgery. The Biological Basis of Modern Surgical Practice,* 14th ed. Philadelphia, PA: WB Saunders; 1989.

Harris ED. The clinical features of rheumatoid arthritis. In Kelly WN, Harris ED Jr, Ruddy S, Sledge CB (eds). *Textbook of Rheumatology.* Philadelphia, PA: WB Saunders; 1989.

Hayes BF. Glucocorticosteroid therapy. In Wyngaarden JB, Smith LH, Bennett JC (eds). *Cecil Textbook of Medicine,* 19th ed. Philadelphia, PA: WB Saunders; 1992.

Hellman DB. Arthritis and musculoskeletal disorders. In Tierney LM Jr, McPhee SJ, Papadakis MA, Schroeder SA (eds). *Current Medical Diagnosis and Treatment.* Norwalk, CT: Appleton & Lange; 1990.

Howell DS. Degenerative joint disease. In Wyngaarden JB, Smith LH, Bennett JC (eds). *Cecil Textbook of Medicine,* 19th ed. Philadelphia, PA: WB Saunders; 1992.

LeRoy EC. Systemic sclerosis. In Wyngaarden JB, Smith LH, Bennett JC (eds). *Cecil Textbook of Medicine,* 19th ed. Philadelphia, PA: WB Saunders; 1992.

Malawista SE. Infectious arthritis. In Wyngaarden JB, Smith LH, Bennett JC (eds). *Cecil Textbook of Medicine,* 19th ed. Philadelphia, PA: WB Saunders; 1992.

McCarren HT. *Compendium of Drug Therapy.* New York: McGraw-Hill; 1993.

Schur PH. Clinical features of SLE. In Wyngaarden JB, Smith LH, Bennett JC (eds). *Cecil Textbook of Medicine,* 19th ed. Philadelphia, PA: WB Saunders; 1992.

Steinburg AD. Systemic lupus erythematosus. In Wyngaarden JB, Smith LH, Bennett JC (eds). *Cecil Textbook of Medicine,* 19th ed. Philadelphia, PA: WB Saunders; 1992.

Turek SL, et al (eds). *Orthopaedics, Principles and Their Application.* Philadelphia, PA: JB Lippincott; 1984.

Wyngaarden JB. Gouty arthritis. In Wyngaarden JB, Smith LH, Bennett JC (eds). *Cecil Textbook of Medicine.* 19th ed. Philadelphia, PA: WB Saunders; 1992.

Subspecialty List: Rheumatology

QUESTION NUMBER AND SUBSPECIALTY

1. Osteoarthritis—stages
2. Osteoarthritis—laboratory and radiology findings
3. Bacterial septic arthritis—characteristics
4. Psoriatic arthritis—characteristics
5. Rheumatoid arthritis—treatment
6. Rheumatoid arthritis—complications
7. Rheumatoid arthritis—criteria
8. Medications
9. Medications
10. Medications
11. Rheumatoid arthritis—characteristics
12. Medications
13. Rheumatoid arthritis—characteristics
14. Rheumatoid arthritis—laboratory evaluation
15. Rheumatoid arthritis—treatment
16. Systemic lupus erythematosus—clinical effects
17. Rheumatoid arthritis—clinical findings
18. Ankylosing spondylitis—clinical findings
19. Gouty arthritis—diagnosis
20. Bacterial septic arthritis—diagnosis
21. Rieter's syndrome—characteristics
22. Progressive systemic sclerosis—characteristics
23. Rheumatoid arthritis—characteristics
24. Systemic lupus erythematosus—characteristics
25. Ankylosing spondylitis—characteristics
26. Osteoarthritis—characteristics

Internal Medicine: Hematology/Oncology
Questions

DIRECTIONS (Questions 1 through 9): Each set of items in this section consists of a list of lettered options followed by several numbered words or phrases. For each numbered word or phrase, select the ONE lettered option that is most closely associated with it. Each lettered option may be selected once, more than once, or not at all.

Questions 1 through 5

Most chemotherapeutic agents share some common toxicities such as nausea and vomiting, neutropenia, hair loss, and painful mouth sores. However, a few agents have special toxicities that target a specific organ or system and require these to be monitored during treatment. Match the side effects listed below with the drug that it is MOST commonly associated.

    (A) bleomycin (Blenoxane)
    (B) cisplatin (Platinol, CDDP)
    (C) cyclophosphamide (Cytoxan, CTX)
    (D) doxorubicin (Adriamycin, Rubex)
    (E) 5-fluorouracil (5-FU)
    (F) vincristine (Oncovin, VCR)

1. Cardiomyopathy

2. Renal insufficiency

3. Pulmonary fibrosis

4. Peripheral neuropathy

5. Hemorrhagic cystitis

Questions 6 through 9

The complete blood count (CBC) and reticulocyte count can provide valuable diagnostic clues when evaluating patients with a low hemoglobin and hematocrit (anemia). Many specific anemias have characteristic CBC patterns. Match the following CBC patterns with the MOST likely underlying cause for anemia.

    (A) anemia of chronic disease
    (B) aplastic anemia

    (C) hemolytic anemia
    (D) iron deficiency anemia
    (E) pernicious anemia

6. Hemoglobin and hematocrit decreased

    WBC and platelet count normal
    MCV decreased
    RBC morphology—microcytic hypochromic
    Reticulocyte count decreased

7. Hemoglobin and hematocrit decreased

    WBC and platelet count decreased
    MCV normal
    RBC morphology—essentially normal
    Reticulocyte count decreased

8. Hemoglobin and hematocrit decreased

    WBC and platelet count normal
    MCV increased
    RBC morphology—macrocytosis
    Reticulocyte count decreased

9. Hemoglobin and hematocrit decreased

    WBC and platelet count normal
    MCV normal
    RBC morphology—target cells or bizarre RBC shapes
    Reticulocyte count increased

DIRECTIONS (Questions 10 through 22): Each of the numbered items or incomplete statements in this section is followed by answers or by completions of the statement. Select the ONE lettered answer or completion that is BEST in each case.

Questions 10 through 22

10. Obtaining a biopsy and pathologic diagnosis is an essential step in the evaluation of cancer. The histologic type of a tumor can be an important prognostic factor, as well as a determinant in planning

treatment. Regarding lung cancer, in which of the following histologic subtypes would chemotherapy be the initial choice of therapy versus surgery or radiation therapy?

(A) squamous cell

(B) adenocarcinoma

(C) small cell

(D) mesothelioma

(E) cystic adenoid carcinoma (cylindroma)

11. Alpha-fetoprotein and beta-HCG are tumor markers useful in monitoring patients treated for

(A) testicular cancer

(B) breast cancer

(C) prostate cancer

(D) uterine cancer

(E) lung cancer

12. A 33-year-old Filipino female is found to have anemia during a pre-employment physical examination. She is asymptomatic except for occasional fatigue. Her past medical history is unremarkable except for a history of having to receive iron during each of two normal pregnancies. She uses no medication and denies alcohol use. She also denies any gynecologic or gastrointestinal symptoms. Physical examination (including a stool hemoccult) and vital signs are normal. CBC confirms a mild decrease in hemoglobin (10.7 g/dL) and hematocrit (34.8). Her MCV, however, is very low (68 fl). Erythrocyte sedimentation rate, serum ferritin, serum iron, and TIBC are all normal. What is the MOST likely explanation for this patient's anemia?

(A) early iron deficiency

(B) anemia of chronic disease

(C) occult hemorrhage

(D) thalassemia

(E) folate deficiency

13. The CBC picture of iron deficiency anemia and anemia of chronic disease may occasionally look very similar. Which of the following distinguish anemia of chronic disease from iron deficiency anemia?

(A) increased MCV

(B) decreased total iron-binding capacity

(C) increased reticulocyte count

(D) decreased serum ferritin

(E) increased platelet count

14. Excessive bleeding due to coumadin overdose may be corrected by the administration of

(A) factor VIII concentrate

(B) aminocaproic acid (Amicar)

(C) protamine sulfate

(D) pyridoxine

(E) vitamin K

15. A 54-year-old white male is being evaluated because he was recently rejected as a blood donor due to a low hemoglobin and hematocrit (10.2 grams/dL/32%). He tells you that except for some fatigue and a 5 to 6 pound weight loss over the past 3 months, he has not been feeling ill. You repeat the CBC and confirm that the patient has a microcytic hypochromic anemia. You suspect iron deficiency. At this point, which of the following would be your BEST course of action?

(A) Start oral ferrous sulfate and have the patient return to see you in 4 to 6 weeks for a repeat CBC.

(B) Obtain more history and perform a physical examination including a rectal exam and test for stool occult blood.

(C) Refer the patient to a hematologist for bone marrow aspiration and biopsy.

(D) Admit the patient to the hospital for blood transfusion.

(E) Arrange for intramuscular iron therapy.

16. All of the following clinical signs and symptoms may be seen with thrombocytopenia EXCEPT

(A) bleeding into the knee joint

(B) prolonged bleeding occurs immediately after minor tissue injury

(C) petechiae

(D) bleeding controlled by local pressure

(E) gastrointestinal bleeding

17. All of the following hemostatic disorders are associated with a prolonged PTT EXCEPT

(A) disseminated intravascular coagulation (DIC)

(B) heparin anticoagulation

(C) Von Willebrand's disease

(D) hemophilia A

(E) immune thrombocytopenic purpura (ITP)

18. Initial therapy of idiopathic thrombocytopenic purpura (ITP) most commonly consists of

(A) splenectomy

(B) immunosuppressive agents

(C) B_{12} injections

(D) IV gamma globulin

(E) corticosteroids

19. Transfusion of fresh frozen plasma (FFP) is the therapy of choice in controlling acute bleeding episodes in all the following coagulopathies EXCEPT

   (A) hemophilia B
   (B) factor XI deficiency
   (C) vitamin K deficiency
   (D) hemorrhagic diathesis of liver disease
   (E) hemophilia A

20. All of the health problems below are commonly associated with homozygous sickle cell anemia EXCEPT

   (A) cholelithiasis
   (B) CHF
   (C) aseptic necrosis of the femoral head
   (D) gout
   (E) hepatic infarct

21. All of the following statements regarding polycythemia vera (PV) are true EXCEPT

   (A) erythropoietin levels are increased in PV
   (B) PV can progress to myelofibrosis
   (C) PV can progress to other hematological neoplasms
   (D) splenomegaly is commonly seen in PV
   (E) pruritis and hyperuricemia are common findings in PV

22. All of the following statements regarding chronic lymphocytic leukemia (CLL) are true EXCEPT

   (A) CLL and diffuse well-differentiated lymphocytic lymphoma are both neoplasms of B-cell origin and are so similar that they follow essentially the same clinical course.
   (B) CLL, which presents with massive splenomegaly, lymphadenopathy, and lymphocytosis, has a median survival of 5 years.
   (C) Combination chemotherapy for CLL is routinely initiated at the time of diagnosis in an attempt to achieve decreased tumor load and possible remission as early in the disease process as possible.
   (D) A Coombs' positive hemolytic anemia occurs in up to 20% of patients with CLL.
   (E) Patients who demonstrate anemia and/or thrombocytopenia at the time of diagnosis of CLL have a 2-year median survival.

DIRECTIONS (Questions 23 through 35): For each of the items in this section, ONE or MORE of the numbered options is correct. Choose answer

   (A) if only (1), (2), and (3) are correct,
   (B) if only (1) and (3) are correct,
   (C) if only (2) and (4) are correct,
   (D) if only (4) is correct,
   (E) if all are correct.

Questions 23 through 35

23. A prolonged bleeding time is found in which of the following clinical settings?

   (1) aspirin ingestion
   (2) Von Willebrand's disease
   (3) thrombocytopenia
   (4) hemophilia A

24. Which of the following side effects commonly occur as complications of radiation therapy for cancer?

   (1) infertility
   (2) neutropenia and thrombocytopenia
   (3) diarrhea
   (4) painful swallowing

25. Regarding long-term survival of patients with breast cancer, which of the following have the greatest prognostic value?

   (1) tumor size
   (2) status of tumor estrogen and progesterone receptors
   (3) number of lymph nodes with tumor cells
   (4) history of early menarche or late menopause

26. Which of the following are risk factors associated with an increased incidence of colon cancer?

   (1) history of Crohn's disease or ulcerative colitis
   (2) colon cancer in a first-degree relative
   (3) family history of familial polyposis coli
   (4) diet high in fat and low in fiber

27. In Hodgkin's disease, the presence of so-called "B symptoms" is associated with an unfavorable prognosis. Which of the following are B symptoms?

   (1) night sweats
   (2) lymphadenopathy
   (3) fever
   (4) chest pain and dyspnea

28. Which of the following clinical findings might be expected in a patient with acute leukemia?

   (1) abnormal bruising or bleeding
   (2) anemia and low WBC count

(3) splenomegaly

(4) sternal tenderness

29. Regarding the anemia associated with folate deficiency, which of the following is/are true?

(1) The MCV is usually normal.

(2) Alcoholics are at increased risk for this disorder.

(3) Associated neurologic symptoms such as peripheral neuropathy are common.

(4) The CBC picture may be similar to that seen in vitamin B_{12} deficiency.

30. Treatment of the underlying disease/precipitating factor is essential to successful management of disseminated intravascular coagulation (DIC). Common situations triggering this disorder include

(1) bacterial sepsis

(2) disseminated malignancy

(3) catastrophic obstetrical event

(4) massive trauma

31. Which of the following are associated with B_{12} deficiency?

(1) anticonvulsant therapy

(2) partial gastrectomy

(3) lead poisoning

(4) Crohn's disease

32. Work-up for iron deficiency (Fe def.) anemia should include

(1) UGI series

(2) stool for guaiac and O&P

(3) proctosigmoidoscopy and BE

(4) thyroid function studies

33. Problems common to multiple myeloma include

(1) pathological fractures

(2) hypercalcemia

(3) spinal cord compression

(4) hyperviscosity syndrome

34. Which of the following statements about chronic myelogenous leukemia (CML) is/are true?

(1) Combination chemotherapy is used to achieve remission in the chronic phase of CML.

(2) Presentation of CML commonly includes splenomegaly, leukocytosis, and symptoms of hypermetabolism.

(3) The Philadelphia chromosome (Ph1) is present in 20% to 30% of CML patients.

(4) The majority of CML patients progress to a blastic phase that can be either myeloid or lymphoid.

35. Therapy and prognosis of lymphocytic ("non-Hodgkin's") lymphoma are determined more by histology than staging. High-grade, or aggressive, lymphomas include

(1) Burkitt's lymphoma

(2) diffuse lymphoblastic lymphoma

(3) diffuse, histiocytic (large cell, immunoblastic) lymphoma

(4) diffuse, well-differentiated, lymphocytic lymphoma

Answers and Explanations

1–5. 1. (D); 2. (B); 3. (A); 4. (F); 5. (C) Cardiomyopathy or myocarditis-pericarditis is associated with doxorubicin used in doses above 550 mg/m². Clinical manifestations include signs and symptoms of CHF, ECG changes, and arrhythmias. Many oncologists assess ejection fraction by MUGA scan before and after doxorubicin therapy, especially in older patients. Cisplatin is associated with a cumulative renal insufficiency manifested by rising BUN and creatinine. The risk of renal insufficiency is greatly reduced by adequate IV hydration and use of Lasix diuresis prior to administration of the drug. Cisplatin may also cause ototoxicity and other signs of peripheral neuropathy. Bleomycin causes pneumonitis and pulmonary fibrosis, especially when the total dose exceeds 400 units. Cough and dyspnea are common symptoms. Pulmonary function abnormalities include decreases in total lung volume, forced vital capacity, and DLCO. Bleomycin has also been associated with a fatal anaphylaxis-like reaction. For this reason, test doses of 2 units of the drug are often given prior to beginning therapy. Vincristine very commonly produces peripheral neuropathy manifested by some combination of paresthesias, decreased DTRs, muscle weakness, or cranial nerve dysfunction. Paralytic ileus may also occur. Hemorrhagic cystitis (occasionally massive) has been reported with cyclophosphamide therapy, especially when used in high doses. Adequate hydration and the occasional use of Mesna may prevent this complication. Ifosfamide, which is related to cyclophosphamide, is also associated with hemorrhagic cystitis. *(Holland et al, pp. 689–693)*

6–9. 6. (D); 7. (B); 8. (E); 9. (C) The most common cause for microcytic, hypochromic anemias is iron deficiency. The decreased reticulocytes are due to inadequate erythropoiesis. Other causes of microcytic anemias (low MCV) include thalassemia and lead poisoning. Anemia of chronic disease can resemble iron deficiency; however, serum iron, TIBC, and ferritin can help differentiate the two. A normocytic anemia associated with decreases in WBCs and platelets (pancytopenia) is the classic picture of aplastic anemia. Bone marrow aspira-

tion and biopsy must be done in these cases to rule out leukemia or bone marrow infiltration by metastatic tumor. Macrocytic anemias (increased MCV) are most commonly associated with vitamin B_{12} and/or folate deficiency. Because these vitamins are co-factors for DNA synthesis, erythropoiesis is affected (low reticulocyte count) along with the nuclear maturation of other cells like WBCs. Serum B_{12} and folate levels should be obtained in patients with macrocytic anemia. B_{12} deficiency may be due to lack of intrinsic factor (pernicious anemia), dietary B_{12} deficiency (rare in the U.S.), or ileal malabsorption. Other causes for anemia with increased MCV are recent hemorrhage or hemolysis. The increased MCV is due to the numbers of reticulocytes in these latter two conditions. Normocytic anemia with increased reticulocytes is the classic CBC picture of hemolytic anemia. In many cases, there is often abnormal RBC morphology on smear (target cells, spherocytes, sickle cells, etc). Other laboratory clues to hemolysis include decreased serum haptoglobin, increased serum LDH, and indirect bilirubin. The Coombs' test may be positive in autoimmune hemolytic anemias. *(Williams et al, pp. 163–164,454–455,488–495, 668–669)*

10. (C) Small-cell lung cancer (also called oat cell) represents approximately 20% of all lung cancers. It is an aggressive disease that is rapidly fatal if not treated in a timely fashion. Fortunately, tumor regression occurs in about 75% of patients treated with combination chemotherapy. The other neoplasms are treated with surgery or radiation therapy. Their response to chemotherapeutic agents has been disappointing. *(Holland et al, pp. 1308–1310)*

11. (A) Some tumors secrete biochemical products that are useful as diagnostic markers for disease, and for following patients for relapse after initial treatment. Alpha-fetoprotein and beta-HCG are produced by many germ cell tumors and are, therefore, valuable laboratory indicators of this disease. Among the germ cell tumors of the testis, seminomas produce these hormones least often;

embryonal, choriocarcinoma, and yolk sac tumors most often. Primary hepatocellular carcinoma is also associated with increases in alpha-fetoprotein. *(Holland et al, pp. 1436,1599)*

12. (D) This clinical picture is most consistent with beta-thalassemia. The combination of Oriental race and an MCV disproportionately low to the level of anemia is a tipoff to the diagnosis. Diagnosis may usually be confirmed by demonstrating an elevated hemoglobin A$_2$ on hemoglobin electrophoresis. An MCV less than 75 fl is unusual with iron deficiency anemia. The normal serum iron and ferritin also rule out this diagnosis. While anemia of chronic disease may present with a microcytic picture, there is often a history of underlying chronic infection, renal disease, endocrine disease, or malignancy. Additionally, patients with anemia of chronic disease usually have low serum iron with normal or increased serum ferritin. The erythrocyte sedimentation rate is very often increased with anemia of chronic disease. Hemorrhage should be evident from history and physical. Additionally, microcytic anemias resulting from hemorrhage are usually due to iron deficiency. Folate deficiency produces a macrocytic anemia. *(Williams et al, pp. 523–530)*

13. (B) Unlike iron deficiency which characteristically has an increased TIBC, anemia of chronic disease has a decreased TIBC. Apparently this is due to decreased transferrin synthesis, which occurs in many chronic conditions. Anemia of chronic disease may have a decreased MCV; however, it most commonly presents as a normocytic anemia. Decreased reticulocyte count and normal or increased serum ferritin are also typical of anemia of chronic disease. Platelet counts are usually not affected. *(Williams et al, p. 543)*

14. (E) Coumadin produces anticoagulation by interfering with the synthesis of the vitamin K-dependent coagulation factors (II, VII, IX, and X). Vitamin K will normalize hemostasis in 1 to 2 days. Fresh frozen plasma will also restore vitamin K-dependent factors to hemostatic levels in more emergent situations. Reversal of heparin is achieved with protamine sulfate. Factor VIII concentrate is used for correcting the hemostatic defect of hemophilia A. Aminocaproic acid is a fibrinolytic inhibitor that interferes with plasminogen activation. It is most frequently used as adjunctive therapy in hemophilia. Pyridoxine has no effect on hemostasis. *(Williams et al, pp. 1459–1460,1575–1576)*

15. (B) Iron deficiency anemia in a middle-aged adult is most commonly caused by occult bleeding. Before prescribing iron replacement in such patients, it is mandatory to rule out bleeding—especially from a GI site, such as a colon cancer. In ad-

dition to digital rectal examination and testing stool for occult blood, a barium swallow, barium enema, or colonoscopy may be indicated. *(Williams et al, pp. 494–495)*

16. (A) Hemarthrosis almost always indicates a coagulation factor deficiency rather than a problem with formation of the primary hemostatic platelet plug. The remaining clinical signs are not unusual with thrombocytopenia or disorders of platelet function. *(Williams et al, pp. 1456,1498,1525–1526)*

17. (E) The PTT is prolonged in disorders affecting the intrinsic coagulation cascade (factors XII, XI, IX, and VIII), as well as from defects in the common coagulation pathway. Hemophilia A (factor VIII deficiency) is the most common intrinsic pathway disorder encountered clinically. DIC is associated with the consumption of multiple coagulation factors. The effects of heparin result partly from its interference with the synthesis of many of the intrinsic and common pathway factors. Additionally, since factor VIII requires von Willebrand's factor to be functionally active, von Willebrand's disease is often associated with a mildly increased PTT. ITP affects the formation of the primary hemostatic plug and is not associated with coagulation factor deficiency. *(Williams et al, p. 1767)*

18. (E) A significant percentage of patients with ITP will normalize their platelet counts on high-dose prednisone, which is tapered after several weeks of therapy. If there is no response to this treatment regimen, or relapse occurs during or after tapering the steroids, splenectomy is usually considered. This is effective in significantly raising platelet counts in a high percentage of patients. Immunosuppressive agents (drugs such as cyclophosphamide, azathioprine, and vincristine) are generally considered only when both the above have failed, due to serious potential toxicities. IV gamma globulin is used for temporary phagocytic blockade in situations such as impending surgery or ITP in late pregnancy. Its value is limited because improvement is usually limited to approximately 4 weeks' duration. B$_{12}$ is of no value in treating ITP. *(Williams et al, p. 1384)*

19. (E) The therapy of choice in hemophilia A (factor VIII deficiency) is infusion of partially purified factor VIII concentrate when available, or cryoprecipitate if it is not (this contains 50% of the factor VIII of FFP in 10% of the volume). Hemophilia B (factor IX deficiency) and factor XI deficiency must be differentiated from hemophilia A, because cryoprecipitate and factor VIII concentrate do not supply these factors effectively, whereas FFP does. FFP, rather than vitamin K, is the therapy of choice for acute bleeding in vitamin K deficiency (as well as oral anticoagulant overdose) because it immediately supplies the diminished prothrombin factors (II, VII, IX, X, and proteins C and S) needed for hemostasis. Purified prothrombin complexes are avoided because these entail a high risk of thrombotic events. Administration of vitamin K (parenterally) requires 8 to 10 hours to permit normal factor synthesis. The hemorrhagic diathesis of liver disease involves vitamin K deficiency, decreased production of multiple coagulation factors, and increased production of coagulation inhibitors. Only FFP can immediately supply enough of the deficient factors to control acute hemorrhage, although vitamin K administration may be helpful in long-term management. *(Williams et al, pp. 1659–1669)*

20. **(D)** Gout has no specific association with sickle cell anemia. Cholelithiasis is commonly associated with sickle cell anemia because of the icterus that occurs secondary to chronic hemolysis, and must always be kept in mind when evaluating the sickle cell patient with abdominal pain (ie, one cannot automatically assume that such pain is due to sickle cell crisis). Chronic anemia and hypoxemia often lead to a chronic hyperdynamic cardiac state and later to CHF. Skeletal infarction can readily lead to aseptic necrosis of the femoral head. Hepatic infarcts are common and can lead to significant hepatic parenchymal damage. *(Williams et al, pp. 618–621)*

21. **(A)** In *secondary* polycythemia, erythropoietin is increased in an effort to compensate for chronic hypoxia (as in chronic pulmonary diseases, high-altitude dwelling, congenital heart disease, Pickwickian syndrome, increased methemoglobin or sulfhemoglobin states), or due to conditions such as Cushing's syndrome and tumors (particularly renal). In PV, erythropoietin is *decreased* or absent, leukocyte alkaline phosphatase is increased, B_{12} is WNL or increased, and hyperuricemia, thrombocytosis, and leukocytosis are common. Clinical features, mostly due to increased blood viscosity, may include plethora, headaches, gout, fatigue/malaise, pruritis, edema, thrombotic or bleeding events, splenomegaly, and acne rosacea. Approximately 30% of patients with PV go on to develop myelofibrosis, and up to 15% may develop leukemias (or, less commonly, lymphomas). Intermittent phlebotomy is a safe mode of therapy. Myelosuppression is recommended in the advent of symptomatic thrombocytosis, rapidly enlarging spleen, or symptoms of hypermetabolism. This can be achieved with radioactive P32 every 3 months as needed, or chemotherapeutic agents such as melphalan, busulfan, chlorambucil, or hydroxyurea. There is fear that myelosuppressive therapy may increase the risk of later leukemia or lymphoma, so phlebotomy alone is usually tried as initial therapy. *(Williams et al, pp. 193–200)*

22. **(C)** Chronic lymphocytic leukemia is a disease that usually appears in the fourth or fifth decade of life, or later, and is characterized by increased mature-appearing lymphocytes in the peripheral blood, associated with spleen, node, and bone marrow infiltration by a B-cell neoplasm. It is clinically indistinguishable from diffuse, well-differentiated, lymphocytic lymphoma. It is a relatively indolent disease that often presents with massive hepatosplenomegaly, peripheral lymphocytosis, and occasionally with lymphadenopathy, with surprisingly few symptoms. It is often picked up on routine exam or CBC. Stage A—lymphocytosis ± mild lymphadenopathy—has a median survival of more than 7 years. Stage B—lymphocytosis, larger lymphadenopathy and hepatosplenomegaly—has a median survival of 5 years. Stage C—Stage B findings plus anemia and/or thrombocytopenia—has a 2-year median survival. No potentially curative therapy regimen has been found. Single alkylating agents, such as low-dose daily or pulse high-dose chlorambucil, or pulse cyclophosphamide, are indicated to palliate hemolytic anemia, symptomatic organomegaly or lymphadenopathy, or systemic symptoms (such as fever, weight loss, fatigue, night sweats). Steroid therapy may be of value in instances of hemolytic anemia, which occurs in about 20% of CLL patients, or autoimmune thrombocytopenia (differentiated from thrombocytopenia secondary to neoplastic marrow invasion by presence of antiplatelet antibodies and increased megakaryocytes in the marrow). Splenectomy may be helpful if such problems fail to respond to steroids, but is not otherwise indicated. Radiation therapy may control localized symptomatic disease; interferon is of no value. Hairy cell leukemia, another adult lymphoid leukemia (seen predominantly in males over 40 years old) must be differentiated from CLL, as interferon *is* very effective in such patients with progressive disease, and alkylating agents are poorly tolerated. As in the other leukemias, infection is a major problem in patients with progressing disease; thus, early diagnosis of infection and initiation of appropriate therapy is essential. *(Williams et al, pp. 1005–1021)*

23. **(A)** The bleeding time is a sensitive screening test for defects in primary hemostasis—the formation of an adequate platelet plug. Aspirin interferes with platelet aggregation, and von Willebrand's disease affects platelet adhesion. With thrombocytopenia, the risk of minor spontaneous hemorrhage increases when the platelet count falls below 50,000. More serious bleeding occurs at platelet counts below 20,000. With hemophilia A, primary hemostasis is not affected, and the bleeding time is normal. The defect in hemophilia A prevents the formation of an adequate fibrin clot (secondary hemostasis). *(Williams et al, pp. 1341, 1775–1776)*

24. **(E)** Ionizing radiation affects cells that are actively replicating. In addition to neoplastic cells, this includes normal hematopoietic stem cells in the bone marrow, the mucosal lining of the mouth and gastrointestinal tract, gonadal germ cells, and hair follicles. Pulmonary fibrosis, cataracts, and secondary malignancies (especially leukemia) can also complicate radiation therapy. *(Holland et al, p. 557)*

25. **(A)** The larger the diameter of tumor at diagnosis, the greater the risk of recurrence. Patients who do not have tumor in axillary lymph nodes have a better prognosis than node-positive patients. Among node-positive patients, recurrence rate increases with the numbers of positive nodes. Tumors that express estrogen and progesterone receptors on their cell surface are associated with a somewhat more favorable course than those that are ER and PR negative. While prolonged exposure of breast tissue to physiologic levels of estrogen (menarche before age 12 or menopause after the age of 55) doubles the risk for breast cancer, they are not very important prognostic factors after disease has developed. *(Holland et al, pp. 1716–1719)*

26. **(E)** All of the listed factors are associated with an increased incidence of colon cancer. The role of fat may be related to increased caloric intake or due to increased secretion of bile acids which may have carcinogenic properties on the colonic mucosa. Dietary fiber may protect against colon cancer by increasing the transit time of stool in the bowel or by binding potential carcinogens. *(Holland et al, pp. 1494–1496)*

27. **(B)** B symptoms include drenching night sweats, unexplained fever (greater than 38°C) and unexplained loss of 10% or more of body weight in the 6 months prior to diagnosis. While lymphadenopathy is an important manifestation of the disease, it is not a B symptom. *(Williams et al, p. 1045)*

28. **(E)** Most clinical manifestations of acute leukemia are due to infiltration of bone marrow or other organs, such as the spleen, with leukemic cells. Crowding out of normal hematopoietic cells in the bone marrow can result in anemia; granulocytopenia and associated bacterial or fungal infection; or thrombocytopenia with ecchymoses and bleeding. Rapid expansion of leukemic cells in the marrow can cause bone pain and tenderness. Metabolic abnormalities secondary to rapid cell turnover include increased uric acid and hyperkalemia. Neurologic symptoms or intracranial hemorrhage secondary to obstruction of capillaries in the CNS by greatly increased numbers of WBCs may also occur. *(Williams et al, pp. 242–243)*

29. **(C)** The anemia of folate deficiency is associated with an increased MCV and is indistinguishable from the CBC picture of vitamin B_{12} deficiency. Dietary deficiencies in the alcoholic can lead to folate deficiency. B_{12} deficiency is associated with demyelinating neuropathies manifested by paresthesias, decreased vibratory sense, ataxia, or dementia. Folate deficiency is not associated with neurologic disease. This can be used clinically to differentiate folate deficiency from B_{12} deficiency. *(Williams et al, pp. 456–459)*

30. **(E)** Management of DIC has several components: (1) Control of major symptoms. Administration of fresh frozen plasma, cyroprecipitate, and/or platelets to replace depleted blood components and prevent exsanguination, and heparin when thrombosis and/or incipient gangrene are evident. (2) Treatment of the triggering disorder. Broad-spectrum antibiotic therapy after appropriate cultures are obtained in suspected sepsis, prompt delivery of fetus and placenta in the event of abruptio placenta, extraction of a retained dead fetus, surgical intervention after trauma, aggressive antitumor therapy (if possible) in the setting of malignancy, etc; and (3) Heparin prophylaxis where (2) is not rapidly manageable and chronic DIC is likely, for example, in acute promyelocytic leukemia, unresectable or disseminated malignancy, when surgical intervention must be postponed, and fat or amniotic fluid embolus. (Automatic initiation of heparin therapy, other than in the above situations, is controversial.) *(Williams et al, pp. 1526–1527)*

31. **(C)** General causes of B_{12} deficiency include: gastric malabsorption due to diminished or absent intrinsic factor after partial or total gastrectomy or in pernicious anemia; intestinal malabsorption, as in Crohn's disease, blind loop syndrome, chronic pancreatitis, fish tapeworm, strict vegetarian diet (B_{12} is found only in animal products); and abnormal metabolism, which can be congenital or acquired (secondary to nitrous oxide exposure). Therapy consists of B_{12} intramuscularly (there are several dose/frequency regimens). Anticonvulsant therapy can cause a macrocytic anemia due to *folate* deficiency. Lead poisoning causes a hypochromic anemia by interfering with hemoglobin synthesis, and some degree of hemolysis. *(Williams et al, pp. 454–456)*

32. **(A)** Thyroid function has no specific relationship to Fe deficiency. The most common cause of Fe deficiency is gastrointestinal (GI) blood loss, so thorough GI evaluation is essential. Common etiologies include hookworm infestations (common in underdeveloped nations), hiatal hernia, peptic ulcer disease, inflammatory bowel disease, neoplasms, chronic ASA ingestion, esophageal varices, telangiectasia, diverticular disease, angiodyspla-

sia, and, occasionally, severe hemorrhoids. Other causes include pregnancy (due to Fe transfer to the fetus), uterine bleeding (menorrhagia, antepartum and postpartum bleeding), hemosiderinuria, malabsorption (seen in atrophic gastritis, celiac disease, after partial gastrectomy), dialysis, hematuria, and pulmonary hemosiderosis. *(Williams et al, pp. 494–495)*

33. **(E)** Multiple myeloma is a malignant neoplasm of the plasma cell, usually producing a monoclonal immunoglobulin increase (seen on protein and/or urine electrophoresis). This disease tends to create multiple osteolytic lesions (best demonstrated on skeletal survey rather than bone scan), which are often very painful and can lead to pathological fractures, increased osteoporosis, hypercalcemia, and spinal cord compression. The excessive protein production can cause CNS symptoms due to hyperviscosity (confusion, paresthesias, somnolence, headache, and hemiplegia or coma when severe), amyloid deposition in (and failure of) multiple organs, and proteinuria/nephrotic syndrome. Tumor invasion of the bone marrow can cause depression of WBC, RBC, and/or platelets, hypogammaglobulinemia, and markedly increased susceptibility to infection. Cryoglobulin production and platelet dysfunction are common, and renal failure can occur as a result of amyloidosis, urate nephropathy, and other disorders. Radiation therapy may be of great value in controlling painful bone symptoms or impending cord compression. Chemotherapy is used to treat the systemic disease, usually consisting of pulse therapy with an alkylating agent (melphalan, cyclophosphamide, or chlorambucil) plus a steroid, and can achieve remission (although not cure). Allopurinol helps minimize hyperuricemia, and good hydration assists clearance of calcium and light protein chains. Plasmapheresis may be appropriate in severe hyperviscosity syndrome, and prompt assessment and treatment of infection is essential. *(Williams et al, pp. 1120–1123)*

34. **(C)** Chronic myelogenous leukemia (CML) is a neoplasm of the multipotent hematopoietic stem cell, which most commonly is found in middle-aged patients. The chronic phase is characterized by an elevated total WBC, predominantly granulocytic (but it is not uncommon to have increased eosinophil and/or basophil counts), with less than 5% blasts in blood and marrow, low or absent leukocyte alkaline phosphatase (LAP), and presence of a specific chromosome marker called the Philadelphia (Ph1) chromosome (a translocation of chromosomes 22 and 9) in 80% to 95% of patients. These studies are valuable in differentiating CML from leukemoid reactions (such as LAP, no Ph1 chromosome), myelofibrosis (such as normal LAP, no Ph1 chromosome), and other myeloproliferative

disorders. Presentation often includes splenomegaly, leukocytosis with anemia (platelet counts are variable), hypermetabolism (weight loss, fever, hyperuricemia, sweating), and arthralgias; lymphoadenopathy may be present, and thrombohemorrhagic events may occur. Single-agent therapy (busulfan, cyclophosphamide, melphalan, or hydroxyurea) may be used to decrease the leukocytosis and symptomatology. It does not clear the Ph1 chromosome abnormality from the marrow—it simply diminishes tumor load enough to remove the immature cells from the blood. It has not been demonstrated that conventional combination chemotherapy improves survival, although promising results are being achieved with intensive chemotherapy and radiation therapy followed by HLA-matched bone marrow transplantation early in the chronic phase. Allopurinol decreases the hyperuricemia, which often otherwise increases on initiation of chemotherapy. Splenectomy is helpful only in relieving symptoms of hypersplenism, and does not change the overall course of the disease. Approximately 50% of patients will accelerate to a blastic phase or crisis, resembling acute leukemia within 3 to 4 years, with almost all patients ultimately continuing on to this state. Blastic crises may be myeloid in origin in two-thirds of cases, and lymphoid in one-third, consistent with the stem cell level of disease process. The blastic phase is usually very resistant to treatment, including bone marrow transplantation, and most patients die within 6 weeks of diagnosis of conversion to this phase, although the lymphoid cases may briefly respond. *(Williams et al, pp. 202–206)*

35. **(A)** Low-grade lymphomas are relatively indolent; high-grade lymphomas are more aggressive, and therapy varies accordingly. Low-grade includes small lymphocytic/plasmacytoid, consistent with CLL (diffuse, well-differentiated, lymphocytic); follicular, small, cleaved cell/diffuse areas, sclerosis (nodular, poorly differentiated, lymphocytic) and follicular mixed, small cleaved, and large cell/diffuse areas of sclerosis (nodular, mixed, lymphocytic-histiocytic). Intermediate-grade includes follicular, large cell/diffuse areas, sclerosis (nodular, histiocytic); diffuse, small, cleaved cell (diffuse, poorly differentiated, lymphocytic); diffuse, mixed small and large cell sclerosis, epithelioid cell component (diffuse, mixed, lymphocytic-histiocytic; and diffuse, large cell, cleaved and noncleaved cell sclerosis (diffuse histiocytic). High grade includes large cell immunoblastic plasmacytoid, clear cell, polymorphous, epithelioid component (diffuse histiocytic); lymphoblastic convoluted and nonconvoluted cell (diffuse lymphoblastic); and small noncleaved cell Burkitt's follicular areas (diffuse, undifferentiated)—"Burkitt's" lymphoma. Although low-grade lymphomas are more indolent in progression, the higher-grade lymphomas are actually more readily

cured with intensive initial chemotherapy; the low-grade lymphomas have a relatively high relapse rate. Therefore, intensive combination chemotherapy, ± radiation, is clearly indicated in initial therapy of high-grade lymphomas. Therapy of low-grade lymphomas is more controversial, with many electing to treat only as needed to achieve local control of disease (regional radiation therapy, less intensive chemotherapy). Single-agent chemotherapy has fallen into disfavor, except in diffuse, well-differentiated lymphoma/CLL. Intensive chemotherapy plus total body irradiation followed by autologous bone marrow transplantation is being investigated in patients who have failed to benefit from chemotherapy (the bone marrow is harvested after second remission is achieved and purged of lymphoma cells with monoclonal antibodies, then reinfused after the patient undergoes further intensive therapy). *(Williams et al, pp. 1070–1074)*

REFERENCES

Babior BM, Bunn HF. Megaloblastic anemia. In Wilson JD, Braunwald E, Isselbacher KJ, Petersdorf RG, Martin JB, Fauci AS, Root RK (eds). *Harrison's Principles of Internal Medicine,* 12th ed. New York: McGraw-Hill; 1991.

Bunn HF. Disorders of hemoglobin. In Wilson JD, Braunwald E, Isselbacher KJ, Petersdorf RG, Martin JB, Fauci AS, Root RK (eds). *Harrison's Principles of Internal Medicine,* 12th ed. New York: McGraw-Hill; 1991.

Champlin R, Golde DW. The leukemias. In Wilson JD, Braunwald E, Isselbacher KJ, Petersdorf RG, Martin JB, Fauci AS, Root RK (eds). *Harrison's Principles of Internal Medicine,* 12th ed. New York: McGraw-Hill; 1991.

Cooper RA, Bunn HF. Hemolytic anemia. In Wilson JD, Braunwald E, Isselbacher KJ, Petersdorf RG, Martin JB, Fauci AS, Root RK (eds). *Harrison's Principles of Internal Medicine,* 12th ed. New York: McGraw-Hill; 1991.

Handin RI. Disorders of the platelet and vessel wall. In Wilson JD, Braunwald E, Isselbacher KJ, Petersdorf RG, Martin JB, Fauci AS, Root RK (eds). *Harrison's Principles of Internal Medicine,* 12th ed. New York: McGraw-Hill; 1991.

Holland JF, Frei E, Bast RC, et al (ed). *Cancer Medicine,* 3rd ed. Philadelphia, PA: Lea & Febiger; 1993.

Williams WJ, Beutler E, Erslev AJ, et al (eds). *Hematology,* 4th ed, New York: McGraw-Hill; 1990.

Subspecialty List: Hematology/Oncology

CHAPTER 5

Pharmacology
Questions

DIRECTIONS (Questions 1 through 18): Each of the numbered items or incomplete statements in this section is followed by answers or by completions of the statement. Select the ONE lettered answer or completion that is BEST in each case.

Questions 1 through 18

1. Which of the following topical antifungal agents is contraindicated in infants?

    (A) undecylenic acid
    (B) clotrimazole
    (C) boric acid
    (D) tolnaftate
    (E) miconazole

2. The first-line drugs presently used against tuberculosis include

    (A) isoniazid and streptomycin
    (B) isoniazid, ethambutol, rifampin, and streptomycin
    (C) isoniazid, streptomycin, cycloserine, and rifampin
    (D) isoniazid, ethambutol, and cycloserine
    (E) isoniazid, viomycin, and cycloserine

3. Antihistamines are contraindicated in all the following medical conditions EXCEPT

    (A) glaucoma
    (B) hypertension
    (C) asthma
    (D) enlarged prostate
    (E) pregnancy

4. The mainstay of therapy for all lipid disorders is

    (A) diet
    (B) Questran
    (C) Lopid
    (D) Mevacor
    (E) niacin

5. When propranolol is to be used in the treatment of sinus tachycardia, the presence of another disease may be a relative contraindication or at least a precaution to its use. All the following are considered such precautions EXCEPT

    (A) congestive heart failure
    (B) asthma
    (C) hypertension
    (D) type I diabetes mellitus
    (E) A-V block

6. Which of the following micronutrients is considered to have the narrowest therapeutic index?

    (A) zinc
    (B) molybdenum
    (C) selenium
    (D) manganese
    (E) magnesium

7. All the following agents are used to manage asthmatics EXCEPT

    (A) theophylline
    (B) cromolyn sodium
    (C) nadolol
    (D) terbutaline
    (E) albuterol

8. All the following statements are true regarding the use of acyclovir in the treatment of herpes simplex EXCEPT

(A) acyclovir ointment is used for the treatment of HSV-1 only

(B) the infusion of IV acyclovir should be given slowly over 1 hour to prevent renal tubular damage

(C) headache and gastrointestinal discomfort are the most frequent adverse reactions to continuous acyclovir

(D) the dosage for chronic suppressive therapy is 200 mg three to five times per day

(E) absorption of oral acyclovir is unaffected by food

9. Mr. Brown has developed itching, crusted lesions in his beard area. New lesions develop each time he shaves. A bacterial culture from a lesion showed *Staphylococcus aureus* (coagulase positive) and beta-hemolytic *Streptococcus*. Mr. Brown is allergic to penicillin. The appropriate course of therapy would be to start the patient on

(A) Burow's compresses and topical steroids

(B) topical antibiotics and wait for the report of antibiotic sensitivity

(C) Burow's compresses, topical steroids, and dicloxacillin 250 mg four times a day

(D) Burow's compresses, topical steroids, and erythromycin 250 mg four times a day

(E) Burow's compresses and wait for report of antibiotic sensitivity

10. Which of the following antibiotics would be useful in treating a beta-lactamase producing staphylococcus skin infection?

(A) penicillin
(B) nafcillin
(C) mezlocillin
(D) amoxicillin
(E) ampicillin

11. Excessive doses of which vitamin may cause infantile idiopathic hypercalcemia?

(A) vitamin A
(B) vitamin B_{12}
(C) vitamin C
(D) vitamin D
(E) vitamin E

12. The antidepressant with the most sedative and anticholinergic effects associated with its use is

(A) amitriptyline
(B) nortriptyline
(C) imipramine
(D) desipramine
(E) amoxapine

13. Which of these antibiotics is a second generation cephalosporin?

(A) cefuroxime (Ceftin)
(B) cephalexin (Keflex)
(C) cefadroxil (Duricef)
(D) cefixime (Suprax)
(E) cephradine (Velosef)

14. Retrobulbar neuritis with typical central scotoma may be caused by pernicious anemia. This is associated with a deficiency of

(A) vitamin A
(B) vitamin B_{12}
(C) vitamin C
(D) vitamin E
(E) vitamin B_1

15. A new patient is referred to your office by her hometown pharmacist. She has requested the refill of two prescriptions from out of state: digoxin 0.25 mg daily, and furosemide 40 mg three times a day. You immediately recognize the potential for a problem which is

(A) hypovolemia; administer IV solution and terminate furosemide use

(B) hyperkalemia and digitoxicity; terminate both drugs until labs are ordered

(C) hypokalemia; order serum potassium and add supplements if value is low

(D) drug seeking behavior; alert the local authorities

(E) an impending MI; send to the emergency room

16. You have a 3-year-old, 38-pound child with asthma who requires treatment with theophylline. What is the appropriate dose for him?

(A) 5 mg/kg/24 hours
(B) 5 mg/kg/6 hours
(C) 10 mg/kg/24 hours
(D) 10 mg/kg/6 hours
(E) 15 mg/kg/6 hours

17. Which of these third generation cephalosporins can be administered orally?

(A) ceftriaxone (Rocephin)
(B) cefoperazone (Cefobid)
(C) ceftizoxime (Cefizox)

(D) cefixime (Suprax)

(E) cefotaxime (Claforan)

18. Which of the following antibiotic regimens would you prescribe for an individual with suspected chlamydia infection?

(A) tetracycline 500 mg qid for 10 days

(B) penicillin 500 mg qid for 10 days

(C) ampicillin 250 mg qid for 7 days

(D) kefzol 500 mg bid for 7 days

(E) rocephin 2 g IM as a single dose

DIRECTIONS (Questions 19 through 28): For each of the items in this section, ONE or MORE of the numbered options is correct. Choose answer

(A) **if only (1), (2), and (3) are correct,**

(B) **if only (1) and (3) are correct,**

(C) **if only (2) and (4) are correct,**

(D) **if only (4) is correct,**

(E) **if all are correct.**

Questions 19 through 28

19. Phenobarbital and phenytoin are effective for generalized motor seizures. Which drugs are effective for absence seizures?

(1) ethosuximide

(2) phenobarbital

(3) valproic acid

(4) diazepam

20. A frightened mother phones you stating that her 5-year-old has ingested about 20 of her synthroid 0.1 mg tablets. What is your advice to the mother?

(1) Observe the child closely; should any symptoms occur, call back for instructions.

(2) Your child will go to sleep and sleep soundly for several hours; check on her periodically.

(3) Have the child eat some bread to "bind up" the drug particles and bring her to the emergency room.

(4) Induce emesis by using syrup of ipecac and bring her to the emergency room.

21. The mother of the child in Question 20 brings her daughter to the emergency room about 1 hour later because the child has convulsed. You receive a call that the child is gravely ill. Your examination reveals her to be comatose. She has lost the gag reflex, has bibasilar rales and a temperature of 101°F. Labs revealed a serum glucose of 50 mg. Which of the following procedures are considered correct medically for this patient?

(1) begin an IV solution of D5W

(2) maintain ventilation and administer oxygen

(3) administer digitalis glycosides and glucocorticoids

(4) administer cholestyramine

22. Which of the following can interfere with interpretation of ovulation prediction kits?

(1) phenytoin

(2) amitriptyline

(3) nitrofurantoin

(4) oral contraceptives

23. Which of the following are useful in the treatment of migraine headaches?

(1) tenormin

(2) vicodin

(3) midrin

(4) sansert

24. Aminoglycosides are associated with

(1) nephrotoxicity

(2) neurotoxicity

(3) ototoxicity

(4) hepatotoxicity

25. A single, 25-year-old black woman was admitted to the hospital with classic symptoms of pelvic inflammatory disease (PID). The patient had been sexually active, using an IUD for contraception. A laparoscopy with subsequent cultures grew *Haemophilus influenzae, Chlamydia trachomatis,* and *Bacteroides oralis* from the endometrium, and *Trichomonas vaginalis* from the vagina. The most appropriate therapy would include

(1) doxycycline

(2) ampicillin

(3) metronidazole

(4) erythromycin

26. Self-blood glucose testing over urine glucose testing by the diabetic patient may offer the following advantage:

(1) tests are more accurate; results are quantitative

(2) detects glucose concentration at levels below the renal threshold value

(3) provides immediate confirmation of hypoglycemic reactions

(4) allows the clinician to alter treatment without the patient being hospitalized

27. Which of the following adverse reactions represents a contraindication to further administration of pertussis-containing vaccines?

    (1) fever of 40.5°C or greater within 48 hours

    (2) hypotonic-hyporesponsive episode within 48 hours

    (3) persistent inconsolable crying lasting 3 or more hours

    (4) a swollen area of 2 cm at the injection site within 48 hours

28. The discomfort of oral ulcerations caused by HSV-1 may be relieved by

    (1) holding and swishing diphenhydramine elixir in the mouth for several minutes

    (2) holding and swishing diphenhydramine elixir mixed with an equal amount of Kaopectate Concentrate in the mouth for several minutes

    (3) applying lidocaine hydrochloride 2% viscous to the lesions

    (4) swishing warm salt water in the mouth for several minutes

DIRECTIONS (Questions 29 through 48): Each set of items in this section consists of a list of lettered options followed by several numbered words or phrases. For each numbered word or phrase, select the ONE lettered option that is most closely associated with it. Each lettered option may be selected once, more than once, or not at all.

Questions 29 through 32

For each drug, select its most common usage.

    (A) fluphenazine (Prolixin)
    (B) oxybutynin (Ditropan)
    (C) tamoxifen (Nolvadex)
    (D) triazolam (Halcion)
    (E) astimazole (Hismanal)

29. Allergic rhinitis

30. Psychotic disorders

31. Neurogenic bladder

32. Insomnia

Questions 33 through 36

For each condition, select the drug most useful in its treatment.

    (A) hypertension
    (B) peptic ulcer disease
    (C) asthma
    (D) nausea
    (E) diabetes mellitus

33. Glyburide (Micronase)

34. Promethazine (Phenergan)

35. Enalapril (Vasotec)

36. Famotidine (Pepcid)

Questions 37 through 40

    (A) sedation
    (B) excitation
    (C) both
    (D) neither

37. Terfenadine (Seldane)

38. Flurazepam (Dalmane)

39. Methyldopa (Aldomet)

40. Diphenhydramine (Benadryl)

Questions 41 through 44

    (A) bronchodilation
    (B) vasodilation
    (C) both
    (D) neither

41. Ranitidine (Zantac)

42. Theophylline (Theo Dur)

43. Trazodone (Desyrel)

44. Hydralazine (Apresoline)

Questions 45 through 48

    (A) angina
    (B) hypertension
    (C) both
    (D) neither

45. Diltiazem (Cardizem)

46. Propranolol (Inderal)

47. Nicardipine (Cardene)

48. Guanethidine (Ismelin)

DIRECTIONS (Questions 49 and 50): Each of the numbered items or incomplete statements in this section is followed by answers or by completions of the statement. Select the ONE lettered answer or completion that is BEST in each case.

Questions 49 and 50

49. Trimethoprim-sulfamethoxazole (Bactrim) is useful for all of the following EXCEPT

    (A) prostatitis
    (B) *Pneumocystis carinii* pneumonia
    (C) nongonococcal urethritis
    (D) *Shigella* enteritis
    (E) urinary tract infections

50. A potential complication of antibiotic use is antibiotic-associated colitis. Which of the following is the treatment of choice?

    (A) clindamycin
    (B) vancomycin
    (C) metrinidazole
    (D) neomycin
    (E) erythromycin

Answers and Explanations

1. **(C)** It is possible that any agent may be absorbed through damaged skin. Some, however, are more readily absorbed than others. Boric acid is a weak fungistat and bacteriostat. Unfortunately, it is absorbed significantly through damaged skin, thus leading to possible systemic toxicity. Because of their underdeveloped drug metabolizing systems, infants may be especially sensitive to this agent. *(Katzung, p. 691)*

2. **(B)** Isoniazid, ethambutol, rifampin, streptomycin, and pyrazinamide are the first-line drugs presently utilized for the chemotherapeutic treatment of tuberculosis. Isoniazid is the most commonly used drug for tuberculosis. This should not be used for active tuberculosis as a single agent, since this favors the resurgence of drug-resistant TB. Cycloserine is a second-line agent generally reserved for highly resistant *M. tuberculosis*. Significant side effects include CNS dysfunction, as well as psychotic reactions. Streptomycin, like other aminoglycosides, may damage the eighth cranial nerve and induce nephrotoxicity. All patients must be well monitored with appropriate laboratory tests. *(Goodman and Gilman, pp. 1146–1159; Tierney et al, pp. 1201–1203)*

3. **(B)** Antihistamines possess anticholinergic activity that may pose a potential hazard to patients with an enlarged prostate and those with acute narrow-angle glaucoma. These agents have an atropine-like effect and can precipitate an acute episode of glaucoma or urinary retention. Teratogenic effects have been noted with some agents, and their use during pregnancy is contraindicated. They may also be contraindicated in persons with asthma, but data supporting this potentially adverse effect for all asthmatics are not uniformly agreed upon. The incidence of anticholinergic side effects are diminished with terfenadine (Seldane) and astemizole (Hismanal). *(Goodman and Gilman, pp. 582–588; Katzung pp. 230–237)*

4. **(A)** Treatment of hyperlipoproteinemia is indicated both for the relief of presenting symptoms and as part of the effort to decrease the risk of cardiac disease. Treatment begins with dietary restrictions. If triglycerides are elevated, weight reduction and alcohol eliminations are indicated and a low-fat diet is instituted. Other risk factors in cardiac disease, such as stress, smoking, or lack of exercise, may need to be addressed concurrently. Questran, Lopid, and Mevacor are lipid-lowering agents that are added if diet alone is insufficient therapy. *(Goodman and Gilman, pp. 880–881; Katzung, pp. 482–483)*

5. **(C)** Propranolol is a nonselective, beta-adrenergic receptor blocking agent. Blocking of beta receptors in the heart may worsen cardiac failure when sympathetic stimulation is often a vital component supporting circulatory function. Beta-receptor blockade in the lungs can lead to bronchoconstriction. Further, beta blockade may mask certain premonitory signs and symptoms (those that are adrenergically mediated) of acute hypoglycemia, thus making insulin dosage more difficult and predisposing the patient to the possibility of hypoglycemic attacks. *(Goodman and Gilman, pp. 229–241; Katzung, pp. 131–136)*

6. **(C)** Twenty to forty micrograms daily of selenium as selenious acid is recommended for maintenance, and up to 100 ng/day for 4 weeks is needed for repletion. It is noted to be a toxic trace element. Suggested maintenance doses of the other trace elements are zinc, 15 mg/day; molybdenum, 20 to 120 ng/day; and manganese, 2.5 to 5.0 mg/day. *(Goodman and Gilman, pp. 1523–1529)*

7. **(C)** Nadolol is a beta-adrenergic blocking agent, and blocking beta receptors in the lungs may cause bronchoconstriction. Theophylline and terbutaline cause bronchodilation, whereas cromolyn is used prophylactically in the treatment of asthma. Cromolyn inhibits both the immediate and nonimmediate bronchoconstrictive reactions to inhaled antigens. *(Goodman and Gilman, pp. 232–233, 618–635)*

8. **(A)** Acyclovir ointment appears to have some value in reducing healing time and duration of

pain in HSV-1 and HSV-2 infections. Its overuse can lead to resistant strains of the herpes virus. The usual dose is 200 mg orally five times daily. *(Goodman and Gilman, pp. 1184–1186; Katsung, pp. 676, 677,876)*

9. **(D)** *S. aureus* (coagulase positive) and beta-hemolytic *Streptococcus* organisms cause the majority of skin infections. These organisms may invade through breaks in the stratum corneum, through the hair follicles, or through the bloodstream. Both organisms are sensitive to erythromycin, certain penicillins, and cephalosporin antibiotics. Systemic therapy is combined with topical therapy. Compresses with Burow's solution are used for impetigo. As long as systemic antibiotics are being used, topical steroids may be applied to reduce inflammation and speed restoration of the stratum corneum barrier. Solid clinical evidence shows that topical steroids enhance the rate of recovery and do not spread infection. Topical antibiotics are not needed when systemic antibiotics are employed. *(Goodman and Gilman, 1573; Tierney et al, pp. 88,98)*

10. **(B)** Nafcillin is resistant to beta-lactamase, as is oxacillin and dicloxacillin. The other choices are all susceptible to breakdown by beta-lactamase. The combination of amoxicillin with clavulanate does provide beta-lactamase protection in the product Augmentin. *(Katsung, pp. 629–636)*

11. **(D)** The absorption of calcium is influenced by vitamin D. Excessive doses of vitamin D are manifested as hypercalcemia with numerous clinical consequences, such as demineralization of bones, renal calculi, and metastatic calcifications in soft tissues. Additionally, hypercalcemia is associated with weakness, vomiting, diarrhea, and lack of muscle tone. Vitamins A, B_{12}, and C are not required for calcium absorption. *(Goodman and Gilman, pp. 1510–1517)*

12. **(A)** These antidepressant agents are all in the tricyclic group. They have been widely used in the treatment of depression, pain syndromes, and panic disorders. They have sedative and anticholinergic side effects, and amitryptyline has the greatest incidence of these. Care should be taken in the elderly with glaucoma or in males with prostatic hypertrophy. *(Goodman and Gilman, pp. 405–414; Katsung, pp. 414–418; Tierney et al, pp. 796–797)*

13. **(A)** Cefuroxime is a second-generation cephalosporin. Cephalexin, cephradine, and cefadroxil are first-generation agents and cefixime is a third-generation medication. The second-generation medications have expanded the broad gram-positive coverage of the first-generation cephalosporins with greater gram-negative coverage. Certain agents

such as cefuroxime are active against beta-lactamase positive *H. influenzae*. *(Katsung, pp. 632–634)*

14. **(B)** Vitamin B_{12} is released from food in the stomach and becomes attached to a glycoprotein called gastric intrinsic factor. This complex is absorbed with greater efficiency than B_{12} alone. The most common cause of B_{12} deficiency is inadequate production of intrinsic factor. This form of B_{12} deficiency anemia is called pernicious anemia. Severe B_{12} deficiency causes two principal symptom clusters—megaloblastic anemia and neuropathy. Retrobulbar neuritis is one form of neuropathy. Vitamins A, C, and E are absorbed independent of intrinsic factor. *(Goodman and Gilman, pp. 1298–1301; Tierney et al, pp. 405–407)*

15. **(C)** The potential problem is hypokalemia caused by furosemide. A serum potassium level should be taken. Hypokalemia can lead to the potentiation of the digitalis glycosides and to digitalis toxicity. The preventive measure is to use potassium supplements along with the diuretic. If the measured potassium is not very low, recommending foods high in potassium, including fresh fruits and vegetables, may be useful in preventing hypokalemia and may obviate the need for potassium supplements. *(Goodman and Gilman, pp. 722–725,729–730, 834–835)*

16. **(B)** The recommended daily dose for a child of 19 kg is about 0.8 mg/kg/hr or 15 mg/hr. This times 24 hours equal 360 mg, which is almost identical to 5 mg/kg every 6 hours. The slight difference in calculation has to do with rounding off of kilograms to the nearest whole number. *(Goodman and Gilman, pp. 628–629; Hathaway et al, p. 948)*

17. **(D)** Cefixime (Suprax) is available only as an oral agent. The remaining agents are administered parenterally. Cefixime is usually given as 400 mg twice daily for respiratory or urinary tract infections. This group of cephalosporins has expanded gram-negative coverage but limited activity against gram-positive species, such as staphylococci and streptococci. *(Katsung, pp. 634–637)*

18. **(A)** Tetracycline is the drug of choice for the treatment of chlamydial infections, including sexually transmitted diseases. The usual side effect is nausea, vomiting, or diarrhea. Also of note is photosensitivity, particularly in fair-skinned individuals. Tetracycline should not be administered to pregnant women or children under the age of six, since it is associated with discoloration of teeth and can cause bony deformity or growth inhibition. *(Katsung, pp. 641–644; Tierney et al, pp 208–209, 1181)*

19. **(B)** Absence seizures, also known as petit mal epilepsy, differ considerably from generalized or grand mal seizures. They occur mostly in children; the attacks are of short duration and consist of syncope, or temporary clouding of consciousness during which the individual may stare blankly or exhibit minor movements of the head and limbs. Ethosuximide and valproic acid are generally used to control absence seizures. Diazepam is used in status epilepticus. *(Goodman and Gilman, pp. 436–439,458; Hathaway et al, pp. 688–689)*

20. **(D)** Obviously, this would represent a huge overdose with a central nervous system stimulant. The child requires immediate medical attention. Use of ipecac syrup to induce vomiting is advocated as long as the child is alert enough to protect her airway. If not, gastric lavage may be used to remove the poison and subsequently the use of activated charcoal to bind the medication. The addition of 70% sorbitol to the activated charcoal will act as a cathartic and increase GI motility. Because thyroxin is a CNS stimulant, it is unlikely the child would go to sleep and sleep it off. She may become comatose, however, because of hypoglycemia, hyperpyrexia, and cardiac problems. *(Goodman and Gilman, pp. 1361–1373; Saunders and Ho, pp. 730–738)*

21. **(E)** Because the child is comatose, ventilation must be maintained. She may have congestive heart failure as evidenced by the bibasilar rales. Therefore, digitalis glycosides may be of benefit to improve cardiac motility and slow down the tachycardia. D5W will provide dextrose, which is needed to maintain her serum glucose. Larger concentrations of dextrose, ie, D50 may be needed if a significant hypoglycemia exists. Further, cholestyramine may be administered to interfere with thyroxine absorption. The addition of glucocorticoids will inhibit the peripheral conversion of T4 to T3. *(Goodman and Gilman, pp. 1361–1373; Saunders and Ho, pp. 730–738)*

22. **(D)** Ovulation is the release of an egg from the ovary. This event is caused by a sudden surge in the level of luteinizing hormone (LH). Ovulation prediction tests try to determine this initial surge so that intercourse can follow to maximize the chances for fertilization. The progestin component of oral contraceptives produces feedback suppression of the hypothalamic-pituitary axis but primarily affects LH. This would inhibit growth of the expelled follicle, but in most cases the follicle is not released because of the action of the estrogen component. Dilantin, Elavil, and Macrodantin do not interfere with ovulation. *(Goodman and Gilman, pp. 1384–1412)*

23. **(E)** The exact mechanism of anti-migraine action of beta-blockers has not been proven, but abun-dant evidence supports their beneficial effects. Vicodin is a combination of hydrocodone and acetaminophen, both analgesics whose effects are additive. Hydrocodone, a narcotic, suppresses the affective component of pain. Midrin is also a combination product containing acetaminophen plus a sympathomimetic amine that acts by constricting dilated cranial and cerebral arterioles. Sansert is methysergide, which inhibits the effects of serotonin, a substance that may be involved in the mechanism of vascular headaches. *(Tierney et al, pp. 729–730)*

24. **(A)** Aminoglycosides include gentamicin, tobramycin, amikacin, streptomycin, neomycin, kanamycin, and others. As a group they are associated with nephrotoxicity, neurotoxicity, and ototoxicity. The renal and hearing deficits are the most common. Neurotoxicity is rare; however, it has been associated with aminoglycoside use, particularly in conjunction with anesthesia or the use of muscular blocking agents. The presentation is that of an acute neuromuscular blockade that may result in respiratory paralysis. *(Katzung, pp. 645–651; Goodman and Gilman, pp. 1104–1108)*

25. **(B)** Sexually transmissible agents of importance in PID are *Neisseria gonorrhoeae* and *Chlamydia trachomatis*. Treatment of nongonococcal PID requires an antibiotic directed at the agents of nongonococcal urethritis, combined with an antianaerobic agent such as a combination of doxycycline and metronidazole. Doxycycline will cover *Chlamydia*. Metronidazole will cover the *Trichomonas* and *Bacteroides*. If there is a treatment failure, a broad spectrum penicillin or cephalosporin may have to be added to cover the *Haemophilus influenzae*. *(Mandell et al, pp. 743–744,1079)*

26. **(E)** All these statements are true. Home glucose monitoring allows the patient to maintain records that facilitate better insulin management. This will lessen the likelihood of developing diabetic complications. *(Tierney et al, pp. 917–919)*

27. **(A)** Pertussis is a bacterial infection that presents with the clinical features of whooping cough. The primary problem associated with the vaccine is central nervous system irritation. The absolute contraindications to the future use of the vaccine are an acute neurologic illness within 7 days; a convulsion within 3 days; persistent, severe, and inconsolable crying for over 3 hours; or a high-pitched cry within 48 hours. It is also contraindicated in the presence of a hyporesponsive or hypotonic episode, fever to 40.5°C within 48 hours, or an anaphylactic reaction to the vaccine. *(Hathaway et al, p. 217)*

28. (A) Diphenhydramine elixir, alone or mixed with an equal amount of water, or Kaopectate Concentrate held and swished around in the mouth for several minutes often relieves the discomfort of oral ulcerations. Lidocaine viscous is also effective as this is a topical anesthetic. Using warm salt water would irritate the vesicles even more and increase the discomfort. *(Scott et al, pp. 23–26)*

29. (E) Astimazole is a new once-a-day antihistamine released in 1989. It has shown good effects in the treatment of allergic rhinitis. It has less sedative side effects than older histamine blockers. *(Goodman and Gilman, pp. 585–586)*

30. (A) Fluphenazine (Prolixin) is a phenothiazine that has activity at all levels of the central nervous system as well as on multiple organ systems. It has been used extensively to manage the manifestations of psychotic disorders. This medication has a side effect of extrapyramidal reactions such as acute dystonia. *(Goodman and Gilman, pp. 386–401)*

31. (B) Oxybutynin (Ditropan) exerts a direct antispasmodic effect on smooth muscle and inhibits the muscarinic action of acetylcholine on smooth muscle. As such, it has wide usage in managing patients with voiding difficulties. The anticholinergic effect of Ditropan is minimal. *(Goodman and Gilman, p. 160)*

32. (D) Triazolam (Halcion) is a type of benzodiazepine. It is a hypnotic with a short duration of action. It increases the duration of sleep and decreases the frequency of nocturnal awakenings. It is recommended for short-term management of insomnia characterized by difficulty in falling asleep, frequent nocturnal awakenings, and/or early morning awakenings. *(Goodman and Gilman, pp. 346–358)*

33. (E) Glyburide is a second generation oral sulfonylurea. These agents are used in the treatment of Type II diabetics, along with dietary restrictions to control the serum glucose levels. The mechanism of action is believed to involve increase in the production of insulin from the pancreatic beta cells and an increase in the sensitivity of peripheral tissues to insulin. *(Goodman and Gilman, pp. 1484–1487)*

34. (D) Promethazine (Phenergan) is a phenothiazine derivative that has many uses, some of which include treatment of allergic rhinitis, urticaria, and nausea, and as a preoperative sedative. *(Goodman and Gilman, p. 585)*

35. (A) Enalapril (Vasotec) is a newer antihypertensive agent belonging to the category of ACE inhibitors and is similar to captopril. It is indicated for the control of mild to moderate hypertension and chronic congestive heart failure. It has the convenience of once-a-day dosing. *(Goodman and Gilman, pp. 760–761)*

36. (B) Famotidine (Pepcid) is classified as an H2 receptor antagonist. It, as well as cimetidine and ranitidine, is useful in the treatment of peptic ulcer disease by inhibiting gastric acid secretion. *(Goodman and Gilman, pp. 899–902)*

37. (D) Terfenadine (Seldane) is a relatively new antihistamine that is chemically and pharmacologically distinct from other antihistamines. It is very well tolerated and causes little, if any, sedation because of minimal to no anticholinergic activity. This has been a point in favor of this drug over conventional antihistamines. *(Goodman and Gilman, p. 587)*

38. (A) Flurazepam (Dalmane) is a sedative hypnotic of the benzodiazepine group. It has its major use as a sleeping aid; however, the prolonged half-life may create a "hung over" sensation. Other benzodiazepines, such as triazolam (Halcion) have shorter half-lives and reduce this side effect. *(Goodman and Gilman, pp. 346–358)*

39. (A) Methyldopa (Aldomet) is an antihypertensive agent belonging to the centrally acting sympatholytic group of drugs. Its major side effect is drowsiness. Other less common side effects include hemolytic anemia and hepatitis. About 20% of patients on methyldopa for a year will develop a positive Coombs' test. *(Goodman and Gilman, pp. 789–791)*

40. (A) Diphenhydramine (Benadryl) is an antihistamine belonging to the ethanolamine group associated with the highest incidence of drowsiness as a side effect. In fact, Benadryl is often used as a hypnotic, especially in hospitalized patients. *(Goodman and Gilman, p. 585)*

41. (D) Ranitidine (Zantac) is an H2 receptor blocker used in the treatment of peptic ulcer disease and gastroesophageal reflux disease. This occurs by diminishing the secretion of gastric acid. Other agents in this class include cimetidine (Tagamet), famotidine (Pepcid) and nizatidine (Axid). *(Goodman and Gilman, pp. 899–902)*

42. (A) Theophylline competitively inhibits phosphodiesterase, the enzyme that degrades cyclic AMP, thus elevating cyclic AMP levels. In bronchial smooth muscle cells, cyclic AMP produces relaxation of muscle fibers. *(Goodman and Gilman, pp. 619–629)*

43. **(D)** Trazadone (Desyrel) is a second-generation tricyclic antidepressant. It has a short half-life that mandates divided dosing throughout the day for greatest efficacy. Less sedative and autonomic side effects have been seen with the second-generation agents. *(Goodman and Gilman, pp. 405–413; Katzung, pp. 410–418)*

44. **(B)** Hydralazine (Apresoline) is an antihypertensive that lowers blood pressure by exerting a peripheral vasodilating effect through a direct relaxation of vascular smooth muscle. It is used after trial of diuretic and beta-adrenergic agents have failed to control blood pressure. *(Goodman and Gilman, pp. 799–801)*

45. **(C)** Diltiazem is a calcium antagonist that is most effective in angina due to coronary artery spasm. It is also used to treat elevated blood pressure. Toxicity is manifest as hypotension, dizziness, flushing, and bradycardia. *(Goodman and Gilman, pp. 774–780; Katzung, pp. 168–172)*

46. **(C)** Propranolol has long been used to treat both angina and hypertension. It also has many other uses, such as the treatment of cardiac arrhythmias and migraine headaches, to mention only two. It is the oldest of the beta-adrenergic blocking agents. There are more selective agents, such as atenolol. These agents do not have intrinsic sympathomimetic activity. *(Goodman and Gilman, pp. 229–240,780)*

47. **(C)** Nicardipine is a new calcium channel blocker currently approved for treatment of angina. It is similar to nifedipine; however, it may have some evidence of coronary artery selectivity. It also causes smooth muscle relaxation and, hence, reduction in systemic blood pressure with associated increase in cardiac output. *(Goodman and Gilman, p. 777)*

48. **(B)** Guanethidine is an older drug not often used any longer, partly because of the way it is metabolized, but primarily because of side effects, the most notable of which are orthostatic hypotension and impotency in males. It remains an effective blood pressure lowering agent; however, far better tolerated antihypertensive drugs are available. *(Goodman and Gilman, pp. 794–795)*

49. **(C)** Bactrim is a treatment of choice for pneumocystis pneumonia and is beneficial in treatment of urinary tract infection as well as prostatitis. Nongonococcal urethritis is not treated with Bactrim. This is frequently caused by *Chlamydia* and responds to doxycycline. *(Katzung, pp. 664–665; Tierney et al, p. 1183)*

50. **(C)** Metronidazole is the treatment of choice for antibiotic-associated colitis. The usual dose is 500 mg three times daily for 7 to 10 days. This is much more cost effective than the use of vancomycin, which can be used for persistent infection. The usual dose is 125 mg four times daily for 10 days. *(Katzung, p. 685; Tierney et al, p. 492)*

REFERENCES

Gilman AG, Rall TW, Nies AS, Taylor P. *The Pharmacological Basis of Therapeutics,* 8th ed. New York: Pergamon Press; 1990.

Hathaway WE, Hay WW Jr, Groothuis JR, Paisley JW. *Current Pediatric Diagnosis and Treatment,* 11th ed. Norwalk, CT. Appleton & Lange; 1993.

Katzung BG. *Basic and Clinical Pharmacology,* 5th ed. Norwalk, CT: Appleton & Lange; 1992.

Mandell GL, Douglas RG Jr, Bennett JE (eds). *Principles and Practice of Infectious Disease,* 3rd ed. New York: Churchill Livingstone; 1990.

Saunders CE, Ho MT. *Current Emergency Diagnosis and Treatment,* 4th ed. Norwalk, CT: Appleton & Lange; 1992.

Tierney LM Jr, McPhee SJ, Papadakis MA, Schroeder SA. *Current Medical Diagnosis and Treatment.* Norwalk, CT: Appleton & Lange; 1993.

Subspecialty List: Pharmacology

QUESTION NUMBER AND SUBSPECIALTY

1. Antifungal medications
2. Antituberculosis medications
3. Antihistamines
4. Lipid therapy
5. Contraindications of beta-blockers
6. Nutrition
7. Asthma
8. Acyclovir
9. Staphylococcal and streptococcal infections
10. Staphylococcus infection
11. Vitamin overdose
12. Antidepressant side effects
13. Cephalosporins
14. Pernicious anemia
15. Medication interaction
16. Theophylline dosage
17. Cephalosporins
18. Chlamydia infection
19. Absence seizures
20. Synthroid overdose
21. Synthroid overdose
22. Ovulation predictors
23. Treatment of migraine headache
24. Aminoglycoside toxicity
25. Pelvic inflammatory disease
26. Home glucose monitoring
27. Adverse reactions to DPT vaccine
28. Treatment of oral herpes lesions
29. Allergic rhinitis
30. Psychotic disorders
31. Neurogenic bladder
32. Insomnia
33. Diabetes
34. Antiemetics
35. Antihypertensives
36. H2 blockers
37. Pharmacologic action, indications and side effects
38. Pharmacologic action, indications and side effects
39. Pharmacologic action, indications and side effects
40. Pharmacologic action, indications and side effects
41. Pharmacologic action, indications and side effects
42. Pharmacologic action, indications and side effects
43. Pharmacologic action, indications and side effects
44. Pharmacologic action, indications and side effects
45. Pharmacologic action, indications and side effects
46. Pharmacologic action, indications and side effects
47. Pharmacologic action, indications and side effects
48. Pharmacologic action, indications and side effects
49. Antibiotic use
50. Antibiotic-associated colitis

CHAPTER 6

Psychiatry
Questions

DIRECTIONS (Questions 1 through 23): For each of the items in this section, ONE or MORE of the numbered options is correct. Choose answer

> **(A) if only (1), (2), and (3) are correct,**
> **(B) if only (1) and (3) are correct,**
> **(C) if only (2) and (4) are correct,**
> **(D) if only (4) is correct,**
> **(E) if all are correct.**

Questions 1 through 23

1. The schizophrenic premorbid personality is often noticeable in childhood and adolesence and is distinguished by

    (1) deficiency of social skills with development of small social network

    (2) impaired self-confidence in relationships with the opposite sex

    (3) episodes of neurotic-like illness such as anxiety, obsessions, and phobias

    (4) a tendency to confine close relationships to family members

2. An acute manic episode is characterized by a mood that is elevated, expansive, or irritable. Associated symptoms include

    (1) hyperactivity, reduced need for sleep, and poor concentration

    (2) religious preoccupation, spending sprees, and the playing of word games

    (3) increased self-esteem (grandiosity), pressure of speech, and poor social judgment

    (4) increased productivity, elevated frustration tolerance, and good humor

3. A major depressive episode is usually associated with which symptoms in addition to depressed mood?

    (1) reduced ability to feel pleasure

    (2) decreased interest in activities

    (3) diminished energy

    (4) insomnia, appetite changes, and feelings of guilt

4. The following is/are true about insomnia:

    (1) When found, it is always indicative of an underlying disorder.

    (2) Its significance is dependent upon its timing in the usual pattern of sleep.

    (3) It is unaffected by times of going to bed, waking, working, and exercise.

    (4) It can be associated with the use of alcohol or other drugs.

5. Recommended sleep hygiene methods for patients complaining of insomnia include

    (1) avoiding caffeine, nicotine, and alcohol

    (2) avoiding prolonged naps

    (3) establishing a set wake-up time

    (4) establishing a set time of going to sleep

6. Which of the following are characteristics included in the criteria for diagnosing attention deficit hyperactivity disorder in children?

    (1) an inability to remain seated in the classroom

    (2) difficulty following instructions or completing tasks

    (3) intrusiveness and frequent interruptions into conversations or activities of others

    (4) marked distress over minor changes in environment or schedule

7. Which of the following are commonly abused prescription drugs?

    (1) methamphetamine (Dexedrine), alprazolam (Xanax)

    (2) imipramine (Tofranil), carbamazepine (Tegretol)

    (3) chlordiazepoxide (Librium), meperidine (Demerol)

    (4) bethanechol (Urecholine), buspirone (Buspar)

A 8. Which of the following are true of alcohol withdrawal syndrome?

(1) It causes elevated blood pressure with orthostatic drop.
(2) Patients are in serious danger of seizures.
(3) It can cause hallucinations and delirium.
(4) It is not a frequent cause of mortality.

B 9. Withdrawal from sedative/hypnotic types of drugs

(1) resembles alcohol withdrawal syndrome
(2) resembles opiate withdrawal syndrome
(3) can produce seizures
(4) resembles cocaine withdrawal syndrome

tx: pentobarbitol or chlordiazepoxide

C 10. Which of the following are true regarding opiate withdrawal syndrome?

(1) It carries a risk of status epilepticus.
(2) Patients have observable piloerection, dilated pupils, and diarrhea.
(3) It causes auditory hallucinations.
(4) Patients usually complain of physical discomfort such as joint pain and muscle cramping.

A 11. The DSMIII-R criteria for the diagnosis of schizophrenia include

(1) the presence of psychosis persisting at least 1 week
(2) impairment in the level of functioning in general lifestyle areas
(3) persisting signs of illness for at least 6 months
(4) pervasive signs of a mood disorder persisting throughout the illness

E 12. Psychosis is a symptom of an underlying disorder. When an acutely psychotic patient is encountered, the differential diagnosis should include

(1) acute drug reaction
(2) bipolar (manic/depressive) disorder
(3) major depression
(4) schizophrenia

B 13. Simple phobias must be distinguished from panic disorder which

(1) often causes panic attacks in public places
(2) consists of a persistent fear of a specific object
(3) generally results in marked impairment in function
(4) is very common in the general population

A 14. Somatiform disorders are characterized by

(1) symptoms that suggest a physical ailment
(2) negative physical and laboratory findings
(3) a concomitant physical ailment
(4) intentional patient malingering

B 15. Reversible causes of dementia in the elderly include

(1) a major depressive episode
(2) vitamin deficiency
(3) prescription medication effects
(4) hydrocephalus

E 16. Common causes of irreversible, chronic, progressive dementia include

(1) Alzheimer's disease
(2) Parkinson's disease
(3) multiple small strokes
(4) alcoholism

17. In addition to a complete history, physical, and neurologic examination, a work-up of the patient presenting with dementia should include

(1) laboratory studies including thyroid function and serum B_{12} and folate determination
(2) abdominal x-rays and complete genitourinary evaluation
(3) CT scan and electroencephalograph
(4) lumbar puncture and cerebrospinal fluid examination

A 18. Imipramine (Tofranil) is a tricyclic antidepressant that commonly causes side effects including

(1) orthostatic hypotension — *spec. to imipramine*
(2) dry mouth
(3) blurred vision   } *anticholinergic*
(4) diarrhea

C 19. Lithium carbonate, a salt commonly used to treat bipolar affective (manic/depressive) illness, can cause

(1) dry mouth
(2) tremor   *at therapeutic*
(3) constipation   *or toxic levels*
(4) diarrhea

C 20. Caution must be used in prescribing benzodiazepines, such as alprazolam (Xanax), because of

(1) jitteriness
(2) drowsiness
(3) abnormal motor movements
(4) impaired motor control

21. Antipsychotic medication, such as haloperidol (Haldol), can cause such neurologic side effects as

  (1) acute dystonia
  (2) abnormal motor movements
  (3) motor agitation
  (4) parkinsonism

22. The borderline personality is characterized by

  (1) manipulative behavior, including suicidal threats
  (2) tempestuous interpersonal relationships
  (3) impulsivity and frequent mood shifts
  (4) persistent psychotic thinking

23. Personality disorders are

  (1) caused by biological factors exclusively
  (2) often occur with a patient meeting criteria for more than one disorder
  (3) often associated only with discrete episodes of mental illness
  (4) maladaptive traits that cause impairment or emotional distress

DIRECTIONS (Questions 24 through 32): Each set of items in this section consists of a list of lettered options followed by several numbered words or phrases. For each numbered word or phrase, select the ONE lettered option that is most closely associated with it. Each lettered option may be selected once, more than once, or not at all.

Questions 24 through 27

  (A) anxiolytic
  (B) tricyclic antidepressant
  (C) sedative/hypnotic
  (D) antipsychotic
  (E) MAO inhibitor

24. Amitriptyline (Elavil)

25. Lorazepam (Ativan)

26. Flurazepam (Dalmane)

27. Thioridazine (Mellaril)

Questions 28 through 30

  (A) generalized anxiety disorder
  (B) panic disorder
  (C) both
  (D) neither

28. Discrete spontaneous episodes

29. Sustained state of tension and irritability

30. Depression

Questions 31 and 32

  (A) preoccupation with body size and weight
  (B) binge eating accompanied by some extreme measure to prevent weight gain
  (C) both
  (D) neither

31. Anorexia nervosa

32. Bulimia nervosa

DIRECTIONS (Questions 33 through 40): Each of the numbered items or incomplete statements in this section is followed by answers or by completions of the statement. Select the ONE lettered answer or completion that is BEST in each case.

Questions 33 through 40

33. The prevalence of schizophrenia, which has been relatively constant across cultural boundaries, is approximately

  (A) 1%
  (B) 5%
  (C) 0.25%
  (D) 8%
  (E) 10%

34. "What brought you in to see me?" is an example of what type of question?

  (A) direct
  (B) closed-ended
  (C) open-ended
  (D) confrontive
  (E) structured

35. When lithium is used to treat bipolar affective illness, which lab tests are used in routine monitoring of the patient for side effects?

(A) uric acid, WBC

(B) CBC, liver enzymes

(C) T_3 uptake, liver enzymes

(D) TSH, creatinine

(E) electrolytes, glucose

36. Which of the following is true of alcohol withdrawal?

(A) Tremor is the most common manifestation of withdrawal.

(B) Seizures are the most serious manifestation.

(C) Seizures related solely to alcohol withdrawal do not benefit from anticonvulsant prophylaxis.

(D) Patients will frequently exhibit "morning shakes."

(E) All of the above.

37. Hallmark features of narcolepsy include

(A) daytime "sleep attacks"

(B) cataplexy

(C) sleep paralysis

(D) hypnogogic hallucinations

(E) all of the above

38. What diagnosis should be strongly suspected in an overweight, hypertensive, middle-aged male who complains of sleepiness and whose wife complains that he snores?

(A) coronary artery disease

(B) chronic obstructive pulmonary disease

(C) obstructive sleep apnea syndrome

(D) major depression

(E) narcolepsy

39. Many of the most common side effect complaints of tricyclic antidepressants are related to their anticholinergic effects and include

(A) blurred vision

(B) urinary retention

(C) constipation

(D) dry mouth

(E) all of the above

40. Which of the following medications is frequently used in the treatment of children with attention deficit hyperactivity?

(A) amitriptyline (Elavil)

(B) phenelzine (Nardil)

(C) methylphenidate (Ritalin)

(D) carbamazepine (Tegretol)

(E) lorazepam (Ativan)

DIRECTIONS (Questions 41 through 44): Each set of items in this section consists of a list of lettered options followed by several numbered words or phrases. For each numbered word or phrase, select the ONE lettered option that is most closely associated with it. Each lettered option may be selected once, more than once, or not at all.

Questions 41 to 44

Choose one of the following diagnostic categories that BEST describes the patient example.

(A) affective disorder

(B) bipolar affective disorder

(C) schizophrenia

(D) dementia

(E) none of the above

41. A 50-year-old white male presents to your office with a history of gradual decline in memory for major events, expresses an inappropriate affect, oriented only to person, and family reports that the symptoms get worse at night. You initially would consider what diagnostic category?

42. You are on call to the ER when you are asked to evaluate a new arrival. You obtain a history from the nurse of a 42-year-old male who was brought in by the family in the past for treatment of depression; however, over the last 2 weeks he has had increased energy, decreased need for sleep, excessive spending, and increased risk-taking behavior. On mental status exam, you see a black male oriented to person, place, time, and date. He is overactive with elevated mood, push of speech, distractability, and tangentiality. What would you suspect as the likely diagnosis?

43. Your first patient of the day while in a family clinic is an 18-year-old male you have never seen before. He is sitting in the exam room alone. His mental status exam reveals he is fully oriented, but his affect is inappropriate to the conversation. He indicates a belief that people are trying to harm him, that he is seeing people that you do not see, and he has bizarre hand gestures. He also indicates that people can read his mind and insert thoughts. This could be a presentation of what diagnostic category?

44. A 32-year-old female was referred to your office for evaluation of an unknown problem. Upon entering the room you see a tearful, slow to react female who reports a gradual worsening in feelings of worthlessness and inability to derive pleasure from usual activities for the last month. She has paid less attention to her dress and grooming. She is fully oriented. What diagnostic category does this scenario fit?

DIRECTIONS (Questions 45 through 60): Each of the numbered items or incomplete statements in this section is followed by answers or by completions of the statement. Select the ONE lettered answer or completion that is BEST in each case.

Questions 45 through 60

45. Cocaine is a stimulant drug that has become a common drug of abuse. A prominent feature of cocaine withdrawal is

  (A) somnolence
  (B) depression
  (C) psychosis
  (D) muscle cramping
  (E) abdominal pain

46. Psychotropic drug use in the elderly

  (A) is contraindicated
  (B) must be closely monitored for side effects
  (C) should always be in low doses
  (D) should not be a first-line approach to treatment
  (E) none of the above

47. Which of the following antidepressant medications would be the safest in a patient with compromised cardiac status?

  (A) Prozac (fluoxetine)
  (B) Elavil (amitriptyline)
  (C) Tofranil (imipramine)
  (D) Nardil (phenelzine)
  (E) Mellaril (thioridazine)

48. Individuals with antisocial personality disorder are

  (A) responsive to rehabilitation measures and psychotherapy
  (B) generally males with a lifelong pattern of irresponsible and often criminal behavior
  (C) not likely to risk their own safety when engaging in antisocial behavior

  (D) often improved in their behavior when forced to take responsibility, as in becoming a parent
  (E) rarely dangerous to others in their behavior

49. Clozaril (clozapine) is an antipsychotic used for treatment of resistant schizophrenia. What potentially life-threatening side effect needs to be monitored for?

  (A) extrapyramidal symptoms
  (B) development of movement disorders
  (C) agranulocytosis
  (D) hypersalivation
  (E) dysgustia

50. The Minnesota Multiphasic Personality Inventory (MMPI)

  (A) is used in place of a lengthy psychiatric interview to assess patients
  (B) is an old test of personality function that is rarely used today
  (C) can be used as a measure of intelligence
  (D) is a self-report test used to assess symptoms of mental illness and personality dysfunction
  (E) can easily be manipulated by an intelligent patient wishing to present a positive picture

51. A neurotransmitter that has been implicated as a causative factor in depression is

  (A) epinephrine
  (B) serotonin
  (C) amphetamine
  (D) tryramine
  (E) phenylalanine

52. Psychiatric conditions associated with HIV infection include which of the following?

  (A) depression
  (B) acute psychosis
  (C) mania
  (D) delirium
  (E) all of the above

53. A personality pattern characterized by excessive inflexibility and perfectionistic views is called

  (A) narcissistic personality disorder
  (B) an unclassified personality problem
  (C) oppositional defiant disorder
  (D) passive-aggressive personality disorder
  (E) obsessive-compulsive personality disorder

54. A number of medical disorders can cause alteration in mood and can mimic a major depressive episode including

(A) hypothyroidism
(B) hyperthyroidism
(C) systemic lupus erythematosus
(D) brain tumor
(E) all the above

55. The most common neurologic problem in AIDS is

(A) AIDS dementia complex
(B) peripheral neuropathy
(C) cerebrovascular accident
(D) transient ischemic attacks
(E) carpal tunnel syndrome

56. Initial management of the acutely suicidal patient should include

(A) psychotherapy
(B) antidepressant medication
(C) hospitalization and close observation
(D) antianxiety medication
(E) electroconvulsive therapy (ECT)

57. Mental retardation is classified in four levels: mild, moderate, severe, and profound, and is caused by

(A) congenital abnormalities
(B) genetic abnormalities
(C) trauma

(D) nonorganic etiology
(E) all the above

58. A patient is determined to be "incompetent" if he/she

(A) is psychotic
(B) is disoriented
(C) is dangerous to himself/herself and others
(D) is unable to make decisions in his/her own best interest
(E) is unable to determine right from wrong

59. Closed head injury can cause a variety of psychiatric syndromes, both temporary and permanent, including

(A) personality changes
(B) psychosis
(C) depression
(D) disruption of sleep patterns
(E) all the above

60. Chronic heavy metal poisoning is an often overlooked syndrome that can cause symptoms resembling

(A) schizophrenia
(B) depression
(C) Parkinson's disease
(D) panic disorder
(E) all the above

Answers and Explanations

1. **(E)** It has long been recognized that schizophrenia occurs in association with many personality types. However, the socially withdrawn type of personality is more strongly represented in schizophrenics and their first-degree relatives. The reason for this is unknown, but it can be a valuable piece of historical information when forming a differential diagnosis. *(Kendell, p. 7)*

2. **(A)** The manic does have an elevated mood, increased energy, and rapid thought processes, with a reduced need for sleep. However, his/her energies are poorly focused, and his/her judgment is impaired to such a degree that activities are often disorganized and counterproductive. He/she generally has little tolerance for interference, and while such a person can be in an expansive mood when things go well, he/she can abruptly become hostile and even violent. *(Dunner, p. 2)*

3. **(E)** The presence of melancholia (the loss of pleasure in activities) associated with at least three of the following: sleep disturbance, eating disturbance or weight change, reduced energy, inappropriate guilt, loss of libido, reduced concentration, morbid or nihilistic thoughts, or psychomotor changes, which fulfill the criteria for diagnosis of major depression. *(Dunner, p. 3)*

4. **(C)** Insomnia is a symptom, a subjective complaint requiring evaluation, and carries a broad differential diagnosis. It can be the result of bad habits; for example, no exercise, alcohol, tobacco or caffeine use, or working and worrying right until bedtime. A careful history must be obtained, including whether the sleeplessness includes difficulty falling asleep, waking during the night, or waking in the early morning hours. Fragmented sleep can be a symptom of depression, alcohol abuse, or medication effect, among other things. Major primary sleep disorders must be ruled out. All-night polysomnography in a sleep lab is sometimes needed for a definitive diagnosis. *(Aldrich, p. 314)*

5. **(A)** When bad habits are affecting a patient's sleep, he/she needs to be encouraged to keep a more structured schedule. Getting up at the same time each morning tends toward becoming sleepy at the same time each night. Getting up at the same time is easier to achieve than controlling falling asleep. Habits that interfere with efficient sleep, namely daytime naps or drug and alcohol use, should be discouraged. *(Zarcone, pp. 490–493)*

6. **(A)** Children with attention deficit hyperactivity disorder (ADHD) often tend to move excessively, are intrusive in their behavior, and are unable to focus their attention on tasks. Rigidity of behavior is more indicative of pervasive development disorder or in its extreme, autistic disorder. *(APA, pp. 50–53)*

7. **(B)** Alprazolam and chlordiazepoxide are benzodiazepines, which are the most commonly prescribed class of psychoactive medications. They can cause tolerance, intoxication, and withdrawal. Meperidine, a synthetic opioid with morphine-like action, is a frequently abused pain reliever. Methamphetamine is a stimulant and is commonly abused for weight control or to combat fatigue. The other agents do not produce tolerance, intoxication, withdrawal symptoms, or the maladaptive behavior symptoms associated with substance abuse. *(APA, pp. 165,175–176,182–183,184–185)*

8. **(A)** Elevated blood pressure with an orthostatic drop is an easily observable sign of alcohol withdrawal syndrome. Seizures, and even status epileptiform, are dangerous and potentially fatal complications of withdrawal from alcohol. Hallucinations and delirium are additional complications and complete the picture of delirium tremens or "DTs." *(Ellinwood et al, pp. 6–11)*

9. **(B)** Drugs, including benzodiazepines (Valium, Librium, Dalmane, etc), and barbiturates are cross-tolerant with alcohol and produce the same withdrawal syndrome. It should be kept in mind that some of the longer-acting agents, such as diazepam (Valium), can cause a delayed syndrome

several days after discontinuation of the drug. It is important to recognize and promptly treat withdrawal before it progresses with an appropriate cross-tolerant agent such as pentobarbital or chlordiazepoxide. *(Ellinwood et al, pp. 6–11)*

10. **(C)** Gooseflesh, markedly dilated pupils in diffuse light, and diarrhea are easily observable signs of acute opiate withdrawal. Opiate withdrawal can cause severe discomfort but is not life-threatening, as is sedative/hypnotic/alcohol withdrawal. The necessity of using objective signs in the treatment of opiate addiction is obvious, due to the tendency of these patients toward drug-seeking behavior. *(Ellinwood et al, pp. 3,7,12)*

11. **(A)** By definition, symptoms of illness existing for less than 6 months cannot be called schizophrenia, and are diagnosed as schizophreniform disorders. The total time of mood disturbance must be less than that of thinking disturbances, or another diagnosis such as schizoaffective or major depression with psychotic features should be made. *(APA, pp. 187–195)*

12. **(E)** Psychosis is an indication of a brain chemical malfunction. Many different causes must be entertained. The first step in narrowing a differential diagnosis is to take a careful history, including the duration of symptoms and the patient's premorbid level of functioning. One must, of course, rule out nonpsychiatric causes of brain dysfunction. *(Davidson, pp. 1–14)*

13. **(C)** Panic disorder causes discrete episodes of panic that occur spontaneously and often become psychologically linked with the circumstances in which they occur. A phobia is the fear of a single distinct object, such as cats. As opposed to panic disorder, simple phobias are common, result in little debilitation, and do not, in themselves, cause patients to seek treatment. *(APA, pp. 243–245)*

14. **(A)** Somatiform disorders present in many forms. Symptoms occur in many body systems, commonly gastrointestinal, cardiovascular, or genitourinary. Often, pain is experienced that cannot be correlated with the anatomic distribution of the nervous system. Occasionally, they occur concurrently with, or subsequent to, a genuine physical ailment or trauma. The patient is not conscious of the production of his/her symptoms. To him/her they are felt as "real." *(APA, pp. 263–267)*

15. **(E)** Although Alzheimer's disease and multi-infarct disease are the leading causes of dementia in the elderly, there are numerous causes that can be treatable. Careful evaluation must be undertaken to rule out metabolic causes, including drug interactions, overmedication, vitamin deficiencies,

and thyroid disease. Primary psychiatric disease can cause reversible dementia. In the condition of normal-pressure hydrocephalus, shunting can alleviate symptoms. *(Jenike, pp. 117–121)*

16. **(E)** The cause of progressive dementia must be carefully evaluated. Although it may be irreversible, the course can sometimes be modified by treatment, enabling the patient continued function at a certain level and perhaps remaining longer at home. Psychotropic medications used judiciously, and treatment of the underlying disorder, can be helpful. *(Jenike, pp. 117–121,126–136)*

17. **(B)** Complete and careful evaluation of the patient with dementia should be undertaken with the goal of discovering possible treatable etiology. In the absence of gastrointestinal or genitourinary symptoms, work-up of these systems is not indicated. Lumbar puncture is not routinely indicated and should not be a part of the initial examination. *(Jenike, pp. 117–121)*

18. **(A)** Imipramine is a tricyclic antidepressant that, in addition to the usual anticholinergic side effects, can produce a significant drop in standing blood pressure. This may require discontinuation of the drug and use of another antidepressant. It must be used with particular care in the elderly because of the hazard of falls. *(Baldessarini, pp. 178–179,182–183)*

19. **(C)** Diarrhea and tremor are common side effects of lithium treatment. They can occur at therapeutic or toxic levels. When they occur, a serum lithium level should be obtained, as the symptoms can precede more dangerous consequences of lithium toxicity. *(Baldessarini, pp. 117–118)*

20. **(C)** Alprazolam (Xanax), a commonly prescribed anxiolytic, has a side effect profile typical of the benzodiazepines. Care must be taken to caution patients in its use while operating heavy machinery or a motor vehicle, as it can markedly slow motor speed as well as cause drowsiness. *(Baldessarini, pp. 256–257)*

21. **(E)** Neuroleptically induced neurologic side effects are common. They usually occur in the first weeks of treatment and may not be dose-related. Anticholinergic medication or amantadine (Symmetrel) may relieve symptoms. The offending agent may have to be discontinued and an alternate treatment chosen. Of particular importance are the movement disorders indicative of tardive dyskinesia, which may be irreversible. *(Baldessarini, pp. 68–80)*

22. **(A)** A borderline personality is distinguished by a great deal of character dysfunction. Their lives

are generally marked by one crisis after another, to which they respond in impulsive ways. They do have periods when reality testing is impaired, but this generally is limited to times of crisis. *(APA, pp. 346–347)*

23. **(C)** Personality disorders are characterological flaws that impair a person's ability to function in society. A patient may exhibit traits of more than one described disorder. It has been believed by some that environment plays a part in shaping the personality. *(APA, p. 335)*

24. **(B)** The general term *tricyclic* antidepressants has been used for the group of antidepressant agents having a three-ring type structure. These agents have similar properties and side effects and are distinguished from the monoamine oxidase inhibitor type. Imipramine (Tofranil) was the first tricyclic antidepressant to be used. There are now several agents that do not fit into either of these categories and sometimes are referred to as "atypical" antidepressants. *(Baldessarini, pp. 131–135)*

25. **(A)** Lorazepam is a relatively short-acting benzodiazepine. Its lack of active metabolites and low tissue accumulation make it a favored drug for anxiety treatment. *(Baldessarini, p. 250)*

26. **(C)** Flurazepam is also a benzodiazepine. It has relatively greater sedating effects and thus is used more commonly to induce sleep rather than to treat daytime anxiety. *(Baldessarini, pp. 250–251)*

27. **(D)** Thioridazine is a relatively low-potency antipsychotic agent. It has high sedative effects and a low tendency to cause extrapyramidal side effects. The choice of an antipsychotic agent must be individualized to the patient. *(Baldessarini, pp. 22,25)*

28. **(B)** Panic disorder is characterized by sudden onset of pounding heart, shortness of breath, dizziness, and extreme anxiety. Patients often feel as though they are about to die. The initial attack often occurs in young adulthood. In severe forms, it can progress to development of phobias associated with situations in which panic attacks have previously occurred. *(Gorman and Liebowitz, pp. 1–4)*

29. **(A)** Generalized anxiety disorder is characterized by the development over time of chronic feelings of tension, anxiety, and restlessness. Discrete episodes of frank panic do not occur. Abuse of alcohol or sedatives often occurs in an attempt to self-medicate. *(Gorman and Liebowitz, pp. 4,10–11,32)*

30. **(C)** The difference between major depression disorder, generalized anxiety disorder, and panic disorder can often be quite blurred. In all three disorders, depressed mood and anxiety can coexist. In anxiety and panic disorders, the onset of tension or panic attacks often precedes the onset of depressed mood by a significant period of time. *(Gorman and Liebowitz, pp. 4,10–11)*

31. **(A)** Anorexia nervosa is a disorder characterized by a refusal to maintain a normal body weight. The person has a distorted body image and sees herself/himself as fat even when severely undernourished. Such persons are preoccupied with body size and shape. *(APA, pp. 65–67)*

32. **(C)** Bulimics have a disorder characterized by binge eating during which they feel a lack of control over their eating behavior. Bulimics, like anorexics, have a preoccupation with their weight and body features. They engage in means to prevent weight gain, such as self-induced vomiting, abuse of laxatives, fasting between binges, or overly strenuous exercise. *(APA, pp. 67–69)*

33. **(A)** Various studies conducted by researchers in numerous developed and developing countries have shown rates approximating 1% or 10 per 1000 population. There have been some inconsistencies in uniformity and diagnostic criteria and data collection, but it is obvious that the disorder occurs in all populations and has a historical basis. *(Helzer, pp. 4–5)*

34. **(C)** In clinical interviews the manner of questioning can be important. Open-ended questions should be used for neurotic, verbal, and normal IQ patients. Structured and closed-ended questions are best used when time is limited or if the patient has a psychosis, delirium, or dementia. *(Kaplan and Sadock, p. 7)*

35. **(D)** Lithium is excreted by the kidneys; thus, blood levels are dependent upon renal function. Lithium can also have long-term effects on renal and thyroid function. Lithium-induced hypothyroidism can be a side effect of lithium treatment and is treated with thyroid replacement. Thus, in addition to routine lithium blood levels, renal and thyroid function should be monitored. *(Baldessarini, pp. 115,119–121)*

36. **(E)** Tremors are part of the uncomplicated alcohol withdrawal. Less common and more severe is alcohol delirium. If seizures occur, they always occur before delirium. Typically the use of anticonvulsants for purely withdrawal seizure is not beneficial. *(Kaplan and Sadock, pp. 54–55)*

37. **(E)** Narcolepsy is a disorder involving more than just excessive daytime sleepiness. Hypersomnolence is more commonly caused by other disorders or poor habits. The diagnosis of true narcolepsy, which is relatively rare, can be made only in the

presence of at least one of the other symptoms. Sleep attacks plus cataplexy is considered pathognomonic of narcolepsy. An all-night polysomnograph and daytime sleep latency testing are confirmatory. *(Guilleminault, pp. 338–341)*

38. **(C)** Obstructive sleep apnea is a common cause of excessive daytime somnolence. Snoring is a common observable sign of upper airway obstruction. This is not a benign condition. In addition to sleepiness being quite debilitating and potentially dangerous, lowered pO_2 during sleep and other physiologic changes can lead to hypertension and potentially fatal cardiac arrhythmias. *(Lugaresi et al, p. 498)*

39. **(E)** Tricyclic antidepressants vary in their potency of anticholinergic effects. The patient's underlying medical status must be taken into account in choosing an antidepressant. Conditions such as benign prostatic hypertrophy can worsen markedly. *(Baldessarini, p. 183)*

40. **(C)** Methylphenidate (Ritalin), along with methamphetamine (Dexedrine), and pemoline (Cylert) are stimulants commonly used to treat children with attention-deficit hyperactivity disorder. Amitriptyline and phenelzine are antidepressants. Carbamazepine is an anticonvulsant with several psychiatric uses. *(Baldessarini, pp. 126–219)*

41. **(D)** Dementia has disturbances to both short- and long-term memory, and interference with social and occupational functioning. Care should be taken to rule out the reversible causes of delirium, such as medication interaction or metabolic derangements. *(Kaplan and Sadock, pp. 24–25)*

42. **(B)** Bipolar affective disorder exhibits erratic and disinhibited behavior. Patients are frequently overextended in their activities and responsibilities. They exhibit low frustration tolerance and vegetative symptoms such as diminished need for sleep, as well as changes in diet and weight. *(Kaplan and Sadock, p. 85)*

43. **(C)** In schizophrenia, one can see psychotic symptoms that impair function and affect feelings, thinking, and behavior. These might include hallucinations involving auditory, tactile, visual, or olfactory senses. *(Kaplan and Sadock, p. 57)*

44. **(A)** Affective disorders are characterized by abnormal feelings of depression or euphoria. These disorders can be divided into unipolar or bipolar. They respond well to mood-stabilizing agents, ie, antidepressants or membrane-stabilizing agents, such as lithium. *(Kaplan and Sadock, p. 81)*

45. **(B)** The most common symptom of acute cocaine withdrawal after heavy use is depression. This can also be accompanied by anxiety and irritability. Often, cocaine abusers also abuse sedative medications or alcohol in an attempt to self-medicate these feelings. Cocaine does not produce a physical withdrawal syndrome as do opiates, sedative/hypnotics, or alcohol. *(APA, pp. 142–143,177–179)*

46. **(B)** When psychoactive drugs are used in the elderly, care must be taken to closely monitor response to the drug. Impaired gastrointestinal, liver, and/or renal function can alter absorption and elimination patterns. Interactions with other prescribed or over-the-counter medications can occur. Psychotropic drugs can be effectively and safely used in the elderly when precautions are taken, and can enhance and even prolong life. *(Jenike, pp. 6–7,9–14)*

47. **(A)** Prozac is a serotonin reuptake inhibitor, as is Paxil and Zoloft. In general these agents have no significant cardiac conduction delay and do not produce orthostatic hypotension. No adverse cardiovascular effects have been noted in cases of overdose. *(Kaplan and Sadock, p. 258)*

48. **(B)** Antisocial personalities do not respond well to treatment. They do not learn from their mistakes and tend to blame others for their misfortunes. Statistically, they are predominantly males and are well represented in prison populations. *(APA, pp. 342–346)*

49. **(C)** A special concern with the use of clozapine is agranulocytosis which occurs in about 1% to 2% of patients. If not detected early this can be fatal. If detected within one to two weeks the medication can be discontinued, and the process usually reverses. Once a patient recovers from the agranulocytosis, he/she cannot be restarted as it will recur. The manufacturer recommends that weekly CBCs be obtained on all patients while on clozapine. *(Kaplan and Sadock, p. 248)*

50. **(D)** The MMPI is a well-standardized test that has been used extensively for more than 40 years. It does not take the place of a careful psychiatric examination, but augments it. It includes sophisticated internal validation factors that point out certain patterns of manipulation on the part of the patient. *(Clarkin and Sweeney, p. 5)*

51. **(B)** Some of the new antidepressants have potent serotonin uptake blocking effects. Amphetamine was once used as an antidepressant, with limited results. Phenylalanine and tyrosine are amino acid precursors of centrally active catecholamines. *(Baldessarini, pp. 151–155)*

52. (E) Organic mental disorders are associated with HIV infection and manifest as psychiatric symptoms. Periodic assessment of mental status in HIV-positive patients is important as these symptoms may be managed with appropriate agents. *(Kaplan and Sadock, pp. 299–300)*

53. (E) A tendency towards perfectionism and minute attention to detail can be desirable in certain occupations. The obsessive-compulsive is, however, impaired in his/her ability to discriminate what is important. Taken to the extreme, the patient is so preoccupied with details, he/she cannot complete the task at hand. *(APA, pp. 354–356)*

54. (E) It is very important to rule out nonpsychiatric causes of a psychiatric-appearing presentation. Many metabolic dysfunctions may cause brain dysfunction and mimic symptoms of psychiatric illness. At times, there may be an underlying life-threatening situation that is potentially correctable. *(Dunner, p. 12)*

55. (A) AIDS dementia complex is also known as AIDS encephalopathy. The major clinical manifestations are gradual onset of memory deficits, diminished concentration, apathy, social withdrawal, psychomotor retardation, and depression in an HIV-positive patient. Some of these symptoms can be improved with psychotropic medications. *(Kaplan and Sadock, pp. 299–300)*

56. (C) A statement of suicidal intent by a patient must be taken very seriously. An actively suicidal patient is not a candidate for outpatient treatment because of the potential lethality of an overdose of many psychiatric medications. Initiation of treatment and stabilization is best accomplished in an inpatient setting and can generally be done in 1 week to 10 days. *(Baldessarini, pp. 195–197)*

57. (E) Mental retardation varies widely in cause and degree of impairment. Causes can be genetic, such as Down syndrome; congenital, as in fetal alcohol syndrome; traumatic, as a result of childhood head injury; or have no readily identifiable cause. *(APA, pp. 28–33)*

58. (D) Competency is a legal term used to define the ability of a person to make decisions based on his/her own best interest. It is further broken down to pertain to the specific task at hand, such as competency to draw up a will, make a contract, or participate in a legal defense. A person may be deemed competent to perform some tasks and not others. *(Baldessarini, p. 280)*

59. (E) A closed head injury causes trauma to the brain by creating shear forces and contusions within the skull. Depending upon the force of the blow and the movements of the brain within the skull, many different brain functions may be impaired. Healing and accommodation of the remaining intact brain can bring about the return of some functions within about 2 years of injury. *(APA, pp. 4–8)*

60. (B) Lead, cadmium, and mercury are commonly encountered potential poisons. They each can have neurobehavioral effects with chronic exposure that can mimic psychiatric illness. The complaints are usually subtle and include tremor, fatigue, memory loss, mood changes, insomnia, and others. Once again, when encountering a depressed patient, rule out other medical causes first. *(Molinaro, pp. 261–269)*

REFERENCES

Aldrich MS. Cardinal manifestations of sleep disorders. In Kryger, Roth, Dement (eds). *Principles and Practice of Sleep Medicine.* Philadelphia, PA: WB Saunders; 1989.

American Psychiatric Association. *Diagnostic and Statistical Manual of Mental Disorders,* 3rd ed. Washington, DC: American Psychiatric Association; 1987.

Baldessarini RJ. *Chemotherapy in Psychiatry,* 2nd ed. Cambridge, MA: Harvard University Press; 1985.

Clarkin J, Sweeney J. Psychological assessment. In Michels R (ed). *Psychiatry,* vol. I. Philadelphia, PA: JB Lippincott; 1988.

Davidson K. Symptomatic psychoses. In Michels R (ed). *Psychiatry,* vol. I. Philadelphia, PA: JB Lippincott; 1988.

Dunner DL. Affective disorder: Clinical features. In Michels R (ed). *Psychiatry,* vol. I. Philadelphia, PA: JB Lippincott; 1988.

Ellinwood E, Woody G, Krichnan R. Treatment for drug abuse. In Michels R (ed). *Psychiatry,* vol. II. Philadelphia, PA: JB Lippincott; 1988.

Gorman J, Liebowitz M. Panic and anxiety disorders. In Michels R (ed). *Psychiatry,* vol. I. Philadelphia, PA: JB Lippincott; 1988.

Guilleminault C. Narcolepsy syndrome. In Kryger, Roth, Dement (eds). *Principles and Practice of Sleep Medicine.* Philadelphia, PA: WB Saunders; 1989.

Helzer JE. Schizophrenia: Epidemiology. In Michels R (ed). *Psychiatry,* vol. I. Philadelphia, PA: JB Lippincott; 1988.

Jenike M. *Handbook of Geriatric Psychopharmacology.* Littleton, MA: PSG Publishing Co; 1985.

Kaplan HI, Sadock BJ. Pocket Handbook of Clinical Psychiatry. Baltimore, MD: Williams & Wilkins; 1990.

Kendell E. Schizophrenia: Clinical features. In Michels R (ed). *Psychiatry.* vol. I. Philadelphia, PA: JB Lippincott; 1988.

Lugaresi E, Cirignotta F, Montagna P. Snoring: Pathogenic, clinical, and therapeutic aspects. In Kryger, Roth, Dement (eds). *Principles and Practice of Sleep Medicine*. Philadelphia, PA: WB Saunders; 1989.

Molinaro J. *A Primary Care Approach to Heavy Metal Poisoning*. Journal American Academy of Physician Assistants. July/August 1989.

Zarcone P. Sleep hygiene. In Kryger, Roth, Dement (eds). *Principles and Practice of Sleep Medicine*. Philadelphia, PA: WB Saunders; 1989.

Subspecialty Listing: Psychiatry

QUESTION NUMBER AND SUBSPECIALTY

1. General psychiatry
2. General psychiatry
3. General psychiatry
4. Sleep disorders medicine
5. Sleep disorders medicine
6. Child psychiatry
7. Substance abuse
8. Substance abuse
9. Substance abuse
10. Substance abuse
11. General psychiatry
12. General psychiatry
13. General psychiatry
14. General psychiatry
15. Geriatric psychiatry
16. Geriatric psychiatry
17. Geriatric psychiatry
18. General psychiatry
19. General psychiatry
20. General psychiatry
21. General psychiatry
22. General psychiatry
23. General psychiatry
24. General psychiatry
25. General psychiatry
26. General psychiatry
27. General psychiatry
28. General psychiatry
29. General psychiatry
30. General psychiatry
31. Eating disorders
32. Eating disorders
33. General psychiatry
34. Interview skills
35. General psychiatry
36. Alcohol withdrawal
37. Sleep disorders medicine
38. Sleep disorders medicine
39. General psychiatry
40. Child psychiatry
41. Psychiatric diagnosis
42. Psychiatric diagnosis
43. Psychiatric diagnosis
44. Psychiatric diagnosis
45. Substance abuse
46. General psychiatry
47. Antidepressants
48. General psychiatry
49. Antipsychotic side effects
50. General psychiatry testing
51. General psychiatry
52. Psychiatric manifestations of AIDS
53. General psychiatry
54. General psychiatry
55. Psychiatric manifestations of AIDS
56. General psychiatry
57. Child psychiatry
58. Forensic psychiatry
59. General psychiatry
60. General psychiatry

CHAPTER 7

Obstetrics and Gynecology
Questions

DIRECTIONS (Questions 1 through 21): For each of the items in this section, ONE or MORE of the numbered options is correct. Choose answer

    (A) if only (1), (2), and (3) are correct,
    (B) if only (1) and (3) are correct,
    (C) if only (2) and (4) are correct,
    (D) if only (4) is correct,
    (E) if all are correct.

Questions 1 through 21

1. Which of the following mothers' offspring would require treatment with hepatitis B immune globulin and hepatitis B vaccine at birth?

    (1) mother with active hepatitis B in last month of pregnancy
    (2) mother with active hepatitis A
    (3) mother who is HBsAg positive
    (4) mother with convalescent titers for hepatitis A

2. Endomyometritis commonly occurs after cesarean section (less common after vaginal delivery); factors involved in the pathogenesis of endomyometritis are

    (1) history of previous episode of pelvic inflammatory disease
    (2) presence of normal cervical and vaginal flora that become pathogenic in the upper genital tract
    (3) the presence of anemia or other chronic diseases prior to delivery
    (4) the ideal medium of the postpartum endometrial cavity for proliferation of bacteria

3. A patient was delivered by forceps and is presently 2 days postpartum. She is found to have a swollen, erythematous right leg with a positive Homan's sign. Which of the following contributed to her present postpartum complications?

    (1) decreased blood flow from her lower extremities during the last weeks of pregnancy

    (2) hypercoagulable state of pregnancy
    (3) decreased activity secondary to postpartum state
    (4) use of oxytocin to stimulate labor

4. A patient develops mastitis postpartum. Which of the following would be signs and symptoms?

    (1) chills and fever
    (2) engorgement of breast within 48 hours after onset of lactation
    (3) areas of inflammation, redness, and induration of one breast
    (4) green discoloration of breast milk

5. A woman presents in labor at 5 cm dilated in breech presentation. Which of the following causes a higher incidence of breech presentation?

    (1) fetal anomalies
    (2) uterine anatomic abnormalities
    (3) premature onset of labor
    (4) grandmultiparity

6. A 28-year-old female presents to the emergency room with a four-day history of swelling and pain in her vagina. On examination she has a right Bartholin's abscess: the abscess is 4 cm in size, fluctulant, and erythematous. Additionally, she has right inguinal adenopathy. Which of the following would be correct emergent and long-term therapy?

    (1) incision and drainage in the emergency room
    (2) PO antibiotics and local treatment with warm soaks
    (3) outpatient surgical correction by marsupialization
    (4) admission to hospital for IV antibiotics and definitive surgery

7. A 25-year-old patient has undergone a rapid, spontaneous vaginal delivery followed by a prolonged third stage of labor, and an eventual manual removal of the placenta. She continues to bleed heavily after placental removal, with an estimated blood loss of greater than 1000 ml. What are the subsequent steps to control the hemorrhage?

   (1) exploration of the uterus for retained products
   (2) administration of methylergonovine (Methergine)
   (3) vigorous fundal massage
   (4) packing of the uterus

8. An 18-year-old G2P0 presents for her first prenatal visit at 16 weeks' gestation. Routine cervical cultures are performed for gonorrhea, and a monoclonal antibody test for chlamydia is obtained. The chlamydia test is positive. Which of the following are the best means of treatment?

   (1) doxycycline 100 mg PO bid for 10 days
   (2) Bactrim DS one tab PO bid for 10 days
   (3) ceftriaxone 250 mg IM
   (4) erythromycin 500 mg PO q6 hours for 7 days

9. A 35-year-old patient presents to labor and delivery at 18 weeks' gestation, complaining of fullness in her vagina. On pelvic exam, the cervix is 6 cm with ballooning of the membranes into the vagina. Additional information you might obtain from the patient that would explain her present condition would be

   (1) history of previous septic abortion
   (2) previous second trimester abortion that was without contractions
   (3) a known balanced chromosomal abnormality in the patient
   (4) history of patient's mother receiving DES during her pregnancy

10. A woman has undergone a suction curettage for a hydatidiform mole. What subsequent steps should be done to ensure she does not develop choriocarcinoma?

    (1) Serial serum beta HCG levels should be obtained every 1 to 2 weeks until negative.
    (2) Prophylatic chemotherapy should be administered.
    (3) The patient should be advised not to become pregnant for at least 1 year.
    (4) The patient should undergo a radical hysterectomy and bilateral salpingo-oophorectomy.

11. At 34 weeks' gestation, a patient's fundal height measures 40 cm. The sonogram at that time reveals polyhydramnios. What else may be found on ultrasound at this time?

    (1) large ovarian cyst
    (2) calcification of the placenta
    (3) placenta previa
    (4) fetal congenital anomalies

12. Preterm labor occurs more frequently in twin gestations. What other antenatal complications occur at a greater frequency in twin gestations?

    (1) fetal anomalies
    (2) preeclampsia
    (3) intrauterine growth retardation
    (4) gestational diabetes

13. Respiratory depression is a known side effect of intravenous magnesium sulfate (a medication commonly used in pregnant women). Which of the following are a means of monitoring the amount of magnesium administered and preventing this complication?

    (1) observing changes in the fetal heart rate
    (2) checking maternal deep tendon reflexes
    (3) monitoring blood pressure
    (4) serum magnesium

14. A 32-year-old patient presents to labor and delivery at 37 weeks' gestation with a complaint of vaginal bleeding. Her history includes two previous cesarean sections. A sonogram performed showed the following (see Figure 7–1). Which of

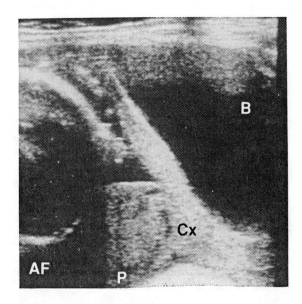

Fig. 7–1. A 32-year-old patient at 37 weeks' gestation. AF, amniotic fluid; B, maternal bladder; Cx, cervix; P, placenta.

the following procedures should not be performed on this patient?

→ (1) bimanual pelvic exam
→ (2) bedrest with IV fluids *IV not necessary*
→ (3) attempted vaginal delivery *no time for placenta to migrate back*
(4) repeat cesarean section

15. At 36 weeks, a 28-year-old patient presents with a complaint of leaking fluid from her vagina. How would you determine whether this was amniotic fluid? *Lecithin/Sphingo-myelin* C

(1) obtain a specimen of fluid and send it for L/S ratio *fetal lung maturity*
→ (2) place some fluid on a glass slide and check for "ferning" under the microscope
(3) estimate amniotic fluid volume on ultrasound
→ (4) test fluid with nitrazine paper

16. A patient has documented spontaneous rupture of membranes at 32 weeks' gestation. It has been decided to manage the patient conservatively with bed rest and monitoring white blood cell count and maternal temperature. What are the major risks to the mother and fetus when conservative management is followed?

— (1) development of neonatal sepsis once delivery occurs
(2) development of late decelerations on non-stress testing *→ variable*
✓ (3) onset of chorioamnionitis
(4) onset of vaginal bleeding secondary to placenta previa *not possible*

17. Which of the following medications are commonly used to arrest preterm labor?

— (1) magnesium sulfate
(2) indomethicin *– ↑ fetal effects*
— (3) ritodrine
(4) ethanol

18. Pregnancy complicated by insulin-dependent diabetes prior to gestation has the following additional complications:

— (1) increase in fetal congenital anomalies
— (2) increased cesarean section rate
— (3) increased incidence of preeclampsia/eclampsia
— (4) increase in fetal respiratory distress syndrome

19. In caring for a mother with diabetes, which of the following are important means of fetal surveillance? B

→ (1) accurate dating of pregnancy
✗ (2) fasting serum glucose at 100 mg/dL *60-90 mg/dL*
→ (3) biweekly NSTs after 34 weeks
✓ (4) maternal 24-hour urinary estriol excretion

20. A 32-year-old woman has been followed by her gynecologist for secondary infertility, her last pregnancy having been 8 years earlier. Her preliminary infertility work-up reveals she is ovulating and her husband's fertility work-up is within normal limits. Her history reveals a past use of an intrauterine device (IUD) that was removed 2 years previously because of an episode of PID. She undergoes a laparoscopy. What would be the expected findings at the time of surgery? C

(1) pelvic endometriosis
— (2) peritubular adhesions
(3) ovarian cysts *– doesn't cause infertility*
— (4) bilateral hydrosalpinx

21. A 35-year-old woman undergoes a dilation and curettage for irregular menstrual bleeding. The endometrial curettings are consistent with the secretory phase of the menstrual cycle. With this information, which of the following is a correct statement about this patient? D

(1) The patient is entering premature menopause.
(2) The endometrium is under predominantly estrogen stimulation.
(3) The patient is taking oral contraceptives.
→ (4) The patient has ovulated.

DIRECTIONS (Questions 22 through 44): Each of the numbered items in this section is followed by answers or by completions of the statement. Select the ONE lettered answer or completion that is BEST in each case.

Questions 22 through 44

22. When reviewing the events of a patient's labor, what is the most predictive factor in determining whether she will develop a postoperative infection after cesarean section?

(A) history of previous cesarean section
(B) whether cesarean section was an emergency
(C) duration of labor prior to cesarean
(D) presence of medical complications, such as preeclampsia or diabetes
(E) malpresentation of fetus, such as breech or transverse lie

Would be early 7 decels

23. On postop day number 5, a patient has persistent spiking temperature despite triple antibiotics for 48 hours. She is also found to be tachypneic and tachycardic. What is the most important postop complication to rule out?

    (A) pneumonia
    (B) tubo-ovarian abscess
    (C) endomyometritis
    (D) sepsis
    (E) pulmonary embolus

24. A 36-year-old woman with two previous full-term pregnancies presents for her first prenatal visit at 12 weeks' gestation. What tests must she be advised to undergo?

    (A) immediate high-resolution ultrasound
    (B) genetic amniocentesis
    (C) maternal serum alpha-fetoprotein at present visit
    (D) amniocentesis for chromosomal abnormalities at 24 weeks
    (E) chromosomal analysis of herself and of the father of the baby

25. A 27-year-old black female with chronic hypertension is being monitored during the active phase of labor. Late decelerations are noted on the monitor. What can be summarized from such a fetal heart rate pattern?

    dx'd by- hyperreflexia & - proteinuria - generalised edema

    (A) The patient has developed superimposed preeclampsia.
    (B) The patient has placenta previa. *fetal bradycardia + vag bld'g*

    (C) The decelerations are secondary to head compression and are of no significance.
    (D) There is evidence on the fetal heart tracing of placental insufficiency.
    (E) The patient should undergo a pelvic exam to rule out cord prolapse. *variable (4 cord pattern)*

26. The tracing shown in Figure 7–2 was obtained on a 23-year-old woman at 41½ weeks during antepartum testing. The tracing can be described as

    (A) suspicious for fetal compromise
    (B) a reactive nonstress test
    (C) a negative oxytocin challenge test
    (D) a fetal heart pattern consistent with a cord pattern
    (E) an indication that the patient must be wrong on her dates of conception

27. A patient is admitted to labor and delivery with contractions every 4 minutes, lasting 45 seconds. On admission, her pelvic exam revealed a 4 cm dilated cervix. One hour later, her cervix was 5 cm dilated. Which of the following is an accurate statement about her labor pattern?

    (A) The fetal presentation should be determined because breech presentation progresses rapidly.
    (B) An intrauterine pressure catheter should be placed to determine intensity of uterine contractions.
    (C) If this is a first pregnancy, she is making good progress.

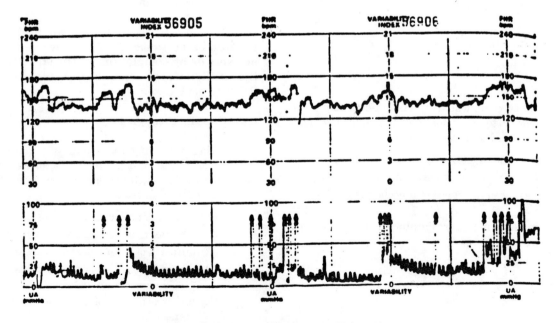

Fig. 7–2. A 23-year-old woman at 41½ weeks.

(D) This is adequate progress for the latent phase of labor.

(E) She has entered her second stage of labor.

28. A 38-year-old female presents to her family practitioner with complaints of irritability, weight gain, lower abdominal swelling, and difficulty concentrating, which she notes occurs 7 to 10 days before her period begins and resolves on the second or third day of her cycle. She stopped using birth control pills at age 35 and she feels the symptoms have gotten progressively worse since that time. When symptomatic, she is not able to function on her job. Her periods have remained regular every 28 days. What is the most likely cause of her symptoms?

(A) premature ovarian failure

(B) secondary dysmenorrhea

(C) polycystic ovary syndrome

(D) premenstrual syndrome

(E) depression

29. A large baby, 9½ pounds, is delivered with midforceps to a 32-year-old patient. The placenta delivered spontaneously without difficulty. The uterus appears to be well contracted with pitocin, but the patient continues to bleed vaginally, presenting bright, red blood. What is the most likely cause of this persistent bleeding?

(A) retained placental products

(B) lacerations of the cervix or vagina

(C) previously undiagnosed coagulopathy

(D) bleeding is from a rectal tear, secondary to the forceps

(E) uterine atony

30. A 27-year-old woman presents in labor at term with a history of a previous cesarean section for cephalopelvic disproportion. What is the most important historical information needed prior to attempting vaginal delivery after a cesarean?

(A) birth weight of previous baby

(B) length of labor in previous pregnancy

(C) strength of contractions in present labor

(D) uterine incision in previous cesarean section

(E) the number of previous cesarean sections

31. At 11 weeks' gestation, a patient presents to the emergency room with a complaint of vaginal bleeding and lower abdominal cramping. On pelvic exam, there is a large amount of blood in the vagina, and placental tissue present in the os. This describes which kind of spontaneous abortion?

(A) inevitable

(B) septic

(C) missed

(D) incomplete

(E) induced

32. A 17-year-old female presented at the GYN clinic, requesting an abortion. She is presently 10 weeks pregnant. What would be the safest, most efficient means of abortion at this time?

(A) intra-amniotic saline injection

(B) suction curettage after cervical dilation with prostaglandin suppository

(C) hysterotomy

(D) dilation and curettage

(E) administration of IV oxytocin

33. At 16 weeks' gestation, a patient presents with a complaint of vaginal bleeding. Her quantitative beta-HCG is higher than expected at 16 weeks' gestation, and her fundal height is approximately 16- to 18-week size. Although she denies a past history of hypertension, her blood pressure is 140/90. No fetal heart sounds can be heard on doptone and there is no sign of a fetus on ultrasound. What would be her most likely diagnosis?

(A) threatened abortion

(B) incomplete abortion

(C) hydatidiform mole

(D) fetal demise at 16 weeks

(E) twin gestation

34. A 28-year-old patient presents to labor and delivery at 38 weeks with a history of sudden onset of sharp pain in her lower abdomen and back, which has since subsided. On evaluation, her blood pressure is 150/100, and there is no detectable fetal heart movement on ultrasound. She also complains of profuse vaginal bleeding. As observed on the fetal monitor, she is having frequent contractions. What is the most likely cause of fetal demise?

(A) placenta previa

(B) gestational diabetes

(C) disseminated intravascular coagulopathy

(D) placental abruption

(E) chronic renal failure

35. A woman at 20 weeks' gestation is diagnosed with fetal demise. She has elected to await the onset of spontaneous labor. What blood test should be drawn at this time to avoid a major complication of intrauterine fetal demise?

(A) beta-HCG

(B) PT, PTT, and fibrinogen

(C) liver function test

(D) CBC

(E) prolactin level

36. At 42 weeks' gestation, a patient's labor is induced. At 5 cm dilated, she undergoes an artificial rupture of membranes with very little fluid present. What other characteristic of a postdate pregnancy might be present at the time of rupture of membranes?

(A) chorioamnionitis
(B) blood-tinged fluid
(C) vernix present in fluid
(D) meconium-stained fluid
(E) hyperstimulation of uterine contractions

37. At a prenatal clinic, a 32-year-old patient presents at 26 weeks' gestation. On history, you find her first child weighed 9½ pounds. Her second child was stillborn. What screening test would you order at this time?

(A) alpha-fetoprotein
(B) VDRL
(C) blood type and Rh
(D) 50-g glucose challenge
(E) toxoplasmosis titers

38. A 29-year-old patient presents to the emergency room at 17 weeks' gestation with a complaint of right upper quadrant and right lower quadrant pain of 6 hours duration. The pain is associated with nausea and vomiting. On exam, she has diffuse abdominal tenderness and decreased bowel sounds, and her fundal height is consistent with dates and is nontender. She has no CVA tenderness. Her temperature is 102.4°F and the WBC count on CBC is 18,000. Her urinalysis shows no WBCs or proteinuria. What is the most likely diagnosis?

(A) hyperemesis gravidarm
(B) acute appendicitis
(C) pylonephritis
(D) unilateral PID
(E) degenerating myomata

39. Complications secondary to anesthesia are one of the most common causes of maternal mortality. The most life-threatening complication of general anesthesia in the pregnant woman is

(A) hypotension
(B) atelectasis
(C) aspiration
(D) uterine atony
(E) eclampsia

40. A 24-year-old patient presents to a GYN clinic for a routine exam. Her OB/GYN history is significant for having her first child at age 16 and her second at age 18. Since separation from her husband at age 19, she has had several sexual partners. On pelvic exam, she has condylomata acuminata on her labia. What gynecologic neoplasm is this woman at risk for?

(A) ovarian cancer
(B) AIDS
(C) endometrial cancer
(D) cervical cancer
(E) cancer of the labia

41. A 23-year-old patient presents to planned parenthood, requesting birth control. Her GYN history is significant for several sexual partners, a recent episode of PID secondary to chlamydia, and one induced abortion. Which of the following forms of birth control would you be least likely to recommend for her use?

(A) contraceptive sponges
(B) intrauterine device
(C) oral contraceptives
(D) diaphragm
(E) condoms

42. A 30-year-old patient complains of progressively worse dysmenorrhea. Her pain begins 2 to 4 days prior to onset of bleeding and is associated with spotting. Additionally, she complains of pain on intercourse (dyspareunia). You think the patient may have endometriosis. What is the best way to make the diagnosis?

(A) a 6-month course of danazol (Danocrine) to see whether the symptoms subside
(B) pelvic ultrasound
(C) treatment with prostaglandin synthetase inhibitors to see if the symptoms abate
(D) diagnostic laparoscopy
(E) diagnostic hysteroscopy

43. Which menstrual irregularity would most likely occur in a woman suffering from anorexia nervosa or in a woman who is a marathon runner?

(A) menorrhagia
(B) amenorrhea
(C) oligomenorrhea
(D) polymenorrhea
(E) metrorrhagia

44. A 25-year-old woman presents with a history of prolonged episodes of amenorrhea followed by prolonged bleeding. She has been sexually active for 6 years and has never conceived. On physical exam, she is obese and somewhat hirsute. On pelvic exam, her ovaries are enlarged bilaterally. The most likely diagnosis is

   (A) progesterone-secreting tumor on the ovaries
   (B) hyperprolactinemia syndrome
   (C) congenital adrenal hyperplasia
   (D) polycystic ovary syndrome
   (E) hypothyroidism

DIRECTIONS (Questions 45 through 52): Each set of items in this section consists of a list of lettered options followed by several numbered words or phrases. For each numbered word or phrase, select the ONE lettered option that is most closely associated with it. Each lettered option may be selected once, more than once, or not at all.

Questions 45 through 48

For the number of weeks of gestation, match the events of pregnancy that occur at the time of pregnancy.

   (A) 6 weeks
   (B) 28 weeks
   (C) 20 weeks
   (D) 16 to 20 weeks
   (E) 14 weeks

45. Fundal height at umbilicus C

46. Fetal movements first perceived by mother D

47. Gestational sac first seen on sonogram (abdominal) A

48. Optimal time to draw maternal serum alpha-feto-protein D

Questions 49 through 52

The following are a list of drugs. Match the known side effects if ingested by a pregnant woman.

   (A) alcohol
   (B) nitrofurantoin
   (C) coumadin
   (D) cocaine
   (E) phenytoin *DILANTIN - Seizure med.*

49. Anomalies are caused by the drug's effect on the fetal clotting factors C

50. Higher incidence of stillborns secondary to placental abruptions when this drug is used during second and third trimesters

51. Taken in large amounts causes definitive syndrome in the fetus, but unsure if occasional use causes fetal harm A

52. The maternal benefits of this drug outweigh the known fetal effects E

DIRECTIONS (Questions 53 through 73): For each of the items in this section, ONE or MORE of the numbered options is correct. Choose answer

   (A) if only (1), (2), and (3) are correct,
   (B) if only (1) and (3) are correct,
   (C) if only (2) and (4) are correct,
   (D) if only (4) is correct,
   (E) if all are correct.

Questions 53 through 73

53. A 62-year-old female who is 12 years postmenopausal complains of urinary urgency, frequency, and occasional incontinence. On pelvic exam, she has a urethral carbuncle and her vaginal mucosa appears atrophic: shiny, pale pink with white patches, and bleeds slightly to touch. Her urinalysis and urine cultures are negative. How would you best treat this patient?

   (1) antibiotic by mouth
   (2) testosterone cream to be applied to affected areas
   (3) vaginal suppositories containing sulfa antibiotics
   (4) estrogen-containing cream per vagina

54. A 26-year-old female who is G2P2 and whose LMP was 8 weeks earlier presents to the emergency room with a complaint of lower abdominal pain and vaginal bleeding described as spotting. Her vital signs are stable and on abdominal exam she has good bowel sounds and no tenderness. On pelvic exam, she has mild cervical motion tenderness and a 6- to 8-week size uterus. Her serum beta-HCG is positive and her hematocrit is 39. You suspect a threatened abortion but want to rule out ectopic pregnancy. What would be the next appropriate step?

   (1) pelvic ultrasound with vaginal probe (if available)
   (2) diagnostic laparoscopy
   (3) serial quantitative beta-HCG
   (4) exploratory laparotomy

55. A 31-year-old female G1P1 presents to the emergency room with lower abdominal pain, vaginal bleeding, and a 6-week history of amenorrhea. Her GYN history is significant for history of oral contraceptive use in the past and having undergone an uncompleted induced abortion. Additionally, she has had an episode of PID and subsequent secondary infertility. Eight months prior to admission, she underwent a laparotomy for microsurgery on her fallopian tubes in an attempt to correct her infertility. A culdocentesis performed in the emergency room was positive for blood, and exploratory laparotomy revealed an ectopic pregnancy. What risk factors did this patient have for developing an ectopic pregnancy?

(1) a history of an induced abortion

(2) a history of PID

(3) a history of oral contraceptive use

(4) a history of tubal surgery

56. A 19-year-old G0P0 female presents to the emergency room with a complaint of lower abdominal pain, vomiting, and fever of 2 days' duration. Her last period was normal and ended 3 days prior to the onset of pain. On physical exam, her temperature was 103°F, and she had decreased bowel sounds and bilateral lower abdominal tenderness with rebound tenderness. On pelvic exam, she had marked cervical motion tenderness and bilateral adnexal tenderness. The diagnosis of PID was made and the patient was admitted for IV antibiotic therapy. Which of the following organisms could be responsible for the infection?

(1) *Neisseria gonorrhoeae*

(2) anaerobic bacteria such as *Bacteroides*

(3) *Chlamydia trachomatis*

(4) *Clostridium difficile*

57. A 22-year-old G2P2 presents to the GYN clinic with a history that her boyfriend had a positive culture for gonorrhea. She complains only of a vaginal discharge. On abdominal exam, she has mild bilateral lower abdominal tenderness, and on pelvic exam, a mucopurulent discharge from the cervix and mild cervical motion tenderness. She appears to have mild PID and because she could tolerate medication by mouth, she is treated on an outpatient basis. Which of the following regimens are adequate treatment for outpatient PID?

(1) vibramycin 100 mg bid PO

(2) 2.4 million U procaine penicillin IM with probenicid and erythromycin 25 mg PO for 7 days

(3) trimethoprim-sulfamethoxazole, 2 tabs PO bid for 7 days

(4) ceftriaxone 250 mg IM for one dose, and doxycycline 100 mg PO bid for 10 days

58. A 29-year-old G3P1Ab2 female is seen in the emergency room with a 24-hour history of bilateral lower abdominal pain, right greater than left. She complains of slight nausea and has had one episode of vomiting. She is sexually active and uses only condoms for birth control. Her last period was lighter than normal. Her past gynecologic history is significant for one previous episode of PID. Her abdominal exam reveals slightly decreased bowel sounds and mild bilateral tenderness without rebound tenderness. On pelvic exam, she has moderate cervical motion tenderness and fullness in her right adnexa. Her temperature is 38.2°C, and WBC on CBC is 14,000. She is admitted with a diagnosis of PID, but which of the following should also be considered in this patient?

(1) acute appendicitis

(2) adenexal torsion

(3) ectopic pregnancy

(4) ruptured tubal ovarian abscess

59. A 24-year-old female presents with a complaint of labial bumps that are painful when she urinates. On questioning the patient, she reveals she has felt feverish and has had generalized malaise. On pelvic exam, she has several vesicular lesions on the labia and a few ulcerative lesions. The lesions are painful to touch. Which of the following could be the cause of this patient's symptoms?

(1) condylomata acuminata

(2) secondary syphilis

(3) lymphogranuloma venereum

(4) herpes

60. A 42-year-old G2P2 female has a known history of uterine myomata that are approximately 14-week size. Within the past year, her periods have become progressively heavier and longer. A dilation and curettage performed 6 months earlier showed normal pathology and failed to decrease the bleeding. Which of the following are acceptable indications for hysterectomy in the patient?

(1) heavy uterine bleeding causing anemia

(2) the possibility of myomatas developing into cancer

(3) inability to adequately evaluate the size of the ovaries

(4) prevention of the development of pelvic adhesions

61. Endometrial hyperplasia is a pathology found in women with irregular menstrual bleeding. It is characterized by excessive growth of the endometrium, which is usually a result of a persistently high level of estrogen that is unopposed by progesterone. Which of the following women are likely to have endometrial hyperplasia?

    (1) a young woman suffering from anorexia nervosa

    (2) a 35-year-old woman with a long history of anovulatory cycles

    (3) a woman with a 10-year history of oral contraceptive use

    (4) an obese woman who has postmenopausal bleeding

62. On a routine pelvic examination, a 5-cm cystic mass is palpated on the left side of a 22-year-old female. Her last menstrual period was approximately 13 days prior to the exam. It is decided to give her birth control pills in an attempt to suppress ovarian function. Six weeks later, she is reexamined and the cyst is 10 cm in size. Which of the following would be the next step in treating this patient?

    (1) Continue birth control pills and reexamine the patient in 8 weeks.

    (2) Perform laparoscopy to determine whether the cyst is functional versus neoplastic.

    (3) Obtain ultrasound to rule out endometrioma.

    (4) Perform exploratory laparotomy in order to remove cyst.

63. A 19-year-old female who is sexually active and uses no form of birth control presents to the emergency room with a complaint of severe abdominal pain. Her last menstrual period (LMP) was approximately 6 weeks before the onset of the pain. She has a history significant for irregular periods. On abdominal exam, she has decreased bowel sounds and rebound tenderness. On pelvic exam, she has a small amount of dark red blood in her vagina and marked tenderness to cervical motion. Prior to bringing the patient to the operating room for an exploratory laparotomy, which tests below would be helpful in differentiating whether this patient has a ruptured corpus luteal cyst versus ectopic pregnancy?

    (1) hemoglobin and hematocrit

    (2) urinary pregnancy test sensitive to 25 mIU beta-HCG

    (3) white blood cell count on CBC

    (4) serum pregnancy test

64. A 63-year-old female who has had four spontaneous deliveries and a total abdominal hysterectomy for fibroids 15 years earlier, presents with a complaint of fullness in her vagina. Additionally, she has noted loss of urine with coughing or sneezing, which is getting progressively worse. On pelvic exam, she has a second-degree cystocele and when asked to valsalva, loses small amounts of urine. Which of the following would be adequate therapy for this patient?

    (1) Marshall–Marchetti–Kranz

    (2) placement of a vaginal pessary

    (3) anterior vaginal repair

    (4) repair of vesicovaginal fistula

65. A 40-year-old G3P3 woman goes to her gynecologist for a routine GYN exam. Which of the following are part of a routine gynecologic exam?

    (1) bimanual pelvic exam

    (2) breast exam

    (3) speculum exam of the cervix and vagina

    (4) abdominal exam

66. When performing a pelvic exam, it is important to

    (1) adequately drape the patient to avoid excessive exposure

    (2) insist that family members, including the patient's husband, leave the examining room

    (3) explain to the patient each step of the procedure

    (4) refrain from informing the patient that a particular part of the exam will be painful

67. When performing a pelvic exam, which cervical changes would be indicative of pregnancy?

    (1) a multiparous cervix

    (2) softening of the cervix

    (3) presence of Nabothian cysts on the cervix

    (4) bluish discoloration of the cervix

68. When obtaining a menstrual history, which of the following are important questions to ask?

    (1) duration and amount of menstrual flow

    (2) age of onset and frequency of menses

    (3) date of last menstrual period and whether it was normal

    (4) presence of intermenstrual bleeding

69. A 42-year-old female with a known history of uterine myomata presents with a complaint of increased bleeding during menses and spotting 4 to 5 days prior to onset of period. On pelvic exam, she has a 14-week size irregular uterus, consistent with fibroids. On speculum exam, there is a small polyp that can be seen in the endocervical canal. Which of the following would be an appropriate procedure for this patient to undergo next?

(1) endometrial biopsy with endocervical curettage

(2) ultrasound of the pelvis

(3) fractional dilation and curettage

(4) CAT scan of the pelvis

70. A 23-year-old crack abuser presents to the emergency room with a complaint of vaginal spotting and no period for 6 weeks. A pregnancy test is positive and her pelvis is consistent with a 6-week gestation. She is discharged with the diagnosis of threatened abortion. Two days later, she returns and miscarries. A VDRL drawn at the time of the initial visit is found to be positive. Upon questioning, the patient then remembers having a bump on her vulva approximately 4 weeks earlier. If the patient failed to get treatment at this time, which of the following symptoms would she then develop?

(1) maculopapular skin rash, often on the palms of the hands and soles of the feet

(2) generalized malaise, headaches, and anorexia

(3) condylomata lata on the vulva, thighs, and buttocks

(4) signs of PID

71. A 27-year-old G2P1Ab1 at 32 weeks' gestation presents to her obstetrician with a complaint of not feeling the baby move for 24 hours. On ultrasound, intrauterine fetal demise is confirmed: there is no sign of fetal movement and there is no fetal cardiac motion. The patient is induced and delivers spontaneously approximately 12 hours later. Which of the following are appropriate means of helping parents deal with the loss of the child?

(1) Allow the parents to hold and examine the stillborn child, if they choose.

(2) Heavily medicate the mother during labor and particularly the delivery, so she will have no recollection of the delivery.

(3) Photographs of the child should be taken and either given to the parents or kept on file for future viewing.

(4) Discourage the father (or other support person) from being present during labor and delivery to spare him the pain.

72. A 32-year-old G3P2Ab1 female at 40 weeks' gestation is being monitored in labor and develops the fetal heart rate depicted in Figure 7–3. Which of the following is true about this patient's tracing?

(1) These are late decelerations.

(2) It is indicative of a cord compression pattern.

(3) It shows fetal tachycardia.

(4) These are variable decelerations.

73. A 16-year-old female is seen in the emergency room as a rape victim. She undergoes a physical and pelvic exam. Prior to being discharged from the emergency room, she should be offered which of the following?

(1) follow-up visit in order to be tested for pregnancy and obtain a repeat VDRL

(2) information on how to contact a rape crisis counselor

(3) treatment for gonorrhea and chlamydia

(4) medication to prevent pregnancy

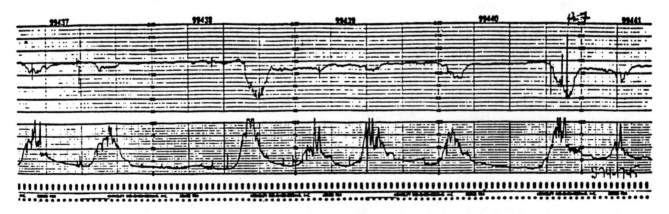

Fig. 7–3. A 32-year-old G3P2Ab1 female at 40 weeks' gestation.

Answers and Explanations

1. **(B)** Babies born to mothers with active hepatitis B and babies born to mothers who are chronic carriers (chronic HBsAg positive) have a high incidence of developing acute and chronic hepatitis, hepatoma, and cirrhosis. Treatment of these neonates is, therefore, necessary. Treatment consists of hyperimmune serum globulin (HBIG) and the hepatitis B vaccine (HBvac). These are both given at birth and the HBvac is given in two more doses, beginning at 1 month of age. *(Burrow and Ferris, p. 332)*

2. **(C)** Organisms that normally colonize the cervix and vagina act as pathogens in the upper genital tract postpartum or postop cesarean section. These organisms gain entrance to the upper tract during labor because of prolonged ruptured membranes and repetitive pelvic exams. The upper genital tract, primarily the endometrial cavity, is dark, vascular, and has necrotic decidua. It becomes, therefore, the ideal media for bacterial growth. *(Burrow and Ferris, p. 350; Hacker and Moore, pp. 295–297)*

3. **(A)** The patient's symptoms are describing a deep vein thombosis (DVT), a known complication in the pregnant and postpartum patient. The factors that increase the risk of DVT in a pregnant or recently pregnant woman are the hypercoagulable state of pregnancy. A number of blood coagulation factors rise during pregnancy. These include fibrinogen, factor VIII, factor VII, and other vitamin K-dependent clotting factors. During pregnancy, depression of the systemic fibrinolytic activity occurs, which returns to normal after delivery of the patient. In the puerperium, however, there are secondary rises of fibrinogen and circulatory platelets. Answers 2 and 3 are anatomical/mechanical reasons for increased chance of DVT Decreased blood flow from the lower extremities occurs secondary to the enlarged uterus and, because of decreased patient mobility, secondary to an operative delivery, such as forceps or cesarean section. *(Cunningham et al, p. 478; Hacker and Moore, p. 201)*

4. **(B)** Chills and fever occur with mastitis, as does the localization of an area of redness, hardening, and induration on the breast. Mastitis typically occurs during the third and fourth week postpartum. Postpartum breasts do become engorged within 24 to 48 hours, but it is bilateral without localized induration or erythema. Postpartum engorgement resolves spontaneously with support and application of ice packs. Mastitis does not cause breast milk to change color but the offending organism, *Staphylococcus aureus,* can be cultured from the breast milk. Treatment consists of an oral (or if necessary, parenteral) penicillinase-resistant antibiotic for 10 days. If an abscess has formed, incision and drainage may be necessary. *(Cunningham et al, p. 485)*

5. **(E)** As term approaches, the fetus assumes the longitudinal lie in the vertex presentation. The reason for vertex predominance is the piriform shape of the uterus. Although the fetal head is larger at term than the podalic pole, the breech and flexed extremities are bulkier and, therefore, adapt to the fundus better. Congenital anomalies, particularly anencephalic and hydrocephalic babies, will present more commonly as breech. Presumably, this is because the piriform-shaped uterus accommodates these anomalies more efficiently. Uterine anomalies such as bicornate and septate uterus predispose to breech presentation. Prior to 32 weeks, the amniotic cavity is larger and the amount of amniotic fluid is greater; therefore, more fetuses are in the breech presentation. Breech presentation is more common in grandmultiparous women because of relaxed uterine musculature. *(Cunningham et al, pp. 178–180,349)*

6. **(A)** Bartholin's glands are bilateral vulvovaginal glands which open into the posterolateral aspect of the vagina. When infected, it is often unilateral, the causative agent frequently being gonococcus. After the initial infection, the duct to the gland becomes scarred, and subsequently asymptomatic mucoid-filled cysts will recur or the duct will become reinfected. When a patient presents to the ER with acute swelling and severe pain, incision

and drainage can be performed in order to relieve the patient's discomfort. If the patient is not excessively uncomfortable, local treatment with warm soaks or ice can be attempted, with PO antibiotics. Definitive treatment is marsupialization of the gland, which is a means of creating a fistulous tract between the cyst and the skin. This will prevent the development of the chronic mucoid-filled cysts or possible reinfection. Marsupialization can be performed as an outpatient procedure in an operating room and is usually done after the acute episode has subsided, either due to I and D or local therapy. In hospital, IV antibiotics are never needed for Bartholin's abscess. *(Hacker and Moore, pp. 4,343; Jones et al, pp. 589–590)*

7. **(A)** There are several things the practitioner should do once it appears that the patient is bleeding heavily postdelivery. The first is to examine the patient for retained products by exploring the uterus manually and then examining the cervix and vagina for lacerations. Once lacerations have been ruled out, the practitioner should then attempt manually to contract the uterus and to administer medication that will cause uterine contractions. Oxytocin is usually given first and if the uterus does not respond, ergonovine or methylergonovine should be administered. The ergotrates cause sustained uterine contractions and are, therefore, more efficacious but can cause hypertension and hence are contraindicated in some cases. A prostaglandin derivative, prostaglandin F2 alpha, has recently been used intramuscularly (or intrauterine) and has been found to be efficacious once oxytocin and ergotrates have failed. Packing of the uterus had been used as a means of controlling postpartum hemorrhage but was found to be ineffective and dangerous because of concealed hemorrhage. As with any situation when there is the potential for shock to develop, the patient's cardiovascular status should be monitored. At least one, if not two, large-gauge IV catheters should be placed, and specimens for blood cross-match should be obtained. *(Cunningham et al, 417–419; Hacker and Moore, pp. 292–293).*

8. **(D)** *Chlamydia trachomatis* is an obligate intracelluar bacterium. It is very difficult to culture; therefore, monoclonal antibody tests are performed and are felt to be almost as accurate as cultures. Cervical infection at the time of delivery will often result in neonatal chlamydial conjunctivitis or neonatal pneumonia. Chlamydial infection in the mother has also been implicated in the development of preterm birth and preterm premature rupture of membranes. It is, therefore, important to test every patient on her first prenatal visit and to treat positive results. Chlamydia is very sensitive to tetracycline and doxycycline but these medications are never used during pregnancy

since they are teratogenic. Erythromycin is the drug of choice; it is safe to use in pregnancy and the organism is sensitive to it. Bactrim has some effect on chlamydia but is not used as a first-line medication in pregnancy. Ceftriaxone is not very effective against chlamydia. Women at greater risk for having chlamydia are young women under the age of 20, those of lower socioeconomic status, patients with several sexual partners, and patients who have or have had other sexually transmitted diseases. *(Cunningham et al, pp. 853–854; Gabbe et al, pp. 1274–1275; Hacker and Moore, p. 185)*

9. **(C)** The patient's condition is describing an incompetent cervix. Patients with an incompetent cervix typically present in the second trimester with the complaint of spotting and a bulging feeling in their vagina. They do not complain of painful contractions. On pelvic exam, there is cervical dilation with the membranes bulging through the os in an hourglass configuration. Although the exact cause of incompetent cervix is not known, it has been associated with previous cervical trauma, including dilation and curettage, conization, and cautery of the cervix. Abnormal cervical development has been noted as one of the genital tract abnormalities that occur in women whose mothers were exposed to diethylstilbestrol (DES). Incompetent cervix is known to occur in these women. A previous first trimester abortion is not associated with a higher incidence of incompetent cervix. Babies born to women with incompetent cervix do not have a chromosomal abnormality. *(Cunningham, pp. 498–499)*

10. **(B)** Gestational trophoblastic neoplasia (GTN) consists of benign GTN, most often hydatidiform mole, and malignant GTN, which includes nonmetastatic and metastatic GTN. Approximately 20% of women who have a hydatidiform mole will go on to develop some form of malignant GTN, one of which is choriocarcinoma. To best detect these patients, serum beta-HCG tests are drawn every 1 to 2 weeks until they are negative. Additionally, a woman who has had a mole should not become pregnant for 1 year, as pregnancy would interfere with the means of following the trophoblastic disease. Oral contraceptives are a safe and most efficient means of preventing pregnancy. Once beta-HCG levels are negative, the patient needs to be followed monthly for 6 months and then every 2 months for 1 year. Should the level of HCG plateau or begin to rise, the patient should undergo further work-up and eventually receive chemotherapy. In nonmetastatic GTN, single-agent chemotherapy is effective with either methotrexate or actinomycin D. Prophylactic chemotherapy was considered a possibility in some centers, but morbidity and mortality associated with therapy did not outweigh the benefits. A radical hysterec-

tomy is not indicated for any stage of GTN, but hysterectomy at the time of diagnosis of a hydatidiform mole is acceptable for a woman who has finished childbearing. It is not necessary to remove the adnexa, but it is still necessary to follow beta-HCG levels to detect possible metastatic trophoblastic tissue. *(Cunningham et al, pp. 540–553; Neshein, pp. 1–7)*

11. (D) Polyhydramnios or hydramnios is excessive amniotic fluid. In most cases of mild polyhydramnios, there is no etiology, but moderate to severe hydramnios is usually associated with fetal anomalies. The anomalies are primarily those of the central nervous system, which includes anencephaly and gastrointestinal anomalies, such as esophogeal atresia. These anomalies are easily diagnosed on ultrasound. Other conditions in which hydramnios occurs are diabetes, immune and nonimmune hydrops, and in one twin of a twin gestation. A large ovarian cyst may be found in a woman with a greater than expected fundal height, but would not be found concurrently with polyhydramnios. Calcification of the placenta occurs with postdate pregnancy or in intrauterine growth retardation, both of which are usually associated with oligohydramnios. *(Cunningham et al, pp. 554–556)*

12. (A) It is more likely that preeclampsia will develop in twin gestations; it usually occurs earlier in gestation and is more severe. Congenital anomalies of one or both twins is more common in multiple as compared to single gestations. Frequently, hydramnios accompanies the anomalous twin. Intrauterine growth retardation occurs secondary to intrauterine crowding and subsequent placental insufficiency. The growth retardation can be in both twins or one alone. When there is a significant difference in the growth of a twin, it is called discordancy. Because of the higher perinatal mortality rate in discordant twins, nonstress testing and frequent ultrasound examinations are performed in order to detect discordant growth at an early stage. Other complications of twin gestation are a higher incidence of cesarean section secondary to malpresentation, postpartum hemorrhage secondary to uterine atony, maternal anemia, and a higher incidence of spontaneous abortion. *(Cunningham et al, pp. 629–647; Hacker and Moore, pp. 244–249).*

13. (C) Magnesium plasma levels of 4 to 7 mEq/L are known to prevent eclamptic seizures. When the levels are above 10 mEq/L, respiratory depression develops. It is, therefore, advantageous to follow plasma levels periodically, approximately every 8 hours, to prevent toxicity. A clinical means of monitoring magnesium levels is to follow the intensity of patellar deep tendon reflexes. Preeclampsia tends to be a hyperstimulatory state;

thus, the deep tendon reflexes tend to be hyperreflexic. Magnesium sulfate has a depressive effect upon this hyperreflexia; it, therefore, becomes a good bedside means of monitoring magnesium levels. If patellar reflexes return to normal, it can be presumed that the magnesium levels are within the therapeutic but not toxic level. Loss of patellar reflexes is associated with plasma levels of greater than 10 mEq/L and impending respiratory depression. Although administration of MgSO4 will cause decreased fetal heart rate variability, this is not an adequate or consistent means of monitoring plasma levels. Because MgSO4 has only a minimal effect on lowering blood pressure, it is not a good means of monitoring levels. *(Cunningham et al, pp. 681–682)*

14. (A) The figure in the sonogram is showing a complete placenta previa. The sonogram is the most definitive means of diagnosing a placenta previa. A bimanual exam would be completely contraindicated, as it would result in severe hemorrhage secondary to digital disruption of the placental site. A sterile speculum exam can be performed if done in an environment where emergency cesarean section is readily available. Because the patient is 37 weeks, there would be no reason to treat the patient conservatively with IV fluids and bedrest. If the patient is preterm and active bleeding has subsided, it is possible to treat conservatively. The patient would then remain on strict bedrest, avoid use of tampons and douching, and refrain from sexual intercourse. If the previa is partial or low-lying and the patient is preterm, conservative treatment may result in avoiding cesarean section; as gestation progresses, the placenta may move away from the cervical os. A vaginal delivery would be completely contraindicated in the instance presented in the question because it is a complete previa at 37 weeks and there is no chance that the placenta would migrate upwards. A repeat cesarean section would be the only reasonable course of action in this case. The patient's history of previous cesarean is the probable etiology of the placenta previa. Previas are more common in women who have undergone previous cesarean sections, multiparous patients, and patients of advanced maternal age. *(Cunningham et al, pp. 712–714)*

15. (C) The accurate diagnosis of spontaneous rupture of membranes is important to ascertain if the patient has not yet begun labor (premature rupture of membranes) or if the patient is in premature gestation, prior to 37 weeks (preterm premature rupture of membranes). In order to evaluate a patient for spontaneous rupture of membranes, the patient must be in the dorsal lithotomy position. A sterile speculum examination is performed. Evidence of rupture of membranes would be clear or blood-tinged fluid in the posterior fornix of the vagina, or "pooling," and escape of clear fluid from the cervical os when the patient coughs. The fluid is then checked with nitrazine paper. Because amniotic fluid is basic with a pH of approximately 7.0 to 7.5 and vaginal secretions are 4.5 to 5.5, it can be surmised that if fluid obtained from the vagina turns nitrazine paper blue (indicative of a higher pH), it is amniotic fluid. Ferning is also a phenomenon of the basic amniotic fluid in the acidic vagina. A ferning pattern is seen on the glass slide when placed under the light microscope. Although in preterm rupture of membranes, it is important to obtain amniotic fluid from the vaginal fornix for lecithin/sphingomyelin (L/S) ration, L/S is an indication of fetal lung maturity, not a test for the presence or absence of ruptured membranes. Ultrasound determination of amniotic fluid volume is an important means of evaluating premature and preterm rupture of membranes, but it is not a means of diagnosing rupture of membranes. (For instance, in postdate pregnancies, intrauterine growth retardation, and fetal congenital anomalies, amniotic fluid is decreased but is not secondary to rupture of membranes.) (Cunningham et al, pp. 309,557–558; Gregg, pp. 241–247)

16. **(B)** The major risk involved in conservative management of preterm rupture of membranes is the onset of chorioamnionitis, which increases both maternal and fetal morbidity and mortality. Babies born after the onset of chorioamnionitis have a higher rate of respiratory distress, neonatal sepsis, and intraventricular hemorrhage. The maternal complications are endomyometritis and sepsis. Vaginal delivery is the preferred route of delivery, but because of malpresentation of the preterm fetus, there is usually a higher incidence of cesarean section. The diagnosis of chorioamnionitis is difficult. Usually by the time the mother has developed a fever greater than 38°C, the infection is already well established. An increase in the maternal white blood cell count on CBC is also used to predict the onset of chorioamnionitis, but has not been found to be a consistent indicator of the development of infection. In preterm premature rupture of membranes, premature delivery and the subsequent complications of hyaline membrane disease and intraventricular hemorrhage, are the most common causes of fetal morbidity and mortality. Therefore, in the absence of labor, obvious signs of infection, or fetal distress, conservative management is recommended. Since approximately one half of cases of neonatal sepsis occurs without overt signs of chorioamnionitis, maternal and fetal surveillance should be performed daily during conservative therapy. Fetal surveillance should include nonstress test (NST) and biophysical profile. A cord pattern or variable decelerations, not late decelerations, would be a likely find-

ing on NST. A sustained fetal tachycardia and/or a nonreactive NST are indicative of chorioamnionitis and ominous fetal outcome. Loss of fetal breathing movements, and severe oligohydramnios on biophysical profile are also predictive of chorioamnionitis and neonatal sepsis. Spontaneous rupture of membranes is not possible with a complete previa, as the os is covered with placenta. (Cunningham et al, p. 751; Klein, pp. 265–276; Vintzileos, pp. 281–307)

17. **(B)** Magnesium sulfate and ritodrine are two of the more commonly used tocolytic agents. The presumed effect of magnesium is that it works as an antagonist to calcium at the myometrial level. MgSO4 is given in the same dose for preterm labor as in preeclampsia: a 4-g loading dose followed by 2 g/hr. Obviously, it also has the same side effects, primarily respiratory depression. Ritodrine is a beta-adrenergic agonist. Its effect is on the adrenergic receptors of the smooth muscle of the myometrium to decrease its contractile potential. Ritodrine also has some beta-one activity; it, therefore, can cause maternal tachycardia and subsequent chest pain, and ECG changes consistent with ischemia. It can also cause pulmonary edema and hyperglycemia. Terbutaline, another beta-adrenergic agonist, is also very commonly used as a first-line drug for tocolysis; it has similar side effects as ritodrine but these side effects tend to be clinically less severe. Since a significant number (approximately 20%) of patients with preterm contractions respond to bedrest and hydration, these measures should be instituted prior to the use of medications. Additionally, the presence of a UTI should be ruled out. If the UA is positive or signs and symptoms are present, antibiotics should be started. Cervical cultures should also be performed, since group B beta streptococcus, chlamydia, and possibly ureaplasma are implicated as causal factors to the onset of preterm labor. The ability to actually stop preterm labor with these tocolytic agents has been questioned. Some studies have shown no significant difference in preterm delivery when use of tocolytic agents is compared to conservative therapy of bedrest and hydration. Because prostaglandins are involved in the initiation of myometrial contractions and, therefore, of labor, the use of prostaglandin synthetase inhibitor drugs (such as indomethacin) can be used to arrest preterm labor. These medications have significant fetal effects and are, therefore, never used as initial means of tocolysis. The side effects are premature closure of the fetal ductus arteriosus and the development of oligohydramnios. Such medications are used only for short periods of time and only after other medications have been tried and failed. Additionally, patients must be followed with frequent sonographic evaluation of amniotic fluid and fetal echocardiogram.

Ethanol was once used intravenously to arrest labor, but its effect of intoxication, lethargy, and respiratory depression in the mother and fetus have since discouraged its use. *(Cunningham et al, pp. 756–758; Hacker and Moore, pp. 270–275).*

18. **(E)** Congenital anomalies are increased threefold in fetuses born to women who are diabetic prior to pregnancy. Clinicians feel that this rate is greatly decreased if the mother is in excellent diabetic control prior to conception. Congenital heart defects are the most common anomalies, followed by neural tube defects. Women with diabetes have a higher incidence of cesarean section delivery. A primary reason is the higher incidence of macrosomia and subsequent cephalopelvic disproportion as well as the possibility of shoulder dystocia. There is general disagreement about the timing of delivery of a diabetic woman. Many centers feel that women should be delivered prior to 40 weeks because of the higher incidence of intrauterine fetal demise after 36 weeks. Elective induction, especially with an unfavorable cervix, often leads to cesarean section. The cesarean section rate for diabetic women (gestational and pregestational) is approximately 50%. There is a fourfold increase in preeclampsia/eclampsia in women with overt diabetes and gestational diabetics with fasting hyperglycemia. Because the lungs of babies born to diabetic mothers mature at a later gestational age, they have an approximately five times greater chance of having respiratory distress syndrome. This makes elective delivery prior to 38 weeks a very difficult decision. Amniocentesis for lung maturity is often performed prior to elective delivery. An L/S ratio of greater than 2 has been found to be inaccurate in predicting fetal lung maturity in diabetic mothers. If present, phosphatidylglycerol (PG) is the best indicator of fetal lung maturity in diabetics. *(Cunningham et al, pp. 816–822)*

19. **(B)** Accurate dating of a pregnancy is very important in both gestational and overt diabetes. This is because of the need to begin fetal surveillance in the third trimester, the incidence of fetal macrosomia, the higher incidence of fetal respiratory distress syndrome, and the greater possibility of elective induction. An accurate LMP, pelvic exam in the first trimester, and early sonogram for dating purposes are helpful in accurately assessing gestational age. Because of the higher incidence of stillbirths, prenatal surveillance is begun as early as 28 to 30 weeks in diabetic mothers. This testing is usually in the form of nonstress test (NST), followed by an oxytocin challenge test if the NST is nonreactive. NST in diabetic pregnancy is found to be predictive of fetal well-being for only approximately 4 to 5 days and, therefore, is done on a biweekly basis. There is controversy over which means of fetal surveillance is most accurate

in diabetics; some centers advocate OCTs or biweekly biophysical profiles instead of NSTs. A fasting glucose of 100 mg/dL is too high for a diabetic mother. A fasting glucose should be between 60 and 90 mg/dL in order to maintain good control. The 1-hour postprandial glucose should be below 120. Twenty-four-hour urinary estriol determinations were previously used to monitor fetal well-being antenatally. It has been subsequently found to be an inaccurate and costly means of fetal surveillance. *(Cunningham et al, pp. 816–822; Hacker and Moore, pp. 204–208)*

20. **(C)** Laparoscopy is one of the final steps in a fertility work-up. Although tubal occlusion secondary to PID can be diagnosed on hysterosalpingogram, additional infertility-causing problems can be diagnosed on laparoscopy, particularly when dye (usually methylene blue or indigo carmine) is injected at the time of surgery. IUDs may cause peritubular adhesions that are responsible for decreased tubal functioning and, therefore, infertility. These adhesions can be seen only on laparoscopy. Because of this patient's history of PID, it is very likely that bilateral hydrosalpinx is the cause of secondary infertility diagnosed at laparoscopy. Pelvic endometriosis can only be diagnosed on laparoscopy and does cause peritubular adhesions and tubal occlusion. However, this patient's past history of PID makes endometriosis a less likely cause of infertility. Simple ovarian cyst seldom causes infertility. *(Jones et al, pp. 293–294)*

21. **(D)** In the normal menstrual cycle, the endometrium undergoes hormonal stimulation in preparation for implantation of the fertilized ovum. During the first half of the cycle, the endometrium is under the influence of estrogen, which is secreted from the developing follicle. This estrogen causes cellular proliferation of the endometrium, termed the proliferative phase. After ovulation, progesterone is secreted from the corpus luteum, and the effect of this hormone on the endometrium is to cause secretion of glycogen and mucus from the glandular cells. This phase is termed the secretory phase and is dependent upon the occurrence of ovulation with the subsequent development of a corpus luteum. This patient could not be going through premature menopause because she has ovulated. Because a secretory endometrium is secondary to progesterone stimulation, this patient's endometrium could not be predominantly under estrogen stimulation. The second choice is therefore incorrect. The third choice is also incorrect because oral contraceptives prevent ovulation and therefore the development of the corpus luteum and secretion of progesterone. *(Hacker and Moore, pp. 454–456; Jones et al, pp. 68–78)*

22. (C) Duration of labor prior to cesarean section is the most predictive factor in whether a patient develops a postoperative infection. It was previously believed that the number of pelvic exams while in labor and duration of rupture of membranes were equally predictive, but controlled studies showed that it was the length of labor that determined the number of pelvic exams and the possibility of ascending infection secondary to rupture of membranes. Although diabetes and other medical complications do affect incidence of postoperative infection, they are not the most causative. *(Burrow and Ferris, p. 350)*

23. (E) The diagnosis of pulmonary embolus is very difficult to make. The most common sign present is tachypnea. Pulmonary embolus is the most dangerous complication of DVT. It occurs approximately 5 to 7 times more frequently in women who have undergone cesarean section. A ventilation–perfusion scan is often the means of diagnosing a PE and is accurate, except in cases of obstructive or constrictive lung disease, heart failure, and pulmonary infiltrate. The definitive diagnosis can best be made on pulmonary angiography. An arterial blood gas is helpful in making the diagnosis. (A) would be a good possibility except that the patient with pneumonia should be responding to triple antibiotics. Tubo-ovarian abscess is infrequent as a complication of cesarean section. It is more commonly seen in PID that failed to respond to triple antibiotics after 48 hours. A patient with sepsis should respond to triple antibiotics. *(Cunningham et al, pp. 479–480; Hacker and Moore, pp. 201–202)*

24. (B) Age 35 has been arbitrarily designated as the age at which a mother must be advised to undergo genetic amniocentesis to rule out Down syndrome. The risk of an offspring with Down syndrome at age 30 is 1 in 885, whereas at age 35, it is 1 in 365; at age 40, it is 1 in 100, and at age 45, it is 1 in 35. Although a woman may decide against amniocentesis, it is the practitioner's responsibility to advise her of the incidence of Down syndrome in her age group and to refer her to available genetic counseling. Additional indications for genetic counseling and possible amniocentesis are previous history of a child born with a chromosomal abnormality; family history of a chromosomal abnormality or Down syndrome; high-risk for neural-tube defect: previous child or family member with NTD, elevated maternal serum alpha-fetoprotein, and family history of serious X-linked hereditary disorder. Chorionic villus sampling (CVS) can also be used for prenatal genetic diagnosis. It is performed between 9 and 12 weeks' gestation, thus allowing for earlier diagnosis, but it cannot be used to diagnose neural

tube defects. *(Cunningham et al, pp. 570–587; Hacker and Moore, pp. 94–101)*

25. (D) Late decelerations are a result of uteroplacental insufficiency. A late deceleration occurs when the fetal heart rate begins to slow after the onset of the contraction and returns to baseline after the contraction is completed. Late decelerations by definition must be repetitive and are often the consequence of fetal hypoxia and subsequent acidosis. Many maternal factors cause uteroplacental insufficiency and, therefore, intrauterine growth retardation. Some of these factors are severe preeclampsia, chronic hypertension, chronic renal disease, severe diabetes with vascular involvement, and heavy maternal smoking. Although it is very likely that a patient with chronic hypertension with superimposed preeclampsia might develop late decelerations, the diagnosis of superimposed preeclampsia cannot be made solely on a fetal heart rate pattern. The diagnosis would instead be made if the patient developed hyperflexia, proteinuria, and generalized edema, in addition to her chronic hypertension. A patient with placenta previa would more than likely develop vaginal bleeding and fetal bradycardia. Decelerations that are secondary to head compression are early decelerations and if they are not severe are of no consequence. A prolapsed cord would typically show a cord pattern (variable deceleration) or bradycardia on fetal monitoring. *(Cunningham et al, pp. 291,298,764–765)*

26. (B) A nonstress test is called reactive if there are two fetal heart rate accelerations accompanying a fetal movement within a 20-minute period. The fetal heart rate accelerations should be 15 beats per minute above the baseline, lasting for 15 seconds. A reactive nonstress test is a means of assuring fetal well-being in the antepartum period in a high-risk pregnancy. Indications for conducting antepartum testing are gestational or insulin-dependent diabetes, postdate pregnancy (starting between $40\frac{1}{2}$ weeks and 41 weeks), intrauterine growth retardation, preeclampsia, chronic hypertension, history of previous preterm delivery or stillbirth, and multiple gestations (ie, twins, triplets). Because this pattern is reactive, it is, therefore, not suspicious for fetal compromise. An oxytocin challenge test entails administration of oxytocin in order to cause contractions. There are no contractions on this tracing. A positive oxytocin challenge test is one in which late decelerations occur consistently with contractions and is indicative of some degree of fetal compromise. A negative OCT is one in which late decelerations do not occur consistently. Oxytocin challenge tests are performed when the NST is nonreactive or if on NST there are spontaneous contractions with late or suspicious decelerations. There is no way on fe-

nullip - 20h →4cm → 1.2/hr
multip - 14h →4cm → 1.5/hr

tal heart rate tracings to determine fetal age. A cord pattern would show variable decelerations, which do not appear on the above tracing. (*Cunningham et al, pp. 291–292,1291–1292*)

27. **(C)** A woman in labor with her first pregnancy should dilate 1.2 cm per hour once she has entered the active phase of labor. The active phase of labor is defined as the onset of rapid change in cervical dilation and usually occurs after reaching 4 cm dilation. A multiparous patient usually dilates 1.5 cm in the active phase. The latent phase precedes the active phase and is defined as the onset of regular uterine contractions, but with slow dilation of the cervix. In a nulliparous patient, the latent phase should last no longer than 20 hours; in multiparous women, approximately 14 hours. (A) is incorrect because it implies the situation is describing more rapid progress than normal, which is not true. (B) implies that progress is inadequate and therefore necessitating an intrauterine pressure catheter. (D) is also incorrect because the question does not describe the latent phase. (E) is incorrect because the second stage of labor is determined from full dilation until delivery of the baby. (*Burke, p. 31*)

28. **(D)** Premenstrual syndrome is made up of many different symptoms that are both physical and psychological. The most common symptoms are feeling bloated, weight gain, loss of efficiency, irritability, difficulty concentrating, tiredness, mood swings, and depression. A woman will experience the symptoms cyclically, in a repetitive relationship to her menses; they will also subside at the same time in her cycle. Symptoms can begin as early as the day of ovulation and end by at least the fourth day of menstrual flow. Women at risk for developing the syndrome are those with a family history, ages 35 to 45, and a history that the symptoms subsided during pregnancy or while taking ovulatory inhibiting medications such as birth control pills. Premenstrual syndrome is associated with ovulation; therefore, it would not occur in premature ovarian failure or polycystic ovary syndrome, both of which are anovulatory cycles. Secondary dysmenorrhea is pain which occurs with menses, but not exclusively. It often occurs in women in their thirties and forties, and is associated with clinical entities such as endometriosis, chronic PID, and adenomyosis. It does not have the behavioral and psychological features that premenstrual syndrome does. Clinical depression can be misdiagnosed as PMS; the primary means of differentiating the two is the association of PMS symptoms to the menstrual cycle. Women with a primary diagnosis of depression will have their symptoms throughout the cycle but can get worse just prior to menstruation. (*Hacker and Moore, pp. 334–337; Johnson, pp. 637-643*)

29. **(B)** The information in the question gives numerous reasons for postpartum bleeding. They are uterine overdistention secondary to a large baby, midforceps delivery and therefore the possibility of cervical tears, and multiparity, which predisposes to a less contractive uterus. The information given states, however, that the uterus is well-contracted; thus uterine atony would be an incorrect answer, as would retained products, because the placenta delivered spontaneously. Midforceps delivery is associated with a higher incidence of cervical and vaginal lacerations; therefore, careful inspection of the cervix and vagina should follow such a delivery. In the above incident, lacerations would be the most likely answer. Causes of excessive postpartum bleeding (postpartum hemorrhage) are overdistention of the uterus secondary to a large infant, polyhydramnios or multiple gestation, midforceps and rotation forcep delivery, delivery through an incompletely dilated cervix, the use of halothane anesthetics, which cause uterine relaxation, and finally, women who had very rapid or very slow dilation. Retained placenta and abnormally adherent placenta, such as placenta accreta, increta, or percreta are also causes of postpartum hemorrhage. Because the question states that the placenta delivered spontaneously, accreta could not be a likely cause. Previously undiagnosed coagulopathy might be a cause for postpartum hemorrhage but, in the above case, not the most likely. Rectal tears or fourth-degree lacerations are more common with forceps delivery but are usually easily repairable and, therefore, do not cause much bleeding. (*Cunningham et al, pp. 405–406,415–418,436*)

30. **(D)** Knowledge of the uterine scar is the most important factor in determining whether a patient is a candidate for vaginal delivery after a cesarean section. The safest and most commonly used incision is the lower segment transverse incision. A classical incision on the uterus is known to easily rupture during labor. The low transverse incision ruptures less than 2% of the time. Therefore, VDAC (vaginal delivery after cesarean) is contraindicated in patients who have a classical incision. It is questionable whether patients with a low vertical incision on the uterus should undergo a trial of labor. The incidence of spontaneous rupture is minimal, but greater than low transverse. Studies show there are no increased complications in women who undergo VDAC after more than one previous cesarean section. The indication for the primary cesarean section should not be a deterrent because the success rate of VDAC in patients with a recurrent indication, such as cephalopelvic disproportion or failure to progress, is approximately 60%. Length of labor and intensity of present contractions have no effect on the decision to allow a patient a trial of labor. (*Cunningham et al, pp. 408, 446*)

31. **(D)** Incomplete abortions are characterized by heavy vaginal bleeding and placental tissue present in a dilated cervical os. The bleeding is heavy because there has been incomplete separation of the placenta and, therefore, inadequate myometrial contraction of the blood vessels. Bleeding from an incomplete abortion can be severe enough to cause marked hypovolemia and shock. Inevitable abortion occurs when a patient has crampy abdominal pain and bleeding, and upon pelvic exam, the cervical os is partially open. Leaking membranes may be seen from the cervical os or the vaginal vault. Septic abortion occurs when the signs and symptoms of spontaneous abortion are accompanied by a temperature elevation of greater than 38°C. This diagnosis is made only after other sources of fever have been excluded, such as UTI. A missed abortion is one in which the fetus dies but the products of conception are retained. A patient typically notes loss of pregnancy signs, such as nausea, vomiting, and breast tenderness. On sequential pelvic exams, the uterus fails to enlarge and, in fact, will decrease in size. On ultrasound, there is no evidence of fetal viability, and it is often used to verify the diagnosis. Induced abortion is one in which the mother elects to terminate the pregnancy. (*Cunningham et al, p. 497; Hacker and Moore, pp. 416–421*)

32. **(B)** Suction curettage is the safest means of elective abortion in the first trimester. It is more efficient if preceded by a preliminary means of dilating the cervix. This can be accomplished with prostaglandin suppository in the vagina or with laminaria tents inserted into the cervix. Intraamniotic saline injection is infrequently used and only during the second trimester. Hysterotomy, dilation and extraction, and the use of oxytocin are reserved for second trimester abortions. The use of prostaglandin-induced labor for second trimester terminations has increased in frequency; the prostaglandins used are either E2 or F2 alpha and are used intra-amniotic or intravaginally. This method does entail that the patient go through labor and is associated with a high rate of retained placenta requiring manual removal. (*Cunningham et al, pp. 502–505; Hacker and Moore, pp. 421–424*)

33. **(C)** Hydatidiform mole is one component of gestational trophoblastic neoplasm (GTN). Moles occur in a gestation in which there is a proliferation of trophoblastic tissue. It can be a complete mole, in which there is no sign of a fetus, or a partial mole, in which the fetus may be viable, or there are findings consistent with a nonviable fetus. The most common symptom of hydatidiform mole is several episodes of vaginal bleeding. A size-to-dates discrepancy is also common. Approximately one-half of the patients are larger than dates and one-fourth are smaller. The trophoblast is responsible for production of human chorionic gonadotropin (HCG); therefore, the levels of beta-HCG in the serum are often greater than expected for the weeks of gestation. The occurrence of preeclampsia prior to 20 weeks is highly suggestive of hydatidiform mole. On ultrasound, there are very characteristic findings, and it is the best means of diagnosing a mole. (A) is incorrect because with a threatened abortion at 18 weeks, there should be fetal heart tones. An incomplete abortion usually occurs prior to 12 to 14 weeks and would more than likely have a decreasing beta-HCG level. A fetal demise at 16 weeks would also have decreasing beta-HCG levels and would not be associated with hypertension. In twin gestation, there would be a higher level of beta-HCG and a larger fundal height, but at 16 weeks, fetal heart tones should be heard. (*Cunningham et al, pp. 541–545; Hacker and Moore, p. 15*).

34. **(D)** Placental abruption is the separation of the placenta before delivery of the fetus. Separation can occur in various degrees, and it can be partial or complete. Abruption can be associated with vaginal bleeding or the bleeding may remain hidden within the uterus. If the separation is of a significant degree, the blood loss will be extensive because the uterus cannot contract down upon the torn vessels that supply the placenta. The baby's blood supply is subsequently disrupted and fetal death occurs. The mother is also severely affected. She will develop shock secondary to blood loss and also has a high chance of developing a consumptive coagulopathy. The coagulopathy is most often hypofibrinogenemia with elevation of fibrinogen-fibrin degradation products. Pregnancy-induced and chronic hypertension are often associated with placental abruption. It is also seen in trauma, short umbilical cord, sudden decompensation of the uterus, and uterine anomaly. Placenta previa does present at term with vaginal bleeding, but infrequently with fetal demise, and is not typically associated with hypertension. Gestational and nongestational diabetes is associated with a higher incidence of fetal demise at term, but the patient's presentation is more consistent with an abruption. Disseminated intravascular coagulopathy is a known complication of preeclampsia and abruption, but would probably not cause fetal demise without some other precipitating event, such as abruption. Chronic renal failure is associated with a higher incidence of fetal wastage but the case presented is more consistent with an acute occurrence. (*Cunningham et al, pp. 701–712*)

35. **(B)** A consumptive coagulopathy, primarily hypofibrinogenemia, occurs within 4 to 6 weeks of intrauterine fetal demise. It is felt to be secondary to the release of thromboplastin from the dead fetus. Because the products of conception tend to shrink

postdemise and labor is more effective if initiated on its own, a woman is allowed to await spontaneous labor if she so chooses. She must be monitored for the possibility of coagulopathy with weekly PT and PTT, plus fibrinogen and platelet counts. The use of prostaglandin E2 and F2 alpha has increased the number of women who have elected immediate termination, because it has greatly increased the success of induction of labor. The release of thromboplastin affects only the coagulation factors and, therefore, there should be no change in liver function tests. The hemoglobin and hematocrit levels would fall if the patient went into DIC, but that would occur significantly after the change in coagulation factors. Prolactin levels would have no effect upon the incidence of DIC post-fetal demise. *(Cunningham et al, pp. 716–719)*

36. **(D)** A pregnancy that progresses past 42 weeks is associated with increased fetal morbidity and mortality. One reason for the increased fetal risk is decreased amniotic fluid with subsequent cord compression. Cord compression may result in fetal distress, which in turn causes fetal defecation in utero and subsequently meconium-stained fluid. Because postdate pregnancies are associated with these complications and an increased risk of intrauterine demise, patients are monitored from 40½ weeks. This monitoring can be one or more of the following: nonstress testing, biophysical profile, or oxytocin challenge test. These tests have all been associated with high false-positive and false-negative results. In many cases, induction is performed at 42 weeks regardless of antepartum test results. Babies born after 42 weeks' gestation can either be large for dates, which increases the risk for failed induction, cephalopelvic dysproportion, and shoulder dystocia, or these babies can be growth-retarded. A growth-retarded fetus has a greater chance for stress during labor and, when born, appears as if it has lost weight, particularly muscle mass and subcutaneous fat. Chorioamnionitis does not occur more commonly with postdate pregnancy. In fact, it is more common with preterm delivery. Blood-tinged fluid is sometimes associated with partial placental abruption but is not a common finding in postdate pregnancy. The presence of vernix would indicate a preterm or term fetus. Rupture of membranes, either spontaneously or artificially, is usually followed by a greater intensity of contractions, but usually not hyperstimulation. *(Cunningham et al, pp. 759–763)*

37. **(D)** The optimal time to screen for gestational diabetes is between 24 and 28 weeks. In some patients, pregnancy is a diabetogenic state. Human placental lactogen is a hormone secreted by the placenta, with levels increasing during the latter half of pregnancy. This hormone has an anti-in-

sulin effect in the mother and, in predisposed patients, will cause glucose intolerance. The glucose challenge test (also called the 50-g glucola or O'Sullivan) is the most commonly employed screening test. It consists of taking 50 g of glucola in a nonfasting state, and having a plasma glucose drawn 1 hour later. If the plasma glucose is 135 to 140 mg/dL, the patient then must undergo a 3-hour glucose tolerance test. All pregnant women should undergo routine screening for gestational diabetes by 28 weeks. Women with a significant obstetric or family history should be screened at their first prenatal visit, even if it is before 28 weeks. Criteria for this screening are maternal age greater than 30, a family history of diabetes, a prior macrosomic baby, a baby with a congenital anomaly, or a stillborn. Women who are hypertensive or obese also have a higher incidence of gestational diabetes. Alpha-fetoprotein screening is only accurate between 15 to 20 weeks. Although women infected with syphilis have a high incidence of stillborns, hopefully they have undergone treatment after the first obstetric loss. Additionally, babies infected with syphilis are usually growth-retarded, not macrosomic. Rh-negative women should receive RhoGAM at 28 weeks, but their blood type and Rh should be drawn at the first prenatal visit. Babies that have congenital toxoplasmosis are generally smaller for gestational age, have microcephaly or hydrocephaly. *(Cunningham et al, pp. 617–619,812–816)*

38. **(B)** Acute appendicitis is the most important surgical diagnosis to rule out during pregnancy. It is also one of the most difficult diagnoses because the enlarging uterus displaces the appendix and, therefore, the location of pain. Additionally, many of the presenting complaints of appendicitis are common complaints of pregnancy, such as nausea, anorexia, and vomiting. A mild leukocytosis is also common in pregnancy, particularly during the third trimester. If the diagnosis of appendicitis is a serious consideration, the patient should undergo exploratory laparotomy. To delay would increase the occurrence of severe peritonitis, gangrene, spontaneous abortion, preterm labor, and increased maternal morbidity. Another possible surgical complication of pregnancy that could be present in the above patient is acute cholecystitis. Hyperemesis gravidarum would be an unlikely diagnosis because it is primarily a first-trimester phenomenon and is not associated with a fever or markedly elevated WBC count. If this patient had pyelonephritis, she would probably have costal vertebral angle (CVA) tenderness, and WBCs in the urine. If PID occurs at all during pregnancy, it is extremely rare and only before 12 weeks. Degeneration of uterine myomata does cause pain, mild leukocytosis, and slightly elevated temperature. Usually, however, it is not associated with

decreased bowel sounds, nausea, and vomiting, and ordinarily there is some uterine tenderness and a palpable myomata. *(Cunningham et al, pp. 831–832)*

39. **(C)** The aspiration of acidic gastric contents or undigested food particles will cause severe respiratory distress and possibly death. In order to prevent this complication, the mother should be fasting for 6 to 12 hours prior to general anesthesia, and medication to reverse gastric acidity should be administered immediately prior to intubation. Additionally, intubation should be performed with pressure on the cricoid cartilage to occlude the esophogus, and extubation should be performed with the mother awake and on her side. A true fasting state with minimal gastric contents is extremely difficult to achieve in obstetric patients. A woman seldom knows when she will begin labor and, more importantly, gastric emptying and peristalsis are delayed or inhibited at the onset of labor. Subsequently, all pregnant women should be treated as if they have a full stomach. In the fasting state, the stomach continues to secrete gastric juices that have a very low pH. To neutralize this pH, antacids are administered within 45 minutes of intubation. Maternal hypotension does not accompany general anesthesia, but is the major side effect of spinal and epidural anesthesia. Atelectasis frequently occurs within the first 24 hours after general anesthesia but is not life-threatening. If left untreated, in some instances atelectasis will progress to pneumonia. Three of the inhalation anesthetics used in obstetrics do cause uterine relaxation and in some cases uterine atony. These agents are halothane, enflurane, and isoflurane. They are used in conjunction with nitrous oxide and given in the smallest possible amounts to avoid this complication. Although uterine atony is associated with lower hematocrit postdelivery and greater chance of blood transfusion, these complications are not as life-threatening as aspiration. Eclampsia probably does not occur more with general anesthesia and, in fact, in severe preeclampsia/eclampsia, general anesthesia is the preferred means of anesthesia. *(Cunningham et al, pp. 329–339)*

40. **(D)** Cervical cancer and its precursor, cervical intraepithelial neoplasia (dyplasia), occur more often in women who are sexually active at an early age (before age 20) and who have multiple sexual partners. Originally, women who were married young and had children at a young age were considered at risk, but it is now felt that cervical cancer is due to sexual intercourse at an early age and multiple sexual partners. Women who smoke are also at a higher risk of developing cervical cancer. Infection has been considered a possible etiology of CIN. The most commonly implicated agent is the human papillomavirus (HPV), the same virus that causes condylomata accumulata. HPV types 6 and 11 are usually associated with benign lesions such as condylomata, whereas types 16 and 18 are associated with severe dysplasia and carcinoma in situ (CIN III). Although evidence is strong in suggesting HPV as having either a causative or exacerbative effect on neoplastic changes in the cervix, many women with CIN or invasive carcinoma have no evidence of the virus. Early sexual relationships and multiple partners have not been a historical finding in women who develop ovarian or endometrial cancer. In fact, endometrial cancer is more common in nulliparous women. Labial cancer occurs at a much later age than the above gynecologic neoplasms. AIDS is not considered a cancer but a woman with CIN should be counseled for AIDS, since some of the risk factors for developing AIDS and CIN are the same. *(Hacker and Moore, p. 177; Jones et al, pp. 58–64,643–654)*

41. **(B)** The patient described would not be a good candidate for an IUD for several reasons. She has a history of PID, and intrauterine devices have been associated with a higher risk of developing PID. This risk is particularly high in a patient with multiple sexual partners, a recent episode of PID, and women under the age of 25. The patient is also nulliparous; IUDs are more difficult to tolerate in women who have never had an intrauterine pregnancy. Additionally, since the patient has a greater risk of developing PID, her future fertility should be a factor in the decision. There may also be a higher chance of having an ectopic pregnancy with an IUD in place. The patient in this instance already has one risk factor for an ectopic pregnancy, PID; she does not need a second factor. As long as she was a nonsmoker and had no other contraindications, oral contraceptives could be recommended to this patient. Oral contraceptives have also been found to have a protective effect against the development of pelvic inflammatory disease. If the patient is well motivated, a diaphram could be suggested. Because it is a barrier device, it also has a protective effect against the acquisition of sexually transmitted diseases (except AIDS). The diaphragm also has minimal medical complications and, therefore, few contraindications. The contraceptive sponge has been associated with a slightly higher risk of developing toxic shock syndrome, but it is an acceptable form of birth control. Condoms are a good means of preventing the spread of sexually transmitted diseases, are readily available, and are without significant medical contraindications. Condoms and the contraceptive sponge are not as effective against pregnancy prevention as the pill and the IUD. *(Hacker and Moore, pp. 453–467; Jones et al, pp. 225–231)*

42. (D) Endometriosis is endometrial-like tissues found outside the uterus that responds to cyclic hormonal stimulation. Because this ectopic tissue can be found in various locations, most commonly on the ovaries, tubes, uterosacral ligaments, and posterior cul de sac, symptoms of the disease vary greatly. Progressively worse dysmenorrhea, unresponsive to PG synthetase inhibitors, is a common presenting complaint. Infertility occurs in approximately 20% to 40% of women with endometriosis and is often the reason a woman undergoes a work-up. Frequently, women with endometriosis also complain of dyspareunia. This is considered to be secondary to endometrial implants in the uterosacral ligament. Because of the various ways that endometriosis presents, laparoscopic visualization is the only means of definitively formulating the diagnosis. Endometrial implants are not visualized on ultrasound. However, endometriomas, cysts formed on the ovary secondary to excessive bleeding from endometrial tissue, can be seen on sonography. There is, however, no way of differentiating an endometrioma from a simple ovarian cyst, a dermoid, or other pelvic pathology. Laparoscopic diagnosis should be made prior to the administration of any medical therapy, such as danazol. The absence of response to PG synthetase inhibitors may be a means of making the preliminary diagnosis of endometriosis but not the conclusive diagnosis. Hysteroscopy would be of no help in making the diagnosis, as endometriosis is extrauterine. *(Jones et al, pp. 303–326; Szarzynski, pp. 37–47)*

43. (B) Women who lose 25% of their ideal body weight secondary to anorexia nervosa and women who engage in vigorous or stressful exercise often have secondary amenorrhea. This is probably due to hypothalamic dysfunction. These women typically have low gonadotropin levels and low estrogen levels. Due to their lack of estrogen, findings on physical exam may include decreased breast size, an atrophic vaginal mucosa, and possibly absent cervical mucus. In general, these patients are anovulatory. Weight gain and decreased exercise will often restore normal hypothalamic functioning. Oligomenorrhea or episodic menstrual bleeding occurring at greater than 35-day intervals is due to anovulatory cycles. It is seen in women who engage in moderate exercise but not anorexia, in which complete cessation of menses is more common. Menorrhagia is cyclic menstrual bleeding that is excessive in amount or duration. Polymenorrhagia, which is also often due to anovulatory cycles, is episodic bleeding occurring at less than 21-day cycles. Metrorrhagia is uterine bleeding between periods and is usually due to uterine polyps or carcinoma but can be due to estrogen withdrawal or anovulation. *(Hacker and Moore, pp. 525–527,532–534; Jones et al, pp. 351–375)*

44. (D) The signs and symptoms of polycystic ovarian syndrome (PCO) are due to hyperandrogenism, which is a result of overproduction of androgen by both the ovaries and adrenal gland. Clinically, patients with the syndrome are hirsute, have menstrual irregularity, and are infertile. Approximately 50% of these women are obese, most have acne, and 15% are virilized. The ovaries have multiple follicular cysts, which are arrested in development. The ovarian stroma consists of luteinized thecal cells that produce androgens. This excess androgen plus that produced by the adrenal gland results in increased LH secretions from the pituitary, which in turn continues stimulation of the ovaries and more androgen secretion. The excess androgen is converted peripherally into estrogen. Because women with PCO are anovulatory, this estrogen is unopposed by progesterone. The unopposed estrogen effect on the endometrium places these women at greater risk for development of adenomatous hyperplasia and possibly endometrial carcinoma. The high levels of estrogen also cause the amenorrhea and at other times, excessive bleeding. Congenital adrenal hyperplasia also presents with hirsutism and virilism, but these patients usually have a male body type and do not have enlarged ovaries. Excess androgen production prevents the secretion of progesterone; therefore, this patient's symptoms would not be due to a progesterone-secreting tumor. Patients with hyperprolactinemia are usually amenorrheic but usually have galactorrhea and are not hirsute. Hypothyroidism also causes amenorrhea, but not hirsutism. *(Hacker and Moore, pp. 535–539; Jones et al, pp. 169–174,351–375)*

45. (C) A fundal height at the umbilicus roughly corresponds to 20 weeks' gestation. On physical examination, there are several ways of determining fundal height and, therefore, gestational age. A fundus palpable to the pubic symphysis is 12 weeks; at the umbilicus, 20 weeks. Those weeks between these two landmarks are approximated. After 20 weeks, and before 32 weeks, fundal height is measured with a tape measure in centimeters. Weeks' gestation correspond (± 1 cm) to the measured centimeters from the top of the symphysis to the top of the fundus. *(Cunningham et al, p. 1260)*

46. (D) Women who have previously been pregnant will first feel fetal movement between 16 and 18 weeks. With a first pregnancy, women will usually feel movement between 18 and 20 weeks. Gestational age can be approximated to when fetal movement is first perceived. *(Cunningham et al, p. 218)*

47. (A) At 6 weeks' gestation, a gestational sac can be seen on abdominal ultrasound; at 5 weeks the sac can be seen on transvaginal sonogram. After 8 weeks, the embryo can be seen, and measurements of crown–rump length can be made. A fetal heart can be visualized at 8 weeks on abdominal sonogram and at 6½ to 7 on transvaginal. *(Cunningham et al, p. 284, Hacker and Moore, pp. 15,429)*

48. **(D)**   Maternal serum alpha-fetoprotein is a screening test to detect the presence of numerous fetal abnormalities, the most common of which are neural tube defects. The major protein secreted by the early fetus is alpha-fetoprotein. This protein is secreted into the amniotic fluid and crosses the fetal membranes into the maternal circulation. The level of alpha-fetoprotein is elevated in the amniotic fluid of an abnormal fetus and, therefore, in the maternal serum. This elevation is best detected between 16 and 20 weeks. In addition to open neural tube defects, other abnormalities detected include congenital nephrosis, esophageal and duodenal atresia, exophalos, Turner and Potter's syndromes, fetal death, or fetal blood in amniotic fluid. *(Cunningham et al, p. 277)*

49. **(C)**   Coumadin is a small molecule that easily crosses the placenta and is taken up by the fetus. The anomalies it causes are a result of hemorrhage secondary to its anticoagulant effect. Exposure during the first trimester causes anomalies that are collectively termed fetal warfarin syndrome. Use of coumadin during the second and third trimesters causes optic atrophy, cataracts, microcephaly, microphthalmia, blindness, and mental retardation. Heparin is a large molecule that does not cross the placenta and is, therefore, the drug of choice for anticoagulation. *(Cunningham et al, pp. 565–566)*

50. **(D)**   The use of cocaine during pregnancy causes an increased chance of placental abruption that is most likely secondary to its vasoconstrictive effects. Because of the placental abruption, there is a higher incidence of stillborn fetuses. Use of cocaine is also felt to cause an increase in preterm delivery and intrauterine growth retardation. *(Cunningham et al, p. 568)*

51. **(A)**   Women who are considered alcoholics, who ingest large amounts of alcohol frequently, will very often produce a child with fetal alcohol syndrome. Children born with the syndrome have characteristic cardiovascular, limb, and craniofacial defects. Additionally, they are found to be growth-retarded, have impaired fine and gross motor function, and lower IQs. The effects on a fetus of a small amount of alcohol ingested during pregnancy is still uncertain. It is best to abstain entirely. *(Cunningham et al, pp. 567–568)*

52. **(E)**   Phenytoin (Dilantin) is one of the most commonly used anticonvulsant medications. It is con-

sidered a cause of minor craniofacial and digital anomalies but is not definitive if these are secondary to drug versus a genetic disposition found in women who have a seizure disorder. Nonetheless, the adverse effects of terminating the medication, consequent seizures, and potentially causing maternal and fetal hypoxia outweigh the chance of developing the anomalies. If a patient is already pregnant and is well controlled by Dilantin, she should remain on the medication. *(Cunningham et al, p. 566)*

53. **(D)**   The patient's symptoms are describing postmenopausal atrophic changes affecting the vagina, bladder, and urethra. The patient may also complain of vaginal discharge, itching, burning, and dyspareunia. These symptoms are all due to estrogen depletion and, therefore, are best treated with estrogen replacement. Replacement can be either in the form of systemic estrogen or local application in the form of vaginal creams or suppositories. Estrogen is well-absorbed through the vaginal mucosa; thus, a relatively small dose can be used with minimal systemic effects. Because some estrogen is systemically absorbed, local therapy is still associated with the known complications of estrogen replacement. Oral estrogen with progesterone is effective treatment for atrophic vaginitis/cystitis and has the advantage of also treating osteoporosis. Antibiotics, orally or locally, would not be indicated in the above patient, as the urine culture was negative. Testosterone is not indicated for the treatment of atrophic vaginitis. *(Hacker and Moore, pp. 544–550; Jones et al, pp. 416–420)*

54. **(B)**   On abdominal ultrasound, a gestational sac is visible at 7 weeks' gestation and at 8 weeks, a fetal pole can be seen. Both can be seen more clearly and somewhat earlier on vaginal probe sonography. The presence of a fetal pole and gestational sac within the endometrial cavity would rule out an ectopic pregnancy. Sonographic findings in the presence of an ectopic pregnancy are generally nonspecific. There may be a sonolucency in the endometrial cavity, suggestive of a gestational sac called a pseudogestational sac. The adnexa may contain a mass with a mixed echogenic pattern and there may be fluid in the posterior cul de sac. A gestational sac may be seen in the adnexa and in advanced gestations, an actual fetal pole with visible fetal heart motion is noted. Quantitative levels of beta-human chorionic gonadotrophin (beta-HCG) are known to double within 48 hours in a viable pregnancy. In an ectopic pregnancy, the trophoblastic tissue that produces beta-HCG does not function as adequately as in a normal pregnancy and, therefore, this doubling time will not occur. Instead it will either maintain a plateau or rise only a small degree. Although an ectopic pregnancy must always be suspected when

a pregnant woman presents with abdominal pain and bleeding, the above patient's physical findings are not significant enough to subject the patient to either laparotomy or laparoscopy. If ultrasound failed to show an intrauterine gestation and beta-HCG levels sequentially did not double, then laparoscopy would be indicated. If the patient had rebound tenderness or more severe tenderness on pelvic exam, a culdocentesis would be an appropriate diagnostic procedure. If the patient arrived in the emergency room hypotensive and tachycardic, with a history of amenorrhea or known pregnancy, immediate exploratory laparotomy would be indicated. *(Cunningham, pp. 520–522; Hacker and Moore, pp. 425–435)*

55. **(C)** Ectopic pregnancy is responsible for the greatest number of maternal deaths in the first trimester. The incidence of ectopic pregnancy is increasing in the United States. The increase in sexually transmitted diseases and subsequent tubal damage and pelvic adhesions are primarily responsible for the rise in ectopic pregnancy. A woman who has had PID has a sevenfold increase in her chance of developing a tubal pregnancy. Women who undergo tubal surgery to correct infertility have a 30% to 50% chance of developing a subsequent ectopic pregnancy. The improvement in microsurgical technique and increase in women requiring tubal surgery secondary to PID has increased the number of women undergoing this procedure and has subsequently added to the increased rate of ectopics. Additional factors in the increased prevalence of tubal pregnancy are conservative surgery at the time of laparotomy for an ectopic pregnancy, which results in an 11% chance of developing a second ectopic pregnancy, and the increased number of women requesting a reversal of a bilateral tubal ligation. An induced abortion uncomplicated by PID does not predispose a patient to the development of an ectopic pregnancy. Birth control pills change the cervical mucosa and make it less permeable to the gonorrhea bacteria. Women on the pill are, therefore, somewhat protected against the development of PID. *(Hacker and Moore, pp. 425–428, Jones et al, p. 480)*

56. **(A)** The patient in the questions has many of the classic presenting signs and symptoms of acute PID. Because of her age, the severity of her presenting symptoms, and most importantly, her parity, she is a good candidate for in-hospital treatment. Gonorrhea and chlamydia are the most commonly implicated organisms in PID. Gonococcal PID typically presents with symptoms of fever, lower abdominal pain, and tenderness. Chlamydial PID, on the other hand, is more indolent; symptoms are usually mild tenderness and low-grade temperature. Unfortunately, chlamydia causes as much, if not more, tubal damage as gon-

orrhea, and is, therefore, as likely to cause infertility. Anaerobic bacteria are typically the etiologic agent in a second episode of PID but can occur in a first episode, particularly when gonorrhea or chlamydia has rendered the environment anaerobic. If a patient has been symptomatic for several days, it is probable that she has developed an anaerobic infection, and the choice of antibiotic therapy should address all these bacteria. Two strains of mycoplasma have also been implicated in the etiology of PID: *Mycoplasma hominis* and *Ureaplasma urealyticum*. *Clostridium difficile* is the organism responsible for pseudomembranous enterocolitis, a side effect of antibiotic administration, usually with ampicillin and clindamycin. *(Hacker and Moore, pp. 387–389, Jones et al, pp. 511–522)*

57. **(D)** Forty-five percent of women who culture positive for gonorrhea will have concurrent chlamydia. Antibiotic therapy must, therefore, treat both these organisms. Because of the increasing prevalence of penicillin-resistant strains of *Neisseria gonorrhoeae*, ceftriaxone, which is highly effective against even resistant strains, is presently the drug of choice for gonorrhea. Doxycycline or any of the tetracyclines is the drug of choice for *Chlamydia*, but there are some strains of gonococcus that are resistant to tetracycline. Combined therapy with ceftriaxone and doxycycline is, therefore, the best outpatient treatment for PID. Cefoxitin 2 g intramuscularly, with probenecid 1 g orally, and a tetracycline is an acceptable alternative to ceftriaxone. If a patient is allergic to penicillin and the practitioner is not willing to risk the cross reactivity with cephalosporins, spectinomycin 2 g intramuscularly, can replace the ceftriaxone. Trimethoprim-sulfamethoxazole is effective against both gonorrhea and *Chlamydia*, but resistant strains of both organisms have developed against the drug. If a patient fails to improve within 48 hours on an outpatient basis, she should be admitted for IV therapy. In-hospital therapy should include coverage for gonorrhea, chlamydia, and anaerobic bacteria. No single drug is adequate; the following combinations are all possible choices: cefoxitin or cefotetan with doxycycline; gentamycin and clindamycin (clindamycin does cover some strains of *Chlamydia*) or imipenem/cilastatin with doxycycline. *(Hacker and Moore, pp. 392–393; Jones et al, pp. 518–520)*

58. **(A)** This patient's past history of a previous episode of PID and generally mild symptoms are highly suggestive of recurrent salpingitis. Nevertheless, the other possibilities should be considered and an attempt should be made to rule them out. A serum or urine pregnancy test would be indicated, particularly if there is a history of amenorrhea or abnormal menses. If the pregnancy test were negative, an ectopic condition would not be a

possibility. Acute appendicitis usually presents with a higher fever and a higher WBC count, but in its earlier stages, can present as did the above patient, particularly because her pain is right-sided and her history includes symptoms of nausea and vomiting. Careful observation, surgical consultation, and possible laparotomy may be required to completely rule out appendicitis. An adnexal mass, usually ovarian cyst, can twist and will present as unilateral lower abdominal pain with only mild leukocytosis and fever. These symptoms are secondary to necrosis, due to the torsion and possible rupture of the cyst. Sonogram would be helpful in identifying a pelvic mass, but to definitively diagnose a twisted adnexal mass, laparoscopy/laparotomy would be necessary. Clinically, the pain associated with twisted adnexa is usually colicky in nature. A patient with a ruptured tubo-ovarian abscess is ordinarily acutely ill and can present in septic shock. Typically, these patients have high fever, greater than 38°C, high WBC counts, and on abdominal exam have marked tenderness, rebound, and rigidity. On pelvic exam, severe cervical motion tenderness and possibly a palpable mass is noted. (Hacker and Moore, pp. 392–393).

59. **(D)** Herpes genitalis is a venereal disease caused by the herpes simplex virus. Ninety percent of the time, it is caused by the herpes simplex type II virus and 10% of the time by the herpes simplex type I virus. The initial episode is usually the most severe, although some patients are asymptomatic. The virus can migrate up the nerve fiber and remain dormant: therefore, the patient can develop recurrent episodes. The first episode can be associated with a generalized viremia, and the patient may present with generalized malaise and low-grade fever. Recurrent episodes are usually precipitated by stress, menstruation, and upper respiratory infection. The principal way in which to differentiate this lesion from other labial lesions is that it is painful to touch. The definitive diagnosis is made on culture. Secondary syphilitic lesions are condyloma latum; they are raised, round, plateau-like lesions of various sizes that often occur in clusters. The lesions are extremely infectious and occur on the labia vulva, the surrounding perineum, and inner thigh and buttocks. These lesions are not painful to touch and neither is the chancre lesion that is characteristic of primary syphilis. Condylomata acuminata is caused by the human papillomavirus and is a sexually transmitted disease. These lesions can occur on the vulva, vagina, perineum, or cervix. They are white, verrucous growths that when large and multiple are described as cauliflower-like. The lesion of lymphogranuloma venerum is a painless vulvovaginal ulcer progressing to adenitis, usually to the nodes of the anus and rectum. Chlamydia is the causative agent. (Hacker and Moore, pp. 380–384; Jones et al, pp. 578–584)

60. **(B)** Fibroids, or more correctly, leiomyomata, are abnormal but benign growths of the myometrium. The major indications to perform a hysterectomy for myomata are bleeding severe enough to cause anemia, severe pelvic pain or secondary dysmenorrhea, and urinary tract symptoms of frequency or urinary retention. Probably the most important reason to remove fibroids is the inability to adequately access the adnexa. When the myomata is greater than 12-weeks size, it prevents adequate palpation of the ovaries on bimanual exam. An ovarian cancer may then be missed or the malignant ovary may be mistaken for the known uterine myomata. Additional reasons for hysterectomy would be growth of the myomata following menopause and rapid increase in size in premenopausal women. Leiomyomata develop into malignant lesions (sarcomas) only less than 1% of the time: prophylactic removal of a myomata to prevent cancer is, therefore, not an indication for hysterectomy except in the above-stated conditions of rapid growth and postmenopausal growth. Even with these conditions, malignant leiomyosarcoma are rare. Pelvic adhesions may form on myomata, but in general, they form only after surgical intervention, PID, or endometriosis. (Hacker and Moore, pp. 348–352)

61. **(C)** Endometrial hyperplasia is found on pathologic specimen usually on dilation and curettage or on an endometrial biopsy performed in the office. It is considered a premalignant lesion and in some instances will progress to endometrial cancer. It is found in women who experience abnormal uterine bleeding secondary to overstimulation of the endometrium by estrogen unopposed by progesterone. Premenopausally, endometrial hyperplasia occurs in women who are anovulatory; women who fail to ovulate do not form a corpus luteum and, therefore, do not produce progesterone. These women usually have a less severe form of hyperplasia called simple hyperplasia or cystic glandular hyperplasia. Postmenopausal women with endometrial hyperplasia also have excessive estrogen stimulation of the endometrium without the protective effect of progesterone. This is often seen in women receiving estrogen replacement without progesterone added to the regimen. It is also seen in women who are not taking exogenous estrogen; the source of estrogen in these women appears to be the peripheral conversion of androsteredione (from the adrenal gland) to estrone. This conversion takes place in adipose tissue and consequently occurs at a greater rate in obese women. Adenomatous hyperplasia is a more severe form of endometrial hyperplasia and is more often found in postmenopausal women. Compared with simple

hyperplasia, it is more likely to progress to endometrial carcinoma. In its most severe form, it is called carcinoma in situ. Anorexic women have low levels of both estrogen and progesterone secondary to minimal secretion of FSH and LH. Women on oral contraceptives are anovulatory but the progesterone component and relatively low level of estrogen prevent hyperplasia. *(Hacker and Moore, pp. 352–354,543–546,576–577)*

62. (D) If a patient is less than 40 years of age and an adnexal/ovarian cyst is less than 6 cm in size, the patient can be placed on birth control pills and observed for 6 weeks. A large percentage of patients, 60% to 70%, will respond to such a regimen and no adnexal mass will be palpable at the next examination. If the cyst is between 6 and 8 cm and is unilocular on sonography, it also can be observed. Multilocular or solid cysts between 6 and 8 cm should be explored. In the case presented, the cyst not only did not respond to hormonal treatment, it grew larger. Exploratory laparotomy is the preferred means of treatment for both diagnostic and therapeutic reasons. Although a simple or uniloculated cyst can be differentiated on ultrasound from a multiloculated cyst, differentiating a benign multilocular cyst from a malignant one is impossible on ultrasound. In order to adequately diagnose the etiology of an adnexal mass, removal and pathologic diagnosis is necessary. Laparoscopy is again not adequate means of distinguishing whether an adnexal mass is a functional cyst or malignant lesion. Functional cysts, such as corpus luteal or follicular greater than 8 cm in size, should be removed in order to prevent torsion or rupture that can present as a surgical emergency. *(Hacker and Moore, pp. 356–358)*

63. (C) This patient requires exploratory laparotomy for either ruptured ectopic pregnancy or ruptured hemorrhagic corpus luteum. Because hemoperitoneum causes an elevation of the WBC count, this test would not help in deciding the origin of the peritoneal irritation. A low hemoglobin and hematocrit (Hbg and Hct) would also be expected in both cases. As the presence of a corpus luteal cyst frequently causes prolonged amenorrhea with irregular or nominal bleeding, the only way to determine whether this patient's amenorrhea is secondary to pregnancy is to obtain a pregnancy test. Urinary pregnancy tests that are sensitive to 25 mIU/mL of urinary human chorionic gonadotropin are positive in more than 95% of ectopic pregnancies. Most serum pregnancy tests are sensitive to 10 mIU/mL and are, therefore, very accurate in diagnosing pregnancy. *(Hacker and Moore, p. 428; Jones et al, p. 488)*

64. (A) The patient's clinical symptoms of stress incontinence, physical findings of cystocele, and re-production of incontinence with stress are all indicative of urinary stress incontinence (USI). This type of incontinence occurs when the proximal urethra drops below the pelvic floor secondary to pelvic relaxation. An increase of intra-abdominal pressure such as coughing is therefore not transmitted equally to the bladder and proximal urethra. This unequal pressure results in greater bladder pressure that overrides urethral resistance and causes incontinence of urine. Stress incontinence can be diagnosed clinically on good history and with the stress test as mentioned in the question and with the Q-Tip test. Additional means of diagnosing urinary stress incontinence are cystometrogram, cystourethroscopy, and uroflowmetry. Cystoceles occur when the bladder descends into the upper vaginal wall and are commonly found in women with USI. Kegel exercise, pelvic diaphram exercises, and placement of a pessary are nonsurgical means of correcting stress incontinence. The Kegel exercises are successful only in women with minimal symptoms and few anatomic defects. Pessaries are usually used only in women who are unfit for surgery. An anterior repair or anterior colporrhaphy is done through the vagina and involves plication of the pubocervical fascia to support the bladder and urethra. A Marshall–Marchetti–Kranz is done through a retropubic approach and involves elevating the vesicourethral junction via sutures to the symphysis pubis. An additional surgical procedure, the modified Pereyra method, is a combined abdominal-vaginal approach to correction of the problem. All surgical procedures attempt to return the proximal urethra to its normal position above the pelvic floor, thus correcting the incontinence. *(Hacker and Moore, pp. 395–403; Jones et al, 460–478)*

65. (E) A large percentage of women see their gynecologist only routinely. The general health care of women then falls into the hands of the practitioner who does routine GYN exams. Obviously, a bimanual exam of the pelvic organs (uterus, ovaries, tubes, and bladder) is part of the gynecologic exam, as is inspection of the cervix and vagina on speculum exam. A breast exam and an explanation of self-examination are important. Breast cancer is the most common malignant neoplasm in women. Early detection via routine exam, self-exam, and screening mammography allows for greater cure rates. Screening mammograms should be done first at age 35 to 40 for a base line and then repeated at physician-determined intervals (usually 1- to 2-year interval) between ages 40 to 50. After age 50, it is suggested that women undergo annual mammography. Woman at increased risk for breast cancer should have their baseline mammogram at age 35 and their subsequent mammograms at closer intervals. *(Hacker and Moore, pp. 443–445; Jones et al, pp. 6–13)*

66. (B) The ability of a practitioner to adequately perform a pelvic exam depends on the patient's preparation for the examination. Communication prior to and throughout the exam is extremely important. Patients tolerate such exams much better when they are informed of what the practitioner is doing or about to do. Preparation by adequately draping the patient is a good means of keeping the patient comfortable and somewhat lessens the sense of self-consciousness and loss of control many women experience during a pelvic examination. Although it may make the examiner uncomfortable, allowing one family member to remain in the examination room may help the patient tolerate the procedure better. When the patient is an adolescent, allowing a mother or sister in the room may greatly decrease her anxieties. Some patients will actually feel more uncomfortable with the husband or a family member remaining in the room. Again, good communication with the patient will alert the practitioner to this possibility. The patient should be informed when a part of the exam may be painful. To avoid doing so may prevent the completion of the exam secondary to the patient's mistrust of the examiner and general discomfort. When informing the patient of impending pain, stress that the discomfort will be far reduced if the patient can relax and not tighten up in response to the anticipated pain. *(Jones et al, pp. 3–7)*

67. (C) Generalized engorgement of pelvic organs causes cyanosis and the discoloration of the cervix called Chadwick's sign. The uterus, both the corpus (body) and cervix, undergoes softening during pregnancy; this is termed Hegar's sign. A multiparous cervix is one in which the os is slitlike when compared to a circular os, which is found in a nulliparous woman. A multiparous os is only indicative of a previous pregnancy, not a present one. Because a nulliparous woman is one who has never completed a pregnancy, she in fact could be pregnant. Nabothian cysts can either accompany or follow a chronic cervicitis and have no connection to pregnancy. They appear as translucent nodules on the ectocervix. *(Bates, pp 403–404)*

68. (E) Whether a patient is being interviewed during a routine exam or being seen for a gynecologic emergency, a thorough menstrual history is important. First, the date of the last menstrual period (LMP) should be obtained and whether the LMP was normal in amount, duration, and interval. The patient should also be asked about her two previous periods and whether they were normal. Next, the patient should be asked about her menstrual cycle: Is it regular in interval, and what is the interval? A normal menstrual cycle is 28 to 30 days. A history of irregular cycles is indicative of anovulatory cycles or other endocrine abnormalities. Duration of menstrual flow, presence of clots, and amount of bleeding and associated pain are additional information that should be obtained. Age of menarche and onset of menopause and perimenopausal symptoms are also important in menstrual history. Intermenstrual bleeding can be spotting just prior to menses or at time of ovulation. It can also be indicative of uterine cancer and should always be investigated. Finally, a history of premenstrual syndrome should be elicited. The symptoms are extremely variable and include bloating, painful breast swelling, fatigue, depression, anxiety, irritability, and hostility. *(Hacker and Moore, pp. 15–16,334–336; Jones et al, pp. 5–6)*

69. (B) An endometrial biopsy can be performed in an office or clinic with either local anesthesia in the form of paracervical block or just premedication with analgesics. The endometrium is sampled with an extremely small suction-type curette in several, usually 4 to 6, different sites. In the case of this patient, as in any woman suspected of having cancer, an endocervical curetting should be performed prior to obtaining endometrial samples. In the case where polyps are visualized in the endocervical canal, they can be either of endocervical origin or endometrial. The polyps can often be removed in office if they are small, but if they are of considerable size should be removed in an operating room. Endometrial polyps are seldom malignant in premenopausal women, but in menopausal or postmenopausal women they should be removed in the operating room. This will allow adequate dilation of the cervix in order to remove all the polyps for pathologic diagnosis. A traditional dilation and curettage (D&C) would not only provide the above patient with endometrial sampling and removal of the polyp (which was probably causing the intermenstrual bleeding), it may also be therapeutic. The patient's increased menstrual bleeding is probably secondary to her known myomata. Submucosal myomata will often cause excessive bleeding. Curettage will decrease this bleeding; it thus becomes not only a diagnostic but also a therapeutic procedure. Endometrial sampling, whether by D&C or endometrial biopsy, is indicated in any woman 40 years of age who has intermenstrual bleeding or a marked change in her bleeding pattern. A sonogram would adequately identify myomata but would not be helpful in determining whether there has been malignant endometrial changes. CAT scan provides greater imaging when compared to ultrasound, particularly if pelvic or periaortic nodes are suspected, but it still does not provide the necessary pathologic diagnosis for this patient. *(Hacker and Moore, p. 350; Jones et al, pp. 19–25,723–726)*

70. (A) Syphilis, particularly in people who use IV drugs and crack or cocaine, is greatly increasing in frequency. It is theorized that many women are exchanging sex for drugs and that is why it is increasing in this population. Primary syphilis is characterized by a chancre that is a nontender, ulcerative lesion usually found on the vulva, but it can be also found in the vagina or on the cervix. It will appear between 10 and 60 days from the time of inoculation and spontaneously regress after 4 to 6 weeks. It is usually associated with nontender, inguinal lymphadenopathy. Because serologic tests are usually negative at this time, the primary means of making the diagnosis is by obtaining a specimen from the lesion. The spirochete can be seen on dark-field microscopy. Secondary syphilis that is characterized by the symptoms mentioned in the question occurs anywhere from 3 to 6 weeks after the appearance of the chancre. The condylomata, late lesions, are extremely infectious and, again, the spirochete can be seen under the darkfield microscope. The VDRL is positive at this time and there is also inguinal adenopathy present. Benzathine penicillin G, 2.4 million U in a onetime dose is the treatment for primary, secondary, or latent syphilis (less than 1 year's duration). Tertiary syphilis, which may affect any organ system of the body, particularly the central nervous system, is treated with three doses of benzathine penicillin G at weekly intervals. When it is not possible to document the duration of infection, the treatment of choice is the three doses at weekly intervals. For patients allergic to penicillin, tetracycline, 500 mg orally for 15 days, is given for primary, secondary, and latent syphilis; 500 mg orally for 30 days for tertiary syphilis. There are no signs of PID with syphilis. *(Hacker and Moore, pp. 186–187, 383–384; Jones et al, pp. 577–579)*

71 **(B)** One of the best means of antepartum fetal surveillance is the mother's perception of fetal movement. Whenever a woman complains of decreased fetal movement, she should immediately undergo fetal monitoring to obtain a reactive tracing and ultrasound to document fetal well-being. Intrauterine demise or neonatal death is not only a medical problem, it is also a psychosocial problem. The practitioner who deals with pregnant women must learn how to deal with women who have suffered a stillborn or neonatal loss. Couples should be allowed to see their child and hold or examine the baby. Often the child has undergone maceration or has a disfiguring anomaly. Wrapping the child to conceal or lessen these changes will help reduce the parents' shock. Although mothers and fathers often will not opt to view their dead child, it has been shown that to do so will help the parents accept the death and grieve appropriately. Taking pictures has also been found to help the parents in accepting the child's death. Additionally, many parents who originally could not deal with the demise can later return to view the pictures. Mothers should be appropriately medicated for pain and should not be "snowed." Being knocked out with good amounts of amnesiacs and analgesics will take away the realization that the child was actually born dead. Often, these women will not accept that their babies were stillborn but in fact believe that something was done to kill the child. Again, an awareness of the stillbirth enhances the mother's ability to appropriately grieve. Allowing the father to remain with the mother during the labor and delivery will allow him to better accept the reality of the child's death. It will also allow the couple to provide each other with support and encouragement. Often in our attempt to help the mother with the pain of labor and delivery of a stillborn, we forget that the father too has lost a child. *(Capitulo and Maffia, pp. 81–86)*

72. **(C)** Variable deceleration is caused by umbilical cord compression. The onset of the decelerations varies according to its relationship to the contraction and the shape of the deceleration varies when compared to the other decelerations. Variable decelerations occur when the cord is around the baby's neck or a limb and also occurs when there is oligohydramnios. Changing the mother's position from the right side to left side, or placing her in Trendelenburg or knee–chest position may relieve the pressure on the cord. The variable deceleration then may resolve with position change. Severe variable decelerations, those lasting greater than 60 seconds, often occur during the second stage of labor, as the patient starts to push. Late decelerations begin after the onset of the contractions and occur consistently at the same time of each contraction and appear similar in form. Late decelerations usually are indicative of some kind of uteroplacental insufficiency such as chronic hypertension, pregnancy-induced hypertension, sudden and severe maternal hypotension. Placing the patient on her left side will cause maximum blood flow to the placenta and often alleviates the late decelerations. The baseline fetal heart rate in this tracing is 150 bpm, the normal fetal heart rate is anywhere between 120 and 160. A rate above 160 bpm is considered fetal tachycardia. *(Hacker and Moore, pp. 252–257; Freeman and Garite, p. 75)*

73. **(E)** Rape makes up about 7% of all violent crime in this country. Approximately 3 to 10 times as many rapes are committed than are reported. Practitioners who care for women at some time in their career must deal with a woman who has been raped. Practitioners are called upon to obtain evidence and treat the patient, both medically and psychologically. The patient should be treated for both gonorrhea and chlamydia at the time she is initially seen A baseline VDRL and pregnancy test should also be drawn, and the patient should be seen again in 6 weeks in order to repeat these tests and to repeat GC and chlamydial cultures. The patient must be informed about the possibility of pregnancy. A certain percentage of women are protected against pregnancy with a preexisting form of birth control such as birth control pills, IUD, bilateral tubal ligation, or hysterectomy. In women unprotected by preexisting means of birth control, postcoital contraception should be offered. This is usually in the form of the birth control pill Ovral (ethinyl estradiol 50 mg/dL and norgestrel 0.5 mg) given as two tabs PO immediately and then two tabs in 12 hours. The patients should be instructed that this dose can cause nausea and vomiting. Additionally, the patient should be offered HIV counseling and testing. *(Hacker and Moore, pp. 486–489; Jones et al, pp. 525–533)*

REFERENCES

Acker DB, Sachs BP, Friedman EA. Risk factors for shoulder dystocia. *Obstetrics and Gynecology,* 1985; 66(6):762–767.

Bates B. *A Guide to Physical Examination,* 5th ed. Philadelphia, PA: Lippincott; 1991.

Burke L. The use of the Friedman curve in labor management. *Cinc J Med.* 1975;56:29–36.

Burrow and Ferris. *Medical Complications During Pregnancy.* Philadelphia, PA: WB Saunders; 1988.

Capitulo KL, Maffia A. *The Perinatal Bereavement Team: Development and Function, Women and Loss.* New York: Praeger Publishers; 1985.

Cunningham FG, MacDonald PC, Gant NF. *Williams Obstetrics,* 18th ed. Norwalk, CT: Appleton & Lange; 1989.

Dougherty ML. Refractory dysmenorrhea: Is there a solution? *Clinician Reviews,* vol. 3, no. 6; 1993.

Freeman RK, Garite TJ. *Fetal Heart Rate Monitoring.* Baltimore, MD: Williams & Wilkins; 1981.

Gabbe S, Niebyl J, Simpson J. *Obstetrics: Normal and Problem Pregnancies,* 2nd ed. Churchill Livingstone; 1991.

Gregg AR. Indroduction to premature rupture of membranes. *OB/GYN Clinics of North America,* vol. 19, no. 2; 1992.

Hacker NF, Moore JG. *Essentials of Obstetrics and Gynecology,* 2nd ed. Philadelphia, PA: WB Saunders; 1992.

Johnson SR. Clinician's approach to the diagnosis and management of premenstrual syndrome. *Clinical Obstetrics and Gynecology,* vol. 35, no. 3; 1992.

Jones HW, Wentz AC, Burnett LS. *Novak's Textbook of Gynecology,* 11th ed. Baltimore, MD: Williams & Wilkins; 1988.

Klein JM. Neonatal morbidity and mortality secondary to premature rupture of membranes. *OB/GYN Clinics of North America,* vol. 19, no. 2; 1992.

Neshein BI. Induced abortion by the suction method. *Acta Ob Gynecol.* Scand. 1984;63:591–595.

Szarzynski JE. Endometriosis, a diagnostic and therapeutic challenge. *Physician Assistant,* vol. 17, no. 5; 1993.

Vintqileos AM, Campbell WA, Rodis JF. Tests of fetal well-being in premature rupture of membranes. *OB/GYN Clinics of North America,* vol. 19, no. 2; 1992.

Subspecialty List: Obstetrics and Gynecology

CHAPTER 8

Practice Test
Questions

DIRECTIONS (Questions 1 through 10): For each of the items in this section, ONE or MORE of the numbered options is correct. Choose answer

 (A) if only (1), (2), and (3) are correct,
 (B) if only (1) and (3) are correct,
 (C) if only (2) and (4) are correct,
 (D) if only 4 is correct,
 (E) if all are correct.

Questions 1 through 10

1. Which of the following arrhythmias can cause syncope?

 (1) severe bradycardia
 (2) premature ventricular contractions
 (3) asystole
 (4) premature atrial contractions

2. The following findings are associated with acute pericarditis

 (1) ST elevation
 (2) pericardial friction rub
 (3) dyspnea
 (4) chest pain often aggravated by leaning forward

3. Secondary causes of hypertension include

 (1) pheochromocytoma
 (2) renal parenchymal disease
 (3) use of estrogen-containing oral contraceptive pills
 (4) primary aldosteronism

4. The first heart sound (S1)

 (1) is caused by the closure of the mitral and tricuspid valves
 (2) precedes the palpable upstroke in carotid pulse
 (3) is a high-pitched sound
 (4) is best heard at the 2nd or 3rd intercostal spaces

5. Physical findings associated with heart failure are

 (1) pulmonary rales
 (2) congestive hepatomegaly
 (3) S3 gallop
 (4) S4

6. Causes of ST segment elevation are

 (1) Prinzmetal's angina
 (2) acute pericarditis
 (3) acute myocardial injury
 (4) early repolarization

7. Manifestations of digitalis intoxication include

 (1) prolonged QT interval
 (2) anorexia
 (3) urinary retention
 (4) arrhythmias

8. Endocarditis prophylaxis is recommended for

 (1) cystoscopy
 (2) colonoscopy
 (3) gallbladder surgery
 (4) dental procedures

9. Factors associated with a poor prognosis after an acute myocardial infarction are

 (1) congestive heart failure
 (2) positive stress test after a myocardial infarction
 (3) poor left ventricular systolic function
 (4) ventricular arrhythmias during first 24 hours

10. What are the guidelines for the classification of blood pressure?

   (1) mild hypertension is a diastolic pressure of 90 to 104 mm Hg

   (2) normal systolic blood pressure is < 160 mm Hg

   (3) severe hypertension is a diastolic pressure > 115 mm Hg

   (4) isolated systolic hypertension is systolic pressure > 180 mm Hg with diastolic < 90 mm Hg

DIRECTIONS (Questions 11 through 19): Each of the numbered items or incomplete statements in this section is followed by answers or by completions of the statement. Select the ONE lettered answer or completion that is BEST in each case.

Questions 11 through 19

11. When lithium is used to treat bipolar affective illness, which lab tests are used in routine monitoring of the patient for side effects?

   (A) uric acid, WBC

   (B) CBC, liver enzymes

   (C) T_3 uptake, liver enzymes

   (D) TSH, creatinine

   (E) electrolytes, glucose

12. Hallmark features of narcolepsy include

   (A) daytime "sleep attacks"

   (B) cataplexy

   (C) sleep paralysis

   (D) hypnogogic hallucinations

   (E) all the above

13. What diagnosis should be strongly suspected in an overweight, hypertensive, middle-aged male, who complains of sleepiness and whose wife complains that he snores?

   (A) coronary artery disease

   (B) chronic obstructive pulmonary disease

   (C) obstructive sleep apnea syndrome

   (D) major depression

   (E) narcolepsy

14. Initial management of the acutely suicidal patient should include

   (A) psychotherapy

   (B) antidepressant medication

   (C) hospitalization and close observation

   (D) antianxiety medication

   (E) electroconvulsive therapy (ECT)

15. All the following are true in cases of Lyme disease EXCEPT

   (A) there is an expanding erythematous annular lesion

   (B) the treatment of choice is trimethoprim-sulfamethoxazole

   (C) it is the most commonly reported tick-borne disease in the United States

   (D) it is a disease of stages if left untreated

   (E) if arthritis develops, it primarily affects the knee joint

16. Two consecutive tuberculin skin tests are read in the same individual as negative and positive, respectively. He is considered a "true" converter. The following are true of a converter EXCEPT

   (A) the tests were given within 2 years of each other

   (B) the first test was 7 mm induration and the second test was 14 mm induration

   (C) the person is considered newly infected

   (D) chemoprophylaxis is not necessary if he is less than 25-years-old and has a negative chest x-ray

   (E) he should receive treatment prophylactically if he is a child less than 3 years old

17. Of all hepatitis infections, hepatitis B (HBV) has the "alphabet soup" of lab values. All the following are true regarding these values EXCEPT

   (A) the surface antibody indicates past infection and is considered protective

   (B) the core antibody IgG indicates infection even if the surface antigen is negative

   (C) the E antigen in the presence of the surface antigen can indicate a greater likelihood for chronic disease

   (D) the surface antigen is the first evidence of acute infection

   (E) the core antigen is usually not detected in the serum by conventional lab methods

DIRECTIONS (Questions 18 and 19): Each set of items in this section consists of a list of lettered options followed by several numbered words or phrases. For each numbered word or phrase, select the ONE lettered option that is most closely associated with it. Each lettered option may be selected once, more than once, or not at all.

Questions 18 and 19

   (A) preoccupation with body size and weight

   (B) binge eating accompanied by some extreme measure to prevent weight gain

(C) both

(D) neither

18. Anorexia nervosa

19. Bulimia nervosa

DIRECTIONS (Questions 20 through 29): For each of the items in this section, ONE or MORE of the numbered options is correct. Choose answer

    (A) if only (1), (2), and (3) are correct,

    (B) if only (1) and (3) are correct,

    (C) if only (2) and (4) are correct,

    (D) if only 4 is correct,

    (E) if all are correct.

Questions 20 through 29

20. Which of the following are frequently found in patients with osteoarthritis?

    (1) Heberden's nodes

    (2) swan neck deformities of the fingers

    (3) rest usually decreases joint discomfort in early stages

    (4) morning stiffness

21. Signs of bacterial septic arthritis include which of the following?

    (1) fever and chills

    (2) slow insidious onset

    (3) involves primarily large weight-bearing joints and the wrist

    (4) usually is polyarticular

22. Which of the following are characteristic of rheumatoid arthritis?

    (1) fatigue

    (2) weakness

    (3) morning stiffness

    (4) frequently affects the DIP joints of the hand

23. Somatiform disorders are characterized by

    (1) symptoms that suggest a physical ailment

    (2) negative physical and laboratory findings

    (3) a concomitant physical ailment

    (4) intentional patient malingering

24. A major depressive episode is usually associated with which symptom(s) in addition to depressed mood?

    (1) reduced ability to feel pleasure

    (2) decreased interest in activities

    (3) diminished energy

    (4) insomnia, appetite changes, and feelings of guilt

25. The schizophrenic premorbid personality is often noticeable in childhood and adolescence and is distinguished by

    (1) deficiency of social skills with development of small social network

    (2) impaired self-confidence in relationships with the opposite sex

    (3) episodes of neurotic-like illness, such as anxiety, obsessions, and phobias

    (4) a tendency to confine close relationships to family members

26. Psychosis is a symptom of an underlying disorder. When an acutely psychotic patient is encountered, the differential diagnosis should include

    (1) acute drug reaction

    (2) bipolar (manic/depressive) disorder

    (3) major depression

    (4) schizophrenia

27. Simple phobias must be distinguished from panic disorder and

    (1) often cause panic attacks in public places

    (2) consist of a persistent fear of a specific object

    (3) generally result in marked impairment in functioning

    (4) are very common in the general population

28. Imipramine (Tofranil) is a tricyclic antidepressant that commonly causes side effects including

    (1) orthostatic hypotension

    (2) dry mouth

    (3) blurred vision

    (4) diarrhea

29. The borderline personality is characterized by

    (1) manipulative behavior including suicidal threats

    (2) tempestuous interpersonal relationships

    (3) impulsivity and frequent mood shifts

    (4) persistent psychotic thinking

DIRECTIONS (Questions 30 through 39): Each of the numbered items or incomplete statements in this section is followed by answers or by completions of the statement. Select the ONE lettered answer or completion that is BEST in each case.

Questions 30 through 39

30. All the health problems listed below are commonly associated with homozygous sickle cell anemia EXCEPT

    (A) cholelithiasis
    (B) CHF
    (C) aseptic necrosis of the femoral head
    (D) gout
    (E) hypoxemia

31. A 14-year-old anemic patient has the following findings: gallstones, mild icterus, splenomegaly, elevated reticulocyte count, and decreased serum haptoglobin; yet he feels reasonably well. These findings most strongly suggest

    (A) autoimmune hemolytic anemia
    (B) von Willebrand's disease
    (C) idiopathic hemochromatosis
    (D) B_{12} deficiency
    (E) hereditary spherocytosis

32. All the following statements regarding chronic lymphocytic leukemia (CLL) are true EXCEPT

    (A) CLL and diffuse, well-differentiated, lymphocytic lymphoma are both neoplasms of B-cell origin and are so similar that they follow essentially the same clinical course
    (B) CLL, which presents with massive splenomegaly, lymphadenopathy, and lymphocytosis has a median survival of 5 years
    (C) combination chemotherapy for CLL is routinely initiated at the time of diagnosis in an attempt to achieve decreased tumor load and possible remission as early in the disease process as possible
    (D) A Coombs' positive hemolytic anemia occurs in up to 20% of patients with CLL
    (E) patients who demonstrate anemia and/or thrombocytopenia at the time of diagnosis of CLL have a 2-year median survival

33. A 55-year-old white female presents with nonspecific complaints of anorexia, fatigue, hair loss, and dry skin. Physical exam reveals a pale, fair-skinned woman with dry skin, mild vertigo, and a beefy red tongue. Laboratory values reveal hypothyroidism and macrocytic anemia. Which of the

anemias listed below is most commonly associated with the findings above?

    (A) anemia of chronic disease
    (B) thalassemia minor
    (C) folate deficiency
    (D) pernicious anemia
    (E) iron deficiency

34. A 50-year-old white male presents with complaints of increasing backache, fatigue, and weight loss of at least several weeks' duration, and acute onset 36 hours earlier of fever, loose cough, and dyspnea. Physical exam strongly suggests pneumonia (confirmed on x-ray), and also reveals pallor, petechiae on the face and legs, several recent bruises, mild hepatosplenomegaly, and several small palpable lymph nodes. The LEAST likely diagnosis is

    (A) adult T-lymphocyte leukemia (ATL)
    (B) aplastic anemia
    (C) multiple myeloma
    (D) acute myelogenous leukemia (AML)
    (E) well-differentiated, lymphocytic lymphoma

35. Target lesions are pathognomonic of

    (A) erythema marginatum
    (B) erythema multiforme
    (C) erythema annulare
    (D) erythema nodosum
    (E) erythema gyratum repens

36. The most common skin cancer is

    (A) squamous cell carcinoma (SCC)
    (B) primary melanoma
    (C) actinic keratosis (AK)
    (D) keratoacanthoma
    (E) basal cell carcinoma (BCC)

37. All the following are considered elevated lesions EXCEPT

    (A) plaques
    (B) macules
    (C) wheals
    (D) pustules
    (E) scales

38. The drug of choice in treating uncomplicated erysipelas is

    (A) tetracycline
    (B) cephalothin
    (C) vancomycin
    (D) penicillin
    (E) nafcillin

39. The LEAST likely symptom associated with acute pyelonephritis would be

(A) nausea and vomiting

(B) leukocytosis

(C) CVA tenderness or pain on deep abdominal palpation

(D) cystitis

(E) fever and chills

DIRECTIONS (Questions 40 through 42): Each set of items in this section consists of a list of lettered options followed by several numbered words or phrases. For each numbered word or phrase, choose the ONE lettered option that is most closely associated with it. Each lettered option may be selected once, more than once, or not at all.

Questions 40 through 42

(A) Lyme disease

(B) Rocky Mountain spotted fever

(C) Both

(D) Neither

40. Bell's palsy is a neurological complication

41. Tetracycline is the treatment of choice

42. Vesicular lesions may develop as the disease progresses

DIRECTIONS (Questions 43 through 56): For each of the items in this section, ONE or MORE of the numbered options is correct. Choose answer

(A) if only (1), (2), and (3) are correct,

(B) if only (1) and (3) are correct,

(C) if only (2) and (4) are correct,

(D) if only (4) is correct,

(E) if all are correct.

Questions 43 through 56

43. Which of the following are part of the treatment regimen for an acute episode of cystitis in pregnancy?

(1) repeat culture and sensitivity several days after therapy is complete

(2) ten-day course of antibiotic therapy

(3) repeat urine cultures periodically during remainder of prenatal course

(4) chronic suppressive therapy

44. Which of the following anatomical changes during pregnancy are responsible for a higher incidence of pyelonephritis in pregnant women?

(1) women with at least one previous pregnancy

(2) incomplete bladder emptying that predisposes to vesicoureteral reflux

(3) increased vascular supply to the bladder and ureters

(4) dilation of upper urinary tract, namely, hydronephrosis

45. After delivery of an Rh-positive baby to an Rh-negative mother, the mother is given a RhoGAM shot. When is RhoGAM also indicated in an Rh-negative mother?

(1) after an ectopic pregnancy

(2) following amniocentesis

(3) routinely at 28 weeks

(4) following spontaneous or induced abortion

46. A 21-year-old G3P1011 female reveals at the time of her first prenatal visit that the father of her baby is an IV-drug user. You advise her to be tested for acquired immune deficiency disease (AIDS) and the test results are positive. She is presently 10 weeks pregnant; what additional counseling/testing should you now perform?

(1) The patient should be advised to undergo immediate abortion because of the detrimental effects of pregnancy on AIDS.

(2) She should be counseled about the likely possibility that she will transmit the AIDS virus to her baby.

(3) She should be given antibiotic prophylaxis for *Pneumocystis carinii* pneumonia.

(4) The patient should be tested for hepatitis B, gonorrhea, and chlamydia.

47. A patient is day 3 postoperative following a cesarean section. On two separate occasions her temperature has spiked to greater than 101°F. If the presumptive diagnosis is endomyometritis, which of the following are acceptable antibiotic therapies?

(1) ampicillin, gentamicin, and clindamycin

(2) penicillin and gentamicin

(3) a second- or third-generation cephalosporin

(4) ampicillin and doxycycline

48. A 34-year-old female has a Pap test result that shows CIN II or moderate dysplasia. Which of the following procedures could be performed next to further evaluate the abnormal Pap?

(1) simple hysterectomy

(2) cone biopsy

(3) antibiotic treatment for cervicitis

(4) colposcopic examination

49. A 35-year-old woman requests birth control pills. Before prescribing a combination estrogen/progesterone pill, you must obtain a negative history of

    (1) previous deep vein thrombosis

    (2) smoking

    (3) ischemic heart disease

    (4) migraine headache

50. A patient is considering permanent sterilization by tubal ligation. What important aspects of the procedure and complications should be explained during presurgical counseling?

    (1) the permanent nature of the procedure and poor outcome of reversal

    (2) the possibility of development of PID secondary to the procedure

    (3) the possibility of pregnancy after the procedure with a higher incidence of ectopic pregnancy

    (4) the possibility that menstrual irregularities may occur after the procedure

51. A couple comes to your office with a complaint of being unable to get pregnant. They have been attempting to conceive for greater than 1 year. Your history reveals that the woman has had an irregular menstrual cycle for many years and has had no previous pregnancy. Her husband denies having previously sired any children. After a thorough physical and pelvic exam, what would be the next steps in evaluating this couple's infertility?

    (1) The woman should be instructed to do a basal body temperature chart.

    (2) The woman should undergo a hysterosalpingogram.

    (3) The man should have a semen analysis performed.

    (4) The woman should have a serum estriol drawn at approximately day 14 of her cycle.

52. Varicella (chickenpox)

    (1) has an average incubation period of 14 days

    (2) cannot be transmitted through blood transfusions

    (3) is usually treated symptomatically

    (4) occurs only in children and young adults

53. Bullae on lower extremities suggests the following diagnosis

    (1) pemphigus vulgaris

    (2) epidermolysis bullosa acquisita (EBA)

    (3) bullous diabeticorum

    (4) bullous pemphigoid

54. Viral disease(s) occurring in children is/are

    (1) rubella

    (2) rubeola

    (3) Kawasaki

    (4) scarlet fever

55. The risk of HIV transmission to health care workers

    (1) is greatly reduced when universal precautions are implemented

    (2) is lower than the risk of hepatitis B virus (HBV) transmission

    (3) is approximately 0.5% following a single needlestick exposure to blood from an HIV-infected patient

    (4) has been documented from exposure to body fluids other than blood, such as feces, sputum, urine, or vomitus

56. AIDS-associated Kaposi's sarcoma

    (1) may present in the lung as nodular infiltrates

    (2) is seen primarily in IV-drug users

    (3) may respond to alpha-interferon administration

    (4) when treated with radiotherapy is associated with a high response rate and an improved prognosis

DIRECTIONS (Questions 57 through 69): Each of the numbered items or incomplete statements in this section is followed by answers or by completions of the statement. Select the ONE lettered answer or completion that is BEST in each case.

Questions 57 through 69

57. Which of the following tests is used initially to evaluate the presence of HIV infection in a patient?

    (A) HIV antibody status by ELISA

    (B) HIV serum p24 antigen status

    (C) HIV antibody status by western blot

    (D) T-lymphocyte subset studies

    (E) in vitro culture of HIV from patient's blood

58. All the following statements about patterns of HIV infection in the United States are true EXCEPT

    (A) the cumulative incidence of AIDS cases is disproportionately higher in blacks and Hispanics than in whites

    (B) the highest risk of HIV infection in pediatric patients occurs in children born to women who themselves are at risk of HIV infection

(C) the percentage of reported AIDS cases in New York and San Francisco compared to the total United States population has gradually increased over time

(D) the percentage of reported AIDS cases in men has gradually decreased over time

(E) the percentage of reported AIDS cases in women has gradually increased over time

59. All the following statements regarding PCP are true EXCEPT

(A) the definitive diagnosis is made by obtaining pneumocysts on silver stain of sputum, bronchial washings, or lung tissue

(B) it is the leading cause of death in AIDS patients

(C) it occurs in 80% to 90% of all AIDS patients

(D) treatment failure is defined as lack of clinical improvement after 3 days

(E) most AIDS patients will survive their first episode of PCP

60. Which of the following is the most sensitive indicator of bleeding tendency in a preoperative patient?

(A) prothrombin time (PT)

(B) partial thromboplastin time (PTT)

(C) platelet count

(D) fibrinogen

(E) history and physical

61. Ulcerative colitis most frequently involves the

(A) cecum

(B) ileum

(C) left colon

(D) right colon

(E) rectum

62. Chovstek and Trousseau signs can be seen in patients with

(A) hypercalcemia

(B) hypomagnesemia

(C) hypocalcemia

(D) hypermagnesemia

(E) hypophosphatemia

63. Which of the following is NOT associated with pancreatitis?

(A) alcohol

(B) gallstones

(C) hyperlipidemia

(D) carcinoma

(E) hyperparathyroidism

64. "Apple core" lesions on barium enema are pathognomonic for

(A) diverticulitis

(B) sigmoid volvulus

(C) Gardner's syndrome

(D) carcinoma of the colon

(E) villous adenoma

65. Name the correct sequence of events in thyroid hormone secretion.

(A) TSH-TRH-T4-T3

(B) TRH-TSH-T3-T4

(C) TRH-TSH-T4-T3

(D) TSH-TRH-T3-T4

(E) TRH-T4-TSH-T3

66. Pneumaturia is diagnostic of

(A) rectovaginal fistula

(B) colovesicular fistula

(C) diverticulitis

(D) carcinoma

(E) urinary tract infection

67. Which of the following operations for duodenal ulcer has the best morbidity and mortality?

(A) proximal gastric vagotomy

(B) partial gastrectomy

(C) truncal vagotomy and pyloroplasty

(D) truncal vagotomy and antrectomy

(E) truncal vagotomy and gastrojejunostomy

68. What substance is secreted by the chief cells of the stomach?

(A) gastrin

(B) pepsin

(C) pepsinogen

(D) gastric acid

(E) glucagon

69. Hemorrhage complicating duodenal ulcer

(A) usually is massive secondary to penetration into the gastroduodenal artery

(B) is a more frequent complication than either obstruction or perforation

(C) requires gastric resection for its control

(D) can be controlled by endoscopic techniques with decreased mortality

(E) can be controlled with simple ligation without the risk of recurrent hemorrhage

DIRECTIONS (Questions 70 through 73): Each set of items in this section consists of a list of lettered options followed by several numbered words or phrases. For each numbered word or phrase, select the ONE lettered option that is most closely associated with it. Each lettered option may be selected once, more than once, or not at all.

Questions 70 through 73

(A) esophageal webbing
(B) traumatic esophageal rupture
(C) linear tearing of the gastroesophageal junction
(D) esophageal spasm
(E) associated with long-standing gastroesophageal reflux

70. Barrett's esophagus

71. Boerhaave syndrome

72. Mallory–Weiss syndrome

73. Plummer–Vinson syndrome

DIRECTIONS (Questions 74 through 85): For each of the items in this section, ONE or MORE of the numbered options is correct. Choose answer

(A) if only (1), (2), and (3) are correct,
(B) if only (1) and (3) are correct,
(C) if only (2) and (4) are correct,
(D) if only (4) is correct,
(E) if all are correct.

Questions 74 through 85

74. Which of the following characteristics of gastric ulcers indicate the need for surgery?
    (1) associated with a duodenal ulcer
    (2) reappearance after a period of healing
    (3) large size
    (4) less than 30% healing after 3 weeks of medical therapy

75. What are the most common causes of large bowel obstruction?
    (1) carcinoma
    (2) volvulus
    (3) diverticulitis
    (4) ulcerative colitis

76. Parathyroid physiology is responsible for the metabolic regulation of
    (1) calcium
    (2) magnesium

(3) phosphorous
(4) chloride

77. Which of the following play(s) a prominent role in development of diverticulitis?
    (1) sex
    (2) diet
    (3) familial history
    (4) age

78. Regarding bilirubin, which of the following is/are correct?
    (1) Bilirubin is formed mostly from the breakdown of hemoglobin.
    (2) Once formed, bilirubin joins with albumin to form a stable protein pigment complex.
    (3) Conjugated bilirubin is acted upon by bacteria in the intestine to produce urobilinogen and urobilin.
    (4) The hepatic parenchymal cell is a site of bilirubin conjugation with *glucoronic* acid.

79. Which of the following physical findings is most likely to be associated with bowel obstruction?
    (1) distention
    (2) tenderness
    (3) auscultatory "rushes"
    (4) tympany upon percussion

80. When examining a patient suspected of sustaining vascular injury, the following should be of concern:
    (1) shock
    (2) type of trauma
    (3) fracture
    (4) color of blood

81. Symptoms in classic stroke from unilateral carotid artery disease may include
    (1) ipsilateral hemiplegia
    (2) contralateral hemiplegia
    (3) contralateral blindness
    (4) ipsilateral blindness

82. A fusiform aneurysm
    (1) is usually secondary to trauma
    (2) is usually secondary to atherosclerosis
    (3) can be caused by infection
    (4) involves the entire circumference of the artery

83. For which of the disorders listed below is a pacemaker indicated?

    (1) acquired heart block
    (2) sick sinus syndrome
    (3) Stokes–Adams attacks
    (4) A-V disassociation

84. Which of the following tests are best used to differentiate between restrictive and obstructive pulmonary disease?

    (1) total lung capacity
    (2) ventilation–perfusion scanning
    (3) forced expiratory volume in 1 second divided by the forced vital capacity
    (4) chest x-ray

85. Which of the following are physical findings consistent with a consolidated pneumonia?

    (1) rales
    (2) increased vocal fremitus
    (3) dullness with percussion
    (4) decreased whispered pectoriloquy

DIRECTIONS (Questions 86 through 100): Each of the numbered items or incomplete statements in this section is followed by answers or by completions of the statement. Select the ONE lettered answer or completion that is BEST in each case.

Questions 86 through 100

86. Which of the following is in the correct order for frequency of occurrence in bronchogenic carcinoma starting with the most frequent and progressing to the least frequent cell type?

    (A) adenocarcinoma, small cell anaplastic carcinoma, large cell carcinoma, epidermoid carcinoma
    (B) epidermoid carcinoma, adenocarcinoma, large cell carcinoma, small cell anaplastic carcinoma
    (C) small cell anaplastic carcinoma, large cell carcinoma, epidermoid carcinoma, adenocarcinoma
    (D) small cell anaplastic carcinoma, adenocarcinoma, large cell carcinoma, epidermoid carcinoma
    (E) large cell carcinoma, small cell carcinoma, adenocarcinoma, epidermoid carcinoma

87. Deep regular respirations with periods of apnea best describe which of the following?

    (A) Cheyne–Stokes respiration
    (B) Biot's breathing
    (C) Kussmaul respiration

    (D) stridulous breathing
    (E) apnea

88. A 50-year-old male presents with a history of persistent cough, hemoptysis, and weight loss, and states he has had "several lung infections" over the past 3 to 4 months. The patient is a 30-pack-per-year smoker and also complains of right shoulder and chest pain. The patient is afebrile, pale, and dyspneic with exertion. The chest x-ray suggests mediastinal widening and perihilar adenopathy. Which of the following diagnoses is most consistent with the given history?

    (A) bronchiectasis
    (B) chronic obstructive pulmonary disease (COPD)
    (C) chronic bronchitis
    (D) asthma
    (E) bronchogenic carcinoma

89. A 19-year-old female is involved in an automobile accident; she is hospitalized with a fractured femur, her past medical history is unremarkable. The patient suddenly develops dyspnea, cough, anxiety with retrosternal lateralized chest pain. Vital signs are: pulse, 120; respiration, 32; blood pressure, 120/80; temperature, 100.1°F. Chest x-ray shows mild bilateral atelectasis, and the ECG is normal. The most likely diagnosis is

    (A) pneumonia
    (B) myocardial infarction
    (C) pulmonary embolism
    (D) costochondritis with hyperventilation
    (E) unrecognized pneumothorax

90. Which agent provides the most rapid effect and best therapeutic index in the treatment of asthma?

    (A) inhaled beta-adrenergic agonist medication
    (B) subcutaneous epinephrine
    (C) IV aminophylline
    (D) hydrocortisone
    (E) oral aminophylline

91. Of the following, which is the best of all clinical respiratory measurements for assessing the progress of various types of pulmonary fibrotic diseases?

    (A) arterial blood gases
    (B) vital capacity
    (C) inspiratory reserve volume
    (D) total lung capacity
    (E) tidal volume

92. The most reliable physical finding in acute appendicitis is

    (A) hyperesthesia of the skin overlying the right lower quadrant
    (B) localized right lower quadrant tenderness
    (C) tenderness on rectal examination
    (D) psoas sign
    (E) all the above

93. Which study is most accurate in confirming the diagnosis of venous thrombosis and the extent of involvement?

    (A) impedance plethysmography
    (B) ultrasound
    (C) ultrasound and real-time B-mode imaging
    (D) radiolabeled fibrinogen
    (E) venography

94. Bilateral nonpitting edema is associated with

    (A) cardiac disease
    (B) lymphedema
    (C) renal disease
    (D) cirrhosis
    (E) venous disease

95. Which arteriosclerotic aneurysm is most common?

    (A) abdominal aortic aneurysm
    (B) carotid artery aneurysm
    (C) popliteal aneurysm
    (D) femoral aneurysm
    (E) subclavian artery aneurysm

96. Frequent causes of cardiac arrest or fibrillation include all the following EXCEPT

    (A) acute myocardial infarction
    (B) a serum potassium of 5.0 mEq/L
    (C) anoxia
    (D) a serum potassium of 7.0 mEq/L
    (E) drugs

97. Which of the following statements regarding bladder cancer is true?

    (A) Its most common histology is adenocarcinoma.
    (B) Its most common presenting symptom is painless hematuria.
    (C) Early pulmonary metastases are characteristic.
    (D) Its most common presenting symptom is urinary retention.
    (E) Surgery is the only effective treatment.

98. All the following statements about intermittent claudication are correct EXCEPT

    (A) it is the most common complaint produced by limb ischemia
    (B) the onset of pain occurs at rest
    (C) the onset of pain occurs during exertion
    (D) the cessation of pain occurs after rest
    (E) the symptoms may remain stable for years or improve

99. What is the site of the most common form of extracranial vascular disease?

    (A) external carotid artery
    (B) common carotid artery
    (C) internal carotid artery
    (D) subclavian artery
    (E) vertebral artery

100. Which congenital defect is most often recognized at birth or on the first day of life and is lethal if not corrected?

    (A) tetralogy of Fallot
    (B) transposition of the great vessels
    (C) patent ductus arteriosus
    (D) atrial septal defect
    (E) ventricular septal defect

DIRECTIONS (Questions 101 through 107): For each of the items in this section, ONE or MORE of the numbered options is correct. Choose answer

    (A) if only (1), (2), and (3) are correct,
    (B) if only (1) and (3) are correct,
    (C) if only (2) and (4) are correct,
    (D) if only (4) is correct,
    (E) if all are correct.

Questions 101 through 107

101. Hypercalcemia may be caused by

    (1) primary hyperparathyroidism
    (2) thyrotoxicosis
    (3) humoral hypercalcemia of malignancy
    (4) thiazide diuretics

102. Treatment of hyperthyroidism can include

    (1) steroids
    (2) lithium
    (3) propylthiouracil
    (4) methimazole

103. Complications of iatrogenic Cushing's syndrome include

(1) cataracts

(2) osteoporosis

(3) myopathy

(4) growth spurt

104. Osteoporosis, a disease in total bone mass, may be caused by

(1) menopause

(2) hyperthyroidism

(3) Cushing's syndrome

(4) alcoholism

105. Diabetes mellitus may present with

(1) polyuria

(2) polydipsia

(3) ketosis

(4) blurry vision

106. The appropriate laboratory work-up for a pheochromocytoma would include

(1) serum for metanephrins

(2) serum for VMA

(3) 24-hour urine for prostaglandins

(4) 24-hour urine for fractionated catecholamines

107. Clinical signs of hypocalcemia include

(1) positive Chovstek's sign

(2) cramps and tingling

(3) tetany

(4) negative Trousseau's sign

DIRECTIONS (Questions 108 through 117): Each of the numbered items or incomplete statements in this section is followed by answers or by completions of the statement. Select the ONE lettered answer or completion that is BEST in each case.

Questions 108 through 117

108. Hypercalcemia should be suspected if a patient has a serum calcium level of

(A) 8.0 mg/dL with albumin of 3.0 g/dL

(B) 9.0 mg/dL with albumin of 3.0 g/dL

(C) 10.0 mg/dL with albumin of 4.0 g/dL

(D) 10.0 mg/dL with albumin of 2.0 g/dL

(E) 9.5 mg/dL with albumin of 3.8 g/dL

109. Dexamethasone suppression test is used to aid in the diagnosis of

(A) Graves' disease

(B) Addison's disease

(C) Cushing's syndrome

(D) Reidel's disease

(E) rheumatoid arthritis

110. Kidney stones can have a variety of mineral components. Which of the following is NOT a cause for stones?

(A) cystine

(B) oxalate

(C) magnesium

(D) purine

(E) phosphate

111. Clinical features of Cushing's syndrome include

(A) thick skin

(B) hirsutism

(C) improving strength

(D) hair loss

(E) abdominal pain

112. High-density lipoprotein is associated with

(A) decreased cardiac mortality

(B) increased cardiac mortality

(C) diabetes

(D) hypertension

(E) high saturated fat intake

113. A patient presents with osteolytic lesions on x-ray; bone pain, deformity, bone scan with numerous hot lesions, and bone biopsy demonstrate intense osteoblastic bone resorption and large numbers of osteoclasts. The most likely bone lesion would be

(A) hyperthyroid bone disease

(B) hyperparathyroid bone disease

(C) Paget's disease

(D) metastatic breast cancer

(E) osteoporosis

114. NPH insulin usually has its peak activity at

(A) 4 to 6 hours

(B) 18 to 24 hours

(C) 10 hours

(D) 6 to 14 hours

(E) 16 hours

115. Monitoring adequate blood sugar control in the diabetic would include which of the following tests?

(A) 12 MN blood sugar

(B) glycohemoglobin level

(C) 24-hour urine for glucose

(D) 6 PM blood sugar

(E) 8 AM insulin level

116. Antihistamines are contraindicated in all the following medical conditions EXCEPT
    (A) glaucoma
    (B) hypertension
    (C) asthma
    (D) prostatic hypertrophy
    (E) pregnancy

117. All the following are used in the management of asthma EXCEPT
    (A) theophylline
    (B) cromolyn sodium
    (C) nadolol
    (D) terbutaline
    (E) albuterol

DIRECTIONS (Questions 118 and 119): For each of the items in this section, ONE or MORE of the numbered options is correct. Choose answer

    (A) if only (1), (2), and (3) are correct,
    (B) if only (1) and (3) are correct,
    (C) if only (2) and (4) are correct,
    (D) if only (4) is correct,
    (E) if all are correct.

Questions 118 and 119

118. Phenobarbital and phenytoin are effective in the management of generalized motor seizures. Which drug(s) is/are effective in petit mal or absence seizures?

    (1) ethosuximide
    (2) phenobarbital
    (3) valproic acid
    (4) diazepam

119. Which of the following are useful in the treatment of migraine headache?

    (1) tenormin
    (2) vicodin
    (3) midrin
    (4) sansert

DIRECTIONS (Questions 120 through 122): Each of the numbered items or incomplete statements in this section is followed by answers or by completions of the statement. Select the ONE lettered answer or completion that is BEST in each case.

Questions 120 through 122

120. The evaluation of new onset seizures in an adult should include all the following EXCEPT
    (A) CT scan
    (B) chest radiograph
    (C) HIV testing
    (D) BUN, electrolytes, and creatinine
    (E) fasting blood sugar

121. A 78-year-old male presents with a "classic triad" of dementia, incontinence of urine, and difficulty with gait. What would you expect to see on a CT scan of the head?
    (A) large ventricles
    (B) brain tumor
    (C) cerebral atrophy
    (D) multiple infarcts
    (E) single infarct

122. A 30-year-old patient presents with a waxing and waning diploplia interspersed with periodic vertigo. The character of her symptoms is worrisome for
    (A) posterior fossa lesion involving cranial nerves VI and VIII
    (B) Ménière's disease
    (C) acoustic neuroma
    (D) multiple sclerosis
    (E) myasthenia gravis

DIRECTIONS (Questions 123 and 124): For each of the items in this section, ONE or MORE of the numbered options is correct. Choose answer

    (A) if only (1), (2), and (3) are correct,
    (B) if only (1) and (3) are correct,
    (C) if only (2) and (4) are correct,
    (D) if only (4) is correct,
    (E) if all are correct.

Questions 123 and 124

123. Hematuria

    (1) is not painful except when there is passage of large clots in the ureter or urethra
    (2) occurs in sepsis and other systemic disorders
    (3) occurs in acute interstitial nephritis
    (4) occurs in cystic and inflammatory diseases

124. In the patient with hyperchloremic acidosis you will find

(1) decreased serum bicarbonate

(2) sulfate and phosphate excreted normally

(3) increased reabsorption of chloride ions

(4) renal excretion of acid is reduced

DIRECTIONS (Question 125): Each of the numbered items or incomplete statements in this section is followed by answers or by completions of the statement. Select the ONE lettered answer or completion that is BEST in each case.

Question 125

125. Which of the following symptoms are least likely to be seen in acute pyelonephritis?

(A) nausea and vomiting

(B) leukocytosis

(C) CVA tenderness or pain on deep abdominal palpation

(D) cystitis

(E) fever and chills

DIRECTIONS (Questions 126 through 139): For each of the items in this section, ONE or MORE of the numbered options is correct. Choose answer

(A) if only (1), (2), and (3) are correct,

(B) if only (1) and (3) are correct,

(C) if only (2) and (4) are correct,

(D) if only (4) is correct,

(E) if all are correct.

Questions 126 through 139

126. Proper care of an amputated digit includes

(1) placing the amputated part in a bath of lactated Ringer's solution

(2) perfusing exposed arteries with iced saline solution

(3) placing the amputated part, protected in a bag of crystalloid solution, on ice

(4) avoiding the use of ice and keeping the amputated part at room temperature

127. Hemorrhage in the acute setting is best controlled by

(1) manual compression of vessels proximal to the bleeding site

(2) the use of vascular clamps

(3) tourniquets

(4) direct pressure to the bleeding site

128. Principles of fluid resuscitation in the acute management of hypovolemic shock includes

(1) insertion of large-bore peripheral IVs

(2) rapidly infusing 2 L of lactated Ringer's solution

(3) type-specific blood is preferred for life-threatening shock

(4) immediate insertion of central venous catheters

129. Signs and symptoms of small bowel obstruction include

(1) intermittent, crampy abdominal pain

(2) vomiting

(3) abdominal distention

(4) diarrhea

130. Radiologic studies that are helpful in the diagnosis of acute cholecystitis include

(1) plain KUB

(2) RUQ ultrasound

(3) technetium-99m scans (HIDA)

(4) oral cholecystogram

131. Which of the following are common characteristics of acute mesenteric ischemia?

(1) It is typically a disease of the elderly and infirm.

(2) It often follows a period of hemodynamic instability.

(3) It is often due to embolic or thrombotic events.

(4) Patients complain of pain that is disproportionate to a relatively benign physical exam.

132. The hallmarks of acute arterial occlusion include

(1) pain

(2) pallor

(3) pulselessness

(4) paralysis and paresthesia

133. Certain high-risk patients may require antibiotics in addition to incision and drainage for the treatment of soft tissue abscesses. These include

(1) patients manifesting systemic toxicity

(2) diabetic patients

(3) patients with valvular heart disease

(4) patients with cirrhosis

134. Which of the following statements are characteristic of perirectal abscesses?

    (1) If mistreated they could lead to life-threatening sepsis.
    (2) They form fistulas-in-ano when they drain spontaneously.
    (3) They require general anesthesia for proper drainage.
    (4) They occur with greater frequency in the immunocompromised patient.

135. Clinical findings often seen with mandibular fractures include

    (1) malocclusion
    (2) rhinorrhea
    (3) deviation of the jaw on opening
    (4) raccoon eye

136. When closing lacerations in the emergency room setting, it is important to relieve tension on the wound edges to achieve an optimal result. Techniques to reduce wound tension include

    (1) undermining soft tissues
    (2) splinting the affected part
    (3) closing the wound in layers
    (4) application of adhesive strips

137. Characteristics of full-thickness burn wounds include

    (1) blister formation
    (2) white or charred appearance
    (3) sensitive to pin prick
    (4) will not heal spontaneously

138. Indications that a cast is too tight include

    (1) increasing pain
    (2) poor capillary refill
    (3) paresthesias
    (4) pain on passive extension of the digits

139. Diagnostic peritoneal lavage is extremely useful in determining which trauma patients require urgent exploratory laparotomy. Indication for peritoneal lavage in multisystem trauma include

    (1) patients with altered mental status from head injury or intoxication
    (2) situations in which the patient will have lengthy nonabdominal surgery
    (3) unexplained hypotension
    (4) situations in which CT scanning is not available

DIRECTIONS (Questions 140 through 144): Each of the numbered items or incomplete statements in this section is followed by answers or by completions of the statement. Select the ONE lettered answer or completion that is BEST in each case.

Questions 140 through 144

140. The primary pathologic effect of acetaminophen poisoning is
    (A) bronchospasm
    (B) bone marrow suppression
    (C) reversible mental status changes
    (D) hepatic dysfunction
    (E) cardiac dysfunction

141. The major toxic effect of carbon monoxide is
    (A) hypoxia
    (B) inhibition of surfactant
    (C) primary myocardial depression
    (D) bronchospasm
    (E) hemolysis

142. The proper rate and sequence of ventilation and chest compression in two-person CPR is
    (A) one ventilation after five compressions at a rate of 80 to 100 compressions per minute
    (B) two ventilations after ten compressions at a rate of 80 to 100 compressions per minute
    (C) one ventilation after ten compressions at a rate of 80 to 100 compressions per minute
    (D) two ventilations after three compressions at a rate of 80 to 100 compressions per minute
    (E) three ventilations after three compressions at a rate of 80 to 100 compressions per minute

143. The leading cause of mortality in the first four decades of life is
    (A) congenital defects
    (B) cancer
    (C) infectious disease
    (D) multisystem trauma
    (E) bronchospastic diseases

144. A positive anterior drawer sign is indicative of
    (A) medial collateral ligament tear
    (B) lateral collateral ligament tear
    (C) anterior cruciate ligament tear
    (D) medial meniscus tear
    (E) lateral meniscus tear

DIRECTIONS (Question 145): For each of the items in this section, ONE or MORE of the numbered options is correct. Choose answer

 (A) **if only (1), (2), and (3) are correct,**
 (B) **if only (1) and (3) are correct,**
 (C) **if only (2) and (4) are correct,**
 (D) **if only (4) is correct,**
 (E) **if all are correct.**

Question 145

145. Which of the following statements regarding pelvic fractures are correct?

 (1) Mortality in patients with pelvic fractures can reach as high as 20%.
 (2) A displaced fracture of the pelvic ring indicates that there is at least one other fracture.
 (3) Anterior pelvic fractures are commonly associated with uretheral injuries.
 (4) Few patients with pelvic fractures sustain hemorrhage sufficient to require transfusion.

DIRECTIONS (Questions 146 through 152): Each of the numbered items or incomplete statements in this section is followed by answers or by completions of the statement. Select the ONE lettered answer or completion that is BEST in each case.

Questions 146 through 152

146. Malignant neoplasms of the musculoskeletal system

 (A) generally have a good prognosis
 (B) include osteoblastomas and giant cell tumors
 (C) rarely require surgical excision
 (D) are usually painful
 (E) rarely metastasize

147. Statistically, the most common type of childhood maltreatment seen by health care practitioners is

 (A) nonorganic failure to thrive
 (B) physical abuse
 (C) sexual abuse
 (D) emotional/verbal abuse
 (E) neglect

148. The most common bacterial pathogen for otitis media at all ages is

 (A) Group A beta hemolytic strep
 (B) *E. coli*
 (C) *S. pneumoniae*
 (D) *S. aureus*
 (E) *B. catarrhalis*

149. Asthmatic children

 (A) rarely present before 5 years of age
 (B) have a generally poor prognosis
 (C) rarely require pharmacologic therapy
 (D) present with hyperreactivity of the airways to a variety of stimuli and a high degree of reversibility of the obstructive process
 (E) demonstrate rales as the diagnostic feature on physical exam

150. Which of the following is the most important first step in treating a child who is unresponsive after suspected cardiopulmonary arrest?

 (A) applying cardiac monitor
 (B) initiating closed chest cardiac massage
 (C) determining if patient is having respiratory difficulty and establishing a patent airway
 (D) assessing whether circulatory problems exist by checking brachial, femoral, or carotid pulses
 (E) establishing an IV line

151. The most common type of burn seen in children is

 (A) scald burns
 (B) flame burns
 (C) electrical burns
 (D) flash burns (exploding flammable materials)
 (E) George Burns

152. A patient has a type III epiphyseal fracture (Salter fracture). This type of fracture is described as

 (A) the epiphyseal plate has slipped from its origin and there is a fracture through the metaphysis producing a triangular metaphyseal fragment
 (B) a crushing injury damaging the epiphyseal plate usually producing growth arrest
 (C) the epiphyseal plate has slipped with a fracture involving the epiphysis
 (D) an intra-articular fracture extending through the epiphysis, epiphyseal plate, and metaphysis
 (E) the epiphyseal plate separates from the metaphysis without displacement or injury to the growth plate

DIRECTIONS (Questions 153 through 164): For each of the items in this section, ONE or MORE of the numbered options is correct. Choose answer

> **(A) if only (1), (2), and (3) are correct,**
> **(B) if only (1) and (3) are correct,**
> **(C) if only (2) and (4) are correct,**
> **(D) if only (4) is correct,**
> **(E) if all are correct.**

Questions 153 through 164

153. Painless rectal bleeding in children may be caused by

 (1) Meckel's diverticulum
 (2) rectal fissures
 (3) juvenile polyps
 (4) intussusception

154. Status epilepticus is when a patient has continuous seizures for 20 minutes, or more than two seizures without a lucid period. Which of the following is/are true regarding the cause, management, and outcome of this condition?

 (1) It may be caused by poor compliance in the use of seizure medication.
 (2) Appropriate laboratory studies include determination of blood glucose level, arterial blood gases, electrolytes, and blood level of anticonvulsant medication.
 (3) Treatment includes establishing airway, giving oxygen, intravenous glucose, and consideration of giving naloxone, thiamine, and correction of metabolic abnormalities; use of an anticonvulsant like phenobarbital.
 (4) Complications include death from anoxia, aspiration, or trauma. Encephalopathy from anoxia, acute renal failure due to myoglobinuria, and rhabdomyolysis and respiratory arrest caused by medications.

155. Treatment for an avulsed secondary tooth includes

 (1) cleaning the tooth thoroughly by scrubbing all dirt and foreign matter from the tooth
 (2) inserting the tooth into the open socket or placing the tooth under the patient's tongue until a dentist is seen
 (3) wrapping the tooth in gauze until a dentist is seen
 (4) seeing a dentist as soon as possible

156. A 5-year-old female presents with a single swollen, firm, nontender anterior cervical node. The child has been entirely healthy for the last several months. There has been no known exposure. Your differential diagnosis includes

 (1) beta-streptococcus adenitis
 (2) malignancies atypical mycobacterium
 (3) cat scratch fever
 (4) atypical mycobacterium

157. Acetaminophen is a common ingestion in the pediatric population. Which of the following is/are true for an ingestion of this type in a child older than 1 year of age?

 (1) The local or national poison control number should be called.
 (2) If activated charcoal is administered in the initial treatment, the stomach should be lavaged before administering N-acetylcysteine (Mucomyst).
 (3) Administer N-acetylcysteine (Mucomyst) if serum acetaminophen level is in the toxic range and less than 24 hours have elapsed since ingestion.
 (4) If the initial serum acetaminophen level is in the toxic range, a loading dose of N-acetylcysteine (Mucomyst) should be administered followed by 17 additional doses.

158. Factor(s) tending to increase the suspicion that a physical injury to a child has a nonaccidental etiology include

 (1) a history that does not explain the extent or characteristics of the injury
 (2) an explanation of his/her involvement in the traumatic incident that is not compatible with the child's developmental level
 (3) a long delay in seeking medical help
 (4) parents who seem overly anxious and distraught

159. Adverse reactions to DPT vaccine that occur in more than 5% of vaccine recipients include

 (1) pain or swelling at the site
 (2) fever greater than 38°C
 (3) anorexia or vomiting
 (4) febrile convulsion

160. *Haemophilus influenzae* type B (HIB) frequently causes the following infections in children

 (1) meningitis
 (2) otitis media
 (3) cellulitis
 (4) sinusitis

161. Incidence studies of acute otitis media show that

   (1) the peak incidence is in the 6- to 36-month age group

   (2) in the first 3 years of life, 60% of children will have at least one episode of otitis media

   (3) 40% of children have middle ear effusion that persists for at least 4 weeks

   (4) the incidence declines after about age 6 years

162. Abnormal sexual development is manifested by

   (1) no sign of puberty in a girl of 15

   (2) onset of puberty in a girl age 9

   (3) bilateral/unilateral breast development in a girl prior to age 8

   (4) no sign of puberty in a boy of 13

163. Human breast milk offers which of the following advantages to neonates?

   (1) secretory IgA

   (2) a high vitamin D content

   (3) epidermal growth factor

   (4) higher iron content than formula

164. The Denver Developmental Screening Test (DDST)

   (1) is a screening instrument designed to determine whether a particular child's development falls within the normal range

   (2) is an intelligence test for children

   (3) consists of a progressive sequence of developmental tasks that test personal-social, fine motor/adaptive, language, and gross motor skills

   (4) requires extensive testing material and is difficult and time consuming to administer

165 A newborn infant in the delivery room is commonly evaluated by the Apgar score. The following statement(s) is/are true:

   (1) a score is given at 1 and at 5 minutes

   (2) the 1-minute score is most predictive of neurologic residual and long-term outcome

   (3) signs including heart rate, muscle tone, and color are given a score

   (4) a total score of 5 indicates an infant in the best possible condition

166. Innocent murmurs are characterized by which of the following?

   (1) low intensity

   (2) may have a fixed split S2

   (3) may be systolic in timing

   (4) may be diastolic in timing

DIRECTIONS (Questions 167 through 170): Each set of items in this section consists of a list of lettered options followed by several numbered words or phrases. For each numbered word or phrase, select the ONE lettered option that is most closely associated with it. Each lettered option may be selected once, more than once, or not at all.

Questions 167 through 170

For each description of a skin lesion, select the disease with which it is associated.

   (A) lichen sclerosis et atrophicus

   (B) psoriasis

   (C) eczema

   (D) tuberous sclerosis

   (E) pityriasis rosea

167. Herald patch

168. Hourglass distribution in anogenital area

169. Adenoma sebaceum

170. Lichenification

DIRECTIONS (Questions 171 through 176): For each of the items in this section, ONE or MORE of the numbered options is correct. Choose answer

   (A) if only (1), (2), and (3) are correct,

   (B) if only (1) and (3) are correct,

   (C) if only (2) and (4) are correct,

   (D) if only (4) is correct,

   (E) if all are correct.

Questions 171 through 176

171. The thick ascending limb of the loop of Henle absorbs sodium chloride rapidly and causes

   (1) a decreased osmolality and tubular fluid concentration of sodium chloride to drop to 30 mmol/L

   (2) the voltage across the lumen to become positive

   (3) the tubular fluid to become dilute

   (4) concentration of fluid in the distal loop when it passes through

172. The statement(s) most accurately associated with scleroderma (progressive systemic sclerosis) in renal tissue would be:

(1) renal failure is associated with 40% to 50% of all deaths

(2) renal involvement is rarely the presenting symptom

(3) closely resembles accelerated nephrosclerosis

(4) petechial hemorrhages and wedge-shaped cortical infarcts

173. In adult polycystic kidney disease, you would find

(1) cortical and medullary cysts

(2) renal failure as a newborn

(3) hepatic cysts and intracranial aneurysms

(4) reduced bicarbonate absorption

174. The normal range of serum osmolality is 285 to 295 mOsm/L and is calculated: (1 mOsm glucose = 180 mg/L; 1 mOsm BUN = 28 mg/L)

(1) 2(Na+mmol/L)+glucose mmol/L+BUN mmol/L

(2) 2(Na+mOsm/L)+glucose mOsm/L+BUN mOsm/L 1.8 mmol28 mmol

(3) 2(Na+mEq/L)+glucose mEq/L+BUN mEq/L

(4) $2(Na+mEq/L) + \dfrac{glucose\ mg/dL}{18} + \dfrac{BUN\ mg/dL}{2.8}$

175. 50% to 70% of body weight is composed of water that is

(1) two-thirds intracellular fluid

(2) one-third extracellular fluid

(3) regulated by the amount of solvent in each compartment

(4) not dependent on the amount of adipose tissue

176. The concentration of urine depends largely on

(1) the loop of Henle

(2) large osmotic pressure gradient between the papilla and cortex

(3) the countercurrent system

(4) nephrons

DIRECTIONS (Questions 177 through 185): Each of the numbered items or incomplete statements in this section is followed by answers or by completions of the statement. Select the ONE lettered answer or completion that is BEST in each case.

Questions 177 through 185

177. In rheumatoid disease the majority of clinical and pathological findings are a result of chronic inflammation of

(A) synovial membranes

(B) epiphyseal disc

(C) articular cartilage

(D) periosteal membrane

(E) subchondrial bone

178. A 52-year-old man presents with severe right ankle pain for 2 days and no other complaints. During the exam, the joint is erythematous, warm, and an effusion is noted. The patient is afebrile (WBC, 9000) with normal differential; BUN and creatinine are within normal limits. Uric acid level is 9.6 mg/dL (normal is 2.5 to 8 mg/dL). The most likely diagnosis is

(A) rheumatoid arthritis

(B) osteoarthritis

(C) pseudogout

(D) gouty arthritis

(E) bacterial septic arthritis

179. Which of the following signs and symptoms are most commonly found in a pregnant woman with pyelonephritis?

(A) lower abdominal pain, fever, and chills

(B) premature onset of contractions

(C) fever and chills, nausea and vomiting, and flank pain

(D) urinary frequency, urgency, and dysuria

(E) a brownish discoloration of urine

180. At 10 weeks' gestation, a 23-year-old G1P0 breaks out in a rash that begins first on her face and then spreads downward. One week earlier, she suffered fever, malaise, and myalgias. Which test should be obtained immediately to determine whether her fetus will be affected by an infection resulting in severe congenital abnormalities?

(A) VDRL

(B) cervical cultures for gonorrhea

(C) chlamydial cultures

(D) rubella titers

(E) group B beta-strep cultures

181. At 32 weeks, a 16-year-old G1P0 presents to the obstetric clinic complaining of headache; her blood pressure is 140/85. According to her prenatal chart, her first trimester blood pressures were 100/70. At this time she has 2+ protein in her urine and she is hyperreflexic. What is the most likely diagnosis?

    (A) chronic hypertension
    (B) migraine headache
    (C) eclampsia
    (D) chronic renal disease
    (E) preeclampsia

182. The above patient is admitted to the hospital and placed on bedrest. Instead of improving, her blood pressure increases to 160/100, the proteinuria remains at 2+ to 3+, and she remains hyperreflexic. A decision to deliver her baby is made; what medication must be started at this time?

    (A) hydrochlorothiazide
    (B) hydralazine
    (C) magnesium sulfate
    (D) diazepam
    (E) furosemide

183. When performing a Pap smear you are attempting to obtain cells from the area that undergoes dysplastic changes. This area is called the

    (A) endocervix
    (B) squamocolumnar junction
    (C) posterior vaginal fornix
    (D) exocervix
    (E) internal os

184. The primary means by which oral contraceptives prevent pregnancy is

    (A) inhibition of endometrial implantation of the embryo
    (B) inhibition of the release of prolactin and, therefore, prevention of ovulation
    (C) inhibition of the release of estrogen from the follicle and, therefore, ovulation
    (C) inhibition of the release of estrogen from the follicle and, therefore, ovulation
    (D) inhibition of spermatozoa by pill-induced changes in the cervical mucus
    (E) inhibition of the midcycle gonadotropin surge and, therefore, ovulation

185. A 15-year-old patient presents with a complaint of severe menstrual cramps that prevent her from attending school and maintaining her normal daily activity. The pain usually occurs on the first day of her menses and has gotten progressively worse since the onset of menarche at age 13. Pelvic exam

is without significant findings. You make the diagnosis of primary dysmenorrhea and decide to treat her in the following manner:

    (A) Tylenol with codeine
    (B) oral contraceptives
    (C) prostaglandin synthetase inhibitors
    (D) diagnostic laparoscopy
    (E) tocolytic agents

DIRECTIONS (Questions 186 through 193): Each set of items in this section consists of a list of lettered options followed by several numbered words or phrases. For each numbered word or phrase, select the ONE lettered option that is most closely associated with it. Each lettered option may be selected once, more than once, or not at all.

Questions 186 through 189

Match the following vaginal infections with the appropriate description.

    (A) *Trichomonas vaginalis*
    (B) atrophic vaginitis
    (C) gonorrhea
    (D) candidiasis
    (E) Gardnerella vaginalis

186. Thick white discharge with vaginal itching and burning; marked erythema of vulvovaginal mucous membranes

187. Vaginal itching and burning; thin, blood-tinged discharge; thin, friable vulvar, and vaginal epithelium

188. Soreness with vaginal itching and burning; frothy, yellow-green discharge; diffusely reddened, mucous membranes

189. Musty, malodorous discharge, thin, grayish in color

Questions 190 through 193

For the number of weeks' gestation, match the events of pregnancy that occur at the time.

    (A) 6 weeks
    (B) 28 weeks
    (C) 20 weeks
    (D) 16 to 20 weeks
    (E) 14 weeks

190. Fundal height at umbilicus

191. Fetal movements first perceived by mother

192. Gestational sac first seen on sonogram (abdominal)

193. Optimal time to draw maternal serum alpha-feto-protein

DIRECTIONS (Questions 194 through 198): Each of the numbered items or incomplete statements in this section is followed by answers or by completions of the statement. Select the ONE lettered answer or completion that is BEST in each case.

194. The test of choice for diagnosis of a pericardial effusion is

(A) chest x-ray
(B) CT scan of chest
(C) MUGA
(D) echocardiogram
(E) right heart catheterization

195. All the following physical findings may be associated with mitral stenosis EXCEPT

(A) diastolic apical rumble
(B) Graham–Steele diastolic murmur
(C) opening snap
(D) S3 gallop
(E) loud S1

196. All the following are causes of left ventricular hypertrophy EXCEPT

(A) mitral stenosis
(B) systemic arterial hypertension
(C) hypertrophic obstructive cardiomyopathy
(D) aortic insufficiency
(E) aortic stenosis

197. The electrocardiogram in Figure 8–1 demonstrates

(A) inferior wall myocardial infarction
(B) left ventricular hypertrophy

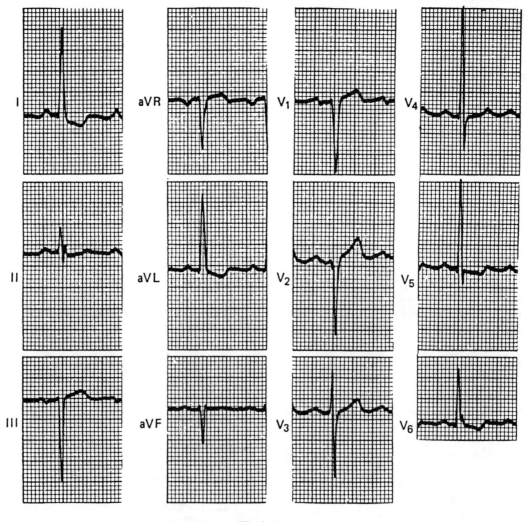

Fig. 8–1

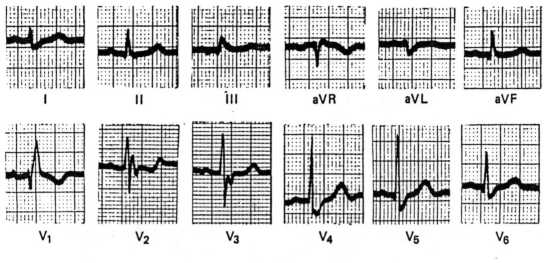

I   II   III   aVR   aVL   aVF

V₁   V₂   V₃   V₄   V₅   V₆

Fig. 8–2

(C) anterolateral ischemia

(D) right bundle branch block

(E) left atrial enlargement

198. The electrocardiogram in Figure 8–2 demonstrates

(A) paced rhythm

(B) left bundle branch block

(C) right bundle branch block

(D) idiopathic subaortic stenosis

(E) posterior wall myocardial infarction

DIRECTIONS (Questions 199 and 200): For each of the items in this section, ONE or MORE of the numbered options is correct. Choose answer

(A) if only (1), (2), and (3) are correct,

(B) if only (1) and (3) are correct,

(C) if only (2) and (4) are correct,

(D) if only (4) is correct,

(E) if all are correct.

Questions 199 and 200

199. Electrocardiographic findings in cardiac tamponade include

(1) diffuse low voltage

(2) prolonged QT interval

(3) electrical alternans

(4) left bundle branch block

200. Risk factors for developing coronary artery disease are

(1) caffeine intake

(2) tobacco smoking

(3) alcohol consumption

(4) high blood pressure

Answers and Explanations

1. **(B)** Syncope can be due to cardiac arrhythmias. The following arrhythmias are associated with syncope: asystole in the presence of complete heart block, paroxysmal ventricular tachycardia or fibrillation, supraventricular tachycardia or bradycardia, and sick sinus syndrome. (*Braunwald, pp. 890–891*)

2. **(A)** Patients with acute pericarditis will have ST-T segment elevation that is concave upward and is usually seen in all leads except aVR and V1. A pericardial friction rub may be heard. It is a scratching, high-pitched sound and classically has three components. A patient may have dyspnea and breathe shallowly as a result of pleuritic chest pain. The chest pain associated with acute pericarditis is increased when supine and is often relieved by leaning forward. (*Braunwald, pp. 1487–1490*)

3. **(E)** Secondary causes of hypertension include pheochromocytoma, renal parenchymal disease, use of oral contraceptive pills, and primary aldosteronism. A pheochromocytoma is a catecholamine-producing tumor that causes paroxysmal hypertension or persistent hypertension with symptoms of headache, palpitations, sweating, nervousness, weight loss, orthostatic hypotension, and hypermetabolism. Renal parenchymal disease is principally caused by chronic glomerulonephritis. As the renal disease worsens, hypertension develops that can lead to renal insufficiency. Estrogen-containing oral contraceptive pills can cause an elevation in blood pressure. The hypertension is often mild but contributes to the cardiovascular complications from the pill. Primary aldosteronism causes hypertension as a result of volume overload, which then converts to increased peripheral resistance. (*Braunwald, pp. 838–848*)

4. **(A)** The first heart sound (S1) is caused by the closure of the mitral and tricuspid valves. It is a high-pitched sound best heard with the diaphragm medial to the apex at the lower sternal border. The S2 is best heard at the 2nd or 3rd intercostal spaces. The S1 precedes the palpable upstroke in the carotid pulse; this can help distinguish it from the S2, which occurs after the peak of the carotid pulse. (*Braunwald, pp. 29–30*)

5. **(A)** Pulmonary rales develop as a result of transudation of fluid into the alveoli and are characteristic of congestive heart failure. Passive congestion of the liver as a result of right heart failure causes hepatomegaly. Congestive hepatomegaly can cause pain, anorexia, and nausea. An S3 gallop is present with left ventricular failure and is best heard at the apex in the left lateral recumbent position. An S4 is not a sign of heart failure but is associated with conditions that cause altered compliance of the ventricle (ie, aortic stenosis, hypertrophic obstructive cardiomyopathy, hypertension). (*Braunwald, pp. 478–482*)

6. **(E)** The most common cause of ST segment elevation is myocardial injury. Injury occurs when there is intense transmural ischemia, which is often caused by narrowing or occlusion of a major coronary artery. Coronary vasospasm can also cause intense transmural ischemia resulting in ST segment elevation. Prinzmetal's angina is caused by coronary vasospasm. In acute pericarditis, the ST segment elevation is usually more generalized and can be seen in many leads. Early repolarization is another cause of ST segment elevation. It is a normal variant and is seen in healthy individuals, particularly blacks, males, and people under 30 years of age. (*Clinical Symposia-CIBA, pp. 21–24; Braunwald, pp. 204–205*)

7. **(C)** Manifestations of digitalis intoxication include anorexia and arrhythmias. Arrhythmias can include many different rhythm disturbances, such as ventricular ectopy, ventricular tachycardia, atrioventricular and junctional escape rhythms. Prolonged QT interval is associated with type Ia antiarrhythmic, such as quinidine, disopyramide, procainamide. Urinary retention can be a side effect of disopyramide. (*Braunwald, pp. 505–506*)

8. **(E)** Endocarditis prophylaxis is recommended for surgery or instrumentation of the genitouri-

nary or GI tract because of the possibility of bacteremia. Prophylaxis is also recommended for dental procedures and surgery of the upper respiratory tract. *(Schulman et al, pp. 1124A–1125A)*

9. **(A)** Factors associated with a poor prognosis after an acute myocardial infarction include congestive heart failure, positive stress test after a myocardial infarction, and poor left ventricular systolic function. The most important factor is the state of the left ventricular function. Ventricular arrhythmias in the first 24 hours after a myocardial infarction are often transient and benign. *(Braunwald, pp. 1271,1291–1293; Rautaharju, pp. 4–52)*

10. **(B)** The Third Joint National Committee on Detection, Evaluation and Treatment of High Blood Pressure have classified mild hypertension as a diastolic blood pressure of 90 to 104 mm Hg. Severe hypertension is a diastolic pressure > 115 mm Hg. Isolated systolic hypertension is commonly seen in the elderly and is classified as a systolic pressure > 160 mm Hg, with diastolic pressure < 90 mm Hg. *(Braunwald, pp. 820–821)*

11. **(D)** Lithium is excreted by the kidneys; thus, blood levels are dependent upon renal function. Lithium can also have long-term effects on renal and thyroid function. Lithium-induced hypothyroidism can be a side effect of lithium administration and is treated with thyroid replacement. Thus, in addition to routine lithium blood levels, renal and thyroid function should be monitored. *(Baldessarini, pp. 96,115,119–121)*

12. **(E)** Narcolepsy is a disorder involving more than just excessive daytime sleepiness. Hypersomnolence is more commonly caused by other disorders or poor habits. The diagnosis of true narcolepsy, which is relatively rare, can be made only in the presence of at least one of the other symptoms. Sleep attacks plus cataplexy is considered pathognomonic of narcolepsy. An all-night polysomnograph and daytime sleep latency testing is confirmatory. *(Guilleminault, pp. 338–341)*

13. **(C)** Obstructive sleep apnea is a common cause of excessive daytime somnolence. Snoring is a commonly observable sign of upper airway obstruction. This is not a benign condition. In addition to the debilitating and potentially dangerous nature of sleepiness, lowered PO_2 during sleep and other physiologic changes can lead to hypertension and potentially fatal cardiac arrhythmias. *(Lugaresi et al, p. 498)*

14. **(C)** A statement of suicidal intent by a patient must be taken very seriously. An actively suicidal patient is not a candidate for outpatient treatment because of the potential lethality of an overdose of many psychiatric medications. Initiation of treatment and stabilization is best accomplished in an in-patient setting and can generally be done in a week to 10 days. *(Baldessarini, pp. 195–197)*

15. **(B)** Lyme disease is the leading cause of tickborne disease in the United States. After the bite of the infected tick, a characteristic expanding annular rash develops, *erythema chronicum migrans.* The rash may resolve spontaneously and advance to a second stage that includes neurologic and cardiac sequelae. A third stage may develop involving arthritis, which primarily affects the large joints, mostly the knees. The treatment of choice is, in order of preference, tetracycline, penicillin, and erythromycin. *(Harrison's Principles of Internal Medicine, pp. 658–659; Cecil, pp. 1726–1727; Merck, p. 1251; Mandell, pp. 1346–1347; Krupp, p. 892; Abramowicz, p. 59)*

16. **(D)** A true converter is one who has 2 consecutive tuberculin skin tests given within 2 years of each other, the first one being read as negative, that is, less than 10 mm induration, and the second one being read as positive, that is, greater than 10 mm induration. The size of the induration must exceed 6 mm between the two readings. The conversion must also not be a result of the "booster" effect. A conversion is an indicator that a new infection has occurred. In any recently infected person, chemoprophylaxis is recommended if the individual is less than 35 years old and has a negative chest x-ray. Household contacts, especially children under 3 years old, are at increased risk for developing the disease, and also should be treated prophylactically. *(Braunwald et al, p. 632; Cecil, p. 1683; Merck, p. 114; Mandell, p. 1389; Krupp, p. 147)*

17. **(B)** Hepatitis B surface antigen (HBsAg) is the first serologic marker of hepatitis B (HBV) infection. It usually occurs during the incubation period and disappears during the recovery phase. The HBV surface antibody (anti-HBs) develops after clinical recovery. It represents past HBV infection. The HBV core antigen (HBcAg) represents the viral inner core. It is not detectable in serum by conventional lab methods, but only by specialized techniques. The HBV core antibody (anti-HBc) is a marker of acute, persistent, or past infection. The anti-HBc (IgM) will be positive for 6 to 18 months after infection, and the anti-HBc (IgG) will remain as the indicator of past infection. There is a "window" period in HBV. This occurs during the transition from the disappearance of HBsAg and the appearance of anti-HBs. Anti-HBc (IgM) will be the only indicator of infection during this time. The HBVe antigen (HBeAg) is only found in HBsAg positive serum. Its presence in the serum, along with HBsAg, for more than 10 weeks, correlates with ongoing viral replication and may be a pre-

dictor of chronic disease. *(Harrison's Principles of Internal Medicine, pp. 1325–1327; Merck, pp. 859–860; Krupp, pp. 397–398)*

18. **(A)** Anorexia nervosa is a disorder characterized by a refusal to maintain a normal body weight. The person has a distorted body image and sees herself or himself as fat even when severely undernourished. Such persons are preoccupied with body size and shape. *(American Psychiatric Association, DSM III, pp. 65–67)*

19. **(C)** Bulimics have a disorder characterized by binge eating during which they feel a lack of control over their eating behavior. Like anorexics, bulimics have a preoccupation with their weight and body features. They engage in means to prevent weight gain such as self-induced vomiting, abuse of laxatives, fasting between binges, or overly strenuous exercise. *(American Psychiatric Association, DSM III, pp. 67–69)*

20. **(B)** Osteoarthritis is the most common disease of axial and peripheral diarthroidal joints. Progressive deterioration and loss of articular cartilage, along with reactive changes at joint margins and subchondral bone, are characteristic. Heberden's nodes are the formation of spurs at the dorsolateral and medial aspects of the distal interphalangeal (DIP) joints, usually developing slowly over months to years. The DIP joints are usually spared in rheumatoid arthritis (RA). The clinical features of osteoarthritis are usually local and, early in the disease, pain occurs after joint use, improving with rest. Later in the disease, pain occurs with minimal motion and even at rest. Morning stiffness and swan neck deformities of the hands are more frequently found in RA. Morning stiffness is thought to be the result of synovial congestion and thickening along with joint effusion. Swan neck deformity is the hyperextension of the PIP joint and flexion of the DIP joint. *(Rodman et al, pp. 40–41,104–108)*

21. **(B)** Septic arthritis is a medical emergency. Failure to rapidly diagnose this condition has the potential to cause permanent damage to the involved joint. Septic arthritis typically affects one joint or a few asymmetrical joints. Patients with septic arthritis usually present with an acute onset of pain, fever, erythema, and swelling of the affected joint; systemic signs of infection are common. Weight-bearing joints (most often the knee) and the wrist are most commonly involved. *(Schwartz, pp. 1983–1984)*

22. **(A)** The onset of RA is frequently heralded by prodromal symptoms such as fatigue, anorexia, weight loss, weakness, generalized aching, and stiffness. Morning stiffness is frequent (see answer to Question 20) in RA. The DIP joints can be involved in RA, but usually are spared and are involved more consistently in osteoarthritis. *(Rodman et al, pp. 40–41)*

23. **(A)** Somatiform disorders present in many forms. Symptoms occur in many body systems, commonly GI, cardiovascular, or genitourinary. Often, pain is experienced that cannot be correlated with the anatomic distribution of the nervous system. They occasionally occur concurrent with or subsequent to a genuine physical ailment or trauma. The patient is not conscious of the production of his or her symptoms; they are felt to be "real." *(American Psychiatric Association, DSM III, pp. 255,263–267)*

24. **(E)** The presence of melancholia (the loss of pleasure in activities) associated with at least three of the following fulfill the criteria for diagnosis of major depression: sleep disturbance, eating disturbance or weight change, reduced energy, inappropriate guilt, loss of libido, reduced concentration, morbid or nihilistic thoughts, or psychomotor changes. *(Dunner, p. 3)*

25. **(E)** It has been recognized for a long time that schizophrenia occurs in association with many personality types. However, the socially withdrawn type of personality is more strongly represented in schizophrenics and their first-degree relatives. The reason for this is unknown, but it can be a valuable piece of historical information when forming a differential diagnosis. *(Kendell, p. 7)*

26. **(E)** Psychosis is an indication of a brain chemical malfunction. Many different causes must be entertained. The first step in narrowing a differential diagnosis is to take a careful history, including the duration of symptoms and the patient's premorbid level of functioning. One must, of course, rule out nonpsychiatric causes of brain dysfunction. *(Davidson, pp. 1–14)*

27. **(C)** Panic disorder causes discrete episodes of panic that occur spontaneously and often become psychologically linked with the circumstances in which they occur. A phobia is the fear of a single distinct object, such as cats. As opposed to panic disorder, simple phobias are common, result in little debilitation, and do not, in themselves, cause patients to seek treatment. *(American Psychiatric Association, DSM III, pp. 243–245)*

28. **(A)** Imipramine is a tricyclic antidepressant that, in addition to the usual anticholinergic side effects, can produce a significant drop in standing blood pressure. This may require discontinuation of the drug and use of another antidepressant. It must be used with care, particularly in the el-

derly because of the hazard of falls. *(Baldessarini, pp. 178–179,182–183)*

29. **(A)** A borderline personality is distinguished by a great deal of character dysfunction. Such lives are generally marked by one crisis after another, to which the patient responds in impulsive ways. There are periods when reality testing is impaired, but this is generally limited to times of crisis. *(American Psychiatric Association, DSM III, pp. 346–347)*

30. **(D)** Gout has no specific association with sickle cell anemia. Cholelithiasis is commonly associated with sickle cell anemia because of the icterus that occurs secondary to chronic hemolysis, and must always be kept in mind when evaluating the sickle cell patient with abdominal pain (ie, one cannot automatically assume that such pain is due to sickle cell crisis). Chronic anemia and hypoxemia often lead to a chronic hyperdynamic cardiac state and later to CHF. Skeletal infarction can readily lead to femoral head aseptic necrosis; hepatic infarcts are common and can lead to significant hepatic parenchymal damage. *(Braunwald et al, pp. 1520–1522)*

31. **(E)** This presentation is consistent with a hemolytic anemia. The presence of gallstones in so young a person and the absence of specific symptoms strongly suggests chronic or congenital hemolysis, such as hereditary spherocytosis, rather than an acute acquired hemolytic process, such as autoimmune hemolytic (immunohemolytic) anemia which generally occurs in adults, is often, although not always, acute in presentation, and has a positive direct Coombs' test. *(Braunwald et al, pp. 1506–1517)*

32. **(C)** Chronic lymphocytic leukemia (CLL) is a disease usually appearing in the fourth or fifth decade of life or later and is characterized by increased mature-appearing lymphocytes in the peripheral blood, associated with spleen, node, and bone marrow infiltration by a beta-cell neoplasm. It is clinically indistinguishable from diffuse, well-differentiated, lymphocytic lymphoma. It is a relatively indolent disease that often presents with massive hepatosplenomegaly, peripheral lymphocytosis, and occasionally with lymphadenopathy, with surprisingly few symptoms. Often it is picked up on a routine exam and through CBCs. Stage A, which is lymphocytosis with or without mild lymphadenopathy, has a median survival of approximately 7 years. Stage B, lymphocytosis, larger lymphadenopathy, and hepatosplenomegaly, has a median survival of 5 years. Stage C, which is Stage B findings plus anemia and/or thrombocytopenia, has a 2-year median survival. No potentially curative therapy regimen has been found.

Single alkylating agents, such as low-dose daily or pulse high-dose chlorambucil or pulse cyclophosphamide, are indicated to palliate hemolytic anemia, symptomatic organomegaly or lymphadenopathy, or systemic symptoms (fever, weight loss, fatigue, night sweats, etc). Steroid therapy may be of value in instances of hemolytic anemia, which occurs in about 20% of CLL patients, or autoimmune thrombocytopenia (differentiated from thrombocytopenia secondary to neoplastic marrow invasion by presence of antiplatelet antibodies and increased megakaryocytes in the marrow). Splenectomy may be helpful if such problems fail to respond to steroids but is not otherwise indicated. Radiation therapy may control localized symptomatic disease; interferon is of no value. Hairy cell leukemia, another adult lymphoid leukemia (seen predominantly in males greater than 40 years of age), must be differentiated from CLL, as interferon *is* very effective in such patients with progressive disease, and alkylating agents are poorly tolerated. As in the other leukemias, infection is a major problem in patients with progressing disease; thus, early diagnosis of infection and initiation of appropriate therapy are essential. *(Braunwald et al, pp. 1548–1550; Eiseman et al, pp. 196–200)*

33. **(D)** A high percentage of patients with PA are of Northern European descent, and are fair-haired and/or prematurely gray. Current thought is that this condition has an immunologic origin, probably an autoimmune response against gastric parietal cells. There is a strong association with other disorders of such origin, including thyroid disorders, Addison's disease, vitiligo, and hypoparathyroidism. Of these, 90% have antiparietal cell antibodies, 50% to 60% have anti-intrinsic factor antibodies. In PA, there is loss of vitamin B_{12} absorption due to the absence of intrinsic factor in the stomach, and gastrin levels are often elevated. Findings may include pallor, slight icterus, smooth (sore) beefy red tongue, mild hepatosplenomegaly, and in more advanced cases, fast pulse, cardiomegaly, CHF, and CNS symptoms (neuropathy, ataxia, weakness, decreased finger coordination, decreased vibratory sense, positive Romberg, Babinski reflexes, and disturbed mentation). CBC and bone marrow demonstrate megaloblastic changes and serum B_{12} levels are low. These patients have a twofold to threefold increased incidence of gastric carcinoma and should be monitored accordingly. *(Braunwald et al, pp. 1499–1501; Hoffbrand and Pettit, pp. 56–57)*

34. **(B)** Thrombocytopenia may be seen in aplastic anemia, leukemias, myelomas, and lymphomas, and may present with petechiae, bruising, purpura, and/or unusual bleeding. All these conditions also cause an increased risk of infection, and

an acute pneumonia (or other infection, such as cellulitis or perirectal abscess) may well be the presenting complaint. Fever is a nonspecific symptom, and may be due to neoplastic activity or infection. All these conditions often present with anemia, which causes pallor and fatigue. Hepatosplenomegaly and/or lymphomas, and occasionally myelomas, are generally not found in aplastic anemia. Bone pain may occur in leukemias due to increasing activity of neoplastic cells in the marrow, and in myeloma due to skeletal destruction; retroperitoneal lymphadenopathy often causes back pain in lymphoma patients. Bone pain is not a specific common finding in aplastic anemia. Weight loss is common in most neoplastic processes, but not in aplastic anemia. Initial work-up for this patient should include CBC, platelet count, ESR, chemical panel, U/A, protein electrophoresis, and bone marrow aspiration/biopsy, with further work-up to be based on these results (CT scans, lymph node biopsy, lumbar puncture, skeletal survey, etc). *(Eiseman et al, pp. 193–228)*

35. **(B)** Erythema multiforme is an acute, self-limited eruption of the skin and the mucous membranes. The target or iris lesion, the most characteristic feature of this disease, develops abruptly and symmetrically on extensor surfaces, as well as on the palms and soles. Erythema marginatum is a specific skin manifestation of rheumatic fever. The lesion may start as an erythematous papule or blotch, spreading peripherally. Lesions may appear on the trunk and the limbs with some pigmentary changes. Eruptions with erythema annulare centrifugum begin as erythematous or urticaria-like papules. These spread to form large rings with central clearing. Etiology appears to be related to underlying disease. Erythematous, tender nodules, usually on the anterior tibia, are typical lesions of erythema nodosum. New lesions may be accompanied by fever, chills, and malaise. Numerous etiologies are attributed to this disease. Spontaneous resolution usually occurs. The lesions of erythema gyratum repens are rapidly growing, scaly, erythematous, concentric bands that may involve the entire body. Underlying malignancy appears to be etiology of this condition. *(Fitzpatrick, pp. 555–556, 1010–1012, 1142–1143, 1859)*

36. **(E)** Basal cell carcinoma (BCC) is the most common malignant skin cancer in light-skinned people. The predominant occurrence is on sun-exposed areas seldom observed before age 40. It rarely metastasizes unless treatment is not initiated promptly once the diagnosis has been made. Treatment modalities include excision, electro- or cryosurgery, or radiation. SCC is a skin cancer that develops mostly because of exposure to sunlight and other chemical agents, such as arsenic, coal tar, and creosote oil. Exposure to x-rays and

gamma rays with resulting SCC is experimentally and epidemiologically evident. Treatment of SCC includes electro-, chemo-, and excisional surgery. Radiation therapy may be used where surgical excision may be cosmetically objectionable. Primary cutaneous malignant melanoma is the leading fatal illness arising in the skin with an increased incidence expected every year. It is a highly visible tumor and occurs primarily during the productive years except for the lentigo maligna melanoma, which is predominantly seen in the elderly. Sun exposure has been implicated in the etiology of primary melanoma. Recognition of precursor lesions such as lentigo maligna, congenital melanocytic nevi, and the dysplastic nevi, and changes in their variegation is crucial for the improvement of the survival rate. Surgical excision with the margin of these varying according to the depth of the tumor is the definitive therapy. Actinic keratosis (AK), a precancerous lesion, presents on sun-exposed areas in almost 100% of the elderly white population. It may also be found on other fair-skinned people from teens up. AK may progress into an SCC without therapy. Treatment may include topical chemotherapy, cryotherapy, curettage, and electrodesiccation and surgical excision. A keratoacanthoma is a fast-growing benign skin tumor believed to arise from the hair follicles. It resembles the SCC during the active growth phase with sunlight, chemical carcinogens, trauma, and genetic predilection being factors in this. Forms of therapy include topical or intralesional injections of 5-fluorouracil, curettage, surgical excision, and waiting for spontaneous regression. *(Fitzpatrick, pp. 733–743, 747–756, 759–772, 947–963)*

37. **(B)** Macules are flat, nonpalpable lesions marked by pigment alteration, and varying in size and shape. Café au lait spots and vitiligo are examples of macules. Plaques are palpable, raised plateau-like lesions of variable sizes and thickness. The scaly psoriatic plaques are an example of these. Wheals are inflamed, flat-topped papules or plaques formed by transient and superficial edema. They may appear as small papules or involve areas as large as the entire back; an example of these would be the wheals in urticaria (hives). Pustules are palpable vesicles filled with exudate that contain bacteria as in folliculitis or they may be sterile, as in the lesions of pustular psoriasis. Scales are palpable results of abnormal shedding or the accumulation of the stratum corneum. An increased rate of cell production appearing as scaly plaques in psoriasis or the scaling with a dermatophyte infection such as tinea versicolor are examples. *(Fitzpatrick, pp. 22–37)*

38. **(D)** Penicillin is the drug of choice in the treatment of erysipelas, which is usually a group A streptococcal skin infection. Erysipelas, a superfi-

cial cellulitis, most often occurs in infants and older adults. The source is commonly the upper respiratory tract. As many as 40% of group A streptococci may be resistant to the tetracyclines. Cephalothin may be substituted in the very ill patient with a questionable penicillin allergy. In the case of an immediate type of reaction, the very ill patient may be treated with vancomycin. Nafcillin should be used in the patient with a suspected severe staphylococcal infection. *(Fitzpatrick, pp. 2104–2113)*

39. **(D)** Acute pyelonephritis is associated with nausea and vomiting, fever, chills, leukocytosis, costovertebral angle tenderness, or pain on deep abdominal palpation. The patient may or may not have cystitis, and can be suffering from headaches or malaise. *(Harrison's Principles of Internal Medicine, pp. 1191–1192)*

40–42. **40. (A); 41. (C); 42. (D)** Lyme disease begins with the tick bite from *Ixodes dammini*, which transmits the spirochete *Borrelia burgdorferi*. The classic rash, erythema chronicum migrans, begins as a macular or maculopapular lesion that expands, leaving centralized clearing. This occurs within 1 month of the tick bite in most patients, and can resolve spontaneously. Within a week to months, a second stage of the disease can occur that includes cardiac and neurologic complications. Bilateral Bell's palsy may occur, as well as severe fatigue, peripheral neuropathy, and meningitis. Early manifestations of the disease are treated with tetracycline 250 mg qid for 10 to 21 days, or amoxicillin 250 mg tid for 10 to 21 days. *(Harrison's Principles of Internal Medicine, p. 659, Cecil, pp. 1727–1728; Merck, pp. 1252–1253; Mandell, pp. 1347–1348; Abramowicz, p. 59; Petri, pp. 95–99; Chapel, p. 218)*

Rocky Mountain spotted fever (RMSF) is transmitted by the bite of the dog tick, *Dermacentor variabilis*, or the wood tick, *D. andersoni*. The disease-causing organism is *Rickettsia rickettsii*. The rash of RMSF typically begins as a macular or maculopapular lesion, but progresses to form petechial lesions. The lesions may coalesce to form large hemorrhagic areas. In RMSF, the treatment of choice is either chloramphenicol 50 mg/kg or tetracycline 25 mg/kg divided equally at 6- to 8-hour intervals. *(Harrison's Principles of Internal Medicine, p. 751; Cecil, p. 1743; Merck, p. 151)*

43. **(A)** A repeat culture is necessary to document complete eradication of the bacteria. At least 7 to 10 days of antibiotics are needed to completely treat a urinary tract infection (UTI) in pregnancy. A patient who has had one UTI during pregnancy must be constantly monitored for recurrence, as she is now at high risk for subsequent infection. Repeated periodically during the prenatal course, urine cultures will ensure early detection of infection. Chronic suppressive therapy consists of taking a small dose of an antibiotic every day and is indicated only if the patient has subsequent positive cultures with the same infecting organism. It is not indicated for an initial episode of cystitis, although it may be considered for patients who have had one severe episode of pyelonephritis during pregnancy. *(Burrow and Ferris, p. 348)*

44. **(C)** There are actually three anatomical changes during pregnancy that predispose the patient to a higher incidence of pyelonephritis. The two above (2 and 4) and decreased bladder tone. Hydronephrosis is found to begin in the first trimester and is predominantly right-sided. Its etiology is controversial, but it is felt to be mechanical, that is, due to obstruction of the ureter by the enlarging uterus and hormonal changes that occur in the urinary tract as a consequence of the pregnancy. Mechanical and hormonal etiologies probably explain the other two anatomical changes—decreased bladder tone and incomplete bladder emptying. *(Burrow and Ferris, p. 348)*

45. **(E)** Women who are Rh-negative have an absence of the Rho or D antigen on their erythrocytes. If they have an Rh-positive baby, this child's positive antigen when crossing the placenta will initiate the production of antibodies (by the mother) against the Rh-positive erythrocytes. These antibodies will either affect a subsequent pregnancy with an Rh-positive baby or affect the current pregnancy if there is a significant feto-maternal hemorrhage. Abortions, whether elective or spontaneous, ectopic and molar pregnancies in Rh-negative mothers have been associated with this isoimmunization process. These mothers should all receive RhoGAM at the time of abortion. Because of the possibility of feto-maternal hemorrhage following an episode of vaginal bleeding during pregnancy and following amniocentesis, such women should also be treated with RhoGAM. Finally, because of the possibility of a silent feto-maternal bleed, RhoGAM is given at 28 weeks in all (except previously isoimmunized) Rh-negative mothers. *(Niswander, pp. 599–604)*

46. **(C)** Although the percentage of mothers with AIDS who transmit the virus to their offspring is not yet known, it has been estimated at approximately 50%. Because AIDS is a sexually transmitted disease, the mother should be tested for other sexually transmitted diseases. At this time, the effect of pregnancy on the progression of AIDS, particularly those women who are asymptomatic, is unknown. Advising the patient to abort the pregnancy because AIDS will have a definite detrimental effect on the disease process is therefore invalid. Women who develop *P. carinii* should

definitely be treated, even if the treatment has an adverse affect on the fetus. But there is no reason to treat a woman prophylactically. *(Minkoff, pp. 2714–2717)*

47. **(B)** Endomyometritis, following cesarean section, is primarily polymicrobial. About 70% of the bacteria recovered are anaerobic: they include anaerobic gram-positive cocci, peptococcus, peptostreptococcus and anaerobic gram-negative species such as *Bacteroides.* Less common are aerobic gram-positive cocci, *S. fecalis,* group B beta-strep, *S. aureus, E. coli,* and enterobacteriaceae. Because these bacteria are usually found in combination, antibiotic therapy is, consequently, in combination. Because anaerobic bacteria are so often involved, there is a need for the addition of clindamycin (or Flagyl) to ampicillin and gentamicin. Clindamycin and Flagyl are known to be effective against *Bacteroides* species. The combination of gentamicin and clindamycin is usually effective except in infections in which enterobacteriaceae is one of the causative organisms. Neither gentamicin nor clindamycin is effective against this bacteria; therefore, ampicillin must be added. Second- and third-generation cephalosporins such as Mefoxin and cefotetan are thought to be as effective as triple antibiotics. *(Cunningham et al, p. 464; Niswander, p. 406)*

48. **(C)** CIN II or moderate dysplasia needs to be further evaluated. Colposcopic evaluation allows the examiner to visualize the cervix at 10 to 14× magnification. This allows for directed biopsy of the squamocolumnar junction and the ability to perform an endocervical curettage. The information obtained from colposcopy and from the Pap smear is then used to form the best plan of treatment for the patient. Prior to the extensive use of colposcopy, cone biopsy was a valid step in the evaluation of a moderate dysplasia. It is currently used diagnostically only if colposcopy is not available. At present, cone biopsy is more commonly used if the squamocolumnar junction is not adequately visualized on colposcopy, if the Pap smear and colposcopically obtained biopsy do not correlate, and as a presurgical means of staging microinvasive and invasive carcinoma. Simple hysterectomy is not considered a diagnostic procedure, but in women who do not wish for more children it could be a therapeutic procedure. Although cervicitis may occur concurrently with moderate dysplasia, all CIN II/moderate dysplasia requires further evaluation. If the patient does have a cervicitis, treatment prior to colposcopy will aid in a more accurate exam. *(Hacker and Moore, p. 483; Jones et al, pp. 58–64,671–673)*

49. **(A)** A history of previous thromboembolic disease and the history of ischemic heart disease are absolute contraindications to the use of oral contraceptives (OCPs). Use of oral contraception increases the risk of developing venous thromboembolic disease and subsequent pulmonary embolus. The risk is related to the estrogen component and is definitely decreased with lower estrogen doses (less than 50 mg). Development of cardiovascular complications, such as myocardial infarction, is also increased; the increase is primarily seen in women over the age of 35 and those who smoke. This risk is secondary to the progestational component that increases LDL and lowers HDL. Smoking is not an absolute contraindication to the use of OCPs. However, because the risk of developing cardiovascular and thromboembolic complications is increased in women over the age of 30 who smoke, most practitioners would be extremely reluctant to prescribe birth control pills to such a patient. Use of OCPs has been known to increase the severity and frequency of migraine headaches in some patients. Nonetheless, it is not an absolute contraindication and, if properly supervised, a patient can use the pill if she has a history of migraine. Additional absolute contraindications of OCPs are current pregnancy, cerebral vascular accident, malignant tumor, and abnormal liver function. Patients, especially older women, using OCPs also have a greater risk of developing hypertension. *(Essent, pp. 359–362; Novak, pp. 208–222)*

50. **(B)** It should be explained to a patient contemplating a bilateral tubal ligation that the procedure is permanent. A woman who considers the procedure as reversible has obviously not firmly decided against future childbearing. The success rate of reversal ranges from 30% to 70% and is dependent upon the surgical technique, the original sterilization procedure, and the patient's previous gynecologic history. Laparoscopic ring and clip procedures and minilap suture and ligation procedures both result in the least amount of tubal damage and greatest amount of remaining tube. These procedures are associated with the best success rate at reversal. Although reversal procedures exist, it must be emphasized to the patient that the original procedure is permanent. The failure rate of tubal ligation is very small, but the major complication of failure is pregnancy. Because the tubes have been damaged, the possibility of the pregnancy developing in the tube is greater. Patients should be informed of this procedural complication as part of the precounseling for tubal ligation. Because all bilateral tubal ligation procedures are performed under sterile technique, there is no increased incidence of PID. There was some suggestion that women who undergo bilateral tubal ligation may later develop dysfunctional uterine bleeding, but the relationship has never been substantiated. *(Hacker and Moore, p. 368)*

51. (B) This couple clearly has primary infertility—they have no previous pregnancies and have attempted pregnancy for more than 1 year without success. A thorough history of both the woman and man together and in separate interviews is essential for the initial work-up of infertility. A woman's past obstetric, gynecologic, and medical history is important. Because on history this patient has irregular menses, documenting whether ovulation occurs is an important first step. A basal body temperature chart is an easy and accurate means of doing so; the woman takes her temperature each morning before any activity. The basal temperature rises approximately 0.4°F at ovulation and should remain elevated for at least 11 days. Of all infertile couples, 35% have more than one cause; therefore, the male should also undergo an infertility work-up simultaneous to the woman. A semen analysis is an important first step in determining male fertility. A hysterosalpingogram is not a preliminary step in an infertility work-up. Once the preliminary steps have failed to reveal an etiology, however, it is an important means of diagnosing tubal and intrauterine abnormalities. An attempt to measure estrogen levels daily in order to document the pre-LH surge of estrogen and subsequently predict ovulation is time consuming and costly and is, therefore, not done routinely. *(Hacker and Moore, pp. 444–448; Jones et al, pp. 263–279)*

52. (E) Varicella is an acute, highly contagious disease most often occurring in childhood, but can occur at any age, worldwide. The average incubation period is 14 or 15 days with the main route of transmission through the respiratory tract. Presenting signs and symptoms may include a prodrome with a generalized pruritic rash following. Characteristic lesions may present, progressing from erythematous macules to papules, vesicles, and crusts, at different stages throughout the disease. Constitutional symptoms are usually mild in normal children. Varicella may be associated with more extensive skin lesions, high fever, severe malaise, pneumonia, and other life-threatening complications in adults and immunologically compromised patients of any age. Treatment is usually symptomatic. *(Fitzpatrick, pp. 2314–2340; Lynch, p. 84)*

53. (E) Pemphigus vulgaris may present with flaccid bullae commonly involving the scalp, umbilicus, and other parts of the body, including the mucous membranes. Delay of diagnosis may be life-threatening. EBA, a chronic blistering disease, is characterized by blister formation over joint surfaces. Extensor surfaces of the lower legs and the mucous membranes may also be involved. In general, these bullae are tense. Spontaneous bullae may appear in diabetics, usually on the extremities, particularly the feet. In general, the bullae heal without scaring over several weeks. Large, tense bullae in bullous pemphigoid are characteristic of this disease. The most common sites include the inner thighs, flexor surfaces of the forearms, axillae, abdomen, and other areas of the body, including the mucous membranes. This disease occurs predominantly in the sixth, seventh, and eighth decades of life. *(Fitzpatrick, pp. 572–573,580–581,589, 2075–2076)*

54. (A) Rubella (german measles) is a common viral infection in children and young adults. The rash appears first on the face, then generalizes with discrete erythematous macules and papules clearing within 2 to 4 days, followed by fine desquamation. This is in contrast to rubeola, which persists. Rubeola (measles) is also a highly contagious viral disease in children. Three distinct phases are present in measles: (1) an asymptomatic incubation period of about 10 to 12 days; (2) prodromal period with fever, chills, malaise, coryza, conjunctivitis, and cough; (3) onset of the rash—erythematous macules and papules starting on the face, then spreading downward. Koplik's spots usually appear in the mouth 24 to 48 hours prior to the rash. The average clinical course is about 10 days. Symptomatic therapy is usual unless complications such as encephalitis warrants antibiotic treatment. Kawasaki, a viral illness, has a list of six criteria to establish the diagnosis:

1. The disease begins with a high fever not responding to antipyretics. The fever must last for at least 5 days to be considered compatible with this disease. At the second stage, fever may fluctuate over the next week or two. Often, myringitis and/or diarrhea may follow. A cough may be present as the third manifestation.
2. Conjunctival infection and uveitis may be present in 70% of children.
3. Fissuring red lips and a hypertrophic tongue, as well as small mucosal ulcerations may accompany the illness.
4. Palms and soles that turn bright red and peel as the fever declines.
5. A skin eruption, of which there are several kinds. There is a red, confluent rash with papules or pustules in the diaper area. Another is a scarlatiniform rash. A third type presents with large, annular, brownish lesions such as those associated with erythema multiforme.
6. Cervical adenitis.

There are many more signs and symptoms than those mentioned, such as abdominal pain and, most troublesome of all, cardiovascular disease. No specific form of treatment is available. Scarlet fever is the incorrect answer. It presents with a diffuse, erythematous eruption, having a sandpaper quality, a sequela of a group A streptococcal infection in the pharynx. Desquamation usually occurs within 4 to 6 days, lasting several weeks.

Other clinical findings include enlarged tonsils, strawberry tongue, and generalized lymphadenopathy. It usually occurs in children; only rarely in adults. Early penicillin therapy prevents development of suppurative and nonsuppurative sequelae. *(Fitzpatrick, pp. 2108–2111,2289–2290,2291–2295, 2376–2382)*

55. (A) The risk of HIV transmission to health care workers has been evaluated and demonstrated to be approximately 0.5% (1 in 200) following a single needlestick exposure to HIV-infected blood. Although the incidence of transmission is low, the magnitude of risk emphasizes the need for effective infection control procedures. Universal precautions, treating all blood and body fluids as though infected with HIV, reduces the risk of occupational exposure. Protective measures include handwashing before and after patient contact, proper disposal of sharp objects, no recapping of needles, use of gloves when handling blood or body fluids/tissues, and use of goggles and gowns when splatter of body fluids is anticipated. The use of masks is necessary only with procedures during which there is aerosolization of body fluids or with contagious airborne diseases. No cases of HIV transmission to health care workers from contact with body fluids other than blood have been documented. The potential for hepatitis B virus (HBV) transmission to health care workers after accidental exposure is much greater than HIV transmission. Studies demonstrate that 10% to 30% of health care workers have serologic evidence of past or present HBV exposure. Twelve thousand health care workers become infected with HBV each year, of which 700 to 1200 become chronic carriers. *(Gerberding, pp. 321–328)*

56. (B) Kaposi's sarcoma (KS) is the most frequent AIDS-associated malignancy and is seen primarily in homosexual men. Unlike classic KS, which presents as relatively indolent cutaneous lesions, KS in AIDS patients is often aggressive and can be found as cutaneous lesions, visceral lesions, or both. Cutaneous KS can appear on any body surface, but is commonly seen on the face and in the oral cavity. KS may cause pulmonary disease, GI disease leading to gastric outlet obstruction or GI bleeding, and cause lymphatic obliteration leading to severe lymphedema. Pulmonary KS may be seen on chest x-ray as nodular infiltrates, with or without pleural effusions, and patients often present with shortness of breath, hemoptysis, and dyspnea. Definitive diagnosis of Kaposi's sarcoma is readily made by biopsy. Radiotherapy is effective palliative treatment for KS lesions; however, progression and dissemination are not altered with treatment, and prognosis is not improved. Multiple cytotoxic chemotherapeutic agents have been used in treatment of visceral KS with vary-

ing response rates. Most of these agents, including vincristine, vinblastine, adriamycin, methotrexate, and bleomycin, have been associated with severe toxicities. Alpha-interferon administered parenterally has proven effective against KS, particularly in patients with early disease who do not yet have marked depletion of CD4 cells. *(Mitsuyasu, pp. 511–523)*

57. (A) The first step in evaluating the presence of HIV infection is the HIV antibody status using the enzyme-linked immunosorbent assay (ELISA) technique. HIV antibodies may be detected by this screening method 1 to 2 months after the onset of acute illness. If this test is found to be positive, it is confirmed by the more specific western blot (WB) method of HIV antibody detection. HIV serum p24 antigen may be detected by ELISA in the period prior to antibody seroconversion but is less sensitive than antibody status and may be present in the serum for only a brief period of time. Persistent p24 antigenemia or the reappearance of antigenemia is associated with poor clinical outcome and more rapid progression to AIDS. In vitro culture of HIV is used in clinical trials and research, but is rarely indicated in routine practice. T-lymphocyte subset studies are routinely used only in known HIV infected patients. Major subsets include CD4 (T helper) cells and CD8 (T suppressor) cells. A decrease in absolute number of CD4 cells generally correlates with a decline in function of the immune system and an increase in risk of opportunistic infection. *(Tindall et al, pp. 329–338)*

58. (C) The cumulative incidence of reported AIDS cases in the United States is disproportionately higher in African-Americans and Hispanics. Although 80% of the population in the United States is composed of whites, 53% of all persons with AIDS are white. Conversely, whereas African-Americans and Hispanics compose 12% and 6% of the United States population, they make up 30% and 17% of all AIDS cases, respectively. The geographic distribution of AIDS cases throughout the United States has shifted with time. The percent of AIDS cases in New York and San Francisco, although disproportionately larger than other areas in the United States, has gradually decreased since 1983, and these other areas have seen an increase in cases. The proportion of adult AIDS cases in women has increased over time. As of December 1992, the percentage of reported AIDS cases in women was 13%, and gradually increasing. Close to 90% of HIV infection in children occurs in those born to women at risk for HIV infection. Women at increased risk should be counseled, tested for HIV antibody status, and advised of the risk of HIV transmission to the fetus should pregnancy arise. *(CDCP, HIV/AIDS Surveillance, pp. 1–23)*

59. **(D)** Lack of clinical improvement after 5 to 7 days of treatment indicates therapeutic failure and the need for replacement with alternate therapy. The addition of high-dose corticosteroid therapy to conventional agents may be successful in improving patients failing to respond to treatment. PCP, which occurs in 80% to 90% of all AIDS patients, is the leading cause of death in these patients. Most patients (approximately 60%) survive their first episode of PCP due to early detection and effective treatment. Clinical presentation is characterized by fever, shortness of breath, and cough. Chest x-ray may reveal diffuse patchy infiltrates; however, it may be normal in up to 30% of patients. A definitive diagnosis of PCP is made only by obtaining pneumocysts on silver stain of sputum, bronchial washings, or lung tissue. *(Hopewell, pp. 409–416; Masur and Kovacs, pp. 421–426; Centers for Disease Control and Prevention, pp. 1–38)*

60. **(E)** The most reliable indicator of bleeding potential is an accurate history and physical. One must elicit a history of prolonged bleeding or the presence of easy bruising. History of family members with bleeding disorders is important. None of the assays listed completely evaluates the cascade of events associated with the formation of a blood clot. The prothrombin measures only the integrity of Factors II, V, VII, and X, whereas the partial thromboplastin time will evaluate the function of Factors VIII, IX, X, XI, and XII. The measurement of fibrinogen will detect the presence of hypofibrinogenemia but does not detect abnormalities in fibrinogenolysis. *(Schwartz et al, pp. 87–89)*

61. **(E)** The rectum is the most frequently involved site for idiopathic ulcerative colitis. The disease will often spread proximally, and symptoms can often be confused with hemorrhoidal symptoms. *(Schwartz et al, p. 1171)*

62. **(C)** Hypocalcemia results in increased neuromuscular excitability. Chovstek sign involves percussion over the facial nerve in front of the ear with resultant contraction of the facial muscles. The Trousseau sign is a less reliable indication of hypocalcemia in which a carpopedal spasm results from the inflation of a blood pressure cuff on the arm for 3 minutes. *(Schwartz et al, pp. 1620–1621; DeGowin et al, p. 783)*

63. **(D)** Carcinoma is not associated with pancreatitis, which is a painful inflammation of the gland. Carcinoma of the pancreas is almost always a painless entity until late in its course. Alcohol-induced pancreatitis is caused because of precipitation of protein in the pancreas, which acts as a

nidus for calcium deposition and ductal obstruction. Similar etiology and ductal obstruction occur with elevated lipids and elevated calcium from hyperlipidemia and hyperparathyroidism, respectively. Gallstone pancreatitis occurs without obstruction of Wirsung's duct by stones impacted in the distal common bile duct and the resultant edema. *(Schwartz et al, pp. 1350–1351)*

64. **(D)** An "apple core" lesion is the classic finding of carcinoma on barium enema. The abrupt, annular compromise differs from the gradual compression seen in inflammatory processes such as diverticulitis. *(Schwartz et al, pp. 1188–1200; Squire, pp. 208–209)*

65. **(C)** Homeostatic regulation of thyroid activity begins with thyroid-releasing hormone (TRH), which is secreted by the hypothalamus as the result of negative feedback. This in turn causes the pituitary to release thyroid-stimulating hormone (TSH), which in turn signals the thyroid gland to release T_4. The T_4 is converted peripherally to T_3, the active form of thyroid hormone. *(Schwartz et al, p. 1550)*

66. **(B)** Pneumaturia or air in the urine along with fecaluria is diagnostic of a colovesicular fistula (between bladder and colon). This is a consequence of inflammation and perforation along adjacent organs and may result from carcinoma or diverticulitis. *(Schwartz et al, p. 1190)*

67. **(A)**

Operation	Mortality	Morbidity
Partial gastrectomy	3%	10%
Vagotomy/antrectomy	2%	12%
Vagotomy/pyloroplasty	1%	15%
Vagotomy/drainage	1%	15%
Proximal gastric vagotomy	0.5%	5%

Proximal gastric vagotomy (PGV) leaves vagal innervation to the antral portion of the stomach, and to other intra-abdominal organs intact. This, along with low morbidity and mortality rates, has made PGV the procedure of choice for duodenal ulcers when no drainage procedure is required. However, PGV is associated with a 15% recurrence rate. *(Schwartz, pp. 1170–1173)*

68. **(C)** The chief cells, which are found deep in the glands of the fundus, secrete pepsinogen. Pepsinogen is the inactive precursor of pepsin, which is active in protein breakdown. The G cells secrete gastrin, a hormone. This hormone stimulates the secretion of gastric acid by the parietal cells, and pepsinogen by the chief cells. Glucagon is a hor-

mone secreted by the walls of the stomach and duodenum and also by the alpha cells of the pancreas. Glucagon acts to increase blood glucose levels. (*Schwartz, pp. 1160–1163*)

69. **(B)** The most common complication of duodenal ulcer is bleeding. This is, however, usually minor, and often presents as melena. If bleeding persists despite adequate medical therapy, endoscopic control is appropriate. The mortality rate is unchanged with endoscopic control. Should an operation become necessary, simple suture ligation would control the bleeding but an anti-ulcer procedure should be done to prevent recurrence. Total gastrectomy with its associated high rates of morbidity and mortality is reserved for patients with Zollinger–Ellison syndrome or those with multiple recurrences of their ulcers. (*Schwartz, pp. 1168–1170*)

70. **(E)** Barrett's esophagus is a consequence of the corrosive insult to the lower esophagus as a result of persistent gastroesophageal reflux. A change or destruction of the squamous cell lining of the lower esophagus and a change to columnar epithelial cells is noted. This is also associated with stenosis of the lower esophageal sphincter. These stenotic lesions are readily amenable to esophageal dilation. (*Schwartz et al, p. 1117*)

71. **(B)** Boerhaave syndrome is a traumatic esophageal rupture following intense straining usually associated with retching. This is an uncommon but life-threatening complication. It is usually associated with severe pain, hematemesis, and, if communicating with the pleural cavity, often associated with respiratory findings of dyspnea or cyanosis. (*Schwartz et al, p. 761*)

72. **(C)** The Mallory–Weiss syndrome is a result of retching and involves linear tearing of the mucosal lining at the gastroesophageal junction. This is also associated with pain and hematemesis. The pain is not as severe as the pain associated with Boerhaave syndrome and is generally a self-limiting condition. (*Schwartz et al, pp. 1151,1180*)

73. **(A)** The Plummer–Vinson syndrome is also known as sideropenic dysphagia. This is a condition often seen in middle-aged women who have a long-standing history of iron deficiency anemia. They develop dysphagia, which upon endoscopy is noted to be from a fibrous web extending around the esophagus below the cricopharyngus muscles. This syndrome is readily treated with iron supplementation and esophageal dilation. (*Schwartz et al, p. 1151*)

74. **(E)** Several features of gastric ulcers indicate the need for surgery. Large ulcers (greater than 4 cm) may require extensive resection. These usually oc-

cur in malnourished, elderly patients. Evidence of deep penetration or association with duodenal ulcers are indications for surgery because of suspicion of malignancy and recurrence, respectively. Finally, failure of medical therapy or recurrence after a period of healing should lead one to consider malignancy and are indications for surgery. (*Schwartz, pp. 1176–1177*)

75. **(A)** Carcinoma is the most common etiology of large bowel obstruction. Volvulus, which involves a torsion of either the cecum or sigmoid represents the second most common cause of large bowel obstruction. Finally, diverticulitis is an infrequent cause of bowel obstruction, generally from a significant abscess formation and resultant inflammation. Ulcerative colitis is not a cause of large bowel obstruction. (*Schwartz et al, pp. 1034–1035; DeGowin et al, pp. 553–555*)

76. **(A)** Parathyroid hormones control the metabolic balances of calcium, phosphorous, and magnesium. Chloride metabolism is regulated via the renal system. The serum levels of calcium are controlled via feedback mechanism involving calcitonin produced from the thyroid gland and parathyroid hormone (PTH), which regulate the release of calcium stores. PTH is secreted from the parathyroid gland in response to a decrease in serum calcium. (*Schwartz et al, pp. 1645–1649*)

77. **(C)** Diet and age play prominent roles. Diverticulosis is a disease resulting from highly processed, low-fiber diets of industrialized nations and is rarely seen before the age of 35. The incidence increases with age and by 85, almost 65% of the population will have diverticulosis. (*Schwartz et al, p. 1185*)

78. **(E)** Bilirubin is produced primarily from hemoglobin, but also comes from breakdown products of myoglobin. The liver also synthesizes some bilirubin. From whatever source, once bilirubin is produced, it complexes with albumin to form a stable complex (indirect bilirubin). This complex is not water soluble and therefore is not excreted in the urine. The indirect bilirubin is transported to the hepatic parenchymal cell. Here, the albumin is removed and the bilirubin is conjugated with glucuronic acid to form a diglucuronide that is water soluble (direct bilirubin). Direct bilirubin is excreted into the bile canaliculi, and ultimately makes its way into the intestine where it is acted upon by bacteria forming urobilin and urobilinogen. (*Schwartz et al, pp. 1091–1094*)

79. **(E)** Distention, tenderness, and tympany, as well as auscultation of rushes and/or tinkling are all associated with bowel obstruction. In addition, the

patient may have complaints of nausea and vomiting. Depending upon the level of the bowel obstruction, there may be fecal vomiting and obstipation. *(Schwartz et al, pp. 1034–1038)*

80. **(E)** Shock is usually due to either hemorrhage from the injured arteries or associated injuries. When profound, vasoconstriction may conceal the presence of an arterial injury until blood pressure is restored. The type of trauma (blunt or penetrating) must be known. Blunt trauma can cause multiple organ injuries. In the injured extremity, fractures and nerve injuries are commonly present in both types of trauma. Bright red bleeding suggests arterial injury. *(Schwartz, p. 937)*

81. **(C)** Classic stroke from unilateral carotid disease is ipsilateral blindness and contralateral hemiplegia. The presence of aphasia depends on involvement of the dominant cerebral hemisphere. Fleeting neurologic defects, transient monoplegia or hemiplegia, or transient ipsilateral blindness may clear within minutes or hours and are termed *transient ischemic attacks. (Schwartz, p. 976)*

82. **(C)** Aneurysm can be defined as the inappropriate dilatation of an artery. There are two types of aneurysms. A fusiform aneurysm is usually due to atherosclerosis and involves the entire circumference of the artery. Saccular aneurysms are focal and usually secondary to traumatic injury, infection, and fibromuscular hyperplasia. Fusiform aneurysms require prosthetic replacement to restore or maintain arterial continuity. Saccular aneurysms may be excised and the artery repaired. *(Schwartz, p. 981)*

83. **(E)** Pacemakers are used when there is an abnormality of cardiac conduction. Arrhythmias and impairment of conduction in the atrioventricular node and the His–Purkinje system are the chief reasons for implantation. Acquired heart block, a fibrosis of the conduction system without other significant cardiac disease, "sick sinus syndrome," an alternating bradycardia and tachycardia, Stokes–Adams attacks, intermittent attacks of syncope, and convulsions with heart block, and complete atrioventricular disassociation in which there may be periods of transient ventricular syncope, convulsions, and death, all require permanent pacemakers. *(Schwartz, p. 897)*

84. **(B)** The term *restrictive ventilatory disorder* denotes a pattern of abnormalities in lung function. The word restrictive is employed to indicate a restriction of or limitation to the amount of gas within the lungs. Thus, ventilatory disorders are characterized by reduction in lung volume. The hallmark of restriction is a decrease in the vital capacity. Obstructive ventilatory disorder denotes the constellation of abnormalities that resolves from airway obstruction, regardless of its cause. Obstructive disorders are detected mainly by the tests of the behavior of the respiratory system under dynamic conditions. The FEV_1/FVC (forced expiratory volume in 1 second divided by the forced vital capacity) is the most widely used, although tests of maximal flow volume relationships are being increasingly used. *(Beeson et al, pp. 416–417,427–428)*

85. **(A)** Patients with pneumonia may present with a variety of clinical manifestations. However, findings disclosed by proper physical examination of the lungs should aid in the formulation of the differential diagnosis. Vocal fremitus is increased in consolidated pneumonias and by inflammation surrounding other pulmonary lesions, by transmitting bronchotracheal air vibration with greater efficiency than do the air-filled pulmonary alveoli. Consolidated pulmonary tissue has increased density as opposed to normal lung tissue, therefore yielding impaired resonance, dullness, and flatness to percussion. This consolidated tissue also transmits whispered syllables distinctly, even when the pathological process is too small to produce bronchial breathing. Rales refer to sounds in the lungs from the movements of fluids or exudates in the airways. Although there are different types of rales, they sound like clicks or small bubbles and occur in bronchiectasis, pneumonia, consolidation, infarction, bronchitis, and TB. *(DeGowin and DeGowin, pp. 296–319)*

86. **(B)** The frequency of different cell types of bronchogenic carcinoma varies in the literature. In general, epidermoid carcinoma occurs with the greatest frequency and constitutes approximately 40% to 50% of pulmonary neoplasms. Adenocarcinoma (bronchogenic and bronchoalveolar), large cell carcinoma, and small cell anaplastic carcinoma occur at similar rates between 15% to 20%. *(Beeson et al, pp. 458–459)*

87. **(A)** Cheyne–Stokes respiration is the most common form of periodic breathing. Periods of apnea alternate regularly with series of respiratory cycles. In each cycle, the rate and amplitude of successive respirations increase to a maximum, then decrease progressively until the series is terminated with an apneic period. Kussmaul respiration is applied to deep, regular sighing respirations, regardless of rate. This pattern of breathing is seen in diabetic ketoacidosis, uremia, peritonitis, severe hemorrhage, and pneumonia. Biot's breathing is an uncommon variant of Cheyne–Stokes respiration, in which periods of apnea alternate irregularly with series of breaths of equal depth. This is most often seen in meningitis. Stridulous breathing is a high-pitched whistling or crowing sound

with respirations when the air passes over a partly closed glottis. This occurs with edema of the vocal cords (ie, infection), neoplasm, abscess of the pharynx, and foreign body in the pharynx. Apnea is simply the absence of respiration. *(DeGowin and DeGowin, pp. 270–281)*

88. **(E)** The clinical manifestations of bronchogenic carcinoma can vary, and many patients are asymptomatic when the pulmonary lesion is discovered. Cough usually productive of scant sputum is a common symptom; hemoptysis occurs frequently secondary to ulceration in the pulmonary lesion. Frequently, because of a significant smoking history, patients with carcinoma also have obstructive pulmonary disease and dyspnea with exertion. Weight loss is another common complaint of bronchogenic carcinoma but generally occurs with more extensive disease beyond the time the neoplasm is limited to the lung. Chest pain may be due to pleural involvement but must also suggest metastatic disease. Pulmonary infections occur distal to the bronchial obstruction and can mask the tumor. Any atypical or recurrent pulmonary infection should suggest carcinoma. Chest x-ray may demonstrate hilar and mediastinal lymph node involvement, pleural effusion, rib metastasis, elevation of a diaphragm, tracheal compression or distortion, and pericardial effusion. Although pulmonary diseases, particularly at end stages, present with similar symptoms, the entire history, physical, laboratory, and roentgenographic findings must be correlated to form the correct diagnosis. Asthma and COPD usually reveal hyperinflation of the lungs and flat diaphragms. Bronchiectasis shows coarse lung markings and even honeycombing due to the abnormal dilatation of the bronchial tree. Chronic bronchitis has been used in various ways, sometimes referring to a simple smoker's cough and at other times to severe COPD. It is usually described as a productive cough that is present on most days for at least 3 months of the year. *(Beeson et al, pp. 457–460)*

89. **(C)** People at risk for pulmonary embolism are those in hypercoagulable states. This may arise from the use of birth control pills, local stasis, immobilization that may be the result of an accident or illness, fractures, obesity, and congestive heart failure. Emboli that cause clinically significant pulmonary insult commonly arise in the ileofemoral and pelvic venous beds. Signs and symptoms often begin abruptly and include dyspnea, cough, anxiety, and chest pain (frequently pleuritic in nature). Hemoptysis may occur; tachycardia and tachypnea are common in this illness. A low-grade fever, hypotension, and cyanosis are also signs of pulmonary embolism. The presence of a deep venous thrombosis aids in the rapid clinical diagnosis. Radiographic evidence of consolidation may be present in cases of pulmonary embolism. *(Mills, p. 535; Beeson et al, pp. 442–444)*

90. **(A)** Therapy for asthma can include all the choices, but inhaled beta-adrenergic agonists provide the most rapid effect and, therefore, have the best therapeutic index. Use of epinephrine is contraindicated in patients with known cardiac disease and is not recommended in patients older than 50. Aminophylline, IV and oral, has a slower onset of action, and therapeutic levels must be maintained and monitored. Hydrocortisone also has a delayed onset of action and its use should be limited if possible. *(Beeson et al, pp. 408–410)*

91. **(B)** Vital capacity is the sum of the inspiratory reserve volume, the tidal volume, and the expiratory reserve volume. Any factors that reduce the ability of the lung to expand also reduce the vital capacity. Therefore, fibrotic lung diseases, such as tuberculosis, emphysema, chronic asthma, lung cancer, chronic bronchitis, and fibrotic pleurisy can all reduce pulmonary compliance and the vital capacity. For this reason, the vital capacity is the most important of clinical respiratory measurements in assessment of the progression of these diseases. Arterial blood gases are helpful in the objective determination of the oxygenation of the blood, but are not reliable in the assessment of progression in fibrotic diseases. Changes in tidal volume may not become apparent until late in the disease process. *(Krupp et al, p. 126; Guyton, pp. 470–472)*

92. **(B)** Although the location of maximal tenderness may vary with the position of the appendix, in typical acute appendicitis, tenderness will be maximal in the right lower quadrant, near McBurney's point. The psoas sign or other peritoneal signs of irritation such as Rovsing's sign (pressure in LLQ produces pain in the RLQ) or the obturator sign (pain in RLQ with internal rotation of a flexed right thigh in a supine patient) are indicators of local or retroperitoneal irritation. If an inflamed appendix hangs into the pelvis, there may be no abdominal findings and the diagnosis missed unless a rectal examination is done. Cutaneous hyperesthesia is a frequent but inconsistent finding in acute appendicitis. It may be the first positive sign in early appendicitis. *(Schwartz, p. 1317)*

93. **(E)** Venography, the injection of contrast material for direct visualization of the venous system of an extremity, is the most accurate method of confirming the diagnosis of venous thrombosis and the extent of involvement. Of the noninvasive studies, duplex scanning, combining ultrasound with real-time B-mode imaging, can demonstrate the thrombi within veins only in the extremities, not in the pelvis. Although 95% accurate, imped-

ance plethysmography is unable to detect calf vein thrombosis or differentiate old from new post-thrombotic sequelae. Radiolabeled fibrinogen studies cannot detect thrombi in pelvic veins and cannot be used in the presence of a diseased or injured extremity. *(Schwartz, p. 1015)*

94. **(B)** Lymphedema, resulting from an abnormality of the lymphatic system, is characteristically firm and rubbery, but nonpitting. It may be unilateral or bilateral. Lymph vesicles may be present containing fluid of high protein concentration. In cardiac and renal disease and cirrhosis, bilateral dependent pitting edema may be present. Venous disease will usually produce unilateral edema and other signs such as brawny discoloration varicose veins; stasis ulcers or dermatitis may also be seen. *(Schwartz, p. 1036)*

95. **(A)** Abdominal aortic aneurysms are the most common of the atherosclerotic aneurysms. Men are affected more frequently than women at a ratio approximating 10:1. Except for traumatic and congenital malformations, almost all peripheral aneurysms result from arteriosclerosis. The majority of peripheral aneurysms are in the popliteal artery. Infrequent sites include the femoral, carotid, and subclavian arteries. *(Schwartz, p. 988)*

96. **(B)** A serum potassium of 5.0 mEq/L is normal. Either deficiency or excess of potassium below 4.0 mEq/L or 6.0 mEq/L can be harmful. Coronary occlusion, anoxia, drugs, and arrhythmias, as well as electrolyte abnormalities, are the five frequent causes of cardiac arrest or fibrillation. *(Schwartz, p. 852)*

97. **(B)** Patients with cancer of the urinary bladder usually present with painless hematuria. Hematuria, either gross or microhematuria, is present in 95% of the cases at the time of diagnosis and is usually the initial sign. Histologically, 90% of the tumors are transitional cell in type. Adenocarcinoma occurs infrequently. Metastasis and local extension usually occur late in the course of the disease. Bladder tumors metastasize via the pelvic lymphatics and by hematogenous routes to bone, liver, and lung, as well as to other sites. The prognosis for bladder cancer is related to the histology of the tumor and its staging. Superficial small tumors may be adequately treated with endoscopic resection and electrodesiccation. The treatment for locally invasive, resectable tumors is preoperative radiation followed by cystectomy, with supravesical diversion of urine. *(Schwartz, pp. 1756–1759)*

98. **(B)** Intermittent claudication is the most common complaint produced by limb ischemia. The pain experienced is felt during exertion, not at rest, and gradually disappears within minutes upon cessation of activity. The symptoms may remain stable for years or improve after exercise programs have been initiated to help develop collateral circulation. Chronic arterial occlusion may progress, and intermittent pain involving muscle groups may be supplanted by continuous pain at rest referred to sites most distal to the arterial occlusion. This type of pain worsens with elevation of the extremity and is relieved by placing the extremity in a dependent position. *(Schwartz, p. 948)*

99. **(B)** Atherosclerosis of the origin of the internal carotid artery is the most common form of extracranial vascular disease. Stenosis involving only the vertebral artery is infrequent and significant only when bilateral or if one vertebral is congenitally absent. Atherosclerotic stenosis or occlusion of the subclavian artery proximal to the site of origin of the vertebral artery produces the subclavian steal syndrome. This phenomenon is a frequent finding on angiography, but clinical symptoms are not common because of collateralization. *(Schwartz, pp. 979,980)*

100. **(B)** In transposition of the great vessels, the two basic handicaps are severe anoxia from the inability to transport oxygen from the lungs to the tissues of the body, and progressive cardiac failure. The severe and rapidly progressive cardiac failure results partly from a high cardiac output and partly from the fact that the coronary arteries are filled with unoxygenated blood resulting in myocardial anoxia. A high percentage of infants are cyanotic at birth and have cardiac failure with dyspnea. Atrial septal defect, ventricular septal defect, and patent ductus arteriosus are not lethal disorders. In patients with tetralogy of Fallot, life expectancy is short; approximately 25% die in the first year, 40% die by 3 years of age, and 70% die by the time they are 10 years old without treatment. *(Schwartz, pp. 772,775)*

101. **(E)** Hypercalcemia may have numerous etiologies. Primary hyperparathyroidism, a common cause for hypercalcemia, stimulates $1,25 \ (OH)2D_3$ generation (which increases gastrointestinal (GI) tract calcium absorption), enhances renal calcium reabsorption, and helps mobilize calcium from bone. Approximately 20% of patients with thyrotoxicosis will have hypercalcemia secondary to direct thyroid hormone-induced bone turnover and resorption. Humoral hypercalcemia of malignancy releases a humoral substance PTHRP (parathyroid hormone-related protein) from the malignant cells (usually squamous) that enhances bone resorption. Thiazide-induced hypercalcemia may be due to increased GI calcium absorption, enhanced renal calcium recovery, stimulation of parathyroid hy-

perplasia, and increased bone resorption. *(Williams, pp. 1449–1455)*

102. **(E)** A variety of treatments are available for hyperthyroidism. Steroids can decrease TSH production and acutely decrease T_4 release and are of value in thyroid storm. Lithium can inhibit T_4 release from the gland but is rarely used as an antithyroid drug. Propylthiouracil (PTU) causes iodination defects and prevents T_4 to T_3 conversion in the periphery. Methimazole (Tapazole) causes decreased secretion of T_4 and organification defects of the thyroid gland, but lacks the peripheral effects of PTU. PTU and methimazole are the two most common antithyroid drugs. *(Felig et al, p. 416)*

103. **(A)** Myopathy commonly ensues after long-term steroid therapy. Cataract and osteoporosis (especially that of trabecular bone) are common side effects of steroid therapy. Steroids cause growth retardation, not growth spurts. *(Williams, pp. 570–576)*

104. **(E)** The list for etiologic causes for osteoporosis is quite lengthy and includes all the listed answers. Low estrogen levels accelerate bone loss as well as thyrotoxicosis. Elevated steroid levels seen with Cushing's inhibits calcium absorption and directly affect bone formation. Alcohol is toxic to the bone and marrow. *(Felig et al, p. 1471)*

105. **(E)** Polyuria occurs with uncontrolled diabetes mellitus, as glucose acts as an osmotic agent. Polydipsia is due to dehydration and hyperosmolarity. Ketosis is due to the absence of insulin and fat breakdown. Blurry vision is a manifestation of corneal fluid shifts with changing serum glucose levels, especially with high glucose levels. *(Cahill et al, p. 7)*

106. **(D)** Twenty-four hour collection for catecholamines (fractionated for epinephrine or nonepinephrine totals) would help in the diagnosis towards pheochromocytoma. The laboratory diagnosis can at times be quite difficult. Urine collections for nours for metanephrines or VMA can be used, serum levels cannot. Assay for prostaglandins would not be of benefit. *(Felig et al, pp. 668–671)*

107. **(A)** Hypocalcemia will present with a variety of clinical manifestations including cramps, tingling, overt tetany, seizures, irritability, poor concentration, learning disability, psychosis, and occasionally extrapyramidal symptoms. On physical exam, the Chovstek's sign (twitching of lips produced by tapping the facial nerve) and Trousseau's sign (hand tetany or carpopedal spasm, induced by inflating a blood pressure cuff 20 mm Hg above systolic BP for 3 minutes) are positive. *(Felig et al, p. 1422)*

108. **(D)** Normal serum calcium level is usually 8.5 to 10.5 mg/dL (can be changed to mmd/L by dividing by 4.0). Approximately 40% of serum calcium is bound to protein and 50% is free or ionized. Serum calcium level needs to be corrected for the low albumin. Thus, for each drop in albumin of 1.0, the calcium level should be corrected upward by 0.8 mg/dL. The simplest calculation is total serum calcium minus albumin plus four is equal to the corrected total serum calcium. Thus, for answer (D), it would be $(10 - 2) + 4 = 12$ mg/dL, which is hypercalcemic. *(Felig et al, p. 1363)*

109. **(C)** Overnight low- or high-dose dexamethasone suppression test can be used to help in the diagnosis of Cushing's syndrome. One milligram of dexamethasone is given at 11 PM and a 6 AM serum cortisol should be <140 nmol/L (5.0 µg/dL) because the circadian ACTH surge will have been blocked by the dexamethasone. The absence of ACTH release will then prevent the early morning rise of cortisol. A serum cortisol level of >140–275 nmol/L (5–10 µg/dL) implies absence of the blockade; ACTH is then released even in the presence of dexamethasone and that is suggestive of Cushing's syndrome. False positive results may occur in 10% to 15% of patients due to acute stress from hospitilization, severe depression, alcoholism, high estrogen states, anxiety, and chronic renal failure. If false positive results are suspected then the low-dose dexamethasone test (0.5 mg q6h for 48 hours) should be done. If the low-dose test is positive then a high-dose dexamethasone test (2.0 mg q6h for 48 hours) is done to differentiate from other causes of hypercortisolism. The test has no useful purpose for Addison's, Graves', or rheumatoid arthritis. Reidel's disease does not exist, although there is a Reidel's thyroiditis. *(Williams, pp. 536–562)*

110. **(D)** Cystine oxalate (as calcium oxalate), magnesium (as magnesium ammonia phosphate), and calcium phosphate are components of renal stones. Purine is not a urinary stone component. Purine is a nucleic acid that has uric acid as a metabolic end product. *(Felig et al, p. 1506)*

111. **(B)** Hirsutism has a reported incidence of 64% to 81% with chronically increased adrenal glucocorticoid and androgen production. Cushing's syndrome which may be either ACTH-dependent or -independent (Cushing's disease is ACTH dependent) may also present as myopathy with weakness, obesity, glucose intolerance, hypertension, acne, striae, and easy bruisability. *(Williams, pp. 536–562)*

112. **(A)** High-density lipoprotein is associated with decreased atherosclerosis and is thus felt to be protection against heart disease. It helps remove

LDL (low-density lipoproteins) from the circulation. Elevated HDLs are usually not seen in patients who consume diets high in saturated fats. *(Felig et al, pp. 1274,1280–1282)*

113. **(C)** Paget's disease is an active bone lesion in which large amounts of bone are broken down by osteoclasts and new unorganized weaker bone is laid down. Treatment with calcitonin or diphosphonates can be quite helpful to patients with Paget's. *(Felig et al, pp. 1487–1491)*

114. **(D)** The peak action of NPH insulin is between 6 to 14 hours. Regular insulin will peak within 2 to 4 hours. The combination of these agents can provide for uniformly stable glucose levels. *(Felig et al, p. 1132)*

115. **(B)** Glycohemoglobin (HbA1c) is an assay that allows for measurement of diabetic control over longer periods of time. Glucose can alter the hemoglobin molecule in a nonenzymatic fashion; thus, constant high glucose will increase the HbA1c level and suggest hyperglycemic episodes. Improving glucose control will gradually decrease the HbA1c level over 1 to 2 weeks. *(Felig et al, p. 1112)*

116 **(B)** Antihistamines possess anticholinergic activity that may be harmful to patients with enlarged prostate and those with acute narrow-angle glaucoma. They may also be contraindicated in patients with asthma. Data supporting this are not uniformly agreed upon. *(Goodman and Gilman, pp. 582–587)*

117. **(C)** Nadolol is a beta-adrenergic blocking agent, and in blocking beta receptors in the lungs, bronchoconstriction results. Theophylline, albuterol, and terbutaline cause brochodilation, whereas cromolyn is used prophylactically in the treatment of asthma. Cromolyn inhibits both the immediate and nonimmediate bronchoconstrictive reactions to inhaled antigens. *(Goodman and Gilman, pp. 234–235,619–620,630–631)*

118. **(B)** Absence or petit mal seizures differ considerably from generalized or grand mal seizures. They occur most frequently in children; the attacks are of short duration and consist of syncope or temporary clouding of consciousness during which the individual may stare blankly or exhibit minor movement of the head and limbs. Ethosuximide and valproic acid are generally used to control absence seizures. Diazepam is used in controlling acute grand mal seizures. *(Goodman and Gilman, pp. 449–453; Silver et al, p. 139)*

119. **(E)** The exact mechanism of antimigraine action of beta-blockers has not been proven, although abundant evidence supports their beneficial ef-

fects. Vicodin is a combination of hydrocodone and acetaminophen, both analgesics with additive effects. Hydrocodone, a narcotic, suppresses the affective component of pain. Midrin is also a combination product containing acetaminophen plus a sympathomimetic amine that acts by constricting dilated cranial and cerebral arterioles. Sansert is methylsergide that inhibits the effects of serotonin, a substance possibly involved in the mechanism of vascular headaches. *(Stein, pp. 2183–2184)*

120. **(C)** An adult with no history of seizure disorder should be evaluated for all potential causes of seizures. A CT scan can rule out a mass lesion or lesions that may present with seizure. A primary lung cancer seen on chest radiograph may alter the treatment regimen of cerebral metastases. Severe hypoglycemia induces seizures and is readily treatable, as are other metabolic abnormalities. Seizures secondary to cerebral lesions of AIDS are rarely a presenting symptom. The CT scan will detect the lesions. HIV testing may add information but is not necessary for diagnosis of the space-occupying lesion. *(Weiner and Goetz, pp. 86–90; Braunwald et al, pp. 1921–1926)*

121. **(A)** The classic triad of progressive dementia, urinary incontinence, and gait disturbance is suggestive of normal pressure hydrocephalus. This is one of the treatable causes of dementia. The CT scan may show ventriculomegaly out of proportion to the normal age-related changes associated with cerebral atrophy. Ventriculoperitoneal shunting may be of benefit. *(Swash, pp. 151–164)*

122. **(D)** Multiple sclerosis (MS) can affect any part of the central nervous system. 50% of patients will have initial symptoms referable to a single site or system while the other 50% will have multiple site involvement. The waxing and waning of symptoms warrants an evaluation for MS, particularly in a female in the 20 to 40 age group. *(Swash, pp. 1106–1114)*

123. **(E)** Hematuria (presence of blood in the urine) may be occult or gross. It may result from trauma, bleeding disorders, infections, stones, glomerular disease, or neoplasm. It generally denotes structural genitourinary disease. Its relationship to voiding, onset, and red blood cell morphology may indicate location and type of lesion. It is usually not painful except when large clots are produced. *(Andreoli et al, p. 484)*

124. **(E)** Hyperchloremic acidosis results from impaired renal excretion of acid and decreased serum bicarbonate. Sulfate and phosphate are excreted normally, and there is also increased reabsorption of chloride ions. This form of metabolic acidosis is due to renal insufficiency and results in an increase in the normal anion gap. *(Cox and Kathpolia, p. 1208)*

125. **(D)** Acute pyelonephritis is associated with nausea, vomiting, fever, chills, flank pain, leukocytosis, costovertebral angle tenderness, or pain on deep palpation of the abdomen. The patient may or may not have the classic symptoms of cystitis, such as frequency and dysuria. Acute pyelonephritis frequently requires hospital admission and IV antibiotics. *(Stamm and Turck, pp. 1191–1192)*

126. **(B)** Cooling an amputated part will extend the time to successful replantation from 6 to 12 hours. The amputated part should not be placed directly on ice. Attempts to cannulate or ligate exposed vessels may cause serious intimal damage. The amputated part should be placed in a bag of lactated Ringer's solution, then placed on ice. *(Urbaniak, pp. 1653–1654)*

127. **(D)** Direct pressure to the bleeding site is the most effective method of controlling hemorrhage in the acute setting. Tourniquets can cause distal ischemia. The use of clamps in the acute setting is discouraged, as damage may be done to associated neural structures. *(Committee on Trauma, ACS, p. 15)*

128. **(A)** Hypovolemic shock is best treated by rapid infusion of 2 L of lactated Ringer's solution delivered via large-bore peripheral IVs. The bolus of lactated Ringer's solution serves as both a treatment and a diagnostic movement to access the patient's response. Large-bore peripheral catheters are easy to insert and have flow characteristics sufficient to deliver large volumes of fluid. Central venous lines are time-consuming to insert, carry with them some morbidity, and do not allow for rapid fluid delivery. Type-specific blood is the preferred form of urgent blood replacement. *(Committee on Trauma, ACS, p. 5)*

129. **(A)** Peristaltic abdominal pain, nausea, and vomiting, as well as abdominal distention, are all closely associated with small bowel obstruction. These patients may also report an *absence* of flatus and bowel movements. *(Beal, p. 891)*

130. **(A)** Cholecystitis is obstruction of the cystic duct or ampulla of the gallbladder, usually due to an impacted stone. This leads to ischemia, edema, and necrosis of the gallbladder wall. Plain films will show only a small percentage of radiopaque gallstones, but may help rule out other processes. Ultrasonography will detect the presence of gallstones, but gives only suggestive evidence as to the presence of obstruction. HIDA scans have a high degree of accuracy in demonstrating the presence or absence of flow through the gallbladder and cystic duct, and into the duodenum. HIDA scans

should be considered the gold standard in the diagnosis of this entity. Oral cholecystograms are a poor choice in this setting as the nausea and vomiting that accompany this condition prevent absorption of the contrast material. *(Beal, p. 885)*

131. **(E)** Acute mesenteric ischemia often follows periods of hypotension from myocardial infarctions, arrhythmias, major trauma, sepsis, etc. There is often a discrepancy between a relatively benign physical exam and complaints of severe pain. This is due to the fact that initial colon damage is limited to the mucosa, with peritoneal signs developing only after progression to transmural bowel infarction. *(Williams, p. 474)*

132. **(E)** These symptoms are often referred to as the "5 Ps." Pallor is the result of peripheral vasconstriction. Paresthesias and paralysis are due to severe nerve and muscle ischemia. Pulselessness may be an acute event or a chronic manifestation of peripheral vascular disease. Pain is often continuous and severe, its onset accurately marking the time of the occlusion. *(Simmerman and Fogarty, pp. 698–699)*

133. **(E)** Any patient who is immunosuppressed or exhibits signs of systemic toxicity requires oral broad-spectrum antibiotics. These patients will require close observation. If erythema and swelling increase, admission for IV antibiotics should be considered. *(Warren, p. 983)*

134. **(E)** Perirectal abscesses are formed by communication with the rectosigmoid colon. When these abscesses drain spontaneously, they form fistulas-in-ano. These abscesses should be explored under general anesthesia, as they can be quite extensive and require adequate drainage. *(Warren, p. 992)*

135. **(B)** Mandibular fractures will often produce malocclusion and pain upon opening of the mouth. Broken teeth are often seen. "Raccoon's eyes" and rhinorrhea are indicative of severe midface injury, as is often seen in maxillary or nasoethmoid fractures. *(Georgiade and Manstein, pp. 411–412)*

136. **(B)** Splinting of the body part involved and the use of adhesive strips do little to reduce wound edge tension. The most effective measures are undermining soft tissues to gain length and closure of the wound in layers. *(Lammers, pp. 478–530)*

137. **(C)** Burn wounds are characterized by the depth of tissue penetration achieved by the thermal force (Fig. 3–1). Wounds are classified as partial-thickness superficial, partial-thickness deep, and full-thickness. Partial-thickness superficial wounds occur when only the epidermis and superficial dermal elements are involved. Partial-thickness deep wounds penetrate through the epidermis and into the middermis. These wounds are characterized by blister formation and intense pain. These wounds will heal spontaneously. Full-thickness wounds occur with destruction of all epidermal and dermal cells. These wounds have a dry, pearly white, or charred black appearance. They are insensitive to pin prick. They will not heal spontaneously, but will require skin grafting. *(Zawacki, pp. 26–27)*

138. (E) Circumferential casts that are too tight produce increasing pain, swelling, coolness, decreasing capillary refill, and pain on passive extension of the digits. In this case, the cast should be split, including the cast padding, and wrapped with an elastic bandage. This maintains immobility of the involved extremity while restoring circulation. *(Simon, pp. 13–14)*

139. (A) The important issue this question raises is the role of abdominal CT scanning in multisystem trauma. The issue in question for the ER personnel is whether or not the multiply injured patient has significant bleeding (thus requiring exploration), not the specific organ involved. CT scanning of the abdomen and pelvis should be reserved for the stable patient with unisystem injury. Multi-injured patients should have peritoneal lavage performed as a quick, specific screening test for hemoperitoneum. *(Committee on Trauma, ACS, pp. 117–118)*

140. (D) Acetaminophen toxicity can be divided into four stages:

Stage I—mild, easily dismissed symptoms lasting up to 24 hours

Stage II—RUQ pain and tenderness, elevation of LFTs, oliguria lasting 24 to 48 hours

Stage III—Peak liver function abnormalities, occasional complete liver failure with hepatorenal syndrome, anorexia, nausea, and/or vomiting lasting 72 to 96 hours

Stage IV—Resolution of hepatic insufficiency 4 days to 2 weeks

A high arylating metabolite of acetaminophen is formed during its metabolism that binds to hepatocytes and causes hepatic necrosis. The minimum dose capable of causing hepatic toxicity is estimated to be 140 mg/kg in children and 7.5 g in adults. *(Linden and Romack, p. 721)*

141. (A) Hypoxemia is the primary pathophysiologic event in carbon monoxide (CO) poisoning. CO acts as a competitive inhibitor of oxygen binding by coupling with hemoglobin. The affinity of CO for hemoglobin is 240 times greater than that of oxygen. Myocardial depression is seen in CO poisoning as a function of hypoxemia. Bronchospasm and surfactant inhibition are not characteristics of this disorder. *(Reisdoff and Wiegenstein, pp. 809–810)*

142. (A) The proper sequence of two-person CPR is one ventilation per 5 compressions. A brief pause is made in compressions to allow for adequate ventilation. All PAs should be familiar with current American Heart Association CPR recommendations. *(Standards and Guidelines, JAMA, pp. 2905–2984)*

143. (D) Multisystem trauma accounts for more deaths in persons aged 1 to 33 years than all other diseases *combined*. Trauma is the leading cause of death for all persons aged 1 to 44 years. *(Baker et al, p. 313)*

144. (C) The anterior cruciate ligaments are intracapsular structures that prevent anterior/posterior dislocation of the tibia upon the femur. These ligaments insert onto the inner sides of the femoral condyles. Backward movement of the tibia upon the femur is indicative of posterior cruciate ligament tears. Medial collateral ligament tears would best be demonstrated by valgus stress, lateral ligaments by varus stress. *(Hoppenfeld, pp. 186–187)*

145. (A) Pelvic fractures are exceeded only by skull fractures in terms of associated complications and mortality. Pubic rami and pubic bone fractures account for 70% of all pelvic fractures and are often associated with genitourinary trauma. All patients with pelvic fractures should be assumed to have a urethral or bladder laceration until proven otherwise. Displaced fractures that disrupt the pelvic ring always should be assumed to have associated fractures and fracture dislocations. Up to 50% of patients have a transfusion requirement in association with pelvic injuries. *(Simon, pp. 196–197)*

146. (D) Neoplastic diseases of the musculoskeletal system constitute a serious problem because of the generally poor prognosis of malignant neoplasms in these areas, thus making (A) an incorrect choice. Those listed under (B), osteoblastomas and giant cell tumors, are examples of benign neoplasms and as so are not an appropriate response when discussing the general topic of malignant neoplasms. (C) is false because these malignant neoplasms frequently require surgical excision, and (E) is incorrect because these tumors commonly metastasize. The only correct choice is (D), in that malignant neoplasms commonly include pain as a prominent clinical feature. *(Kempe et al, pp. 624–625)*

147. (B) The most common types of child abuse and neglect seen by physicians are (approximately): physical abuse (70%); sexual abuse (25%); and failure to thrive due to underfeeding (5%). Emotional abuse and neglect may actually be more common, but children are rarely brought to health care providers with symptoms of these diagnoses as a chief complaint. *(Behrman et al, p. 79)*

148. **(C)** *S. pneumoniae* accounts for 30% of organisms cultured from effusions. Group A beta-strep and *S. aureus* occur in 5%. *E. coli* occurs in neonates along with other gram-negative bacilli in about 20% of effusions. *S. aureus* occurs 5% of the time and *B. catarrhalis*, 20%. *(Behrman et al, p. 880)*

149. **(D)** The correct response to this question is (D) because asthmatic children do present with these listed findings. (A) is false because 80% to 90% of asthmatic children have their first symptoms before age 4 to 5 years. (B) is false because, generally, asthmatic children have a favorable prognosis and respond to treatment. (C) is false because pharmacologic therapy is the mainstay of treatment for asthma. There are numerous pharmacologic agents used alone or in combination for effectively relieving the signs and symptoms of asthma. (E) is false because a wheeze is the hallmark sign on physical exam that is associated with asthma; rales are more typical of pneumonia. *(Behrman et al, pp. 495–500)*

150. **(C)** Cardiopulmonary arrest in the pediatric patient is primarily a result of respiratory difficulties resulting from obstruction and hypoxia. Patency of airway should be the first priority of treatment once it is established that the patient is unresponsive or having respiratory difficulty. Airways may be established by the head-tilt and chin-lift method or by gently lifting the occiput of the head off the bed or surface by a towel or hand under the occiput and placing the patient in the "sniffing position." Breathing and circulation should then be evaluated, and cardiac monitors and IVs should be initiated if initial attempts at CPR are ineffective. *(Barkin, pp. 10–19)*

151. **(A)** Scald burns are the most common burns in children. Flame burns are more common in older children who play with matches or flammable material. *(Barkin, p. 237)*

152. **(C)** A type I epiphyseal fracture is a separation of the epiphysis from the metaphysis without displacement or damage to the growth plate. A type II involves slippage of the growth plate with a fracture into the metaphysis of the bone. Type III fracture involves a slippage of the growth plate with a fracture of the epiphysis. Type IV is an intra-articular fracture involving the epiphysis, metaphysis, and epiphyseal plate. Type V is a crush injury to the epiphyseal plate. The higher the number, the more likely there will be a growth disturbance due to the injury. Types III, IV, and V often require surgical reduction. *(Barkin, pp. 391–392)*

153. **(A)** Meckel's diverticulum presents with painless rectal bleeding 40% to 60% of the time. It may cause intestinal obstruction, intussusception, herniation, volvulus, or diverticulitis. Anal fissures are slit-like tears in the anal canal and are usually secondary to passage of large, hard stools. Small amounts of bright red blood may be noted on the stool after defecation. Without a history of pain on defecation, other causes of rectal bleeding should be ruled out. Juvenile polyps are always benign, are rare before age 1, and are seen most commonly between 3 and 5 years of age. They present with small amounts of bright red blood in the stools, intermittent melena, and painless occult GI bleeding with anemia in previously healthy children. Polyps may act as a lead point for intussusception. Intussusception is marked by sporadic, severe abdominal pain, stools with notable blood and mucus, and vomiting. *(Kempe et al, pp. 529–542)*

154. **(E)** All this information is true. Metabolic abnormalities such as hypoglycemia, hypernatremia, hyponatremia, hypocalcemia, and hypomagnesemia should be considered, as anticonvulsants may be ineffective in the presence of metabolic abnormalities. Respiratory status should be monitored with the use of IV anticonvulsants. *(Barkin, pp. 132–134)*

155. **(C)** The avulsed tooth may be rinsed but not scrubbed, because this will remove the cementum that is very important in the success of the tooth reimplantation. Placing the tooth back into the socket or under the tongue is acceptable; gauze will dry out the tooth and decrease success of reimplantation. The dentist should be seen as soon as possible for splinting the tooth in place. *(Barkin, p. 342)*

156. **(E)** Beta hemolytic *Streptococcus* must be considered in the differential, although the finding of a nontender node would tend to rule out this diagnosis. Malignancies are higher on the list of possibilities. The most common site for presentation of Hodgkin's disease is in the cervical glands. The enlargement is firm, nontender, discrete, and may involve one or more nodes. Cat scratch fever usually presents with enlarged, tender nodes within 2 weeks of the primary lesion. The axillary and epitrochlear nodes are most often involved, followed by the cervical nodes. The etiologic agent is believed to be a small gram-negative bacilli. Cat scratch disease is usually self-limiting. Infection with atypical mycobacterium species often presents in 1- to 5-year-old children who have no history of exposure to tuberculosis and usually lack systemic symptoms, although fever has been associated with the disease. Excision of the node is cu-

rative in 95% of lesions and is the treatment of choice. *(Behrman et al, pp. 640,710,1089)*

157. (C) The poison center number should be called after determining the age of the child, the amount ingested, and the current status of the child. Initial serum acetaminophen level should be obtained four hours after ingestion and plotted on the appropriate nomogram or reported to the poison center. If serum acetaminophen level is in the toxic range, or if no levels are available and the ingestion is considered to be toxic, load with 140 mg/kg of N-acetylcysteine (Mucomyst) PO, followed by 70 mg/kg PO q4h for 17 additional doses. If activated charcoal is used in the initial treatment, the stomach must be lavaged prior to initiation of the N-acetylcysteine (Mucomyst) therapy. *(Barkin, pp. 298–299)*

158. (A) Many cases of physical abuse are first suspected because the injury is unexplained. More commonly an explanation is offered but is implausible. Often, there are inconsistencies between the history given of a minor accident and the physical findings of a major injury, or between the history and the child's developmental levels (ie, a 6-month-old baby could not have turned on a hot water faucet that caused burns). In true accidents, parents normally bring their injured children in immediately for examination. Studies have shown that 40% of abused children are not brought to medical attention until the morning after the injury, and another 40% not until 1 to 4 days later. Parents whose children have suffered an accident frequently exhibit a greater degree of emotional turmoil and guilt than do abusive parents. *(Behrman et al, p. 80)*

159. (A) The reported rates of adverse reactions are pain at the site (51%), swelling (8.9%), fever greater than 38°C (47%), anorexia (21%), and vomiting (6%). Febrile convulsions occur after 0.06% of doses. *(Red Book, p. 321)*

160. (B) Unencapsulated *H. influenzae* is the second most common cause of acute otitis media in children, but *Haemophilus influenzae* type B is a rare cause of acute otitis media or sinusitis. Type B is the leading cause of bacterial meningitis in children aged 1 month to 4 years in the United States. Cellulitis due to *Haemophilus influenzae* type B characteristically develops in young children with upper respiratory infection. *(Oski et al, pp. 1087–1089)*

161. (E) The peak incidence for acute otitis media is between 6 and 36 months of age, with 2 out of every 3 children having at least one episode by their third birthday and 1 out of 3 having 3 episodes or more. Forty percent of children have middle ear effusion for at least 3 months. The incidence declines after age 6. *(Oski et al, pp. 898–900)*

162. (B) In a girl, puberty is considered delayed if there is no sign of it by age 13. Puberty in a female is considered precocious if it occurs prior to age 8, so breast development prior to age 8 is considered premature thelarche. Puberty in males is *not* delayed until after age 14½. *(Oski et al, pp. 1799–1800)*

163. (B) Human milk contains secretory IgA along with epidermal growth factor, lactoferrrin, thyroid hormone, gastrin, and prolactin. Vitamin D levels range from 40 to 42 U in most standard formulas while the level in human milk is 2 U. Absorption of the small amount of iron in breast milk is up to 50%, while only 4% is absorbed from both fortified and nonfortified formulas. Formula-fed infants should receive an iron-containing formula from birth in order to prevent an iron deficiency anemia. *(Taeusch et al, pp. 663,713–715)*

164. (B) The DDST can provide a profile of developmental progress and a means of identifying abnormal delays during infancy and the preschool years. (1) is true, with the emphasis that the DDST is a screening instrument, not a diagnostic means. (3) is true, with the emphasis on progressive sequence of developmental tasks that include the listed areas. (2) is incorrect because the DDST is not designed to be an intelligence test; (4) is incorrect because the DDST in fact is administered easily and quickly without extensive testing material. *(Kempe et al, pp. 33–34)*

165. (B) The Apgar method is a practical means for evaluating the status of a newborn infant. In (1), a score of 0 to 10 is assigned to the newborn at both 1 and 5 minutes. In (3), there are 5 objective signs evaluated: heart rate, respiratory effort, muscle tone, response to facial irritation, and color. (2) is incorrect because it is the 5-minute score that is more predictive of death, neurologic residual, and long-term outcome. However, the 1-minute score is an index of asphyxia and of the need for assisted ventilation. (4) is incorrect because each of the five signs receives a possible two points, making a total score of ten the indication of an infant in the best possible condition. *(Behrman et al, pp. 362–363)*

166. (B) Innocent murmurs are systolic and of low intensity and are usually heard at the second left interspace, just inside the apex or beneath either clavicle. Diastolic murmurs are almost always significant. A fixed split-second sound in the pulmonary area indicates an atrial septal defect. *(Oski et al, pp. 38–40)*

167. **(E)** Pityriasis rosea is a common eruption that is thought to be viral in etiology. It is heralded by a patch that is large (1 to 10 cm in diameter) somewhere on the body, often on the chest or upper extremity. In a few days, multiple raised pink lesions appear, mostly on the trunk, but can involve most of the body. The patient is asymptomatic except for mild pruritus. The lesions last from 2 weeks to 3 months. *(Behrman et al, p. 1412)*

168. **(A)** Lichen sclerosis et atrophicus is a skin disorder characterized by white, atrophic thinning of the skin in a figure-eight pattern around the anus and vagina. Excoriations and secondary infections may occur. *(Behrman et al, p. 1418)*

169. **(D)** Tuberous sclerosis is a dominantly inherited condition that causes mental deficiency and intractable convulsions. There are characteristic cerebral lesions throughout the cortical gray matter. Calcium is often deposited in these lesions and may be visible on x-ray. The most characteristic skin lesion is adenoma sebaceum, which consists of small red or brownish nodules in a butterfly distribution on the nose and cheeks. The lesions appear between 2 and 5 years of age and by late childhood are found in 80% of patients. *(Behrman et al, p. 1309)*

170. **(C)** Chronic eczema is characterized by thickened, dry, and scaly lesions with coarse skin markings, lichenification, and altered pigmentation. *(Behrman et al, p. 1404)*

171. **(E)** The loop of Henle lies between the proximal and distal convoluted tubules. The thick ascending limb rises toward the collecting ducts that later form the ureters. This limb of the loop absorbs sodium chloride quickly, causing a decreased serum osmolality and the tubular fluid concentration of sodium drops to 30 mmol/L. The voltage across the lumen becomes positive because of the addition of Na^+ and flux of H^-. The tubular fluid becomes dilute due to Na loss. However, the concentration of fluid increases in the distal loop when it passes through this region. *(Kelly's Textbook, pp. 733–734)*

172. **(E)** Scleroderma (progressive systemic sclerosis) is associated with 40% to 50% of all deaths resulting from renal failure. It closely resembles accelerated nephrosclerosis, usually appears in the third to fifth decade, and renal involvement is rarely the presenting symptom. It is a multi-organ disease that also attacks the heart, lungs, colon, jejunum, and ileum. Dysphagia occurs in 90% of patients. There are petechial hemorrhages, wedge-shaped cortical infarcts in the kidney, and diffuse thickening of the skin with telangiectasia and variable pigmentation. *(Harrison's Principles of Internal Medicine, p. 1202)*

173. **(B)** In adult polycystic kidney disease, there are cortical and medullary cysts. There are also hepatic and intracranial ("berry") aneurysms found during work-up. It is an autosomal dominant disease that can also involve the pancreas. Uremia develops slowly and these patients generally live longer than those with other causes of renal insufficiency. *(Harrison's Principles of Internal Medicine, p. 1206)*

174. **(D)** The normal range for serum osmolality is 285 to 295 mOsm/L. It is calculated by:

$$2(Na+ \text{ mmol/L}) + \frac{\text{glucose mg/dL}}{18} + \frac{\text{BUN mg/dL}}{2.8}$$

The serum osmolarity is a measure of the concentration of solute in serum concentration of solute, in intracellular and extracellular water. Here, 1 mOsm of glucose = 180 mg/L; 1 mOsm of BUN = 28 mg/L.

$$2(140) + \frac{180}{18} + \frac{28}{2.8} = 280 + 10 + 10 = 300 \text{ mOsm/L}$$

(Andreoli et al, p. 536)

175. **(A)** Water comprises 50% to 70% of body weight. Distribution of water is chiefly into two areas of the body, namely, the intracellular and extracellular fluid. The percentage attributed to each region is dependent on the amount of adipose (fat) tissue, which has a certain percentage of water. Two-thirds of body water is located in intracellular fluid, and one-third in extracellular fluid. Extracellular fluid is further divided into plasma and interstitial portions. The total amount of water is regulated by the amount of solvent in each compartment. *(Kelly's Textbook, p. 737)*

176. **(E)** The ability to concentrate the urine is a primary characteristic of the kidney. This is needed to prevent dehydration. This ability is shared by the nephrons, the sodium countercurrent system, the large osmotic gradient between the papilla and cortex, and the loop of Henle. The chief operative ion in water conservation is sodium (Na^+). *(Kelly's Textbook, pp. 734–735)*

177. **(A)** The classic presentation of rheumatoid arthritis is the result of chronic inflammation of synovial membranes. It is the formation of chronic granulation tissue (pannus) resulting from chronic synovitis that produces hydrolytic enzymes. These enzymes are capable of eroding articular cartilage, subchondrial bone, ligaments, and tendons. *(Beeson et al, pp. 1999–2000)*

178. (D) The patient presents with a monoarticular arthritis involving the ankle joint. The laboratory investigation reveals an elevated uric acid level, and synovial fluid exam shows urate crystals classically seen in gouty arthritis. Bacterial septic arthritis is easily ruled out, as the patient has no fever, and one would expect a synovial white cell count in the range of 50,000 to 200,000. In rheumatoid arthritis, a monoarticular presentation is unlikely. Normal x-ray and urate crystals make the diagnosis of osteoarthritis remote. Pseudogout presents similarly, but crystal exam of the synovial fluid yields the rod-shaped crystals of calcium pyrophosphate. Also, one may find cartilaginous calcification on x-ray in pseudogout. Acute gouty arthritis tends to affect the lower extremities, particularly the metatarsal phalangeal (MTP) joint (75% of patients), but also is seen frequently in the tarsal joints and ankle. The joints of the upper extremities can be affected, particularly the elbow, wrist, and metacarpal phalangeal joints. Shoulder, hips, and sacroiliac joint involvement is rare in pseudogout. *(Beeson et al, pp. 1161–1168; Mercier and Pettid, pp. 169–171)*

179. (C) Although pyelonephritis can be asymptomatic during pregnancy, patients are generally fairly sick. They present with fever and chills, nausea, vomiting, and back/flank pain. Often, the typical symptoms of urinary tract infection are not present, such as urinary frequency, urgency, and dysuria. Although premature onset of contractions and, therefore, labor are often the consequence of pyelonephritis in pregnancy, it is not usually the presenting symptom. *(Burrow and Ferris, p. 350)*

180. (D) A mother infected with the rubella virus during pregnancy has a very high chance of having a child with congenital rubella syndrome. A generalized viremia, such as described in the question usually precedes the onset of rash by approximately 1 week. In a nonimmune mother who has been infected with the rubella virus, antibody titers will rise 1 to 2 weeks after the onset of rash and 2 to 3 weeks after the onset of viremia. It is, therefore, important to obtain rubella titers immediately after onset of symptoms in order to determine the immune status of the mother. Ideally, these titers should be obtained at the first prenatal visit or prior to conception in order to avoid confusion should the mother be exposed to the virus during pregnancy. All women who do not have immunity to rubella should be vaccinated prior to pregnancy or postpartum. A VDRL would be the most likely other answer, as syphilis acquired during pregnancy is associated with fetal congenital anomalies. Moreover, although secondary syphilis often presents with a rash, the rash typically occurs on palms and soles and is preceded by a history of chancres, usually in the vaginal and cervical areas. Gonorrhea, *Chlamydia,* and group B beta-streptococcus will cause infection in the fetus in utero and during delivery, but are not associated with congenital anomalies. *(Cunningham et al, pp. 119,131,614–619)*

181. (E) Preeclampsia, or more correctly termed *pregnancy-induced hypertension,* classically presents in young nulliparous women. It is characterized by an elevation in blood pressure of 140/90, on two occasions 6 hours apart, proteinuria and generalized edema (edema found in the face and hands). Pregnancy-induced hypertension occurs primarily past 20 weeks' gestation and involves many organ systems, including cardiovascular, renal, central nervous system, and hematologic. Although the etiology remains unknown, the basic underlying pathophysiology is that of vasospasm. In most cases, the diagnosis is made if the blood pressure is 140/90, but an elevation of 30 mm Hg above baseline for systolic and 15 mm Hg for diastolic is acceptable. Patients typically have only minimal complaints—headache, spots before eyes, blurred or double vision, and upper abdominal pain. Chronic hypertension would be unlikely in a 16-year-old and her first trimester blood pressure was normal. Migraines are not typically associated with hypertension. Although chronic renal disease is a possibility, the combination of hypertension, proteinuria, and hyperreflexia is more likely preeclampsia. Eclampsia, a major complication of pregnancy-induced hypertension, is the development of generalized tonic-clonic seizure. *(Cunningham et al, pp. 653–654)*

182. (C) Treatment of mild preeclampsia prior to term gestation is bedrest; treatment of severe pregnancy-induced hypertension is delivery. To prevent the major and most life-threatening complication of pregnancy-induced hypertension, an eclamptic seizure, magnesium sulfate is administered prior to or concurrent with induction of labor. Although $MgSO_4$ has a slight effect on lowering blood pressure, its primary use is as an anticonvulsant medication. It is used preferentially over other anticonvulsants because of its efficiency in preventing eclamptic seizures and its minimal effect upon the fetus. $MgSO_4$ is usually given in a 4-g bolus, followed by a maintenance dose of 2 g/hour or intramuscular injection of 10 g. Hydrochlorthiazide and furosemide are both diuretics and both previously were used to treat the edema associated with pregnancy-induced hypertension. Subsequently, it has been found that use of diuretics is actually detrimental, because in preeclampsia the intravascular compartment is actually depleted. Lasix (or furosemide) is used in preeclampsia complicated by pulmonary edema. Hydralazine commonly is used in preeclampsia to lower blood pressure, but usually is used only if the diastolic pressure exceeds 110 mm Hg. Diazepam and phenytoin are commonly used antiseizure medications, but their generalized sedative effect on the fetus prevents their routine use. *(Cunningham et al, pp. 627–688; Hacker and Moore, pp. 130–132)*

183. **(B)** Neoplastic changes of the surface epithelium of the cervix are called cervical intraepithelial neoplasm (CIN) or dysplasia. If left untreated, a certain percentage of these neoplastic changes will progress to carcinoma in situ and eventually invasive carcinoma of the cervix. The squamocolumnar junction is the area between the stratified squamous epithelium of the exocervix and the columnar epithelium of the endocervical canal. It is at or very near this junction that the most severe changes of CIN occur. The location of the squamocolumnar junction change with a woman's reproductive stage and age. In women of reproductive age, it is located in the external cervical os. In order to best obtain cells from the squamocolumnar junction for a Pap smear, both the endocervix and exocervix are sampled. After the cervix is cleaned of excessive discharge, a cotton-tip applicator is inserted into the endocervical canal and then twirled to obtain cells from all sides. This is then applied to a glass slide. A second sample is then obtained from the exocervix with a wooden or plastic spatula or another cotton-tipped applicator. This specimen is then placed on the same glass slide and fixed immediately with 95% ethyl alcohol. The squamocolumnar junction does not typically occur as high as the internal os, nor would dysplastic cells often be found in the posterior vaginal fornix. *(Jones et al, pp. 643–657)*

184. **(E)** The primary means by which oral contraceptives prevent pregnancy is by the deference of ovulation. The effect of estrogen/progesterone in oral contraceptives is to inhibit release of the pituitary gonadotropins LH and FSH. This in turn prevents the LH surge and, therefore, ovulation. The actual site of action is probably the hypothalamus: the combination of estrogen and progesterone inhibits hypothalamic release of the gonadotropin-releasing hormone (GnRH) and subsequently the release of the gonadotropins from the pituitary. Because ovulation does not occur, an embryo does not form. Thus, preventing implantation is not a means by which oral contraceptives prevent pregnancy. Inhibiting the release of prolactin has no effect on preventing ovulation. There is a preovulatory rise of estradiol secretion by the developing follicle, which is a result of FSH stimulation on the ovary. This rise in estrogen may cause the LH surge and, subsequently, ovulation. Because, however, the use of oral contraceptives prevents the release of FSH and LH, the rise in estrogen never takes place. Again, it is the effect of oral contraceptives on the release of gonadotropins from the pituitary, not any effect of the pill directly on the ovary that prevents ovulation. Although oral contraceptives do change the cervical mucus and, therefore, cause the cervix to be impermeable to spermatoza, this is not the primary contraceptive action of the pill. *(Hacker and Moore, pp. 358–364, 398–400; Jones et al, pp. 210–215)*

185. **(C)** Primary dysmenorrhea is pain that occurs with menstruation without any identifiable pelvic pathology. It typically begins on the first day of menstrual bleeding and occurs for usually only 12 hours. The pain is due to intrinsic uterine factors: exaggerated uterine contractility that is hormonally stimulated. Prostaglandins, found in the musculature of the uterus are synthesized under the influence of progesterone. Therefore, anovulatory cycles, in which there is no development of the corpus luteum, are generally not associated with dysmenorrhea. Because prostaglandins (PG) cause contractions of smooth muscle, it is the excess production of PG that causes more severe dysmenorrhea. The above patient's history is consistent with primary dysmenorrhea: onset usually 2 to 4 years after menarche, no significant previous gynecological history, pain occurring on the first day of the cycle, and no findings on pelvic exam. Primary dysmenorrhea usually responds well to treatment with prostaglandin synthetase inhibitors such as Motrin, Anaprox, or indomethacin. Examples of secondary dysmenorrhea would be endometriosis, intrauterine demise, adenomyosis, endometrial polyps, or PID. Prior to the development of PG synthetase inhibitors, Tylenol with codeine was used for dysmenorrhea. Because codeine is an addictive narcotic, this medication should not be given, as PG synthetase inhibitors are a better nonaddictive alternative. Because they prevent ovulation, oral contraceptives are acceptable therapy in women with primary dysmenorrhea who are sexually active and require birth control. Nonetheless, the first line of therapy in nonsexually active patients should be PG synthetase inhibitors. Diagnostic laparoscopy would be reserved only for those patients who fail on medication, PG inhibitory and oral contraceptives, and in patients who are strongly suspected of secondary dysmenorrhea. Tocolytic agents should theoretically work, as they are inhibiting uterine contractions, but their side effects and route of administration would mitigate against their usage. *(Gerbie, p. 613)*

186. **(D)** Candida vulvovaginitis is caused by the yeast organism *Candida albicans*. It is characterized by a thick, white "cottage cheese"-like discharge that is pruritic. The hyphae and buds of *C. albicans* can be seen on a KOH wet mount. Treatment consists of clotrimazole (Gyne-Lotrimin) or miconazole nitrate (Monistat). *Candida* vulvo-

vaginitis is more common in diabetics and frequently occurs after systemic antibiotic use and during pregnancy. *(Hacker and Moore, p. 298; Jones et al, pp. 572–573)*

187. **(B)** Atrophic postmenopausal vaginitis occurs when the vaginal mucosa undergoes atrophic changes secondary to absence of estrogen. Because the mucosa is thin and friable, it bleeds easily to the touch and often this is mistaken for postmenopausal bleeding of a more serious origin. In addition to complaints of itching and burning, patients also complain of dyspareunia. Treatment is topical estrogens (suppositories or cream). *(Jones et al, p. 575; Bates, p. 393)*

188. **(A)** *Trichomonas vaginalis* is the protozoan flagellate that causes trichomonas vaginitis. This protozoan is capable of living only in the female vagina and male urethra. It is considered a sexually transmitted disease; the woman's partner should, therefore, be treated. The bubbly greenish-yellow discharge is characteristic of *Trichomonas*. The *Trichomonas* can be seen flagellating on a normal saline wet mount. Treatment is metronidazole (Flagyl) that can be given in a 1-day dose of 2 g or as a 5-to-7-day dose of 250 mg twice daily. It must be remembered that Flagyl has an effect similar to Antabuse. Therefore, when alcohol is ingested while taking Flagyl, violent vomiting may occur. *(Hacker and Moore, p. 298)*

189. **(E)** The gram-negative bacillus *G. vaginalis* is responsible for Gardnerella vaginitis. The most common presenting complaint is the fishy, musty, malodorous discharge. *Gardnerella* can be diagnosed on normal saline wet mount where the bacillus appear as studding on the epithelial cells of the vaginal culture. *(Gerbie, pp. 619–622)*

190. **(C)** A fundal height at the umbilicus roughly corresponds to 20 weeks' gestation. On physical exam, there are several ways of determining fundal height and therefore gestational age. A fundus palpable to the pubic symphysis is 12 weeks; at the umbilicus, 20; those weeks between these two landmarks are approximated. After 20 weeks and before 32 weeks, fundal height is measured with a tape measure in centimeters. Weeks' gestation correspond (± 1 cm) to the measured centimeters from the top of the symphysis to the top of the fundus. *(Cunningham et al, p. 1260)*

191. **(D)** Women who have previously been pregnant will first feel fetal movement between 16 and 18 weeks. With a first pregnancy, a woman will usually feel movement between 18 and 20 weeks. Gestational age can be approximated to when fetal movement is first perceived. *(Cunningham et al, p. 218)*

192. **(A)** At 6 weeks' gestation, a gestational sac can be seen on abdominal ultrasound. After 8 weeks, the embryo can be seen, and measurements of crown-rump length can be made. A fetal heart can be visualized at 7 weeks. *(Cunningham et al, p. 284; Niswander, p. 29)*

193. **(D)** Maternal serum alpha-fetoprotein is a screening test to detect the presence of numerous fetal abnormalities, the most common of which is neural tube defects. The major protein secreted by the early fetus is alpha-fetoprotein. This protein is secreted into the amniotic fluid and crosses the fetal membranes into the maternal circulation. The level of alpha-fetoprotein is elevated in the amniotic fluid of an abnormal fetus and therefore in the maternal serum. This elevation is best detected between 16 and 20 weeks. In addition to open neural tube defects, other abnormalities detected include congenital nephrosis, esophogeal and duodenal atresia, exophalos, Turner and Potter's syndrome, fetal death, or fetal blood or amniotic fluid. *(Cunningham et al, p. 277)*

194. **(D)** Patients suspected of having a pericardial effusion should have a two-dimensional echocardiogram to confirm the presence and size of a pericardial effusion. Echocardiography provides the most accurate and rapid technique available for evaluating an effusion. A chest x-ray will not show an enlarged cardiac silhouette until at least 250 mL of fluid have accumulated in the pericardial sac. A CT scan is complimentary to the echocardiogram and is effective in diagnosing loculated effusions, hemorrhagic effusions, and pericardial thickening. If an effusion is present and tamponade is suspected, a right heart catheterization can confirm the diagnosis. *(Braunwald, pp. 364,1491–1492,1497)*

195. **(D)** An S3 gallop is not present with mitral stenosis. An S3 gallop is associated with rapid ventricular filling and is heard with ventricular dysfunction or with marked left-ventricular volume overload. Mitral stenosis is a low-pitched diastolic murmur heard best at the apex. There may be a loud S1 and opening snap of the mitral valve. The Graham–Steele murmur of pulmonic regurgitation is due to pulmonary hypertension that can occur with mitral stenosis. The Graham–Steele murmur is a high-pitched, blowing, decrescendo murmur best heard along the left sternal border (2nd to 4th intercostal spaces). *(Braunwald, pp. 1027–1028)*

196. **(A)** Left ventricular hypertrophy is caused by conditions that lead to pressure or volume overload of the left ventricle. In systemic arterial hypertension, hypertrophic obstructive cardiomyopathy, and aortic stenosis, left ventricular hypertrophy occurs in response to chronic pressure overload. In

aortic insufficiency, left ventricular hypertrophy is the result of volume overload. Left ventricular hypertrophy is not seen in mitral stenosis because it does not result in left ventricular volume or pressure overload. *(Clinical Symposia-CIBA, pp. 5–7)*

197. **(B)** The electrocardiogram shows left ventricular hypertrophy. The criteria for LVH include:

1. Increased QRS voltage in standards leads—R wave in lead I plus S wave in lead III is greater than 25 mm
2. Increased precordial voltage S wave in V1 plus R wave in V5 or V6 > 35 mm
3. ST segment and T wave abnormalities
4. Left atrial abnormality

(Clinical Symposia-CIBA p. 5)

198. **(C)** The electrocardiogram demonstrates a right bundle branch block (RBBB), hence a delay of right ventricular depolarization. Characteristics of a RBBB include QRS complex greater than 0.12 seconds in duration, terminal broad S wave in lead I and an RSR1 complex in lead V1. *(Clinical Symposia-CIBA, pp. 6–8)*

199. **(B)** Diffuse low voltage and electrical alternans may occur in cardiac tamponade. Diffuse low voltage is caused by the attenuation of the electrical signals by the fluid in the pericardial sac. Electrical alternans is caused by the pendulum movement of the heart within the pericardial sac. *(Braunwald, p. 1496)*

200. **(C)** Tobacco smoking and high blood pressure are major risk factors for the development of coronary artery disease. Nicotine and carbon monoxide affect the heart and coronary arteries by causing an increased myocardial oxygen demand and interfering with the oxygen supply. High blood pressure can result in left ventricular enlargement and dysfunction leading to ischemic heart disease. Caffeine can cause tachycardia and arrhythmias, but there is no proof that it increases the risk of coronary artery disease. Alcohol does not increase the risk of coronary artery disease, and some investigations indicate it may increase HDL-cholesterol levels. *(Braunwald, pp. 1153–1184)*

Subspecialty List: Practice Test

QUESTION NUMBER AND SUBSPECIALTY

1. Cardiology—syncope
2. Cardiology—pericarditis
3. Cardiology—hypertension
4. Cardiology—anatomy and physiology
5. Cardiology—physical diagnosis
6. Cardiology—ECG findings
7. Cardiology—medications
8. Cardiology—prophylaxis
9. Cardiology—prognosis
10. Cardiology—blood pressure classification
11. Psychiatry—medication
12. Psychiatry—narcolepsy
13. Psychiatry—sleep apnea
14. Psychiatry—management
15. Infectious disease—Lyme disease
16. Infectious disease—tuberculosis
17. Infectious disease—hepatitis B
18. Psychiatry—anorexia nervosa
19. Psychiatry—bulimia
20. Rheumatology—osteoarthritis
21. Rheumatology—septic arthritis
22. Rheumatology—rheumatoid arthritis
23. Psychiatry—diagnosis
24. Psychiatry—depression
25. Psychiatry—schizophrenia
26. Psychiatry—psychosis
27. Psychiatry—phobias
28. Psychiatry—medications
29. Psychiatry—borderline personality
30. Hematology/Oncology—sickle cell anemia
31. Hematology/Oncology—hemolytic anemia
32. Hematology/Oncology—chronic lymphocytic leukemia
33. Hematology/Oncology—pernicious anemia
34. Hematology/Oncology—aplastic anemia
35. Dermatology—erythema multiforme
36. Dermatology—skin cancers
37. Dermatology—skin lesion characteristics
38. Dermatology—erysipelas
39. Renal—pyelonephritis
40. Infectious disease—Lyme disease
41. Infectious disease—Rocky Mountain spotted fever
42. Infectious disease—differential diagnosis
43. Obstetrics—infections in pregnancy
44. Obstetrics—infections in pregnancy
45. Obstetrics—RhoGAM
46. Obstetrics—AIDS
47. Obstetrics—endomyometritis
48. Gynecology—Pap smear
49. Gynecology—contraception
50. Gynecology—sterilization
51. Gynecology—infertility
52. Dermatology—varicella
53. Dermatology—bullae differential diagnosis
54. Dermatology—viral diseases
55. AIDS—transmission
56. AIDS—Karposi sarcoma
57. AIDS—HIV testing
58. AIDS—HIV transmission
59. AIDS—*Pneumocyctis carinii* pneumonia
60. Surgery—bleeding
61. Surgery—ulcerative colitis
62. Surgery—hypocalcemia
63. Surgery—pancreatitis
64. Surgery—radiological findings
65. Surgery—thyroid
66. Surgery—pneumaturia
67. Surgery—morbidity and mortality
68. Surgery—physiology
69. Surgery—duodenal ulcers
70. Surgery—esophageal disorders
71. Surgery—esophageal disorders
72. Surgery—esophageal disorders
73. Surgery—esophageal disorders
74. Surgery—gastric ulcers
75. Surgery—large bowel obstruction
76. Surgery—parathyroid physiology
77. Surgery—diverticulitis
78. Surgery—bilirubin metabolism
79. Surgery—bowel obstruction; physical diagnosis
80. Surgery—vascular trauma
81. Surgery—stroke; signs and symptoms
82. Surgery—aneurysms
83. Surgery—pacemakers; indications
84. Pulmonary—restrictive vs. obstructive disease
85. Pulmonary—pneumonia; physical findings
86. Pulmonary—lung cancer
87. Pulmonary—respiratory patterns
88. Pulmonary—lung cancer
89. Pulmonary—pulmonary embolism

90. Pulmonary—asthma treatment
91. Pulmonary—pulmonary function
92. Surgery—appendicitis; physical diagnosis
93. Surgery—venous obstruction; diagnosis
94. Surgery—nonpitting edema; diagnosis
95. Surgery—aneurysms
96. Surgery—causes of atrial fibrillation
97. Surgery—bladder cancer
98. Surgery—claudication
99. Surgery—extracranial vascular disease
100. Surgery—congenital vascular defects
101. Hypercalcemia
102. Thyroid
103. Adrenal
104. Osteoporosis
105. Diabetes
106. Adrenal
107. Hypocalcemia
108. Hypercalcemia
109. Adrenal disease
110. Nephrolithiasis
111. Cushing's syndrome
112. Lipid metabolism
113. Paget's disease
114. Diabetes—insulin properties
115. Diabetic monitoring
116. Pharmacology
117. Pulmonary—asthma
118. Neurology—seizures
119. Neurology—migraine
120. Neurology—seizures
121. Neurology—dementia
122. Neurology—multiple sclerosis
123. Urology—hematuria
124. Renal—metabolic acidosis
125. Renal—pyelonephritis
126. Emergency Medicine—amputation
127. Emergency Medicine—hemorrhage
128. Emergency Medicine—fluid resuscitation
129. Surgery—small bowel obstruction; signs and symptoms
130. Gastroenterology—acute cholecystitis
131. Emergency Medicine—mesenteric ischemia
132. Surgery—peripheral vascular
133. Emergency Medicine—soft tissue infection
134. Emergency Medicine—perirectal abscess
135. Emergency Medicine—facial fractures
136. Emergency Medicine—wound care
137. Emergency Medicine—burns
138. Orthopedics—physical exam
139. Emergency Medicine—paracentesis
140. Emergency Medicine—toxicology
141. Emergency Medicine—toxicology
142. Emergency Medicine—CPR
143. Emergency Medicine—trauma
144. Orthopedics—physical exam
145. Orthopedics—pelvic fractures
146. Oncology—musculoskeletal tumors
147. Pediatrics—child abuse
148. Pediatrics—otitis media
149. Pediatrics—asthma
150. Pediatrics—CPR
151. Pediatrics—burns
152. Orthopedics— Salter fractures
153. Gastroenterology—rectal bleeding
154. Neurology—seizures
155. Emergency medicine—fractured teeth
156. Pediatrics—lymphadenopathy
157. Pediatrics—poisoning
158. Pediatrics—child abuse
159. Pediatrics—immunizations
160. Pediatrics—haemophilus infection
161. Pediatrics—otitis media
162. Pediatrics—sexual development
163. Pediatrics—nutrition
164. Pediatrics—child development
165. Neonatology—physical exam
166. Pediatrics—cardiology
167. Dermatology—physical exam
168. Dermatology—physical exam
169. Dermatology—physical exam
170. Dermatology—physical exam
171. Renal—anatomy and physiology
172. Renal—sclerosis
173. Renal—cysts
174. Renal—osmolality
175. Renal—water metabolism
176. Renal—urine concentration
177. Rheumatology—physiology
178. Rheumatology—gouty arthritis
179. Obstetrics—pyelonephritis
180. Obstetrics—rash
181. Obstetrics—preeclampsia
182. Obstetrics—preeclampsia
183. Gynecology—Pap smear
184. Gynecology—contraception
185. Gynecology—dysmenorrhea
186. Gynecology—vaginal infections
187. Gynecology—vaginal infections
188. Gynecology—vaginal infections
189. Gynecology—vaginal infections
190. Obstetrics—events of pregnancy
191. Obstetrics—events of pregnancy
192. Obstetrics—events of pregnancy
193. Obstetrics—events of pregnancy
194. Cardiology—pericardial effusions
195. Cardiology—physical diagnosis
196. Cardiology—left ventricular hypertrophy
197. Cardiology—ECG
198. Cardiology—ECG
199. Cardiology—cardiac tamponade
200. Cardiology—risk factors